Minimally Invasive and Robotic-Assisted Surgery in Pediatric Urology

Patricio C. Gargollo
Editor

Minimally Invasive and Robotic-Assisted Surgery in Pediatric Urology

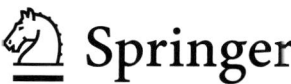 Springer

Editor
Patricio C. Gargollo
Mayo Clinic
Department of Urology
Rochester, MN
USA

ISBN 978-3-030-57221-1   ISBN 978-3-030-57219-8 (eBook)
https://doi.org/10.1007/978-3-030-57219-8

© Springer Nature Switzerland AG 2020
This work is subject to copyright. All rights are reserved by the Publisher, whether the whole or part of the material is concerned, specifically the rights of translation, reprinting, reuse of illustrations, recitation, broadcasting, reproduction on microfilms or in any other physical way, and transmission or information storage and retrieval, electronic adaptation, computer software, or by similar or dissimilar methodology now known or hereafter developed.
The use of general descriptive names, registered names, trademarks, service marks, etc. in this publication does not imply, even in the absence of a specific statement, that such names are exempt from the relevant protective laws and regulations and therefore free for general use.
The publisher, the authors, and the editors are safe to assume that the advice and information in this book are believed to be true and accurate at the date of publication. Neither the publisher nor the authors or the editors give a warranty, expressed or implied, with respect to the material contained herein or for any errors or omissions that may have been made. The publisher remains neutral with regard to jurisdictional claims in published maps and institutional affiliations.

This Springer imprint is published by the registered company Springer Nature Switzerland AG
The registered company address is: Gewerbestrasse 11, 6330 Cham, Switzerland

Preface

Advances in the field of laparoscopic and robotic-assisted surgery have transformed the field of urology in the last 30 years. Although, by nature and training, urologists are "endoscopists," improvements in optics and instrumentation have allowed us to venture outside of traditional cystoscopy and ureteroscopy and into the abdominal and retroperitoneal compartments. Both traditional laparoscopy and now robotic-assisted surgery have allowed the urologist to perform progressively more complex procedures while exploiting the benefits of smaller incisions, less pain, faster recovery, and potentially less blood loss. Laparoscopy, however, is like any surgical tool and there are clear benefits in some cases and questionable benefits in others. While few would argue that a laparoscopic or robotic-assisted nephrectomy or pyeloplasty have clear benefits over their open counterparts (particularly in older patients), the same cannot be said about ureteral reimplantation for example. The purpose of this book is to provide a data-driven analysis of robotic-assisted laparoscopic and endoscopic procedures in children. The introductory chapters lay out the logistics of establishing a dedicated minimally invasive program at your institution and the basics of anatomy, instrumentation, access, and trocar placement. Subsequent chapters are divided by anatomic compartment (upper tract and lower tract) and the final chapters cover oncology special considerations in infants, advanced and future techniques, and complications. The authors chosen for this textbook are all experts and innovators in the field of pediatric urology minimally invasive surgery and have gathered and processed an immense amount of information which will hopefully help you and your residents and fellows understand and maximize the benefits of minimally invasive surgery in pediatric urology.

In the immortal and wise words of many giants in the field of surgery "It's not difficult to learn HOW to operate, it's difficult to learn WHEN to operate."

Rochester, MN, USA   Patricio C. Gargollo, MD

Contents

Part I   Introductory Chapters

1   **History of Minimally Invasive and Robotic Assisted Surgery in Pediatric Urology** 3
Craig A. Peters

2   **Physiologic Considerations in Laparoscopic Surgery** 19
Jonathan A. Gerber, Alexandra N. Borden, and Duong D. Tu

3   **Establishing a Pediatric Robotic Surgery Program**................ 31
Sarah L. Hecht and Vijaya M. Vemulakonda

4   **Relevant Anatomy in Minimally Invasive Surgery** 43
Roxanne E. Haslam and Casey A. Seideman

5   **Robotic and Laparoscopic Instrumentation in Pediatric Urology** ... 51
James T. Rague and Michael P. Kurtz

6   **Patient Positioning, Trocar Placement and Initial Access**........... 69
Fadi Y. Zu'bi and Walid A. Farhat

Part II   Upper Tract Surgery

7   **Pyeloplasty**... 91
Chad Crigger, John Barnard, Daniel J. McClelland, and Michael Ost

8   **Robot Assisted Laparoscopic Heminephrectomy**.................. 101
Geeta Kekre, Arun Srinivasan, and Aseem R. Shukla

9   **Nephrectomy: Minimally Invasive Surgery** 115
Benjamin Whittam, Kahlil Saad, and Matthieu Peycelon

10   **Complex Upper Tract Reconstruction** 139
Angela M. Arlen, Karmon M. Janssen, and Andrew J. Kirsch

Part III Lower Tract Surgery

11 Ureteral Reimplantation 149
Jeffrey Villanueva, Janelle Fox, and Glenn Cannon

12 Management of Duplication Anomalies 163
Paul Kokorowski

**13 Minimally Invasive Techniques for Management of
Urachal Anomalies and Posterior Bladder Pathology** 181
Christopher C. Ballantyne and Sean T. Corbett

14 Robotic Appendicovesicostomy 197
Carlos A. Villanueva Del Rio

15 Complex Bladder Reconstruction 209
Daniel G. DaJusta and Molly E. Fuchs

16 Bladder Augmentation Procedures 223
Brittany L. Adamic, Lakshmi Kirkire, Ciro Andolfi,
and Mohan S. Gundeti

Part IV Endoscopy and Percutaneous Surgery

17 Endoscopic Treatment of Vesicoureteral Reflux 243
Angela M. Arlen and Andrew J. Kirsch

18 PCNL 251
Matthew T. Migliozzi, Mark G. Biebel, and Michael P. Kurtz

Part V Other Procedures and Miscellaneous Topics

19 Laparoscopic Orchiopexy 277
Niccolo M. Passoni and Micah A. Jacobs

20 Laparoscopic Varicocelectomy 291
Christina P. Carpenter and Dana W. Giel

21 Special Considerations in Infants 299
Natalia Ballesteros and Miguel Alfredo Castellan

22 Minimally Invasive Pediatric Oncology for Renal Malignancies 311
Rohit Tejwani and Jonathan C. Routh

**23 The Use of Minimally Invasive RPLND in the Treatment of
Para-Testicular Rhabdomyosarcoma in the Pediatric Population** ... 323
Stephen W. Reese, Emily Ji, Venkat M. Ramakrishnan,
Andrew A. Wagner, and Richard S. Lee

24 Laparoendoscopic Single-Site Surgery 337
Laura B. Cornwell and George Chiang

25	**Robotic Fetal Surgery: The Next Frontier?**	359

Timothy C. Boswell, Edward S. Ahn, Rodrigo Ruano,
and Patricio C. Gargollo

26	**Complications in Pediatric Urology Minimally Invasive Surgery** ...	381

Christina Kim

27	**New Robotic Systems**	405

Marianne M. Casilla-Lennon, Adam Benjamin Hittelman,
and Jose Murillo B. Netto

28	**Education and Simulation in Minimally Invasive Surgery**	419

Claudia Berrondo, Katie L. Canalichio, and Thomas S. Lendvay

Index 437

Contributors

Brittany L. Adamic, MD University of Chicago, Department of Surgery, Section of Urology, Chicago, IL, USA

Edward S. Ahn, MD Mayo Clinic, Department of Neurological Surgery, Rochester, MN, USA

Ciro Andolfi, MD University of Chicago Medical Center, Department of Surgery, Sections of Adult and Pediatric Urology, Chicago, IL, USA

Comer Children's Hospital, Department of Surgery, Section of Urology, Chicago, IL, USA

Angela M. Arlen, MD Yale University School of Medicine, Department of Urology, New Haven, CT, USA

Christopher C. Ballantyne, MD University of Virginia, Department of Urology, Charlottesville, VA, USA

Natalia Ballesteros, MD Nicklaus Children's Hospital, Department of Pediatric Urology, Miami, FL, USA

John Barnard, MD West Virginia University, Department of Urology, Morgantown, WV, USA

Claudia Berrondo, MD Seattle Children's Hospital, Department of Pediatric Urology, Seattle, WA, USA

Mark G. Biebel, MD Boston Medical Center/Boston University School of Medicine, Department of Urology, Boston, MA, USA

Alexandra N. Borden, PA-C Texas Children's Hospital and Baylor College of Medicine, Houston, TX, USA

Timothy C. Boswell, MD Mayo Clinic, Department of Urology, Rochester, MN, USA

Katie L. Canalichio, MD Seattle Children's Hospital, Department of Pediatric Urology, Seattle, WA, USA

Glenn Cannon, MD Children's Hospital of Pittsburgh, Department of Urology, Division of Pediatric Urology, Pittsburgh, PA, USA

Christina P. Carpenter, MD, MS Columbia University Irving Medical Center, New York-Presbyterian Morgan Stanley Children's Hospital, Department of Urology, Division of Pediatric Urology, New York, NY, USA

Marianne M. Casilla-Lennon, MD Yale New Haven Hospital, Yale School of Medicine, Department of Urology, New Haven, CT, USA

Miguel Alfredo Castellan, MD Nicklaus Children's Hospital, Department of Pediatric Urology, Miami, FL, USA

George Chiang, MD University of California San Diego, Rady Children's Hospital, Department of Urology, San Diego, CA, USA

Sean T. Corbett, MD University of Virginia, Department of Urology, Charlottesville, VA, USA

Laura B. Cornwell, MD University of California San Diego, Rady Children's Hospital, Department of Urology, San Diego, CA, USA

Chad Crigger, MD, MPH West Virginia University School of Medicine, Department of Urology, Morgantown, WV, USA

Daniel G. DaJusta, MD The Ohio State University, Nationwide Children's Hospital, Department of Pediatric Urology, Columbus, OH, USA

Walid A. Farhat, MD University of Wisconsin School of Medicine and Public Health, Department of Urology, Madison, WI, USA

Janelle Fox, MD Children's Hospital of Pittsburgh, Department of Urology, Division of Pediatric Urology, Pittsburgh, PA, USA

Molly E. Fuchs, MD The Ohio State University, Nationwide Children's Hospital, Department of Pediatric Urology, Columbus, OH, USA

Patricio C. Gargollo, MD Mayo Clinic, Department of Urology, Rochester, MN, USA

Jonathan A. Gerber, MD Texas Children's Hospital and Baylor College of Medicine, Houston, TX, USA

Dana W. Giel, MD LeBonheur Children's Hospital, University of Tennessee Health Science Center, Department of Pediatric Urology, Memphis, TN, USA

Mohan S. Gundeti, MD The University of Chicago Medicine, Department of Urology, Chicago, IL, USA

Roxanne E. Haslam, MD Oregon Health and Science University, Department of Urology, Division of Pediatric Surgery, Portland, OR, USA

Sarah L. Hecht, MD Oregon Health & Science University, Department of Urology, Portland, OR, USA

Adam Benjamin Hittelman, MD, PhD Yale New Haven Hospital, Yale School of Medicine, Department of Urology, New Haven, CT, USA

Micah A. Jacobs, MD, MPH University of Texas Southwestern Medical Center, Department of Urology, Dallas, TX, USA

Karmon M. Janssen, DO, MS Emory University, Children's Healthcare of Atlanta, Department of Pediatric Urology, Atlanta, GA, USA

Emily Ji, BS Brigham and Women's Hospital, Harvard Medical School, Department of Urology, Division of Urological Surgery, Boston, MA, USA

Geeta Kekre, MS, MCh, DNB Children's Hospital of Philadelphia, Philadelphia, PA, USA

Lokmanya Tilak Municipal Medical College and General Hospital, The Department of Paediatric Surgery, Mumbai, India

Christina Kim, MD University of Wisconsin-Madison, Department of Urology, Madison, WI, USA

Lakshmi Kirkire, MD University of Chicago, Pritzker School of Medicine, Chicago, IL, USA

Andrew J. Kirsch, MD Emory University, Children's Healthcare of Atlanta, Atlanta, GA, USA

Paul Kokorowski, MD, MPH Children's Hospital Los Angeles, Keck School of Medicine, University of Southern California, Division of Pediatric Urology, Los Angeles, CA, USA

Michael P. Kurtz, MD, MPH Harvard Medical School, Boston Children's Hospital, Department of Urology, Boston, MA, USA

Richard S. Lee, MD Boston Children's Hospital, Harvard Medical School, Department of Urology, Boston, MA, USA

Thomas S. Lendvay, MD, FACS Seattle Children's Hospital, Department of Pediatric Urology, Seattle, WA, USA

Daniel J. McClelland, MD West Virginia University, Department of Urology, Morgantown, WV, USA

Matthew T. Migliozzi, MS Boston Children's Hospital, Department of Urology, Boston, MA, USA

Jose Murillo B. Netto, MD, PhD Hospital Universitario da Universidade Federal de Juiz de Fora e Hospital e Maternidade Therezinha de Jesus da Faculdade de Ciências Médicas e da Saúde de Juiz de Fora, Department of Surgery – Urology, Juiz de Fora, MG, Brazil

Michael Ost, MD, MBA West Virginia University School of Medicine, Department of Urology, Morgantown, WV, USA

Niccolo M. Passoni, MD University of Texas Southwestern Medical Center, Department of Urology, Dallas, TX, USA

Craig A. Peters, MD Children's Health Texas and the University of Texas Southwestern, Department of Urology, Dallas, TX, USA

Matthieu Peycelon, MD Riley Hospital for Children at Indiana University, Division of Pediatric Urology, Indianapolis, IN, USA

James T. Rague, MD Ann & Robert H. Lurie Children's Hospital of Chicago, Boston, MA, USA

Venkat M. Ramakrishnan, MD, PhD Brigham and Women's Hospital, Harvard Medical School, Department of Urology, Division of Urological Surgery, Boston, MA, USA

Stephen W. Reese, MD Brigham and Women's Hospital, Harvard Medical School, Department of Urology, Division of Urological Surgery, Boston, MA, USA

Jonathan C. Routh, MD, MPH Duke University Medical Center, Division of Urologic Surgery, Department of Surgery, Durham, NC, USA

Rodrigo Ruano, MD, PhD Mayo Clinic, Department of Obstetrics and Gynecology, Rochester, MN, USA

Kahlil Saad, MD Riley Hospital for Children at Indiana University, Division of Pediatric Urology, Indianapolis, IN, USA

Casey A. Seideman, MD Oregon Health and Science University, Department of Urology, Division of Pediatric Surgery, Portland, OR, USA

Aseem R. Shukla, MD Children's Hospital of Philadelphia, Perelman School of Medicine at the University of Pennsylvania, Division of Urology, Philadelphia, PA, USA

Arun Srinivasan, MD Children's Hospital of Philadelphia, Perelman School of Medicine at the University of Pennsylvania, Division of Urology, Philadelphia, PA, USA

Rohit Tejwani, MD, MS Duke University Medical Center, Division of Urologic Surgery, Department of Surgery, Durham, NC, USA

Duong D. Tu, MD Texas Children's Hospital and Baylor College of Medicine, Houston, TX, USA

Vijaya M. Vemulakonda, JD, MD Children's Hospital of Colorado, Department of Urology, Aurora, CO, USA

Jeffrey Villanueva, MD Children's Hospital of Pittsburgh, Department of Urology, Division of Pediatric Urology, Pittsburgh, PA, USA

Carlos A. Villanueva Del Rio, MD Phoenix Children's Hospital, Phoenix, AZ, USA

Andrew A. Wagner, MD Beth Israel Deaconess Medical Center, Harvard Medical School, Department of Urology, Boston, MA, USA

Benjamin Whittam, MD, MS Riley Hospital for Children at Indiana University, Division of Pediatric Urology, Indianapolis, IN, USA

Fadi Y. Zu'bi, MD The Hospital for Sick Children, Department of Urology, Toronto, ON, Canada

Part I
Introductory Chapters

Chapter 1
History of Minimally Invasive and Robotic Assisted Surgery in Pediatric Urology

Craig A. Peters

The development of minimally invasive surgical (MIS) techniques in Pediatric Urology has been paradoxically both in advance of applications in the adult sphere, as well as lagging behind in many areas. Reflecting on the history of this development may provide some insights into appropriate future directions and themes of useful focus for further growth. The first uses of laparoscopy in Urology were in children for the non-palpable testis with diagnostic techniques reported in 1976 [1]. It would be another 15 years before the next phase of operative laparoscopic orchiopexy began to be actively developed. More complex laparoscopic procedures began to emerge in the early 1990s, generally following the patterns of adult practice [2–7]. While the basis for this slower emergence is multifactorial, key aspects include a greater sense of caution in the Pediatric Urological community and a limited ability to objectively define a reduction in patient morbidity using MIS techniques. This theme continues to the present and the debate continues to challenge the evolution of Pediatric Urological MIS.

The value of any minimally invasive technique must be in the ability to accomplish the surgical goal with less overall morbidity and risk. Due to children's inherently rapid recovery after most surgery, this open vs. MIS morbidity differential can be limited and difficult to prove. With fewer cases in pediatrics, this is further challenged. It is also important to recognize that there is no established and agreed upon degree of benefit that would justify the "costs" of MIS in children. These costs are financial (although difficult to quantify), as well as technical, time-related, and the impact of the learning curve. As with nearly all new technologies, there will be early and late adopters, each with a standard set of usual arguments to support their perspective; this is healthy and appropriate. Overly enthusiastic adoption of new technology can be reckless; some degree of rigor must be present in the

---

C. A. Peters (✉)
Children's Health Texas and the University of Texas Southwestern, Department of Urology, Dallas, TX, USA
e-mail: craig.peters@utsouthwestern.edu

© Springer Nature Switzerland AG 2020
P. C. Gargollo (ed.), *Minimally Invasive and Robotic-Assisted Surgery in Pediatric Urology*, https://doi.org/10.1007/978-3-030-57219-8_1

assessment of these technologies. It is equally important to permit a new technology to mature if there seems some potential benefit. Too early an assessment and judgment can prevent a potentially valuable technology from ever being utilized [8]. With modern regulatory and liability constraints, this can have a truly stifling effect.

The impact on clinical care of Pediatric Urological MIS is difficult to truly assess, as it remains relatively early in its evolution. The introduction of endoscopic injection of a bulking agent for vesicoureteral reflux altered the treatment paradigm for many practitioners, despite results that were statistically inferior to prior interventions. They were so much less morbid, however, that the balance point was markedly altered [9–11]. With the introduction and aggressive marketing of Deflux, interventions for cure of VUR increased significantly [12]. So much so that the insurance companies took note and attempted to exclude payment for this modality. Open repair of VUR declined. Over time this, has leveled out with a spread of endoscopic, laparoscopic/robotic and open surgery continuing to be used. This area is probably most controversial, not in small part due to the underlying controversy as to the indications for intervention for cure in the first place.

This echoes some of the issues that newer technologies have raised related to defining the most appropriate therapeutic intervention; a question that challenges our profession in the care of prostate cancer as well as UPJ obstruction or VUR. If the choice for operative intervention is balanced by the appropriate concern for the morbidity of surgery, reduction in the morbidity, both perceived and real, will alter the risk balance calculus. Of course this was seen in the area of calculus disease with the introduction of extracorporeal shock wave lithotripsy and percutaneous methods. It has become perfectly appropriate to remove stones that in prior decades would have been routinely observed. It is not easy to define the balance point between risk and benefit, however, as the risks are often quite different in the two options. As a result of our lack of robust long-term data on health impact, absence of a consensus of the value of these risks, and evolving surgical outcomes due to new technologies, there is clearly no simple formula to define who "needs" surgery. This issue is obviously true in the arena of VUR and UPJ obstruction, but more recently there is question as to the need for intervention in ureteroceles, previously a straightforward entity that should "always" be corrected. While the technology should not drive the decision to intervene, the morbidity of any intervention is an integral part of its therapeutic value. When a new technology alters that, it must be considered in the clinical decision. It therefore becomes important for those using the technology to rigorously and objectively assess the risk-benefit analysis as carefully as possible.

An unexpected downstream consequence of the emergence of MIS in Pediatric Urology has been the changes it has induced in the practice of those who do not use MIS techniques. Numerous reports of smaller incisions, hybrid techniques involving open and laparoscopic methods, and variations in surgical technique have surfaced in parallel and in direct response to the altered paradigm of MIS [13–16]. While surgeons will generally attempt to limit the invasiveness of their procedures and there has been a steady evolution of less morbid procedures, a great surge in this effort for open surgery emerged as laparoscopy became a common practice. Descriptions of "minimally invasive" open surgery, mini-incisions, and procedures where part of the anatomy is mobilized laparoscopically to permit an open surgery through a smaller incision have become common in the last 20 years. Studies have been reported as to parental preference on incision size and location [17, 18]. These responses to laparoscopy may be seen as secondary effects of the laparoscopic paradigm shift that may be just as impactful on surgical choices as the laparoscopy itself.

Such responses are often, however, apparently driven by the skeptics or late adopters of the newer technologies, and often couched as reasons to justify not using the new technology. While perhaps these are overly conservative, they do indeed provide a useful challenge to the adoption of new technology for technology's sake. It is essential that any new technology be justified in terms of its potential value. Simply being new is not a justification. None-the-less, we cannot ignore potential value, even if not fully developed, and rationalize this with strained modifications of usual approaches that are promoted as acceptable. Taking a conservative approach must be done thoughtfully and with an open mind.

An important element in assessing newer technologies in surgery is the relative valuation of various elements of the surgical experience. Measurements of morbidity are difficult, often subjective, and have never been uniformly agreed upon in the professional community or by the patients (and families) impacted. Typical metrics of length of stay, narcotic dosages, and cost are subject to numerous external factors and may be actually difficult to measure, despite the appeal of being "objective". Even biological parameters have to be balanced against other factors such as cost and patient/family perception. Medical interventions are not done in a social vacuum. It will be essential, as these fields move forward, to develop a consistent, consensus-based measure of value that will permit comparison of various techniques and technologies in a way that true value (benefit / cost) can be assessed Otherwise we will continue to fruitlessly debate one approach over another. Such consensus must come from the key stakeholders, including patients and families, the medical community and societal representatives.

Specific MIS Techniques

Endoscopic Treatment of VUR

The emergence of an endoscopic intervention for reflux in 1983 with Teflon injections (STING) [10] ushered in a decades-long and ongoing effort to simplify reflux treatment. Promoted by Mr. Barry O'Donnell, the success and reduced morbidity was clear and greatly appealing. Concern over the potential negative effect of migrated Teflon particles prevented FDA approval of the material in the US and it was never adopted to any significant degree [19]. There followed multiple attempts to find an equally efficacious but safer product, including cross-linked collagen, blood, fat, detachable balloons, myocytes, and various polymers, including dextranomer – hyaluronic acid (Deflux) [20–29]. Deflux is currently the most commonly used material, although some are still using Macroplastique and hydroxyl appetite. Deflux has a large publication record that demonstrates significant variability in efficacy. Initial FDA approval was based on two small animal studies and a very limited human study from Italy at the time when pediatric drugs and devices were being pushed through the FDA under new rules [30]. The human study was structured in such a way that a benefit was almost inevitable and it had a very limited one-year follow-up. It would be highly unlikely that this material would be approved under current regulatory scrutiny, not for safety but for limited efficacy. This remains the concern for Deflux, even in experienced hands, and user variability has been heavily emphasized in many reports [31]. Initial success may be followed by later recurrence of reflux after prophylaxis has been discontinued. For those patients who truly needed intervention, this may have significant effects. It is apparent by the rapid increase in numbers of patients treated that the indications for using curative intervention (as compared with expectant therapy with prophylactic antibiotics) became much looser due to the reduced morbidity and early enthusiasm for Deflux [12]. As such, it is inevitable that patients who might not have as much risk from reflux were included in the treatment groups. Their outcomes would appear better simply because they were of lower risk. The enthusiasm for Deflux has been waning lately due to the recognition that its long-term utility is less than initially perceived, and due to the evolution of reflux care where we have become more stringent in who is offered curative intervention. There has been limited effort to develop new materials for endoscopic cure of reflux, perhaps due to the changing clinical balance in reflux care. It may also reflect the uncertainty of whether Deflux' limited durability reflects the material or patient dynamics. At present, Deflux represents a potential useful approach in children with low-risk reflux in whom the family seeks some intervention [32]. It remains uncertain how durable the effect will be in any individual patient.

MIS Therapy of Stone Disease

Early use of endoscopic techniques for stone disease in children was largely limited by instrument size. Ureteroscopes were too large for a pre-pubertal child as were percutaneous nephroscopic tools. Perhaps a more important limitation was the lack of experience of the provider, who by nature of caring for children, would see fewer stones needing intervention and thereby had limited experience. As this was relatively new technology, many pediatric urologists had limited exposure to these methods as residents caring for adult patients. This challenge began to shift in the late 1990s concurrent with the emergence of smaller ureteroscopes and nephroscopes and access sheaths. Our first experiences with ureteroscopy in small children was with a rigid 7.5 Fr ACMI hysteroscope that had two working channels of adequate size. EHL was used for fragmentation initially until small lasers were available. This availability was often limited in freestanding children's hospitals where these expensive technologies could not be justified on the basis of limited patient volumes. In some contexts pediatric and adult colleagues partnered to provide care to smaller children. By this means, the pediatric urologists began to develop sufficient experience to feel comfortable with the care of small children with stone disease.

Alternative approaches were driven by the need for smaller instruments, and the "mini-perc" was one such example [33]. In a 2 yo patient with a concomitant urethral and small renal stone, we were unable to perform SWL for the renal stone at the pediatric facility, but could not perform the cystoscopy for the urethral stone at the adult facility with SWL. Rather than use the 24 Fr access sheath and with no ureteroscope small enough for retrograde access, the kidney was accessed with a 10 Fr peel away vascular access sheath through which the 7.5 Fr hysteroscope was passed to remove the renal pelvic stone. The concept was then adapted and used by Jackman and others [34] who modified the access sheath to reduce the tapered end to facilitate renal entry. Need drove the innovation that remains a useful technique in select cases.

As ureteroscopic technology has improved, the use of percutaneous access has diminished and most renal stones are approached retrograde in children. The uncommon large renal stone is still managed percutaneously or with combined approaches. The outcomes have been reported and are parallel to the adult experience where stone burden and location are key predictors of interventional success [35]. In children it has long been my bias to attempt definitive therapy in as few sessions as possible. This may prompt more aggressive measures in some larger stones, but the need for multiple sessions remains in the larger stones. SWL remains a useful technique, but has been much less widely used in recent years due to the reduced power of current systems, as well as concerns regarding fluoroscopic targeting and radiation exposure. Ultrasound guidance is useful in many but not all situations and can limit the utility of modern SWL.

Robotic technology has been applied to pediatric stone disease with large stone burden, but only in uncommon clinical scenarios [36] (Fig. 1.1). When concomitant reconstruction such as a pyeloplasty is needed, this combination is very appropriate and successful. With an increasing incidence of pediatric stone disease and

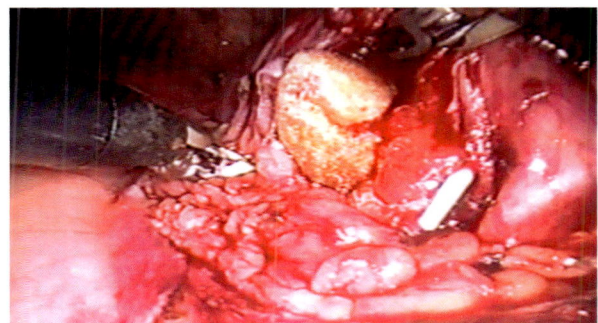

Fig. 1.1 Exposure of a large cystine stone during robotically assisted pyelolithotomy. A double-J ureteral stent has been pre-placed

continued improvement in ureteroscopes and small nephroscopes, stone management in children will become more similar with adult applications. It must be always borne in mind, however, that children are not just small adults and stone care in the child requires dedicated pediatric care.

Laparoscopic and Robotic Surgery

Diagnostic Laparoscopy

The initial usage of laparoscopy in Urology was in the pediatric patient with a non-palpable testis, permitting definitive localization of the testis or verification of absence [1, 37, 38] (Fig. 1.2). Since imaging could not confirm absence with certainty, this provided a more direct and certain means to identify those children in whom further exploration was not needed. When a testis was identified, the surgeon knew the location and could adjust the location of the incision. This was argued to facilitate therapy for the higher intra-abdominal testis. There was no universal acceptance of this presumed advantage and some continued to argue that exploration was just as efficient [39, 40]. This theme has continued even with the advent of operative laparoscopic techniques for orchiopexy of the intra-abdominal testis. The laparoskeptic has continued to argue that there is no advantage, and indeed it is difficult to prove the advantage as most children recover quickly from all of these procedures and we are limited in our ability to objectively assess surgical morbidity. None-the-less, the excellent visualization afforded by laparoscopy, its efficiency in detecting the absent testis, the provision of positional information, and more recently the integration with the definitive orchiopexy in those who need it, seems a strong argument in favor of laparoscopy for the non-palpable testis [41]. Reports of missed

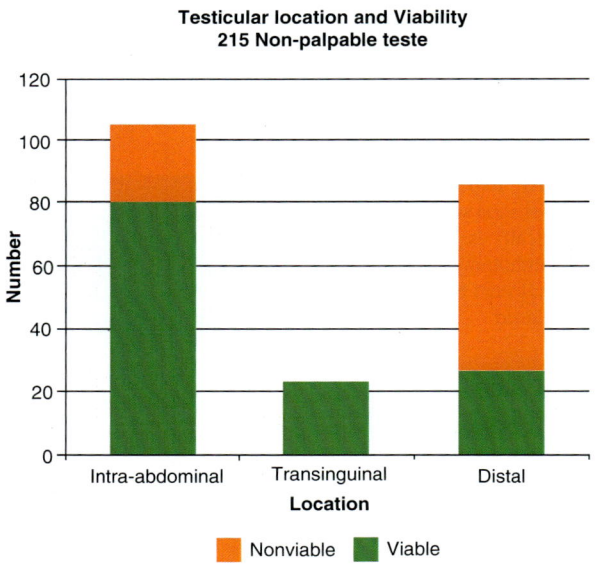

Fig. 1.2 Graph demonstrating the distribution of testicular location and viability at the time of diagnostic laparoscopy for non-palpable testes. (Data from Cisek et al. [41])

intra-abdominal testes after open exploration reinforce this argument as well [42]. At present, diagnostic laparoscopy for the NPT can be seen as the gold standard for these children, and when properly performed, the safety profile is excellent. Having seen experienced surgeons devote up to an hour in futile exploration for an absent testis, it is difficult to rationalize persisting with open exploration.

Operative Laparoscopy

As we gained comfort and familiarity with basic laparoscopic skills, the next step was to begin simple extirpative procedures and nephrectomy was the most obvious first step. At that point in time, removal of the multi-cystic dysplastic kidney was still being performed and this afforded a reasonable procedure to adapt in children. The only available instruments were 10 mm in size and this seemed cumbersome in small children, but the more rapid recovery was readily apparent, even while the procedure was more prolonged. The longer operative times were an obvious target for critics, but it did steadily decline with experience. The value of a wider field of view was appreciated and was highlighted by the honest report of an inadvertent appendectomy during open day surgery nephrectomy in an infant [43].

Another target of criticism was that laparoscopy converted a retroperitoneal procedure into an intra-peritoneal one, although it was uncertain and unproven that this added real risk. None-the-less, development of retroperitoneal techniques emerged in the mid to late 1990s [44–48]. Both lateral and prone techniques were developed and this provided a point of controversy in terms of relative advantages. The retroperitoneal approach did have some advantages, although it is hard to know if it was actually safer. In some ways, it may have been more perceptual, as the intra-peritoneal organs were only a few cells away and indeed were only less visible. Development of the retroperitoneal working space was and remains challenging, but once achieved, the direct visualization of the kidney for extirpative or reconstructive procedures is excellent (Fig. 1.3). Ergonomics were difficult as well, and delicate reconstructive procedures were made even more difficult.

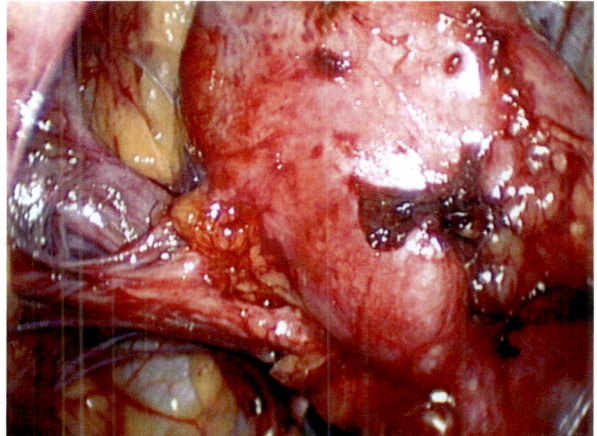

Fig. 1.3 Intra-operative image of a retroperitoneal laparoscopic nephrectomy illustrating the direct view of the renal hilum with the posterior retroperitoneal approach. The anatomically posterior artery is visualized in front of the veins

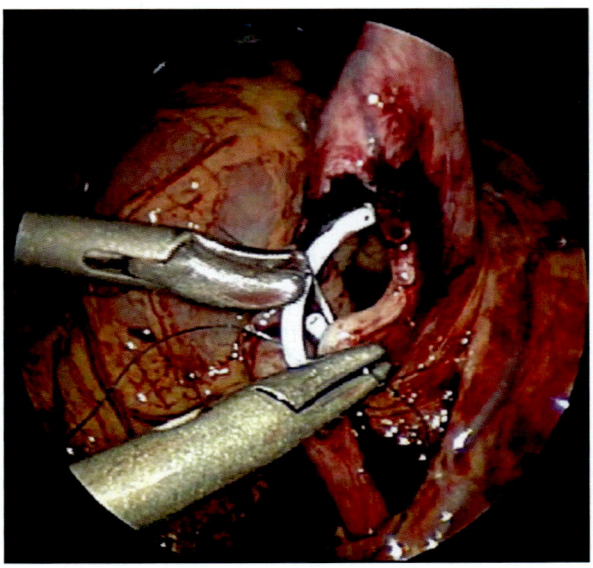

Fig. 1.4 Operative view of laparoscopic pyeloplasty during the anastomosis of the ureter and renal pelvis with a double-J ureteral stent in position for post-operative drainage

With continued experience working around the kidney, pyeloplasty became the next threshold to overcome. After performing relatively few in adults with an adult urology colleague, this was attempted in children, mostly of school age. The author's first case required 7 h, most of which was suturing and knot tying [49, 50] (Fig. 1.4). It was felt that we should reproduce the open procedure as closely as possible and interrupted sutures were used since that was our standard for open surgery at the time. Patients were highly selected with significant discussion with parents recognizing the limited experience with the procedure and its outcomes. Stents were not used, as they were not being used in open surgery, but wound drains were placed. Results were satisfactory but it remained a very challenging procedure and relatively few surgeons were performing it when robotic systems became available in 2002. Laparoscopic pyeloplasty, however, has persisted during the robotic era, largely due to the expense of the robotic system, and most published results show satisfactory results [51]. It does require careful attention to technique and must be performed at reasonable volumes for the surgeon to be efficient. The author's experience has been that after performing many more robotic procedures, he can perform a conventional free-hand laparoscopic pyeloplasty much more effectively than prior to using the robot. Presumably this is due to the development and refinement of the surgical steps, including use of the hitch stitch, stent placement, and exposure.

Partial nephrectomy or hemi-nephrectomy for duplicated systems was reported as well, and this offered several advantages over open surgery, in particular the ability to remove much of the ureter through much smaller incisions, when typically it was performed with a large flank incision or a second lower incision [44, 52, 53]. Retroperitoneal approaches were also described, and were particularly advantageous from the posterior approach. This provided direct vision and access to the polar vessels without having to mobilize the ureter or pelvis first (Fig. 1.3).

Roughly concurrent with the emergence of laparoscopic pyeloplasty and partial nephrectomy, ureteral reimplantation laparoscopically began to be explored. The initial animal study used the Lich-Gregoir extravesical approach that is more of a ureteroplasty than an actual reimplantation [54]. In the pig model, this was very efficient and rather straightforward to accomplish. It was not in the human. The angle of approach to the distal ureter in the human is a tighter space and the bladder wall is oriented almost perpendicular with the laparoscopic instruments. This angle makes dissection and suturing particularly challenging. Initial enthusiastic reports were not followed by widespread applications, despite a well-known admonition to "get on the wagon or become part of the road" at an early presentation [2]. A few persistent practitioners reported early series, but also recognized the limitations and risks [55–57].

A significant paradigm shift came with the report of intravesical laparoscopic ureteral reimplantation using the Cohen technique with the bladder being insufflated (pneumovesicum) as described by Yeung [58, 59]. This is still a technically challenging procedure but results have been very good in the hands of a high volume and experienced surgeon. Several others have taken up this method with similar results [60–62]. Emerging concurrently with increased use of endoscopic anti-reflux procedures and a reduction in surgical interventions, however, this method is not widely used. The challenge remains that to maintain an effective pneumovesicum, one must keep the ports well-secured within the bladder. A similar challenge is present using the robot [63, 64] (Fig. 1.5). and while it is effective in the thin child where the bladder wall can be secured through the skin port site, in heavier children this has proven difficult. The concept is appealing but awaits a better method to secure and close the bladder port sites.

More complex procedures such as augmentation cystoplasty, appendicovesicostomy and bladder neck reconstructions have been reported in limited numbers with conventional laparoscopy. but are not likely to ever be widely used due to inefficiencies and time constraints.

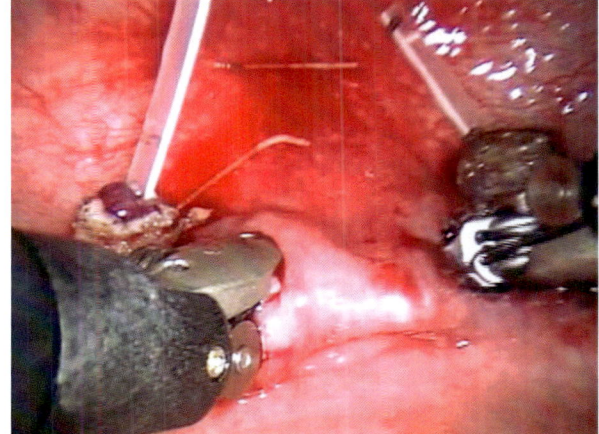

Fig. 1.5 Operative view of an intravesical robotic ureteral reimplantation using a pneumovesicum for exposure. The ureters have been mobilized with 5 French feeding tubes sewn in place and the the cross-trigonal tunnel is being developed with sharp and blunt dissection

Enter the Robot

The introduction of the DaVinci and Zeus surgical systems (it remains controversial as to whether these are true "robots" as this depends on whose definition of robot you subscribe to) coming on the heels of the introduction of operative laparoscopy in Pediatric Urology changed the trajectory of MIS significantly and quickly. Approved by the FDA for adult procedures in 2000, the DaVinci was first used in children in 2002. With the challenge of suturing and knot tying markedly reduced by way of the articulated working instruments, multiple procedures could be approached laparoscopically. Pyeloplasty was in many ways, the perfect test case, and having struggled with these using conventional laparoscopic techniques, it was a real epiphany to have the robotic assistance to complete the procedures in much shorter times and more importantly, with greater assurance of success. With a three dimensional and stable image coupled with precise and smooth instrument control, the technical advantage was more than obvious. Initial applications were successful and it proved useful in multiple procedures. With experience and utilization of dedicated surgical teams, procedure times rapidly declined. Based on contemporaneous comparisons, there seemed to be less post-operative pain, more rapid return to normal activities and equal success [65–67]. What has not improved was cost, and that remains a major limitation of the DaVinci system.

Two systems were initially available and our hospital set up a group to determine which system to purchase. The Zeus (Computer Motion) system had several advantages, including a modular design where the working arms mounted directly to the surgical table and were 5 mm in size. Its visualization system was less robust and used polarized glasses, and the control instruments were much more difficult to use to get the full articulation of the wristed instruments. There was an option for voice-activated controls (Hermes) that had been developed with CM's first system, the Aesop laparoscope controller. On the balance, the DaVinci (Intuitive Surgical (ISC)) seemed to be more flexible and robust for our multispecialty group. This was a fortuitous choice as ISC eventually bought out CM to settle an ongoing intellectual property legal dispute, and the Zeus system was discontinued. The DaVinci has evolved since its introduction and continues to be the most widely used surgical robotic system for Urology. Of course, it was made profitable by way of its application to radical prostatectomy, even though it was initially designed for cardiac surgery. Its applications in adult use are well known and continue to grow. The more recent introduction of the Xi and Single Site systems offer benefits for some applications, but as yet they are not seen to be significantly helpful for pediatric urology use.

While the utility of the robotic system has been shown in numerous surgical procedures and in all ages, the same arguments continue to be leveled against it including no proven benefit, longer surgical durations, and of course cost. Its continued use has prompted changes in surgical technique by the roboskeptics and a push to use even smaller and smaller incisions. It is interesting to have watched the changing value system in response to the increasing use of the robot, including length of stay, incision length, and the need for analgesics. Striving for reduced morbidity these efforts are certainly worthwhile and valuable, but often seem to be largely to justify not adapting robotic technology.

Another shift that has occurred is to minimize some post-operative assessment; for example following ureteral reimplantation for reflux. Many have given up performing post-operative cystography even though there are multiple reports of less than optimal success rates with the robotic approach. This is a risky approach given the limited experience with the technique, and the published reports of surgical failures. It was several decades after the adoption of open surgical reimplants before post-operative cystography was widely seen as of limited benefit. Until there is a solid foundation of proven surgical success, thorough assessment of outcomes should be seen as essential for robotic ureteral reimplantation.

Robotic techniques for pyeloplasty and ureteral reimplantation have been well described and there is continued innovation in terms of approaches and techniques to make these more efficient and effective [68–71]. While robotic pyeloplasty can be seen as achieving parity with open surgery, the same cannot be said for ureteral reimplantation. There have been multiple reports with lesser success and a higher rate of complications [72–75].

Similar concern exists related to augmentation cystoplasty where surgical times have not been able to be significantly reduced despite nearly a decade of application [76–78]. It is also uncertain as to how effective the published approach is, as it uses a different method (no bowel segment reconfiguration) than what most pediatric urologists would consider state of the art. Bowel reconfiguration has been a standard part of augmentation for several decades, having evolved due to unsatisfactory early results in the 1980s. It is difficult to interpret the published results to date. Few surgeons are using the robot for augmentation; as with ureteral reimplantation, complete transparency is essential to allow appropriate adoption of new technologies and techniques.

Future Directions

The main themes that have emerged in the evolution of MIS for pediatric Urology point us to where the field must move. Those who challenge the adoption of these newer technologies, may be seen as the "late adopters" of innovation, yet should also be considered to provide direction for future innovation. Key goals for successful future evolution of Pediatric Urological MIS must include the following:

1. Development of objective methods to assess surgical morbidity
2. Agreement as to the value of various aspects of the surgical experience beyond cost, and how to balance these elements with cost
3. Openness to novel techniques concurrent with standards of rigor and timing for assessment of new technology
4. Development of more collaborative partnerships with industry and regulatory agencies to facilitate truly useful new tools for our field

An overriding aspect of the evolution of MIS in general has been the impact of convergent technology that has permitted much of the modern technological tools we have today. That convergence continues to accelerate and will provide even more potential to enhance surgical care of children. As emphasized by Satava [79], the surgical robot is a digital information platform, and that means it can be linked with other information systems. This will permit more robust surgical planning and modeling, increased autonomy, better quality control and education, and by using artificial intelligence, better surgical decision-making [80].

As we continue to participate in this evolution, it remains critically important to maintain scrupulous integrity of results, and to welcome the skeptic who is critical to effective and dynamic innovation [81].

From CA Peters [82]

> …it is unlikely that we can accurately imagine what form a surgical robot might take in the next decades, yet the glimpse of that potential offered by the early experience with these first-generation systems is compelling indeed.

References

1. Cortesi N, Ferrari P, Zambarda E, Manenti A, Baldini A, Morano FP. Diagnosis of bilateral abdominal cryptorchidism by laparoscopy. Endoscopy. 1976;8(1):33–4.
2. Ehrlich RM, Gershman A, Fuchs G. Laparoscopic ureteral reimplantation for vesicoureteral reflux: initial case reports. J Endourol. 1993;7:S171.
3. Ehrlich RM, Gershman A, Mee S, Fuchs G. Laparoscopic nephrectomy in a child: expanding horizons for laparoscopy in pediatric urology. J Endourol. 1992;6:463–5.
4. Koyle MA, Woo HH, Kavoussi LR. Laparoscopic nephrectomy in the first year of life. J Pediatr Surg. 1993;28(5):693–5.
5. Jordan GH, Robey EL, Winslow BH. Laparoendoscopic surgical managment of the abdominal/transinguinal undescended testicle. J Endourol. 1992;6:157–61.
6. Jordan GH, Winslow BH. Laparoendoscopic upper pole partial nephrectomy with ureterectomy. J Urol. 1993;150(3):940–3.
7. Peters CA. Laparoscopy in pediatric urology. Urology. 1993;41:33–7.
8. Peters C. Laparoscopy in paediatric urology: adoption of innovative technology. BJU Int. 2003;92 Suppl 1:52–7.
9. Kirsch AJ, Arlen AM, Lackgren G. Current trends in dextranomer hyaluronic acid copolymer (Deflux) injection technique for endoscopic treatment of vesicoureteral reflux. Urology. 2014;84(2):462–8.
10. O'Donnell B, Puri P. Treatment of vesicoureteric reflux by endoscopic injection of Teflon. Br Med J (Clin Res Ed). 1984;289(6436):7–9.
11. Stenberg A, Hensle TW, Lackgren G. Vesicoureteral reflux: a new treatment algorithm. Curr Urol Rep. 2002;3(2):107–14.
12. Lendvay TS, Sorensen M, Cowan CA, Joyner BD, Mitchell MM, Grady RW. The evolution of vesicoureteral reflux management in the era of dextranomer/hyaluronic acid copolymer: a pediatric health information system database study. J Urol. 2006;176(4 Pt 2):1864–7.
13. Farhat W, Afshar K, Papanikolaou F, Austin R, Khoury A, Bagli D. Retroperitoneal-assisted laparoscopic pyeloplasty in children: initial experience. J Endourol. 2004;18(9):879–82.
14. Urbanowicz W, Honkisz I, Sulislawski J, Dobrowolska-Glazar B. The retroperitoneal, inguinal approach to distal part of the ureter. Cent European J Urol. 2014;67(1):108–11.

15. Babu R. 'Mini reimplantation' for the management of primary obstructed megaureter. J Pediatr Urol. 2016;12(2):103 e1–4.
16. Yap M, Nseyo U, Din H, Alagiri M. Unilateral extravesical ureteral reimplantation via inguinal incision for the correction of vesicoureteral reflux: a 10-year experience. Int Braz J Urol. 2017;43(5):917–24.
17. Barbosa JA, Barayan G, Gridley CM, Sanchez DC, Passerotti CC, Houck CS, et al. Parent and patient perceptions of robotic vs open urological surgery scars in children. J Urol. 2013;190(1):244–50.
18. Garcia-Roig ML, Travers C, McCracken C, Cerwinka W, Kirsch JM, Kirsch AJ. Surgical scar location preference for pediatric kidney and pelvic surgery: a Crowdsourced survey. J Urol. 2017;197(3 Pt 2):911–9
19. Malizia AA Jr, Reiman HM, Myers RP, Sande JR, Barham SS, Benson RC Jr, et al. Migration and granulomatous reaction after periurethral injection of polytef (Teflon). JAMA. 1984;251(24):3277–81.
20. Tanhaeivash R, Kajbafzadeh AM, Zeinoddini A, Khalili N, Vahidi Rad M, Heidari R. Combination of calcium hydroxyapatite and autologous blood for endoscopic treatment of vesicoureteral reflux in children. Int Urol Nephrol. 2014;46(7):1263–8.
21. Kohri K, Umekawa T, Esa A, Kaneko S, Akiyama T, Kurita T. Long-term results and curative mechanisms of vesicoureteral reflux by endoscopic injection of blood. Urology. 1989;34(5):258–61.
22. Mevorach RA, Hulbert WC, Rabinowitz R, Kennedy WA, Kogan BA, Kryger JV, et al. Results of a 2-year multicenter trial of endoscopic treatment of vesicoureteral reflux with synthetic calcium hydroxyapatite. J Urol. 2006;175(1):288–91.
23. Matthews RD, Christensen JP, Canning DA. Persistence of autologous free fat transplant in bladder submucosa of rats. J Urol. 1994;152(2 Pt 2):819–21.
24. Leonard MP, Canning DA, Peters CA, Gearhart JP, Jeffs RD. Endoscopic injection of glutaraldehyde cross-linked bovine dermal collagen for correction of vesicoureteral reflux. J Urol. 1991;145(1):115–9.
25. Atala A, Peters CA, Retik AB, Mandell J. Endoscopic treatment of vesicoureteral reflux with a self-detachable balloon system. J Urol. 1992;148(2 Pt 2):724–7.
26. Aboutaleb H, Bolduc S, Upadhyay J, Farhat W, Bagli DJ, Khoury AE. Subureteral polydimethylsiloxane injection versus extravesical reimplantation for primary low grade vesicoureteral reflux in children: a comparative study. J Urol. 2003;169(1):313–6.
27. Oswald J, Riccabona M, Lusuardi L, Bartsch G, Radmayr C. Prospective comparison and 1-year follow-up of a single endoscopic subureteral polydimethylsiloxane versus dextranomer/hyaluronic acid copolymer injection for treatment of vesicoureteral reflux in children. Urology. 2002;60(5):894–7; discussion 8.
28. Stenberg A, Lackgren G. A new bioimplant for the endoscopic treatment of vesicoureteral reflux: experimental and short-term clinical results. J Urol. 1995;154(2 Pt 2):800–3.
29. Starmer B, McAndrew F Corbett H. A review of novel STING bulking agents. J Pediatr Urol. 2019;15(5):484–90.
30. Capozza N, Caione P. Dextranomer/hyaluronic acid copolymer implantation for vesico-ureteral reflux: a randomized comparison with antibiotic prophylaxis. J Pediatr. 2002;140(2):230–4.
31. Holmdahl G, Brandstrom P, Lackgren G, Sillen U, Stokland E, Jodal U, et al. The Swedish reflux trial in children: II. Vesicoureteral reflux outcome. J Urol. 2010;184(1):280–5.
32. Lightfoot M, Bilgutay AN, Tollin N, Eisenberg S, Weiser J, Bryan L, et al. Long-term clinical outcomes and parental satisfaction after Dextranomer/hyaluronic acid (dx/HA) injection for primary Vesicoureteral reflux. Front Pediatr. 2019;7:392.
33. Jackman SV, Hedican SP, Peters CA, Docimo SG. Percutaneous nephrolithotomy in infants and preschool age children: experience with a new technique. Urology. 1998;52(4):697–701.
34. Jackman SV, Docimo SG, Cadeddu JA, Bishoff JT, Kavoussi LR, Jarrett TW. The "miniperc" technique: a less invasive alternative to percutaneous nephrolithotomy. World J Urol. 1998;16(6):371–4.

35. Smaldone MC, Cannon GM Jr, Wu HY, Bassett J, Polsky EG, Bellinger MF, et al. Is ureteroscopy first line treatment for pediatric stone disease? J Urol. 2007;178(5):2128–31; discussion 31.
36. Lee RS, Passerotti CC, Cendron M, Estrada CR, Borer JG, Peters CA. Early results of robot assisted laparoscopic lithotomy in adolescents. J Urol. 2007;177(6):2306–9. discussion 9-10
37. Manson AL, Terhune D, Jordan G, Auman JR, Peterson N, MacDonald G. Preoperative laparoscopic localization of the nonpalpable testis. J Urol. 1985;134(5):919–20.
38. Moore RG, Peters CA, Bauer SB, Mandell J, Retik AB. Laparoscopic evaluation of the nonpalpable tests: a prospective assessment of accuracy. J Urol. 1994;151(3):728–31.
39. Belman AB, Rushton HG. Is an empty left hemiscrotum and hypertrophied right descended testis predictive of perinatal torsion? J Urol. 2003;170(4 Pt 2):1674–5; discussion 5–6.
40. Ferro F, Lais A, Bagolan P, Talamo M, Caterino S. Impact of primary surgical approach in the management of the impalpable testis. Eur Urol. 1992;22(2):142–6.
41. Cisek LJ, Peters CA, Atala A, Bauer SB, Diamond DA, Retik AB. Current findings in diagnostic laparoscopic evaluation of the nonpalpable testis. J Urol. 1998;160(3 Pt 2):1145–9; discussion 50.
42. Barqawi AZ, Blyth B, Jordan GH, Ehrlich RM, Koyle MA. Role of laparoscopy in patients with previous negative exploration for impalpable testis. Urology. 2003;61(6):1234–7; discussion 7.
43. Elder JS, Hladky D, Selzman AA. Outpatient nephrectomy for nonfunctioning kidneys. J Urol. 1995;154(2 Pt 2):712–4; discussion 4–5.
44. Lee RS, Retik AB, Borer JG, Diamond DA, Peters CA. Pediatric retroperitoneal laparoscopic partial nephrectomy: comparison with an age matched cohort of open surgery. J Urol. 2005;174(2):708–11; discussion 12.
45. El-Ghoneimi A, Farhat W, Bolduc S, Bagli D, McLorie G, Aigrain Y, et al. Laparoscopic dismembered pyeloplasty by a retroperitoneal approach in children. BJU Int. 2003;92(1):104–8; discussion 8.
46. Borer JG, Peters CA. Pediatric retroperitoneoscopic nephrectomy. J Endourol. 2000;14(5):413–6; discussion 7.
47. Borer JG, Cisek LJ, Atala A, Diamond DA, Retik AB, Peters CA. Pediatric retroperitoneoscopic nephrectomy using 2 mm. Instrumentation. J Urol. 1999;162(5):1725–9; discussion 30.
48. El-Ghoneimi A, Valla JS, Steyaert H, Aigrain Y. Laparoscopic renal surgery via a retroperitoneal approach in children. J Urol. 1998;160(3 Pt 2):1138–41.
49. Peters CA, Schlussel RN, Retik AB. Pediatric laparoscopic dismembered pyeloplasty. J Urol. 1995;153(6):1962–5.
50. Kavoussi LR, Peters CA. Laparoscopic pyeloplasty. J Urol. 1993;150(6):1891–4.
51. Reddy MN, Nerli RB. The laparoscopic pyeloplasty: is there a role in the age of robotics? Urol Clin North Am. 2015;42(1):43–52.
52. Wallis MC, Khoury AE, Lorenzo AJ, Pippi-Salle JL, Bagli DJ, Farhat WA. Outcome analysis of retroperitoneal laparoscopic heminephrectomy in children. J Urol. 2006;175(6):2277–80; discussion 80–2.
53. El-Ghoneimi A, Farhat W, Bolduc S, Bagli D, McLorie G, Khoury A. Retroperitoneal laparoscopic vs open partial nephroureterectomy in children. BJU Int. 2003;91(6):532–5.
54. Atala A, Kavoussi LR, Goldstein DS, Retik AB, Peters CA. Laparoscopic correction of vesicoureteral reflux. J Urol. 1993;150(2 Pt 2):748–51.
55. Lakshmanan Y, Fung LC. Laparoscopic extravesicular ureteral reimplantation for vesicoureteral reflux: recent technical advances. J Endourol. 2000;14(7):589–93; discussion 93–4.
56. Lakshmanan Y, Fung LC. Laparoscopic extravesicular ureteral reimplantation for vesicoureteral reflux: recent technical advances. J Endourol. 2000;14(7):589–93.
57. Janetschek G, Radmayr C, Bartsch G. Laparoscopic ureteral anti-reflux plasty reimplantation. First clinical experience. Ann Urol (Paris). 1995;29(2):101–5.

58. Thakre AA, Yeung CK. Technique of intravesical laparoscopy for ureteric Reimplantation to treat VUR. Adv Urol. 2008;2008:937231.
59. Yeung CK, Sihoe JD, Borzi PA. Endoscopic cross-trigonal ureteral reimplantation under carbon dioxide bladder insufflation: a novel technique. J Endourol. 2005;19(3):295–9.
60. Schober MS, Jayanthi VR. Vesicoscopic ureteral reimplant: is there a role in the age of robotics? Urol Clin North Am. 2015;42(1):53–9.
61. Canon SJ, Jayanthi VR, Patel AS. Vesicoscopic cross-trigonal ureteral reimplantation: a minimally invasive option for repair of vesicoureteral reflux. J Urol 2007;178(1):269–73; discussion 73.
62. Ansari MS, Yadav P, Arora S, Singh P, Sekhon V. Bilateral Transvesicoscopic cross-trigonal ureteric Reimplantation in children: surgical subtleties and a prospective summary. Urology. 2017;101:67–72.
63. Peters CA, Woo R. Intravesical robotically assisted bilateral ureteral reimplantation. J Endourol. 2005;19(6):618–21; discussion 21–2.
64. Yeung CK, Chowdhary SK, Sreedhar B. Minimally invasive Management for Vesicoureteral Reflux in infants and young children. Clin Perinatol. 2017;44(4):835–49.
65. Lee RS, Retik AB, Borer JG, Peters CA. Pediatric robot assisted laparoscopic dismembered pyeloplasty: comparison with a cohort of open surgery. J Urol. 2006;175(2):683–7; discussion 7.
66. Copeland DR, Boneti C, Kokoska ER, Jackson RJ, Smith SD. Evaluation of initial experience and comparison of the da Vinci surgical system with established laparoscopic and open pediatric Nissen fundoplication surgery. JSLS. 2008;12(3):238–40.
67. Lee RS, Sethi AS, Passerotti CC, Retik AB, Borer JG, Nguyen HT, et al. Robot assisted laparoscopic partial nephrectomy: a viable and safe option in children. J Urol. 2009;181(2):823–8; discussion 8–9.
68. Satyanarayan A, Peters CA. Advances in robotic surgery for pediatric ureteropelvic junction obstruction and vesicoureteral reflux: history, present, and future. World J Urol. 2020;38(8):1821–6.
69. Fichtenbaum EJ, Strine AC, Concodora CW, Schulte M, Noh PH. Tubeless outpatient robotic upper urinary tract reconstruction in the pediatric population: short-term assessment of safety. J Robot Surg. 2018;12(2):257–60.
70. Chan YY, Durbin-Johnson B, Sturm RM, Kurzrock EA. Outcomes after pediatric open, laparoscopic, and robotic pyeloplasty at academic institutions. J Pediatr Urol. 2017;13(1):49 e1–6.
71. Finkelstein JB, Van Batavia JP, Casale P. Is outpatient robotic pyeloplasty feasible? J Robot Surg. 2016;10:233–7.
72. Timberlake MD, Peters CA. Current status of robotic-assisted surgery for the treatment of vesicoureteral reflux in children. Curr Opin Urol. 2017;27(1):20–6.
73. Baek M, Koh CJ. Lessons learned over a decade of pediatric robotic ureteral reimplantation. Investig Clin Urol. 2017;58(1):3–11.
74. Weiss DA, Shukla AR. The robotic-assisted ureteral reimplantation: the evolution to a new standard. Urol Clin North Am. 2015;42(1):99–109.
75. Grimsby GM, Dwyer ME, Jacobs MA, Ost MC, Schneck FX, Cannon GM, et al. Multi-institutional review of outcomes of robot-assisted laparoscopic extravesical ureteral reimplantation. J Urol. 2015;193(5 Suppl):1791–5.
76. Murthy P, Cohn JA, Selig RB, Gundeti MS. Robot-assisted laparoscopic augmentation Ileocystoplasty and Mitrofanoff Appendicovesicostomy in children: updated interim results. Eur Urol. 2015;68(6):1069–75.
77. Barashi NS, Rodriguez MV, Packiam VT, Gundeti MS. Bladder reconstruction with bowel: robot-assisted laparoscopic Ileocystoplasty with Mitrofanoff Appendicovesicostomy in pediatric patients. J Endourol. 2018;32(S1):S119–S26.
78. Gundeti MS, Petravick ME, Pariser JJ, Pearce SM, Anderson BB, Grimsby GM, et al. A multi-institutional study of perioperative and functional outcomes for pediatric robotic-assisted laparoscopic Mitrofanoff appendicovesicostomy. J Pediatr Urol. 2016;12(6):386 e1–5.

79. Satava RM. Disruptive visions: a robot is not a machine…systems integration for surgeons. Surg Endosc. 2004;18:617–20.
80. Loftus TJ, Tighe PJ, Filiberto AC, Efron PA, Brakenridge SC, Mohr AM, et al. Artificial intelligence and surgical decision-making. JAMA Surg. 2019;155:148–58.
81. Dimick JB, Sedrakyan A, McCulloch P. The IDEAL framework for evaluating surgical innovation: how it can be used to improve the quality of evidence. JAMA Surg. 2019;154:685–6.
82. Peters CA. Robotically assisted paediatric pyeloplasty: cutting edge or expensive toy? BJU Int. 2004;94(9):1214–5.

Chapter 2
Physiologic Considerations in Laparoscopic Surgery

Jonathan A. Gerber, Alexandra N. Borden, and Duong D. Tu

Introduction

Primitive forms of endoscopy and laparoscopy have been described for centuries. As early as 1805, Bozzini utilized a candle as an external light source with a series of mirrors to internally inspect the rectum and bladder [1]. These initial forays into endoscopic and laparoscopic investigation and intervention took place exclusively in the adult patient. Another century passed before the application of laparoscopic investigation spread to the pediatric population when, in 1923, Kelling described the first laparoscopic endeavor in the pediatric population [2]. These early adventures were limited to accessible orifices, while contemporary laparoscopy is synonymous with the evaluation of naturally inaccessible cavities such as the peritoneal or thoracic cavities. Stephen Gans is credited with performing the first laparoscopy in 1971, which at the time referred to as "peritoneoscopy" [3]. Since inception, significant advancements in technology have allowed for the development and miniaturization of laparoscopic technology and equipment to what is used today.

During the period of laparoscopic development, various insufflation gases have been tried, including room air, nitrogen, helium, and oxygen. Significant issues arose from the use of these gases including venous air embolisms and even spontaneous combustion, which resulted in catastrophic outcomes [4]. The ideal insufflation gas had to be readily available, inexpensive, water soluble (i.e., rapid tissue diffusion), and for obvious reasons, non-combustible. Carbon dioxide (CO_2) met those requirements and is now the insufflation agent of choice. By virtue of its high

---

Jonathan A. Gerber and Alexandra N. Borden contributed equally with all other contributors.

J. A. Gerber · A. N. Borden (✉) · D. D. Tu
Texas Children's Hospital and Baylor College of Medicine, Houston, TX, USA
e-mail: jagerber@texaschildrens.org; anborden@texaschildrens.org; dxtu@texaschildrens.org

© Springer Nature Switzerland AG 2020
P. C. Gargollo (ed.), *Minimally Invasive and Robotic-Assisted Surgery in Pediatric Urology*, https://doi.org/10.1007/978-3-030-57219-8_2

diffusion coefficient, residual CO2 following a laparoscopic procedure is absorbed within 24 hours. In addition, high solubility in blood decreases the risk of gas embolus intra-operatively.

Continued innovation eventually gave rise to the development of robot assisted laparoscopic surgery, which retains the core principles of laparoscopic surgery in addition to improved ergonomics and instrument articulation. A certain level of proficiency in laparoscopic and robotic assisted cases is now required for graduating urology residents. Given this growing prevalence of robot-assisted laparoscopic urologic surgeries, intimate knowledge of the physiologic considerations associated with this technology is essential. Increased intraabdominal pressure, patient positioning, and gas absorption are just some of the components of laparoscopic surgery that affect multiple organ systems. In this chapter we aim to provide the basics of understanding of how these elements of laparoscopy affect various organ systems including the cardiovascular, pulmonary, renal, and central nervous systems. The majority of these physiologic changes can be attributed to one of two reasons: (1) directly from the pneumoperitoneum itself, or (2) indirectly from hypercarbia and neuroendocrine pathways.

Direct Effects of Pneumoperitoneum

Cardiovascular

Cardiovascular effects all ultimately relate to cardiac output, which in turn, relate to heart rate (HR), contractility, preload, and afterload. To facilitate understanding of the cardiac physiology and its practical relevance, cardiac output (CO) can be divided into two main parts based on the formula for calculation: CO = Stroke volume (SV) × Heart rate (HR). Let's examine each component separately in the context of laparoscopic surgery.

Stroke Volume (SV)

Stoke volume is the efficiency of the pump, i.e. the heart, represented by the amount of blood the heart pushes out to the rest of the body (end systolic volume, ESV) relative to the volume of blood that fills the ventricle before contraction (end diastolic volume, EDV). Formulaically, this is represented by SV = EDV − ESV. Conceptually, again returning to the pump analogy, the efficiency (how much blood is pushed out) rests upon the force of the pump (contractility) and how full the pump's tank is at the time of contraction. This "tank" volume is defined as preload. To a certain extent, higher preload increases the stretch on the cardiac muscle, which in turn, augments the force of contraction (contractility).

The other determinant of SV is systemic vascular resistance (SVR). Higher SVR produces lower SV. As the heart pushes out blood, the increased resistance impedes the flow of blood, in turn decreasing the volume of blood pumped for each contraction, decreasing SV, and therefore cardiac output.

In laparoscopic surgery, insufflation increases intra-abdominal pressure (IAP). This effects cardiac output in degree and direction by the amount of pneumoperitoneum (PnP), and the patient's volume status. Initially during insufflation, when IAP is below 5 mmHg, venous return *increases* due to compression of the splanchnic vasculature, resulting in an increase in venous return to the right atrium (increased preload → increased contractility) and an initial increase in cardiac output [5]. As IAP continues to rise to >15 mmHg, venous return is diminished due to inferior vena caval (IVC) compression and lower extremity blood pooling (decreased preload → decreased stroke volume). This is combined with increased arterial resistance due to aortic compression (increased SVR → further decreasing stroke volume) resulting in overall decreased cardiac output [5]. All of these factors lead to a subsequent decline in cardiac output up to 30% [6, 7]. The degree of these physiologic changes are affected by the patient's volume status. If the patient is hypervolemic, there is a protective effect against these changes, and the patient is able to maintain a more stable cardiac output. In other words, the point in which the pressure compresses the IVC and aorta is shifted to the right, and the patient may be able to tolerate higher pressures.

Heart Rate (HR)

To maintain cardiac output in light of decreased stroke volume, the heart rate would have to exhibit a compensatory increase. However, significant bradycardia may occur upon insufflation due to stretching of the peritoneum and stimulation of the vagus nerve [8]. Otherwise, heart rate remains largely unaffected by the direct effects of PnP [9, 10].

Practical Points

Consideration of the patient's preoperative hypovolemia and intended patient positioning is essential. Preoperative fasting and the higher resting metabolic rates in children can result in decreased preload which will require the judicious use of fluids intraoperatively [11]. Fortunately, pediatric cases typically utilize IAP <12 mmHg, thereby minimizing significant and prolonged organ dysfunction or decreased cardiac output [12].

If significant bradycardia due to vagal response occurs with insufflation, IAP should be reduced via opening of the laparoscopic ports for desufflation along with provision of a fluid bolus to increase intravascular volume for the reasons stated above. After recovery of heart rate, repeat attempt at insufflation at a slower rate and lower IAP is typically well tolerated, and there should be no significant change in heart rate with reasonable insufflation pressures (10–15 mm Hg). However, if bradycardia recurs even with slow re-insufflation, conversion to open laparotomy is advised.

Trendelenburg position increases SVR and heart rate, but increases venous return and hence cardiac output, which counters the decreased cardiac output induced by pneumoperitoneum [13, 14].

Together, all of these physiologic changes occur on a spectrum, with the overall effects dependent on the IAP. In summary, maintain euvolemia, if not hypervolemia, and keep the IAP < 15 mm Hg. If there is bradycardia, desufflate until the HR recovers and slow down the insufflation flow.

Respiratory

Increased applied pressure from PnP and Trendelenburg positioning each displace the diaphragm cephalad—increasing airway pressure, and reducing tidal volume and functional residual capacity [15]. This can be seen as increased peak inspiratory pressures, decreased pulmonary compliance, stable or increased alveolar dead space, and decreased peak expiratory flow [16–19]. Potential respiratory consequences include barotrauma, VQ mismatch and resultant hypoxia.

Practical Points

Direct pressure from PnP makes it difficult to expand the lungs enough for both oxygenation and ventilation of excess CO_2 absorbed by insufflation. This scenario is reconciled by either increasing minute ventilation which allows for blowing off CO_2 faster at the same, limited, functional capacity or increasing positive end expiratory pressure (PEEP) to counteract the pressure upon the diaphragm and expand the airways [18]. Maracaja-Neto et al. proposed a PEEP of 10 cm H_2O as the pressure effective in attenuating these respiratory changes [20].

Renal

It has been well established that pneumoperitoneum, particularly with IAP > 15 mm Hg, have significant, albeit, transient effects on the kidneys. Mechanical compression of the renal vasculature and the renal parenchyma lead to decreased renal perfusion, oliguria, and decreased glomerular filtration rate

(GFR) [21]. Pneumoperitoneum greater than 15 mm Hg leads to a direct rise in serum creatinine that normalizes in 24 h after desufflation, again exemplifying the transitory nature of this phenomenon.

It was previously thought that the activation of the renin-angiotensin-aldosterone system (RAAS) was the main cause of oliguria. This was disproved in a 2002 study which found no difference between the levels of antidiuretic hormone, aldosterone, and renin in patients who underwent laparoscopic compared to open gastric bypass surgeries [22].

Rather, as demonstrated in canine and swine studies of induced Page-kidneys and prolonged pneumoperitoneum, compression of both the renal parenchyma itself and the renal vein are the purported etiologies of oliguria in laparoscopic surgery [21, 23]. Postoperative renal function was not diminished, as this compressive state is transient and reversible with desufflation.

Practical Points

All of these renal effects are most notable at IAP > 15 mm Hg. This is the same pressure cut-off that adversely affects cardiac output (CO), as discussed in the previous section. Therefore, the decreased renal perfusion, and its incumbent effects, are accentuated by decreased CO. In general, it is best to keep insufflation pressures below 15 mm Hg for the majority of a laparoscopic surgery, with excursions above this pressure in limited, controlled applications, e.g. momentary increase in insufflation pressure while repairing a bleeding vessel.

To offset the intraoperative and postoperative renal effects of laparoscopic surgery, efforts should be made to provide adequate fluid loading both before and during the procedure while at the same time maintaining a balance that would prevent hypervolemia and subsequent post-operative edema.

CNS

Cerebral hemodynamics are heavily influenced by cardiovascular status, patient positioning, and abdominal pressure. Increased IAP directly increases intracranial pressure (ICP). Halverson et al. demonstrated an increase in ICP with incremental increases (5 mm Hg) in IAP. Increased ICP is exacerbated by Trendelenberg position and is not improved if the patient is repositioned in reverse Trendelenberg. The pattern of increased ICP with elevated IAP was found to be true in both positions. This was persistent even in the presence of relatively low-pressure (5–8 mm Hg) pneumoperitoneum [24]. The likely mechanism causing the increased ICP is impaired venous drainage due to compression of the lumbar venous plexus at elevated IAP. Moreover, cerebrospinal fluid (CSF) reabsorption is impaired by elevated IAP also contributing to elevated ICP [25].

Practical Points

Increased ICP is directly correlated with incremental increases in IAP. This is in concordance with this chapter's overarching theme of judicious insufflation pressure during laparoscopic surgery. Seeing that the effect is present even at low insufflation pressures (5–8 mm Hg), the effect is unavoidable with the working pressures needed for most laparoscopic cases. This increase in ICP is directly correlated with incremental increases in IAP, but may be safe if working pressures reside below 10 mm Hg. Also, an important characteristic of this effect on ICP is that it is transient in nature. The patient population at highest risk are head injury patients, presumably due to the loss of ICP regulatory mechanisms. Laparoscopic surgery in these patients should be avoided [26]. There is no contraindication for laparoscopic surgery in children with ventriculoperitoneal shunts [27].

Indirect Effects of Laparoscopic Surgery

Cardiovascular

Concomitantly, neuroendocrine effects are seen with increased IAP due to catecholamine release along with activation of the Renin-Angiotensin-Aldosterone-System (RAAS) [28]. These effects are known to increase mean arterial pressure (MAP) and SVR due to vasoconstriction resulting in a rise in both heart rate and blood pressure.

Effects of CO2 gas absorption must also be accounted for as hypercarbia can result in an acidosis with cardiovascular consequences. Directly, this acidosis can reduce cardiac contractility and induce systemic vasodilation. However, indirect effects ensue via stimulation of the sympathetic nervous system causing tachycardia and vasoconstriction in direct opposition to the primary vasodilatory effect [29]. This catecholamine induced increase in heart rate and blood pressure can result in arrhythmias [5].

Respiratory

The high solubility of CO_2 and hence, the transperitoneal absorption of it, affects respiration, as the higher levels of circulating CO_2 require an increased minute ventilation to maintain near normal levels. In patients with respiratory compromise, renal failure, or cardiovascular disease, this increased absorption can result in hypercarbia, respiratory acidosis and cardiac arrhythmias, due to the diminished ability to eliminate excess CO_2.

Practical Points

The wide-ranging, multi-system effects of hypercarbia underscores the importance of having a vigilant anesthetic team, one that would effectively monitor for and prevent the accumulation of CO_2. This can be performed through the use of arterial blood gas (ABG) sampling, although in healthy patients with normal lungs and airway, end-tidal CO_2 provides a reasonable estimate of arterial CO_2. Minute ventilation is the tidal volume multiplied by the respiratory rate, therefore, the mechanical ventilator manipulation of either of these two parameters will increase the ventilation or "blowing off" of CO_2. From a surgeon perspective, critical levels should prompt decreasing insufflation pressure or temporary complete desufflation of the pneumoperitoneum.

Renal

Decreased perfusion and function cannot be explained through mechanical compression alone. Although, decreased perfusion as a result of increased IAP leads to the activation of neuroendocrine pathways which significantly impact renal function. The resultant release of renin activates the renin-angiotensin-aldosterone system (RAAS) with subsequent secretion of aldosterone and the release of anti-diuretic hormone (ADH). Both cause water and salt retention, to expand circulating blood volume to compensate for decreased renal perfusion. Additionally, angiotensin II causes systemic vasoconstriction, increasing blood pressure to further compensate for decreased perfusion.

Endothelin, a powerful vasoconstrictor, has been implicated in renal dysfunction induced by pneumoperitoneum. Increased plasma concentrations were first associated with renal compression, both directly and from pneumoperitoneum in a canine model. Endothelin produces renal dysfunction by decreasing renal perfusion, GFR, and sodium excretion [30].

Practical Points

These renal effects have not been studied in the pediatric population, and so may not be clinically relevant in otherwise healthy children. However, many urologic patients will have a level of renal dysfunction that, although perhaps not a contraindication for laparoscopic surgery, may make them more susceptible to the above mentioned effects and would warrant closer monitoring postoperatively with respect to fluid balance, electrolytes, and creatinine.

CNS

Increases in the amount of CO_2 in the blood or the partial pressure of CO_2 ($PaCO_2$) has been shown to increase cerebral blood flow [31]. This is mediated via the vasodilatory effects of hypercarbia on the cerebral vasculature and is an important regulator of maintaining near normal carbon dioxide and related acid levels in the brain. Elevated levels depress neuronal activity, and so the increased blood flow is designed to "wash out" these excesses: a neuroprotective process. Interestingly, hyperventilation and reverse Trendelenburg positioning do not prevent this increased cerebral blood flow [24].

Clinical Summary

Almost all of these physiologic discoveries are exhibited either in the adult population or extrapolated from animal studies. Moreover, multiple studies describing these effects in the pediatric population detail observations in young animals. Therefore, some of these descriptions cannot be fully applied to children, although there should be enough parallels in order to instruct our clinical decision-making.

Throughout this chapter, practical points have been interspersed in an attempt to summarize key concepts into actionable clinical recommendations. This section is designed to consolidate these recommendations.

Typically, pediatric laparoscopic cases utilize pneumoperitoneum (PnP) with pressures of 12 mm Hg or less, preventing the cardiovascular effects of decreased cardiac output (CO) and decreased venous return (VR). In fact, these lower pressures augment CO and VR. The importance of maintaining euvolemia is evident here from not only a cardiovascular standpoint but also a renal one. This becomes even more crucial if intra-abdominal pressures (IAP) rise above 15 mm Hg when CO and VR decrease, systemic vascular resistance (SVR) increases, and oliguria begins to set in. Heart rate (HR) shows no significant changes even at higher IAP, except in the early phase of insufflation (peritoneal stretch and vagal stimulation) when bradycardia can occur. If this is seen, the abdomen should be desufflated until the HR recovers and insufflation restarted at a slower rate. Recurrence warrants strong consideration for abandoning the laparoscopic approach.

To counteract the direct pressure effects of PnP on the diaphragm and lungs, the anesthesiologist should increase the minute ventilation to decrease end-tidal CO_2 and/or increase positive end expiratory pressure (PEEP) to expand the lungs for more effective oxygenation and ventilation.

Cerebral blood flow and intracranial pressure starts increasing from low insufflation pressures of 5–8 mm Hg, incrementally with increases in IAP. Despite the transitory nature of this effect, laparoscopic surgery and PnP should be avoided in head injury patients. There is no contraindication in children with ventriculoperitoneal shunts (Fig. 2.1).

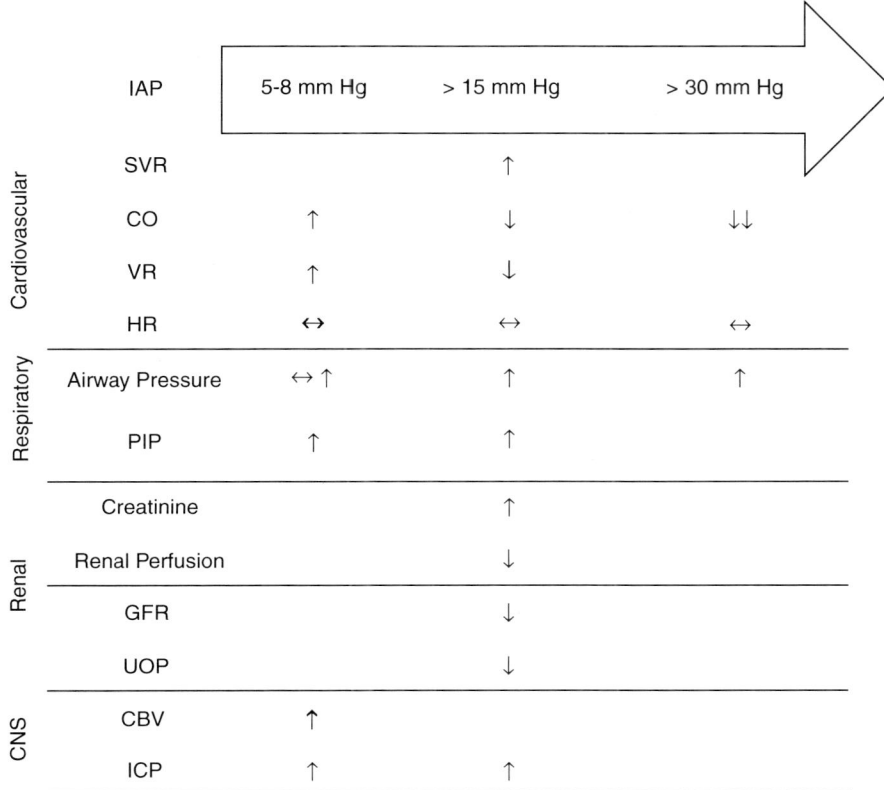

Fig. 2.1 Direct effects of pneumoperitoneum and increased intra-abdominal pressure. SVR = systemic vascular resistance, CO = cardiac output, VR = venous return, HR = heart rate, PIP = peak inspiratory pressure, GFR = glomerular filtration rate, UOP = urine output, CNS = central nervous system, CBV = cerebral blood volume, ICP = intracranial pressure

Many of the indirect effects (Fig. 2.2) of PnP occur as the result of the absorption of CO_2 into the bloodstream with much of the adverse effects related to hypercapnia ($PaCO_2$ > 46 mm Hg). Here, like many things, prevention is the key. The partial pressure of carbon dioxide ($PaCO_2$) can be calculated by an arterial blood gas (ABG), although in healthy patients without pulmonary disease, end-tidal CO_2 is an effective surrogate. A vigilant anesthetic team will monitor for these trends and make ventilator adjustments (increase minute ventilation) to buffer against CO_2 accumulation. Decreasing the insufflation pressure can also serve to de-escalate, but if this is unsuccessful, complete desufflation should be performed until levels normalize.

Children with pre-existing renal dysfunction should have close post-operative monitoring with respect to fluid balance, electrolyte disturbance, and serum creatinine.

Indirect Effects of CO_2 PnP	Hypercapnia $PaCO_2 > 46$ mm Hg	Acidosis	↓ Myocardial contractility ↑Pulmonary vascular resistance Systemic vasodilaton	
		Vasodilation	↑ Cerebral blood flow	
		Sympathetic Nervous System Activation *Via catecholamine release*	↑ HR ↑ BP ↑ Pulmonary artery pressure Arrhythmia Systemic vasoconstriction	
	Neurohormonal Response	RAAS Pathway	ADH Aldosterone	↑MAP ↑SVR ↑ HR ↑ BP
			Angiotensin II	Vasoconstriction ↑ BP
		Endothelin	Powerful vasoconstrictor	↓renal perfusion ↓ GFR ↓ Sodium excretion

Fig. 2.2 Indirect effects of CO_2 pneumoperitoneum

	HR	VR	CO	FRC	PC
Trendelenburg	↓	↑	↑	↓	↓
Reverse Trendelenburg	↑	↓	↓	↑	↑

Fig. 2.3 Cardiopulmonary effects of positioning. HR = heart rate, VR = venous return, CO = cardiac output, FRC = functional residual capacity, PC = pulmonary compliance

Finally, Trendelenburg positioning exerts cardiopulmonary effects (Fig. 2.3) but is often necessary for exposure and efficient completion of the surgery. One needs to have knowledge of these effects so that intra-operative repositioning can be considered if amelioration is refractory to other measures, especially with respect to respiratory ventilation. An effect not altered by repositioning is the increase in cerebral blood flow.

Conclusion

Laparoscopic surgery has become increasingly more popular in nearly all surgical subspecialties and has been associated with numerous benefits such as reduced post-operative pain and decreased hospital stay. Minimally invasive techniques continue to evolve and expand to new areas of medicine and new patient populations. For the patient's safety, it is imperative that the complex physiologic changes brought on by laparoscopic surgery and its pneumoperitoneum are well understood and anticipated.

References

1. Ramai D, Zakhia K, Etienne D, Reddy M. Philipp Bozzini (1773-1809): the earliest description of endoscopy. J Med Biogr. 2018;26(2):137–41. https://doi.org/10.1177/0967772018755587.
2. Kelling G. Zur colioskopie. Arch Klin Chir. 1923;126:226–9.
3. Gans SL, Berci G. Advances in endoscopy of infants and children. J Pediatr Surg. 1971;6(2):199–233. https://www.ncbi.nlm.nih.gov/pubmed/4254542.
4. Shadangi BK, Khanna S, Mehta Y Wrong gas: risk of intra-abdominal fire during laparoscopic surgery. Indian J Anaesth. 2012;56(6):599–600. https://doi.org/10.4103/0019-5049.104598.
5. Ost MC, Tan BJ, Lee BR. Urological laparoscopy: basic physiological considerations and immunological consequences. J Urol. 2005;174(4 Pt 1):1183–8 https://www.ncbi.nlm.nih.gov/pubmed/16145366
6. Westerband A, Van De Water J, Amzallag M, et al. Cardiovascular changes during laparoscopic cholecystectomy. Surg Gynecol Obstet. 1992;175(6):535–8. https://www.ncbi.nlm.nih.gov/pubmed/1448734.
7. McLaughlin JG, Scheeres DE, Dean RJ, Bonnell BW. The adverse hemodynamic effects of laparoscopic cholecystectomy. Surg Endosc. 1995;9(2):121–4. https://www.ncbi.nlm.nih.gov/pubmed/7597577.
8. Spinelli G, Vargas M, Aprea G, Cortese G, Servillo G. Pediatric anesthesia for minimally invasive surgery in pediatric urology. Transl Pediatr. 2016;5(4):214–21. https://doi.org/10.21037/tp.2016.09.02.
9. O'Malley C, Cunningham AJ. Physiologic changes during laparoscopy. Anesthesiol Clin North Am. 2001;19:1–19. https://doi.org/10.1016/S0889-8537(05)70208-X.
10. Kashtan J, Green JF, Parsons EQ, Holcroft JW. Hemodynamic effects of increased abdominal pressure. J Surg Res. 1981;30:249–55.
11. Stringel G. Laparoscopic pediatric surgery. In: Wetter PA, editor. Prevention & management of laparoendoscopic surgical complications. 3rd ed. 2012. https://laparoscopy.blogs.com/prevention_management_3/2010/11/laparoscopic-pediatric-surgery.html.
12. Munoz CJ, Nguyen HT, Houck CS. Robotic surgery and anesthesia for pediatric urologic procedures. Curr Opin Anaesthesiol. 2016;29(3):337–44. https://doi.org/10.1097/ACO.0000000000000333.
13. Falabella A, Moore-Jeffries E, Sullivan MJ, Nelson R, Lew M. Cardiac function during steep Trendelenburg position and CO2 pneumoperitoneum for robotic-assisted prostatectomy: a trans-oesophageal Doppler probe study. Int J Med Robot. 2007;3(4):312–5. https://doi.org/10.1002/rcs.165.
14. Pearle M. Physiologic effects of pneumoperitoneum. St. Louis: Quality Medical Publishing; 1996.
15. Atkinson TM, Giraud GD, Togioka BM, Jones DB, Cigarroa JE. Cardiovascular and ventilatory consequences of laparoscopic surgery. Circulation. 2017;135(7):700–10. https://doi.org/10.1161/CIRCULATIONAHA.116.023262.
16. Means LJ, Green MC, Bilal R. Anesthesia for minimally invasive surgery. Semin Pediatr Surg. 2004;13(3):181–7. https://www.ncbi.nlm.nih.gov/pubmed/15272426.
17. Jo YY, Kwak HJ. What is the proper ventilation strategy during laparoscopic surgery? Korean J Anesthesiol. 2017;70(6):596–600. https://doi.org/10.4097/kjae.2017.70.6.596.
18. Sharma KC, Brandstetter RD, Brensilver JM, Jung LD. Cardiopulmonary physiology and pathophysiology as a consequence of laparoscopic surgery. Chest. 1996;110(3):810–5. https://doi.org/10.1378/chest.110.3.810.
19. Rauh R, Hemmerling TM, Rist M, Jacobi KE. Influence of pneumoperitoneum and patient positioning on respiratory system compliance. J Clin Anesth. 2001;13:361–5.
20. Maracajá-Neto LF, Verçosa N, Roncally AC, Giannella A, Bozza FA, Lessa MA. Beneficial effects of high positive end-expiratory pressure in lung respiratory mechanics during laparoscopic surgery. Acta Anaesthesiol Scand. 2009;53(2):210–7. https://doi.org/10.1111/j.1399-6576.2008.01826.x.

21. McDougall EM, Monk TG, Wolf JS Jr, et al. The effect of prolonged pneumoperitoneum on renal function in an animal model. J Am Coll Surg. 1996;182(4):317–28. https://www.ncbi.nlm.nih.gov/pubmed/8605555.
22. Nguyen NT, Perez RV, Fleming N, Rivers R, Wolfe BM. Effect of prolonged pneumoperitoneum on intraoperative urine output during laparoscopic gastric bypass. J Am Coll Surg. 2002;195(4):476–83. https://www.ncbi.nlm.nih.gov/pubmed/12375752.
23. Razvi HA, Fields D, Vargas JC, Vaughan ED Jr, Vukasin A, Sosa RE. Oliguria during laparoscopic surgery: evidence for direct renal parenchymal compression as an etiologic factor. J Endourol. 1996;10(1):1–4. https://doi.org/10.1089/end.1996.10.1.
24. de Waal EE, de Vries JW, Kruitwagen CL, Kalkman CJ. The effects of low-pressure carbon dioxide pneumoperitoneum on cerebral oxygenation and cerebral blood volume in children. Anesth Analg. 2002;94(3):500–5; table of contents. https://www.ncbi.nlm.nih.gov/pubmed/11867365.
25. Halverson AL, Barrett WL, Iglesias AR, Lee WT, Garber SM, Sackier JM. Decreased cerebrospinal fluid absorption during abdominal insufflation. Surg Endosc. 1999;13(8):797–800.
26. Mobbs RJ, Yang MO. The dangers of diagnostic laparoscopy in the head injured patient. J Clin Neurosci. 2002;9(5):592–3. https://doi.org/10.1054/jocn.2001.1070.
27. Fraser JD, Aguayo P, Sharp SW, Holcomb GW, Ostlie DJ, Peter SDS. The safety of laparoscopy in pediatric patients with ventriculoperitoneal shunts. J Laparoendosc Adv Surg Tech A. 2009;19(5):675–8. https://doi.org/10.1089/lap.2009.0116.
28. Myre K, Rostrup M, Buanes T, Stokland O. Plasma catecholamines and haemodynamic changes during pneumoperitoneum. Acta Anaesthesiol Scand. 1998;42(3):343–7. https://www.ncbi.nlm.nih.gov/pubmed/9542563.
29. Gutt CN, Oniu T, Mehrabi A, et al. Circulatory and respiratory complications of carbon dioxide insufflation. Dig Surg. 2004;21(2):95–105. https://doi.org/10.1159/000077038.
30. Hamilton BD, Chow GK, Inman SR, Stowe NT, Winfield HN. Increased intra-abdominal pressure during pneumoperitoneum stimulates endothelin release in a canine model. J Endourol. 1998;12(2):193–7. https://doi.org/10.1089/end.1998.12.193.
31. De Cosmo G, Iannace E, Primieri P, et al. Changes in cerebral hemodynamics during laparoscopic cholecystectomy. Neurol Res. 1999;21(7):658–60. https://doi.org/10.1080/01616412.1999.11740993.

Chapter 3
Establishing a Pediatric Robotic Surgery Program

Sarah L. Hecht and Vijaya M. Vemulakonda

Introduction

Since the introduction of diagnostic laparoscopy for evaluation of the non-palpable testis, laparoscopic techniques have been widely adopted for a variety of common pediatric urologic procedures [1, 2]. Laparoscopy is now accepted practice for many extirpative procedures and is the standard of care for management of nonpalpable testes. The role of laparoscopy in pediatric urology continues to grow, with laparoscopic pyeloplasty and ureteral reimplantation performed at many pediatric centers of excellence [1].

While more complex reconstructive procedures have been performed [3], these have not gained wide acceptance due to steep learning curves and associated long operative times. Robotic surgery may offer advantages over traditional minimally invasive surgery in children such as articulated instruments, three dimensional vision with greater magnification, operator-controlled camera movement, tremor filtration, and removal of the fulcrum effect [4–7]. These benefits have led to wide adoption of robotic surgery in adults and increasing expansion among pediatric centers [8–10].

Historically pediatric centers have lagged behind their adult counterparts in adopting robotic technology. Prohibitive cost, lower surgical volume, and less dramatic advantages in children have been cited as reasons [7]. Currently, leading tertiary and quaternary referral centers have sustained pediatric robotic surgery programs for over a decade. We are now at an inflection point wherein the availability of technology and robotically trained surgeons will likely push

---

S. L. Hecht (✉)
Oregon Health & Science University, Department of Urology, Portland, OR, USA

V. M. Vemulakonda
Children's Hospital of Colorado, Department of Urology, Aurora, CO, USA
e-mail: vijaya.vemulakonda@childrenscolorado.org

© Springer Nature Switzerland AG 2020
P. C. Gargollo (ed.), *Minimally Invasive and Robotic-Assisted Surgery in Pediatric Urology*, https://doi.org/10.1007/978-3-030-57219-8_3

expansion of robotic surgery into children's hospitals across the country [10, 11]. As with the adoption of any new technique or procedure, it is important to systematically review the published experience and apply lessons learned to minimize preventable delays and errors. In this chapter we will focus on logistics, practicalities, and pearls for successful implementation of a pediatric robotic surgery program.

Mission Statement

Implementation of any new surgical program should be guided by an overarching vision and well-defined purpose. Financial incentive alone will be insufficient to obtain hospital buy-in or to sustain a practice. Each institution should consider its mission independently. Common goals for robotic surgery programs center around offering state-of-the-art surgical options, improving patient safety and perioperative outcomes, decreasing morbidity, inspiring surgical and technological innovation, advancing translational research, expanding surgical education, maximizing departmental or hospital reach, and meeting patient and/or surgeon demands.

Business Plan

Instituting a robotic surgery program necessitates a significant up-front investment. To date, potential decreases in length of stay for children undergoing robotic surgery have not been shown to offset the increased cost of surgery. Seideman et al. modeled cost differences between open and laparoscopic pyeloplasty. Despite shorter operative time and length of stay for robotic pyeloplasty, the cost of robotic surgery remained higher than laparoscopy [12]. This model estimated robotic pyeloplasty times would need to decrease from 210 min to 96 min for the robotic approach to be cost efficient. In a national analysis, Varda et al. found robotic pyeloplasty to be significantly more expensive than either open or laparoscopic pyeloplasty [13]. A similar national evaluation by Bowen et al. showed that despite shorter lengths of hospital stay, robotic ureteral reimplantation cost significantly more than open surgery [11]. The robotic team must accept that a robotic surgery program will not be immediately profitable. A formal business plan is essential, and should be carried out by surgeons aided by hospital administrators. Surgical volume needs to be adequate to offset cost, overcome learning curves, and maintain efficiency. Moreover, the adult literature suggests that high volume surgeons and centers yield better patient outcomes, and surgical volume should be high enough to pass this inflection point [14–19]. The business plan should include a market analysis, cost analysis, and a marketing plan (Fig. 3.1).

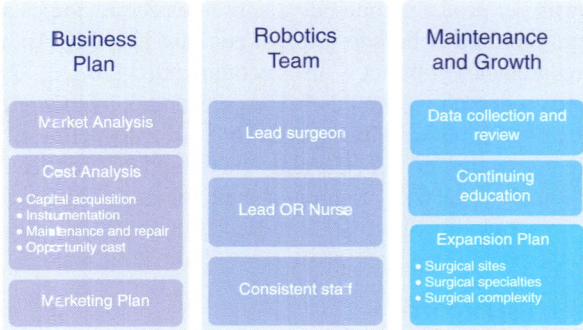

Fig. 3.1 Minimum requirements for launching a robotic surgery program

Market Analysis

A market analysis should assess the patient population, payer mix, procedure reimbursement, healthcare competition, and anticipated growth in surgical volume [20–24]. An initial review of the institution's current surgical volume and potential robotic case volume should be performed. This should include defining what procedures are best suited for a robotic approach given institutional and surgeon experience. In order to ensure a successful launch and minimize the learning curve, surgeons may choose to limit cases to fairly straightforward and common pediatric procedures (e.g., pyeloplasty, ureteral reimplantation, ureteroureterostomy). In a healthcare system within which pediatric urologic case volume is insufficient to offset equipment costs, partnering with an established adult robotics program is a viable startup approach [7, 22, 25, 26]. An expansion plan should be drafted to include interdisciplinary utilization of the robot and progression to include more complex surgical cases.

After program implementation, work closely with your marketing team to advertise the arrival of a new robotic surgery program. The website is the mainstay of marketing and should be continually updated to reflect new offerings and accomplishments. Other avenues include patient education brochures, community outreach, institutional social media accounts, and advertising via local media. The robotic company representative may be a useful resource is funding or providing marketing materials.

Cost Analysis

The da Vinci robotic system currently has no major competitors and has significant costs associated with its purchase, use, and maintenance. The cost of the robot can exceed $2 million USD depending on the type of system purchased [27–30]. An additional console for training purposes adds to this cost, as do simulation programs but may reduce long-term costs by reducing the learning curve. In addition, ongoing costs per procedure include disposable robotic drapes and instruments, adding several hundred dollars to the cost per case [30, 31]. An annual six-figure per system maintenance contract is also recommended [28, 30, 32]. Costs for surgeon training and credentialing should also be considered, including direct costs of robotics training courses as well as opportunity cost of lost clinical revenue as new robotic surgeons overcome the learning curve and experienced robotic surgeons sacrifice clinical productivity to proctor their peers.

Infrastructure

Dedicated OR Space

The hospital should identify a dedicated operating room that can accommodate the robot, console, anesthesia cart, operating bed, nursing tables, and the ancillary supplies necessary, while maintaining enough space to safely and efficiently navigate around the room. LCD monitors should be installed to allow for optimal visualization of the case [33]. Robotic instruments and disposable laparoscopic instruments such as suction irrigation or laparoscopic clips should be stocked in the room to minimize equipment delays. Additionally, instruments should be available in the room to address complications laparoscopically or to convert to an open procedure. Having a sales representative available during the initial cases may be beneficial as the surgical team familiarizes themselves with the equipment and setup [23, 34].

Dedicated OR Team

The importance of a dedicated robotic team cannot be overstated [20, 22–24, 35]. Cases should be scheduled during regular block time to ensure a complete and predictable team and to avoid unexpected staff changes. By working with a consistent team of staff members and limiting the types of cases to be done when beginning a robotics program, the surgeon and the institution may help to build the expertise and confidence necessary for a successful team. The surgeon should take the lead in providing training to his or her identified robotics staff. This should include devising a curriculum of formal training modules (typically offered through the manufacturer) as well as hands-on training with or without the robotic sales representative present. The team should review and practice the basic mechanics of the case, including robotic positioning, docking and undocking, and instrument changes to facilitate preparedness during an actual case [4]. Instrument trays should be standardized, and multiple trays should readily available to reduce equipment delays and turnover times [36]. If feasible, observation of an experienced robotics team at an institution with an established robotics program may provide staff members with a more comprehensive understanding of the challenges facing them during the early implementation of a new program.

Robotic surgery is unique in that the surgeon is away from the operative field. The competence of the first assistant and the nursing staff is thus all the more critical. Given the complexity of robotic procedures, it is often recommended to place an additional staff member in the room during initial cases. This will allow one staff member to focus on the equipment and machinery, while the other two focus on the patient. By taking time to familiarize the team with the basic steps of the case, the surgeon is able to impart a sense of comfort in the team and create an opportunity for the team to become more cohesive and focused during each case. Additionally, creation of a cohesive team empowers team members to express concerns or identify strategies for improvement before and after each case.

Operative Considerations

Personal Preparation

Although robotic-assisted laparoscopy has a shorter learning curve than conventional laparoscopy [4], the laparoscopist incorporating robotic skills into his or her practice should still take time to prepare prior to utilizing these skills in a "live setting". In developing a program with multiple surgeons, a lead surgeon should be identified to coordinate training surgeons and staff and to spearhead development of a cohesive program. This preparation should include ex vivo skills such as instrument transfers, suturing, and knot tying, as well as practice with robotic set up, docking, and undocking to minimize preventable delays or equipment issues during a case [37]. One of the most significant differences in robotics is the lack of haptic feedback. Ex vivo training may help the laparoscopist learn to rely on visual cues rather than haptic feedback when handling suture or tissues during a case. Taking the time to train with the robot as opposed to relying on laparoscopic skills alone has been associated with shorter operating times and improved outcomes during robotic-assisted cases in the adult setting [38]. As a result, a few hours spent familiarizing oneself with these differences may lend to improved efficiency and decreased frustration in the operating room setting.

Intraoperative Checklist (Fig. 3.2)

Creating a standardized checklist may help to minimize preventable errors and facilitate a smooth transition to the live setting [39, 40]. Prior to the start of each case, the surgeon should review with the nursing staff and anesthesia the expected course of the case, including expected positioning of the patient and of the robot,

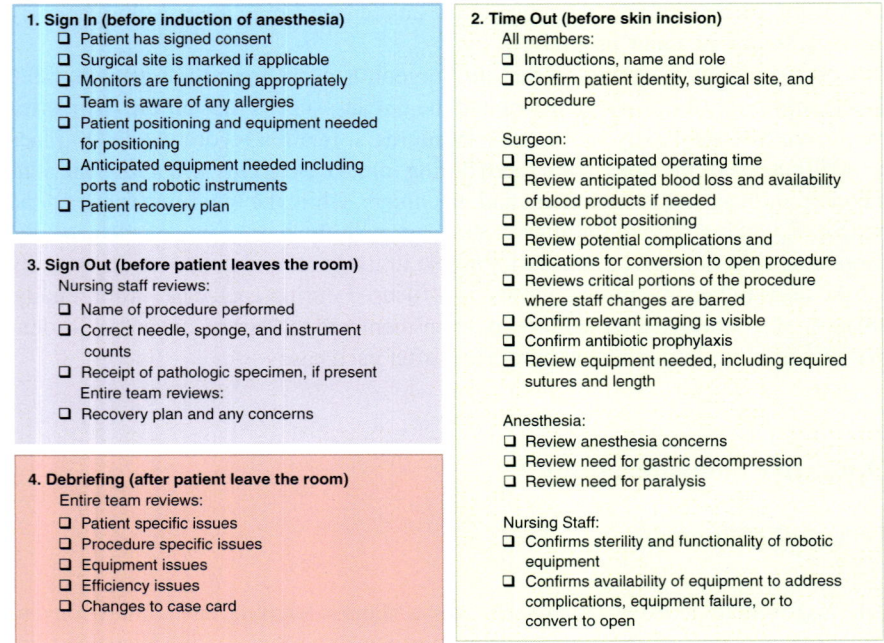

Fig. 3.2 Sample intraoperative safety checklist. (Based on WHO Guidelines for Safe Surgery 2009)

and duration of the case. In determining the expected duration of the case, allot additional time for potential delays in robot docking and instrument exchange as the bedside assistant and staff familiarize themselves with the technique. This discussion with the team should include the sutures to be used and instruments to be used and to be made available. Finally, the robotic console and monitors should be checked to ensure adequate visualization and optimal ergonomics to minimize muscle fatigue during the case. This preoperative briefing should also be used as a venue for staff to raise concerns prior to the start of the case. This review may be formalized by the use of a checklist system.

As initially envisioned in the ICU setting, the checklist includes the basic steps required to set up and to complete procedures in a high acuity setting [41]. This concept has been translated to the operating room in a variety of ways, most notably during the time out process to confirm patient identification and procedure prior to the start of the case. The goal of the checklist is to provide a basic algorithm for each procedure in order to minimize avoidable mistakes. Additionally, use of the checklist requires participation of the entire surgical team, empowering nurses and staff to speak up when an identified essential step is overlooked.

In robotic cases, the checklist provides an opportunity for the robotics team to ensure proper preparation and positioning of the patient, as well as ensuring that all necessary equipment is readily available and functional. The checklist also provides an opportunity for education of the team by providing a roadmap to the procedure

[42, 43]. Finally, utilization of the checklist provides a structure for preoperative and postoperative debriefing to identify opportunities and strategies for improvement during subsequent cases.

Positioning

With early iterations of the da Vinci ® robotic surgical systems (S, SI, SIe), fastidious positioning of the patient, ports, and the robot was paramount. Classically, port placement in robotic surgery differs from laparoscopic port placement in that the surgeon must consider collision of the robotic arms outside the body. The surgeon must also ensure that robotic arms will not contact and injure the patient when operating at the extremes of the target field. Ports should also be "burped" (gently repositioned) after robot docking to ensure no undue traction at the trocar site. With newer robotic systems (da Vinci Xi ®), thinner arms and longer instruments have markedly reduced extracorporeal arm collisions and cosmesis can be more heavily considered. Similarly, new robotic systems have improved range of motion and all ports can accommodate the camera, allowing for multi-quadrant surgery and flexibility in robot docking. Pelvic surgery, for instance, no longer requires the robot to be docked between the legs, yielding lithotomy positioning or a split leg table unnecessary. Additional innovations include an integrated operating table which allows for table rotation and thus less extreme patient positioning, as well as Single Site ® surgery in which surgery is performed through a single umbilical port.

Maintenance and Growth

Data Collection and Review

Documentation and review is an essential step in the growth of the developing robotic surgeon, the developing robotic program, and potential future research endeavors. If possible, early and complex cases should be recorded to allow for later review. Additionally, various metrics should be collected prospectively, including operative times, docking times, turnover times, as well as issues to be addressed at the conclusion of the case, such as equipment malfunctions or unavailability. Areas for improvement should be identified during a post-operative debriefing. Additionally, data should be collected regarding early and late surgical outcomes. These recordings and identified areas of improvement should then be reviewed by the surgeon periodically to identify issues and potential modifications to improve surgical preparation, perioperative communication, and surgical technique [44]. By tracking surgical outcomes using objective measures, the surgeon may determine the feasibility of the robotics program and may identify areas upon which to focus further training. Continued critical assessment lends credibility to the developing

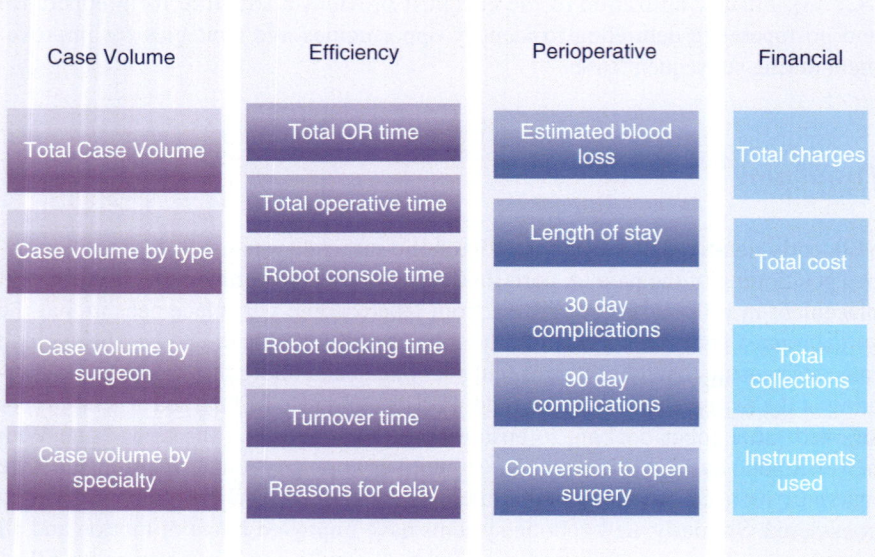

Fig. 3.3 Sample list of metrics to collect for periodic analysis

robotics program and is especially important during the expansion of robotic techniques to more complex and less standard reconstructive procedures. A sample checklist of metrics to be recorded is provided (Fig. 3.3).

Education and Expansion

Expansion of the program should be pursued only after internal review reveals outcomes comparable to the peer-reviewed literature. The robotic surgeon(s) should pursue continuing education through conferences, operative training courses, animal and/or cadaver labs, and literature review. Education and credentialing of additional robotic surgeons, residents, fellows, and bedside assistants should be formalized. A robotic curriculum should include online training modules provided by the robot manufacturer, preoperative didactics, dry labs, initial proctoring, graduated autonomy in the operating room, minimum case volumes, and well-defined milestones [22, 24, 35]. Repeat market analysis may be necessary for expansion to additional specialties or sites, more complex operations, and for recruitment of additional surgeons.

Conclusions

As with any developing technique, the incorporation of robotic-assisted laparoscopic techniques requires extensive preparation and practice prior to implementation in the clinical setting. This requires the dedication of the surgeon to develop his skills outside of the operating room regardless of his prior laparoscopic experience. The surgeon should anticipate issues of fatigue and frustration and should identify collaborators and mentors to assist with early cases to develop a sense of confidence and autonomy. Additionally, a successful robotics program requires a commitment from the institution for both the personnel and the resources necessary to ensure the smooth implementation of a robotics program. The surgeon and the OR staff should work as a team to identify potential issues prior to the start of the case and to review that issues at the conclusion of the case. The surgeon should also devote time to review and critically assess his performance and the performance of the robotics team to continue to improve both the overall efficacy and success of the program. Finally, the surgeon should continue to compare his outcomes to those of his colleagues and to his own outcomes utilizing conventional laparoscopic or open techniques. By employing an intentional, systematic and critical approach to the development and growth of a robotics program, a surgeon can optimize his development of a sustainable robotics practice.

References

1. Kim C, Docimo SG. Use of laparoscopy in pediatric urology. Rev Urol. 2005;7(4):215–23.
2. Sweeney DD, Smaldone MC, Docimo SG. Minimally invasive surgery for urologic disease in children. Nat Rev Urol. 2007;4(1):26–38.
3. Howe A, Kozel Z, Palmer L. Robotic surgery in pediatric urology. Asian J Urol. 2017;4(1):55–67.
4. Ahlering TE, Skarecky D, Lee D, Clayman RV. Successful transfer of open surgical skills to a laparoscopic environment using a robotic interface: initial experience with laparoscopic radical prostatectomy. J Urol. 2003;170(5):1738–41.
5. van Haasteren G, Levine S, Hayes W. Pediatric robotic surgery: early assessment. Pediatrics. 2009;124(6):1642–9.
6. Kant AJ, Klein MD, Langenburg SE. Robotics in pediatric surgery: perspectives for imaging. Pediatr Radiol. 2004;34(6):454–61.
7. Bütter A, Merritt N, Dave S. Establishing a pediatric robotic surgery program in Canada. J Robot Surg. 2017;11(2):207–10.
8. Lee DJ, Kim PH, Koh CJ. Current trends in pediatric minimally invasive urologic surgery. Korean J Urol. 2010;51(2):80–7.
9. Casale P, Kojima Y. Robotic-assisted laparoscopic surgery in pediatric urology: an update. Scand J Surg. 2009;98(2):110–9.
10. Cundy TP, Shetty K, Clark J, Chang TP, Sriskandarajah K, Gattas NE, et al. The first decade of robotic surgery in children. J Pediatr Surg. 2013;48(4):858–65.
11. Bowen DK, Faasse MA, Liu DB, Gong EM, Lindgren BW, Johnson EK. Use of pediatric open, laparoscopic and robot-assisted laparoscopic ureteral reimplantation in the United States: 2000 to 2012. J Urol. 2016;196(1):207–12.
12. Seideman CA, Sleeper JP, Lotan Y. Cost comparison of robot-assisted and laparoscopic pyeloplasty. J Endourol. 2012;26(8):1044–8.
13. Varda BK, Johnson EK, Clark C, Chung B, Nelson CP, Chang S. National trends of perioperative outcomes and cost for open laparoscopic and robotic pediatric pyeloplasty. J Urol. 2014;191(4):1090–5.
14. Begg CB, Riedel ER, Bach PB, Kattan MW, Schrag D, Warren JL, et al. Variations in morbidity after radical prostatectomy. N Engl J Med. 2002;346(15):1138–44.
15. Keller DS, Hashemi L, Lu M, Delaney CP. Short-term outcomes for robotic colorectal surgery by provider volume. J Am Coll Surg. 2013;217(6):1063–9.

16. Yu H, Hevelone Nathanael D, Lipsitz Stuart R, Kowalczyk Keith J, Nguyen Paul L, Hu Jim C. Hospital volume, utilization, costs and outcomes of robot-assisted laparoscopic radical prostatectomy. J Urol. 2012;187(5):1632–8.
17. Bastawrous A, Baer C, Rashidi L, Neighorn C. Higher robotic colorectal surgery volume improves outcomes. Am J Surg. 2018;215(5):874–8.
18. Rashidi L, Neighorn C, Bastawrous A. Outcome comparisons between high-volume robotic and laparoscopic surgeons in a large healthcare system. Am J Surg. 2017;213(5):901–5.
19. Sukumar S, Djahangirian O, Sood A, Sammon JD, Varda B, Janosek-Albright K, et al. Minimally invasive vs open pyeloplasty in children: the differential effect of procedure volume on operative outcomes. Urology. 2014;84(1):180–4.
20. Rocco B, Lorusso A, Coelho RF, Palmer KJ, Patel VR. Building a robotic program. Scand J Surg. 2009;98(2):72–5.
21. Steers WD. Tips on establishing a robotics program in an academic setting. Sci World J. 2006;6:2531–41.
22. Murthy PB, Schadler ED, Orvieto M, Zagaja G, Shalhav AL, Gundeti MS. Setting up a pediatric robotic urology program: a USA institution experience. Int J Urol. 2018;25(2):86–93.
23. Luthringer T, Aleksic I, Caire A, Albala DM. Developing a successful robotics program. Curr Opin Urol. 2012;22(1):40–6.
24. Patel VR. Essential elements to the establishment and design of a successful robotic surgery programme. Int J Med Robot. 2006;2(1):28–35.
25. de Lambert G, Fourcade L, Centi J, Fredon F, Braik K, Szwarc C, et al. How to successfully implement a robotic pediatric surgery program: lessons learned after 96 procedures. Surg Endosc. 2013;27(6):2137–44.
26. Camps JI. The use of robotics in pediatric surgery: my initial experience. Pediatr Surg Int. 2011;27(9):991–6.
27. United States Securities and Exchange Commission Form 10-K for the fiscal year ended December 31, 2017. Intuitive Surgical, Inc. [cited 2019 May 19]. Available from: https://www.sec.gov/Archives/edgar/data/1035267/000103526718000013/isrg-20171231x10k.htm.
28. Turchetti G, Palla I, Pierotti F, Cuschieri A. Economic evaluation of da Vinci-assisted robotic surgery: a systematic review. Surg Endosc. 2012;26(3):598–606.
29. Protyniak B, Jorden J, Farmer R. Multiquadrant robotic colorectal surgery: the da Vinci Xi vs Si comparison. J Robot Surg. 2018;12(1):67–74.
30. Tsuda S, Oleynikov D, Gould J, Azagury D, Sandler B, Hutter M, et al. SAGES TAVAC safety and effectiveness analysis: da Vinci® Surgical System (Intuitive Surgical, Sunnyvale, CA). Surg Endosc. 2015;29(10):2873–84.
31. Rao PP. Robotic surgery: new robots and finally some real competition! World J Urol. 2018;36(4):537–41.
32. Ho C, Tsakonas E, Tran K, Cimon K, Severn M, Mierzwinski-Urban M, et al. Robot-assisted surgery compared with open surgery and laparoscopic surgery: clinical effectiveness and economic analyses. Ottawa: Canadian Agency for Drugs and Technologies in Health; 2011. p. 298.
33. Buzink SN, van Lier L, de Hingh IHJT, Jakimowicz JJ. Risk-sensitive events during laparoscopic cholecystectomy: the influence of the integrated operating room and a preoperative checklist tool. Surg Endosc. 2010;24(8):1990–5.
34. Coon TM. Integrating robotic technology into the operating room. Am J Orthop (Belle Mead NJ). 2009;38(2 Suppl):7–9.
35. Estes SJ, Goldenberg D, Winder JS, Juza RM, Lyn-Sue JR. Best practices for robotic surgery programs. JSLS [Internet]. 2017 [cited 2019 May 11];21(2):e2016.00102. Available from: https://www.ncbi.nlm.nih.gov/pmc/articles/PMC5508805/.
36. van Brenk CM. Setting up a robotic surgery program: a Nurse's perspective. Semin Colon Rectal Surg. 2009;20(4):162–5.
37. Benson AD, Kramer BA, Boehler M, Schwind CJ, Schwartz BF. Robot-assisted laparoscopic skills development: formal versus informal training. J Endourol. 2010;24(8):1351–5.

38. Kwon EO, Bautista TC, Jung H, Goharderakhshan RZ, Williams SG, Chien GW. Impact of robotic training on surgical and pathologic outcomes during robot-assisted laparoscopic radical prostatectomy. Urology. 2010;76(2):363–8.
39. Haynes AB, Weiser TG, Berry WR, Lipsitz SR, Breizat A-HS, Dellinger EP, et al. A surgical safety checklist to reduce morbidity and mortality in a global population. N Engl J Med. 2009;360(5):491–9.
40. Song JB, Vemana G, Mobley JM, Bhayani SB. The second "time-out": a surgical safety checklist for lengthy robotic surgeries. Patient Saf Surg. 2013;7:19.
41. Pronovost P, Needham D, Berenholtz S, Sinopoli D, Chu H, Cosgrove S, et al. An intervention to decrease catheter-related bloodstream infections in the ICU. N Engl J Med. 2006;355(26):2725–32.
42. Verdaasdonk EGG, Stassen LPS, van der Elst M, Karsten TM, Dankelman J. Problems with technical equipment during laparoscopic surgery. An observational study. Surg Endosc. 2007;21(2):275–9.
43. Meijer DW. Safety of the laparoscopy setup. Minim Invasive Ther Allied Technol. 2003;12(3):125–8.
44. Vincent C, Moorthy K, Sarker SK, Chang A, Darzi AW. Systems approaches to surgical quality and safety: from concept to measurement. Ann Surg. 2004;239(4):475–82.

Chapter 4
Relevant Anatomy in Minimally Invasive Surgery

Roxanne E. Haslam and Casey A. Seideman

Abdominal Wall and Access

The anatomy of the abdominal wall and umbilicus is important when obtaining access for minimally invasive surgery. Specific considerations must be made when obtaining laparoscopic access to the pediatric abdomen. The umbilical ring does not typically close for a few years after birth, therefore, in younger children, the abdomen can be entered through the umbilical ring [1]. Entry can also be made through a supraumbilical or infraumbilical incision, and extended through the subcutaneous fascia down to the rectus fascia. The rectus fascia can then be grasped and lifted upward, away from the underlying organs, providing counter tension for insertion of a trocar or Veress needle. In neonates, care must be taken to avoid the piercing the umbilical vein during initial trocar placement and insufflation, this could not only cause bleeding, but also result in a venous air embolus. Some surgeons prefer an open technique because of the shallow depth of the abdomen. Another important consideration during access should be the position of the pediatric bladder, which unlike the adult bladder, is intraabdominally located. When full, the bladder can extend superiorly as far as the umbilicus.

The great vessels are in close proximity to the abdominal wall in pediatric patients, and the right common iliac artery is at particular risk when it crosses the midline (directly under umbilicus). Transillumination of the anterior abdominal wall during placement of the secondary trocars can assist in visualizing and avoiding the inferior epigastric vessels (Fig. 4.1a, b). In the event of injury, a Carter-Thomason needle fascial closure device can be used to place a figure-of-eight suture to ligate the vessel and achieve hemostasis.

R. E. Haslam · C. A. Seideman (✉)
Oregon Health and Science University, Department of Urology, Division of Pediatric Surgery, Portland, OR, USA
e-mail: haslamro@ohsu.edu; seideman@ohsu.edu

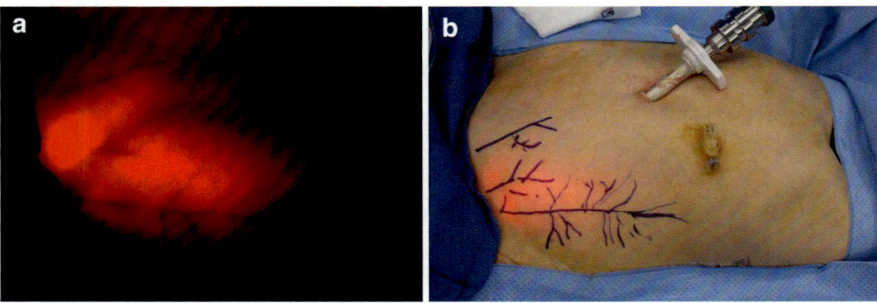

Figs. 4.1 (**a**, **b**) Transillumination of the inferior epigastric vessels. (Courtesy of Patricio C. Gargollo, MD)

After primary trocar placement, direct visualization of a needle injection of local anesthetic transabdominally can be used to identify the site and angle for placement of the secondary trocars. Due to the thin abdominal wall of pediatric patients, a pneumoperitoneum of 8–12 mmHg is often adequate for visualization and allows for better venous return to the heart. Children, especially less than 5 years of age, are at higher risk of port site hernias than adults [2]. Due to the thin abdominal wall, the defect created through the different layers at an oblique angle does not offset the layers as prominently as in adults to prevent herniation. The fascia should be closed for all 5 mm and larger trocar sites.

The Kidney

The kidneys are paired retroperitoneal organs which lie on either side of the lumbar vertebrae. The renal parenchyma is surrounded by a tough capsule, perinephric fat, and enclosed within Gerota's fascia. This fascial plane separates the perinephric fat and the pararenal fat. Gerota's fascia is fused superiorly and laterally, extending over adrenal glands superiorly, the adventitia of the renal vessels, aorta and inferior vena cava medially, and is open inferiorly. This is of clinical relevance because this plane affects the distribution of perinephric fluid collections and has oncologic significance.

Due to the position of the liver, the right kidney is found at the level of L1–L3, whereas the left kidney is slightly higher around T12–L2. The diaphragm lies posterior and superior to the upper poles of the kidneys. The adjacent pleura extends down to the level of the 12th rib posteriorly and the 11th rib anteriorly. The kidney is surrounded by the psoas muscle posteromedially and the quadratus lumborum posterolaterally. The kidneys lie at an oblique angle, making the upper poles more medial and posterior than the lower poles. The subcostal nerve and vessels, iliohypogastric, and ilioinguinal nerves descend obliquely across the posterior surfaces of the kidneys. The renal pelvis is located along the lateral border of the psoas muscle.

Fig. 4.2 View of the left kidney through the colonic mesentery for transmesenteric access

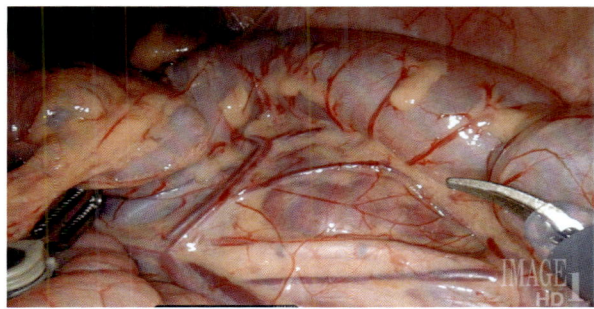

On the left, the spleen, another retroperitoneal organ, lies superolateral. The kidney and the spleen are separated by a folding layer of peritoneum which makes up the splenorenal ligament. Excessive tension on this ligament can cause capsular tearing of the spleen and bleeding. The tail of the pancreas, the stomach, and the splenic flexure of the colon are also in close relation to the left kidney. Transperitoneal access to the kidneys requires mobilization of descending (left) colon or the ascending (right), respectively, at the white line of Toldt, which is the lateral reflection of the posterior parietal peritoneum. The second portion of the duodenum is also retroperitoneal. During right renal surgery this portion of the duodenum must be mobilized anteromedially (Kocherization). While the renal parenchyma, hilum, and pelvis are most commonly accessed via the transperitoneal approach, a transmesenteric approach can be performed if the ureter or renal hilum is visible under the colonic mesentery (Fig. 4.2). Anatomically, the relatively superior location of the splenic flexure and its mesentery in relation to the left kidney (compared to the hepatic flexure) make this approach feasible. Similarly, in malrotated or horseshoe kidneys the anteromedial rotation facilitates visualization of the ureter through the mesentery. Less dissection and bowel manipulation have been shown to decrease operative time and length of hospital stay compared to the transperitoneal approach [3].

The renal hilum is composed of the renal pelvis, artery, and vein. The left and right renal arteries come off the aorta, and as they approach the hilum give off branches to the inferior suprarenal artery, and the ureteric artery, before dividing into anterior and posterior branches. The renal artery lies posterior to the renal vein, and may divide before reaching the kidney. The anterior branch supplies the anterior surface, and a portion of the upper and lower poles via four segmental branches: apical, upper, middle, and lower. The posterior branch supplies the midsegment of the posterior surface, and is typically the first segmental branch, often splitting prior to entering the hilum. A ureteropelvic junction obstruction may occur when the posterior segmental branch passes anterior to the ureter. Of note, injury to segmental vasculature leads parenchymal loss The renal vasculature can be variable, 25–28% of patients have an accessory renal artery, usually extending to the lower pole [4]. In patients with a duplicated collecting system, it is common for each to have its own arterial supply.

The renal veins are found anterior to the renal arteries and aorta. The left renal vein is longer than the right. As the left renal vein crosses over the aorta, compression by an overlying superior mesenteric artery may cause nutcracker syndrome. The left kidney has collateral drainage through the left gonadal vein inferiorly, inferior adrenal vein superiorly, and lumbar vein posteriorly. There is no collateral drainage of the right kidney.

Lymphatic drainage differs between the left and right kidney. The left sided lymphatics drain primarily into the para-aortic lymph nodes, and occasionally into the retrocrural nodes or thoracic duct. The right renal lymphatics drain primarily into the interaortocaval and paracaval lymph nodes.

The Ureter

The ureter descends from the renal pelvis along the psoas muscle to the pelvic brim. Near the bifurcation of the common iliac artery into the internal and external iliac arteries the ureter can be found crossing anterior to the iliac vessels. It then travels alongside the internal iliac artery on the lateral pelvic side wall. At the level of the ischial spine, it courses more medially, then crosses the obturator vessels and nerve. In males, the ureter crosses under the vas deferens prior to passing the seminal vesicle and entering the bladder. In females, the ureter passes behind the ovary, then crosses under the uterine vessels, coursing near the anterior vaginal fornix before its insertion into the bladder (Fig. 4.3).

The fibromuscular layer surrounding the terminal ureter before it enters the bladder is known as the Waldeyer sheath. The ureter then enters the posterolateral wall of the bladder, where it becomes intravesical and extends obliquely (0.5-1 cm in neonates and 1.2–2.5 cm in adults) before terminating internally at the ureteral orifice [5]. It should be noted that the only structures to pass anteriorly over the pelvic ureter is the vas deferens in males and the uterine artery in females.

Duplication of the ureter may be complete or partial. Complete duplication results in two ureteral insertions into the bladder, due to the formation of a second ureteric bud during development. Partial duplication is a result of duplication of a single

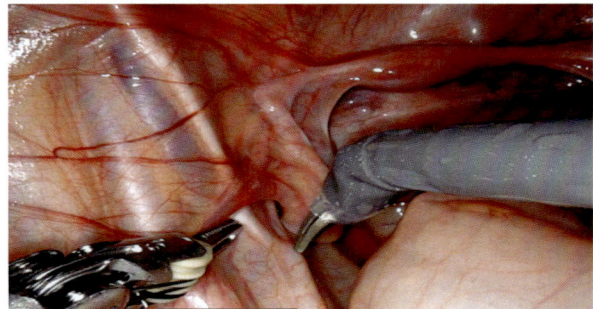

Fig. 4.3 The ureter courses along the common iliac and then crosses under the uterine artery, passing close to the vaginal fornix prior to entering the bladder

ureteric bud, resulting in two proximal ureters, which join distally prior to insertion into the bladder. In complete duplication, the ureter of the upper moiety inserts inferiorly and medially to the lower moiety ureter, this is known as the Weigert-Meyer rule.

The arterial blood supply to the ureter varies along its longitudinal axis. The proximal ureter obtains its blood supply from the aorta and renal artery, these vessels enter the ureter from the medial aspect of the adventitia. After the ureter enters the pelvis and crosses the iliac vessels the blood supply enters the ureter laterally from the branches of the iliac artery, including branches of the internal iliac, vesical, and uterine arteries. Therefore, the pelvic peritoneum should be incised on the medial aspect of the ureter. Intramural vessels primarily run parallel to the longitudinal access of the ureter, but some make plexiform connections. Due to the anastomoses within the periureteral adventitia, surgical mobilization of the ureter can be performed if care is taken to maintain the adventitia.

The Bladder

The bladder is a retroperitoneal organ. The superior posterior aspect of the bladder is covered by the peritoneum. The anterior peritoneal folds are important landmarks during laparoscopy of the pelvis. The medial umbilical ligaments (the obliterated umbilical arteries) lie lateral to the median umbilical ligament. The median umbilical contains the urachal ligament, the remnant of the urachus, which connects the bladder to the anterior abdominal wall at the umbilicus. This contains the paraumbilical veins, which may need to be ligated when mobilizing the bladder. An intraabdominal view of a remnant urachus is shown in Fig. 4.4. The lateral most folds are the umbilical ligaments which contain the inferior epigastric vessels (Fig. 4.5).

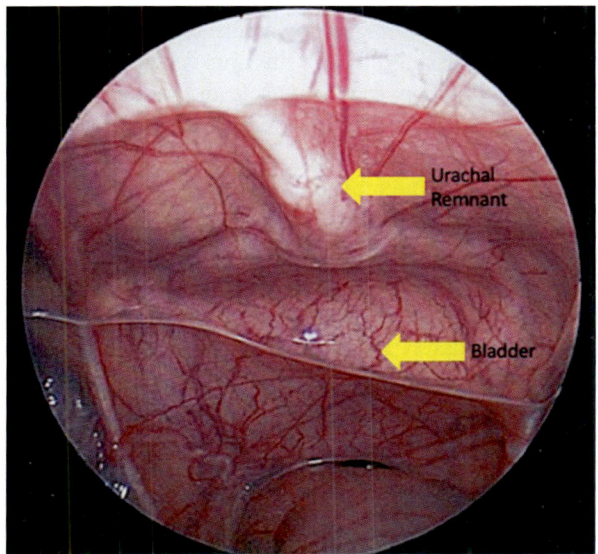

Fig. 4.4 The urachus is an embryological remnant of the allantois, which runs from the urinary bladder to the umbilicus and forms the median umbilical ligament

Fig. 4.5 Intraabdominal view of the inferior epigastric vessels coursing on the abdominal wall

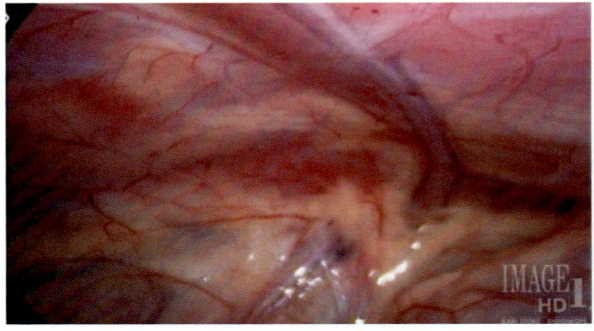

The primary bladder blood supply includes the superior and inferior vesical arteries, which are either directly or indirectly, derived from the internal iliac artery. The superior vesical artery can originate directly from the internal iliac, or indirectly, by branching off the more proximal umbilical artery. The inferior vesical artery branches more distally. Small branches of the obturator and inferior gluteal arteries are a source of collateral flow. In females, the uterine and vaginal arteries also provide additional branches. While the branches of the arteries may be variable, their ultimate course through the lateral and posterior pedicles is more reliable (in females within the cardinal and uterosacral ligaments). The veins of the bladder form into the vesical plexus and drain into the internal iliac veins.

The Deep Inguinal Ring

The inferior epigastric vessels pass over the inguinal ligament anteromedially, branching from the external iliac vessel prior to its passage through the femoral ring. The inferior epigastric vessels course medial to the inguinal ring, and extend superiorly, passing through the transversalis fascia below the linea semicircularis, and traversing between the muscle and posterior lamina sheath of the rectus abdominis. Branches of the inferior epigastric vessels continue superiorly and above the level of the umbilicus, and anastomose with the superior epigastric vessels and the lower posterior intercostal arteries.

The testicular arteries branch off the aorta below the renal arteries. They pass anterior to the psoas muscle and cross over the ureter. The gonadal vessels (laterally) along with the vas deferens (medially) pass through the inguinal ring and exit the abdomen. The course of these structures is especially important during laparoscopic evaluation of cryptorchidism. In the case of a blind ending vas deferens, further exploration is needed to discern the position of the gonadal vessels and accompanying testis. However, blind ending gonadal vessels do not warrant further exploration [6]. The vas deferens, also referred to as the ductus deferens, courses through the retroperitoneal medially passing across the obliterated umbilical artery and then over the distal ureter to reach the posterior prostate and becomes the ampulla before joining the seminal vesicle. During a laparoscopic orchiopexy the vas deferens is at risk for injury because of its retroperitoneal position. The vas deferens is supplied by the concurrent deferential artery, which typically arises from the superior vesical artery, although occasionally from the inferior vesical artery. The concomitant blood supply to the testicle provided by the deferential artery makes it possible to ligate the ligate the testicular artery during a staged orchiopexy. The collateral flow is then allowed to mature over the following 6 months before mobilizing the intraabdominal testicle into the scrotum.

References

1. Hunter JG, Spight DH, Sandone C, Fairman J. Minimally invasive pediatric surgery: general considerations. In: Atlas of minimally invasive surgical operations. New York: McGraw-Hill Education Inc; 2018. [cited 2019 April 25]. Available from: https://accesssurgery-mhmedical-com.liboff.ohsu.edu/book.aspx?bookid=2403#187823106 with authorized username and password.
2. Paya K, Wurm J, Fakhari M, Felcer-Puig R, Puig S. Trocar-site hernia as a typical postoperative complication of minimally invasive surgery among preschool children. Surg Endosc. 2008;22:2724–7.
3. Romero FR, Wagner AA, Trapp C, Permpongkosol S, Muntener M, Link RE, et al. Transmesenteric laparoscopic pyeloplasty. J Urol. 2006;176:2526–629.
4. Wein A, Kavoussi L, Partin A, Peters C. Surgical, radiologic, and endoscopic anatomy of the kidney and ureter. In: Campbell-Walsh urology. 11th ed. Philadelphia: Elsevier; 2016. p. 967–97.
5. Keane TE, Graham SD, Goldstein M. Glenn's urological surgery. 8th ed. Philadelphia: Wolters Kluwer; 2016.
6. Bishoff J, Kavoussi L. Testicular surgery. In: Atlas of laparoscopic and robotic urologic surgery. 3rd ed. Philadelphia: Elsevier; 2017. p. 324–48.

Chapter 5
Robotic and Laparoscopic Instrumentation in Pediatric Urology

James T. Rague and Michael P. Kurtz

History and Iteration

The da Vinci Surgical System (Intuitive Surgical Inc., Sunnyvale, CA, USA) is the current leading system for robot assisted laparoscopic surgery in general and for pediatric urology. Intuitive Surgical International was founded in 1995 with the goal of creating a surgical platform to maintain the benefits of minimally invasive surgery while improving surgeon dexterity, visualization and ergonomics beyond traditional laparoscopy. Since that time there have been great improvements and continued technologic advancement in robotic surgery with four generations of robotic systems having been developed.

The goal of the initial design was to create a system with motion capabilities that could mimic that of its human operator, allowing for excellent hand-eye coordination with natural and intuitive movements. The first produced prototype, known as "Lenny," first showed the benefit of the wristed instruments manipulators in animal studies. The first trial on human subjects began in 1997 with the next design iteration, called "Mona", which allowed for an exchangeable sterile component [1]. This led to the design of the first generation da Vinci Surgical system. The first commercial version was delivered in 1998. During the same period of time Computer Motion Inc. (Santa Barbara, CA, USA) developed the ZEUS telepresence system, a competitor to the da Vinci system The instruments in this system however lacked articulating tips, with surgeon movements mimicking conventional laparoscopy (4 degrees of freedom) [2].

J. T. Rague
Ann & Robert H. Lurie Children's Hospital of Chicago, Boston, MA, USA
e-mail: jrague@luriechildrens.org

M. P. Kurtz (✉)
Harvard Medical School, Boston Children's Hospital, Department of Urology, Boston, MA, USA
e-mail: Michael.Kurtz@childrens.harvard.edu

© Springer Nature Switzerland AG 2020
P. C. Gargollo (ed.), *Minimally Invasive and Robotic-Assisted Surgery in Pediatric Urology*, https://doi.org/10.1007/978-3-030-57219-8_5

The first iteration of the da Vinci system was created in 2000 with three robotic arms mounted on the cart and a closed console with 3D video system and in-line view [2]. In 2004 the two companies (Intuitive and Computer Motion, Inc) merged and with further developments, the "da Vinci S" system was developed in 2006 [3]. This included the cable-driven mechanical EndoWrist technology (6 degrees of freedom, clutch mechanism, loop-like handles) to allow for improved range of motion and dexterity. The development of the da Vinci S system included a fourth manipulator arm, expanded the available working instruments, had slimmer arms to improve reach within the abdomen, and an improved high-definition vision system [1, 3].

In 2009, the "da Vinci Si" was launched with improved high-definition, 3D vision, improved ergonomics with a finger-based clutch mechanism, and the addition of the dual-console mode to allow for two surgeons to share the controls [3]. The development of the Si also allowed for the development of robotic single-port surgery using instruments with only 4 degrees of freedom [4].

In 2014, the 4th generation of the da Vinci platform was released (da Vinci Xi) to support multi-quadrant surgery, easier docking, and improved motion of the patient cart [4, 5]. Instead of mounting on a single central post, the arms are mounted on an overhead boom with 342 degrees of rotation. A laser crosshair on the boom assists with aligning the cart with the designated camera port [6]. The arms are also made slimmer to decrease arm clashing. The endoscope is 8 mm to allow placement into any working robotic port and allow for "camera port hopping" [4]. The Xi is designed for parallel movement, where the instruments work best when working in a near parallel configuration. The ports are therefore placed in a line, as opposed to with the Si where the 4th arm is placed laterally or in an arc. With the Xi, the ports should be 6 cm apart, compared to the traditional 8–10 cm port spacing with the Si. The instruments for the Xi are 1.75 inches longer than instruments for the Si which assists in reach [6].

Instrumentation

The EndoWrist articulation of instruments allows for precise control with ±90 degrees of articulation in the wrist, motion scaling, and hand tremor elimination. There are four degrees of freedom with standard laparoscopic instruments on two axes (moving inward, outward, clockwise and counterclockwise). Robotic platforms may allow up to seven, adding the pitch (up/down), yaw (side-side), and pincer-like movements of the human hand/wrist [7]. The array of available instruments for each system are listed in Table 5.1 and include energy instruments, needle drivers, various forceps, and specialized instruments. Instrument diameter also varies with the two common sizes being traditional 8 mm and 5 mm for smaller access ports.

Each instrument contains multiple components. The tip of each instrument allows for the specific surgical task to be completed (grasper, needle driver, cautery tip, etc.). Some of the specialized instruments do not articulate, such as the Harmonic scalpel [1].

5 Robotic and Laparoscopic Instrumentation in Pediatric Urology

Table 5.1 da Vinci instrumentation by port size and platform

	da Vinci surgical instrumentation by size of trocar required			
	5 mm (Si only)	8 mm (Si or Xi)	Single port (SP)	Xi single site
Scissors	Yes (curved, round tip)	Yes (potts, round tip)	Yes (round tip)	5 mm curved
Monopolar scissors	No	Yes	Not known	No
Monopolar hook	Yes, hook and spatula	Yes, hook and spatula	Yes, hook	Yes, hook
Bipolar instruments	None	Yes (Maryland Forceps, Fenestrated Forceps, Curved Dissector, Micro Forceps, Long Grasper, Vessel Sealer)	Yes (Fenestrated Forceps, Maryland Forceps)	Yes (Maryland, Fenestrated)
Needle driver	Yes	Several options: Large, Large SutureCutTM, Mega, Mega SutureCutTM, Black Diamond Micro Forceps[a]	Yes	Curved
Bowel grasper	Yes	Yes	No known	
Clip applier	No	Yes (Small, Medium, and Large for XI)	No known	Medium-large
Larger graspers	Schertel grasper, bullet nose dissector	Yes (Cobra, Fenstetrated Tip-Up, GraptormTM, Cadiere Long-Tip, Prograsp, Tenaculum)	No known	Crocodile, Cadiere
Debakey	Yes	Yes	No known	No
Maryland	Yes	Yes	Yes	Yes
Harmonic	Yes	Yes	No known	No
EndoWrist Stapler	No	Yes (Xi only) 30 and 45 mm	No known	No
EndoWrist Vessel Sealer	No	Yes	No known	No
EndorWrist Tenaculum	No	Yes	No known	No
Suction/Irrigator	No	Yes	No known	Yes

[a]Black Diamond Micro Forceps are listed as forceps, can be used as needle driver for fine needles

Instrumentation Development and Advantages of Da Vinci Xi

Various authors have sought to assess and compare outcomes in urologic procedures between the two Si and newer Xi system. Patel et al examined their outcomes for nephroureterectomy with the use of the da Vinci Xi compared to the Standard/S/Si to assess whether advances in technology have led to improved outcomes. In their cohort of adult patients, they found decreased operative time with the use of the Xi. EBL and length of hospital stay were similar. They felt that port hopping allowed for a more seamless transition from operating on the upper urinary tract to the lower urinary tract, which is an advantage for nephroureterectomy, specifically. They found overall lower anesthesia costs, likely related to the shorter operative time. Overall, there were no reported additional operative or perioperative advantages [8].

While this comparison has not been performed in pediatric patients to date, the ability to port-hop could also be advantageous in pediatric robotic surgery in order to allow for better visualization of both the upper and lower urinary tract in the case of a nephroureterectomy or combined upper and lower tract procedures. In addition, for the creation of a continent catheterizable stoma with an Si system, we mobilize the right colon (often all the way to the hepatic flexure) laparoscopically, docking only after the upper quadrant procedure is completed. With an Xi system, this can be completed with a single docking, and purely robotically. The slimmer arm construction as well as ability to place ports closer together while minimizing clash may also be advantageous in a smaller abdomen.

Robotic Surgery in Pediatrics

While the benefits of robotic surgery have been clearly shown in the adult population, the role for and benefits of robotic surgery in the pediatric population remains somewhat controversial. The first robotic surgery in a child was a Nissen fundoplication that was performed in July 2000 [9, 10]. Since that time, robotic surgery has in pediatric patients has been slow to take off when compared to the rate of utilization in the adult population. A total of 2393 procedures were performed in 1840 patients during the first 10 years of robotic surgery utilization in pediatrics, as compared to over 400,000 adult robotic procedures performed in 2013 alone [10]. In pediatric urology, the most commonly performed robotic procedure is pyeloplasty for UPJ obstruction, a far less prevalent condition than adult genitourinary malignancy.

There are many challenges associated with robot-assisted surgery (RAS) in the pediatric population, largely based on underlying anatomic features of children. In pediatric patients, there is an overall decreased intraabdominal working space with decreased insufflation capacity. Intuitive Surgical systems recommends a distance of 8 mm between each trocar for the Si system and 6 cm for the Xi system, which may be difficult to achieve in infants. Many therefore place the robotic ports in closer proximity with a distance of only 3–4 cm [11], although we prefer 7 cm with an Si system. Robotic instruments are also not currently manufactured specifically for pediatric populations. The size and length of the instruments can therefore be problematic in smaller children. The 3 mm instruments available for conventional laparoscopy are not available for robotic surgery, where instruments are only available in 8 mm or 5 mm diameter [12].

Decreased work space intra-abdominally also leads to decreased robotic instrument mobility and increase in instrument collisions. Finkelstein et al. demonstrated that with a measured distance of >13 cm between both anterior superior iliac spines (for lower urinary tract procedures) and >15 cm puboxyphoid distance (for upper urinary tract procedures), there was a decreased rate of instrument collision and improved operative times. This suggests that given the limitation of current robotic systems, patient selection is key to assure a safe and effective robotic procedure [13].

Additional challenges such as increased abdominal wall laxity in pediatric patients leads to increased risk of bowel and vascular injury upon trocar placement. Techniques such as the open Hasson technique or intussusception of the trocars during placement are employed to help avoid such injuries [12].

8 mm Versus 5 mm Instrumentation: Success and Limitations

Given the limited working space available in pediatric patients, many authors have sought to assess the role of the available working instruments. While robotic surgery instruments have anecdotally been considered superior to conventional laparoscopic instruments for performance of complex surgical skills in small working spaces, few have compared functional outcomes [14]. The large diameter, articulating design of robotic instruments are bulkier size when compared to conventional laparoscopic instruments may pose a limitation in confined work-spaces. When comparing the 5 mm and 8 mm instruments, there is a clear difference in size and functionality in small spaces, which is at first counterintuitive given the smaller diameter and presumed pediatric application of the smaller instrument. The distances from the instrument tip to the proximal articulation axis are 28 and 18.5 mm for the 5- and 8-mm needle-holder instruments respectively. The 'gooseneck' 5 mm instruments therefore require more room to maneuver and are paradoxically less well suited for small working spaces. The 8 mm instruments possess the standard EndoWrist technology.

To assess the required space necessary for use of 5 mm instruments given the variation of articulation axis, Meehan et al measured instrument-specific parameters. They determined that the tip of the 5 mm needle driver must extend 2.71 cm beyond the intracorporeal end of the trocar in order for all articulations and for the robot to recognize and manipulate the instrument. They next assessed the remote center of the robotic arm. This represents the point in space at which the robotic arm pivots. This point is marked on the trocar with a wide band, and recommended to be visible within the working cavity upon port placement. The remote center is located 2.9 cm from the end of the trocar. Therefore, the sum of the remote center distance and the necessary distance of the tip of the instrument from the trocar measure to 5.61 cm. This distance is therefore the required internal depth necessary for use of the 5 mm instrument. The authors suggest techniques to trick the robot, such as pulling the trocar back such that the remote center is not within the body but instead a few millimeters outside of the body. This allows for a decreased minimal internal depth [15]. This moves the port more with respect to the abdominal wall, which can in theory cause trouble with air leaks.

In addition to necessary depth of working space, total working volume required for instrument manipulation is important. Thakre et al. assessed minimal working volume required for use of 8 mm instruments and discovered that none of their assigned tasks could be performed in the 40 mm edge cube due to severe external collisions, whereas all tasks could be performed in the 60 mm edge cube without collisions. They determined that the smallest workable volume is 125 cm^3, which may provide surgeons with a framework for minimum bladder volume in which one can perform operations such as intravesical reimplantation [16].

Comparative studies were subsequently performed in the 60-mm edged box, using 5 mm and 8 mm instruments [17]. Trainees performed three skills (peg transfer, circle cutting, intracorporeal suturing) in the confined work-space with 5 mm and 8 mm instruments using the da Vinci Si. Performance was analyzed and scored and all trainees scored better on all tasks when using the 8 mm instruments. Most importantly, there was decreased instrument collision and parietal impacts with the walls of the box when using the 8 mm instruments. Study participants included medical students and residents with limited robotic experience and unsurprisingly overall results were better when performed by skilled surgeons regardless of instrument size. This study highlights the space-consuming effect of the 5 mm instruments when compared to the 8 mm instruments.

Similarly, Cundy et al sought to compare the two instruments by having participants perform intracorporeal interrupted suturing in various sized workspaces with various robotic and non-robotic instruments [14]. The cylindrical workspaces had volumes of 50, 113, and 201 cm^3. The 3 mm non-robotic needle driver, the 5 mm and 8 mm robotic needle drivers were used for each task and outcomes were compared. Two-dimensional optics were used for each task to standardize the visual quality. Each participant performed and interrupted suture with all three instruments in all three work space sizes. The primary outcomes were objective task scores, and instrument workspace breaches. The highest task scores were associated with the 3-mm non-robotic instruments in all work-spaces evaluated. The greatest discrepancy came in the smallest work-space where the median scores for the 5 mm and 8 mm instruments were 6.8 and 14.5% lower than the median score with the 3-mm instrument. This however did not represent statistical significance. A higher number of workspace breaches occurred with the robotic instruments in all workspace sizes. Investigators therefore suggest that in the most confined spaces, robotic instruments likely obscure field of view and may be less safe than the 3 mm conventional laparoscopic instruments. Authors suggest that future instrument technology should focus on shortening the articulating segment curve radius length, limiting the degree-of-freedom redundancy and optimizing extracorporeal arm configurations to diminish external collision.

In addition to model-based studies, outcomes in live patients with the use of the 5 mm instruments have been assessed. Baek et al. in 2018 sought to assess the efficacy and safety of RAL pyeloplasty in infants using 5 mm instruments compared to RAL pyeloplasty in older children [18]. Given the aforementioned challenges with 5 mm instruments, most surgeons continue to use the 8 mm instruments. They however hypothesized that the use of 5 mm instruments in infants would improve perioperative outcomes. They found no significant difference in operative time between infants and older children with similar time of port placement. Similar to prior studies, they found that the 5 mm instruments with longer articulating wrist distance requires a longer working distance. Scar size is however decreased with use of smaller ports. Given the limited working space in infants compared to older children, the authors found that decreasing the depth of port insertion with the peritoneal cavity may reduce clashing, but increases risk of dislodgement and camera fogging. Additional highlighted limitations with 5 mm instrumentation include energy delivery, given no available 5 mm bipolar electrocautery instruments or curved scissors with cautery for the S and Si systems. The primary cautery is in the form of a hook [18].

Evolving Technologies

Over the past 15 years various competitors have attempted to create a surgical robot, but until recently have failed to bring a device to market. There are now two new devices that have received regulatory approval for human use in various parts of the world.

Senhance (Transenterix, USA)

Senhance was initially called the ALF-X when developed by the Italian Company, Sofar. This was renamed when purchased by Transenterix (Mooresville, NC). The Senhance system now has FDA approval for performance of laparoscopic colorectal, gynecologic, inguinal hernia and gallbladder surgery [4]. The system has yet to be approved for use in urologic surgery. This system includes a remote-controlled unit known as the cockpit, a 3D HD monitor, infrared Eye Tracking system, foot pedal, keyboard, touch pad and up to four independent robotic arms (they are not attached to a single cart). The open console requires the use of polarized glasses for the 3D display. The eye tracking feature allows the camera to be controlled by viewing various parts of the operative field. The camera follows the surgeon's eyes if two handles are being clutched. The camera will zoom in and out with the movement of the surgeon's head backward and forward. The handles of the operating instruments have haptic feedback which aids in dissection and suturing. This is an improvement over the Da Vinci system, where the surgeon must rely on visual cues to infer tissue handling force. The surgeon is seated upright in an adjustable chair with a viewing screen. This allows for others to view the main surgeon screen and allows for greater interaction with other surgeons in the room. The optics require a 10 mm trocar with all other instruments besides needle holders being accommodated by 5 mm port. The articulating needle holder requires a 10 mm port. There is currently no articulating cutting tool. These instruments are reusable and attached by magnets which facilitates replacement during surgery. In total, there are 22 different instruments available. All are resterilizable. The camera options include bot the 0-degress and 30-degree options, similar to the Da Vinci system [4].

Safety tools include a go/no-go foot pedal to control movements, sensitive grip for precise manipulation, restricted movement speed, emergency stop with warning lights and sounds. The separate arms may be an advantage in cases for multi-quadrant surgery, however can be cumbersome and restrict access to the patient or OR table in case of emergency [4].

In October 2018, TransEnterix received FDA 510(k) clearance for 3 mm diameter instruments as well as additional 5 mm Senhance System instruments, to become the first robotic system to offer 3 mm instruments. This is promising for robotic surgery in the pediatric population in order to allow for smaller incisions and potentially reduce the risk of port hernia. As we have seen above, details regarding working length beyond the trocar will be even more important than the port diameter itself.

Clinical trials with this robotic system have been performed in Germany including 116 robotic-assisted cases over a 6-month period [19]. Operations ranged from transabdominal preperitoneal (TAPP) inguinal hernia, upper GI cases including cholecystectomies, and colorectal procedures. Complications included bleeding, inguinal hernia repair, and conversion to conventional laparoscopy due to severe adhesions in a thoracic gastric surgery case. They determined that the system was safe for general and visceral surgery and highlighted the fast docking time, manual tremor control, and easy access to the operating table due to non-restrictive positioning [19].

The ALF-X system had been tested in porcine models for partial nephrectomy [20]. The authors felt that the system was versatile for performing RALPN with reduction in operative times along the learning curve. They feel it to be safe and feasible.

The system has also been used in a heterogenous series of gynecologic procedures. In 2016, Fanfani et al reported their data from their Phase II study of 146 patients undergoing surgery for presumed benign or borderline adnexal disease, and benign and early stage malignant uterine disease. They found successful completion of procedures without conversion in 95.2% of cases. They found similar operative time and EBL when compared to other MIS on the adnexa. They felt that future developments for this platform should be availability multifunctional graspers and 3 mm instruments, which have since been FDA approved [21].

The 3 mm instruments have been used for robot assisted hysterectomy by surgeons in Italy. From July to September 2017, four patients underwent hysterectomy with bilateral salpingo-oophorectomy. All procedures were performed successfully without major complications, and all patients were discharged home on postoperative day 1. The authors note that there was no increased learning curve with the use of smaller instruments. The haptic feedback of the Senhance system allowed surgeons to experience flexibility of the thinner 3 mm instrument. They felt the greatest limitation to be the absence of a bipolar grasper. Further clinical testing will be required as this platform continues to grow in order to assess its feasibility and safety for the use in adult and pediatric patients [22].

The first clinical experience in the US was published in 2018 [23]. Colorectal and general surgery cases were performed for a total of eight cases. The surgeons noted learning curve with the eye-tracking feature, suggesting 45–60-min preoperative training prior to starting the case. The haptic feedback of the device was comparable to laparoscopic surgery and the ergonomic upright position of the surgeon console was felt to be favorable.

Disadvantages over prior robotic platforms were also noted, including lack of articulating instruments, restricted variety of instruments, no energy or stapling devices, and large independent arm booms that are highly space occupying. Authors also noted that the eye-tracking calibration must be performed prior to each session, which is time consuming [23].

REVO-I

Introduced in 2015 and approved by Korean FDA in 2017, it is now available for use in South Korea [24]. This system consists of a closed console similar to the Da Vinci system, a four-armed robotic operation cart, an HD vision cart, and reusable endoscopic instruments. Instruments are re-usable 20 times compared to 10 times with da Vinci system. The latest version includes haptic feedback similar to the Senhance surgical robot. Monopolar and bipolar energy are available, without additional special instruments such as the Harmonic scalpel. The camera is slightly smaller than the da Vinci Si camera, measuring 10 mm compared to 12 mm [4].

The first human trial was published in 2018 assessing the Revo-I for use in Retzius-sparing robotic radical prostatectomy in patients with localized prostate cancer [25]. A total of 17 procedures were performed, with the goal of assessing intra-operative performance and safety of the new platform. All procedures were completed successfully without conversion to open or laparoscopic surgery. One patient required intraoperative transfusion due to blood loss, and two patients required post-operative transfusion. There were no additional major complications reported. Physician questionnaires were administered after surgery to assess factors such as ease of docking, convenience of instrument insertion and removal, and convenience of the console and video monitor. Survey results demonstrated physician comfort with performing port placement and docking and found the console and video monitor to be convenient.

Physician's in this human study did report a variety of differences between this system and the Da Vinci system. They noted that the scissors were less sharp, making tissue cutting more difficult. At times, the operations were interrupted when the surgeons hand movement speed exceeded the optimum speed adjusted for the robot. The robot arms of the Revo-I system are also larger, requiring greater care by the bedside assistant to avoid external collisions [25].

Laparoendoscopic Single-Site Surgery (LESS)

Laparoendoscopic single-site (LESS) surgery has been used in pediatric urology for the past 10 years for a variety of procedures including inguinal hernia repair, varicocelectomy, orchiopexy, nephrectomy, and reconstructive procedures. LESS offers potentially improved cosmesis with fewer sites of potential hernia. Despite these advantages, a single operative port also leads to decreased maneuverability and instrument control, as well as longer operative time. Triangulation, tissue, handling and suturing are all more difficult when compared to conventional laparoscopy. To help combat these difficulties, a multitude of new technologies have been developed including multi-channel access ports and articulating instruments, leading to improved vision, less instrument class and improved suturing.

In addition to improvement in LESS, robotic laparoendoscopic single-site (R-LESS) has been developed. The Robotic da Vinci Single-Site system was developed with the goal of improving traditional single-incision laparoscopic surgery (SILS) with the improved ergonomics and precision of the robotic instruments. SILS is general is limited due to difficulty with instrument triangulation, camera/view quality, poor ergonomics and difficult learning curve [26].

Many of the hurdles in performing LESS remain present in R-LESS with robotic arm collision, and inadequate triangulation. Since 2009, there have been numerous studies reporting on R-LESS [27]. While the original R-LESS technique required a "chopstick"-like movements of instruments, with lack of wrist articulation, the development and use of the GelPort decreased arm clashing and allowed for improved triangulation. The da Vinci Single-Site Port (Intuitive Surgical Inc.) includes five openings: two for the robotic arms, one for the assistant's instrument, one for the robotic camera, and one for insufflation. The port is folded, clamped with an atraumatic clamp and lubricated with water to facilitate its introduction. The silicone port is deployed into the abdominal wall, and the carbon dioxide insufflation is begun (at 12–15 mmHg).

Robotic instrument advancements have also been made with the addition 5-mm, flexible instruments with articulating wrists. With these advancements, a variety of urologic procedures have become more feasible including complex partial nephrectomy, dismembered pyeloplasty and radical prostatectomy in adults [28].

Single-site robotic surgery has been reported for various procedures including cholecystectomy. Schraibman et al. present their experience of four patients, comparing it to SILS. All patients had a single port placed via a 2.5 cm incision. The da Vinci Si system was used in all cases. They found the robotic platform to be advantageous with a better aesthetic result, less post-operative pain, precise dissection with improved visualization when compared to SILS [29]. Low rates of conversion to open procedures have been reported. Gonzalez et al in their larger series of 465 patients undergoing single-incision robotic cholecystectomy reported success in 97.8% of cases. There were six cases requiring additional ports and 4 cases that required conversion to traditional laparoscopy [30].

The use of R-LESS in the pediatric literature however remains sparse. While conversion from a single incision has been reported to be low, there is worry about the ease of conversion if necessary in a pediatric population. It seems that conversion to additional robotic ports would be prohibitive, requiring the availability and maneuvering of two robotic systems. It is a reasonable question as how best to proceed if single-port surgery is not feasible, and in our opinion the ability to proceed with non-robot-assisted laparoscopic instruments would be the most expeditious. This is what was performed in cases of cholecystectomy that required conversion from a single-port.

Da Vinci SP

The latest technologic advancement currently in pre-clinical trials is the new single-port robotic SP 1098 by Intuitive Surgical [26]. Da Vinci SP earned FDA 510(k) clearance for pyeloplasty, nephrectomy, partial nephrectomy, and prostatectomy, with the first being the most likely common use for pediatric urology. This platform accommodates three working instruments all with articulation, adequate triangulation, and 7 degrees of freedom as well as an 8 mm articulating camera all through a single 25 mm working port. The surgeon console is identical the standard da Vinci system with the addition of a separate foot clutch allowing for simultaneous movement of the instruments and camera. The side cart for the SP system uses the same base and column as is used for the Si and Xi systems (IS3000 model) with alteration in the surgical arms and manipulators for use with a single port. The surgical instruments used for this system have the standard EndoWrist function with 7 degrees of freedom as well as an added joint, providing an "elbow" for adequate triangulation through a single port. These instruments are also longer with a snake-like wrist, which is similar to the 5-mm multi-port instruments. EndoWrist SP instruments include needle driver, round tip scissors, monopolar cautery hook, Maryland bipolar forces and fenestrated bipolar forceps [26].

The SP platform has been deployed in pre-clinical cadaver studies for the performance of transvesical partial prostatectomy (TVPP) [31] After gaining access to the space of Retzius through a single 3-cm, midline, suprapubic incision, an access mini device (GelPOINT) was introduced in to the bladder. The da Vinci SP system was then docked to the GelPOINT by inserting the SP cannula through the GelSeal Cap. The authors found many advantages with the use of the SP device when compared to the traditional approach. The ability to use the GelPOINT device and gain intravesical access allowed for avoidance of the traditional transperitoneal approach and pneumovesicum. The device allowed for sufficient triangulation in a small working space. The intravesical approach also allowed for adequate device seal and lack of need of pneumoperitoneum. In these cadaver studies, there was no need for conversion to open procedure or intra-operative complications reported [31].

This system was first applied to genitourinary surgery in a clinical trial in adult patients in the United States and France. A total of 11 radical prostatectomies were performed, and 8 patients underwent renal surgery (4 partial nephrectomies, 2 radical nephrectomies, and 2 simple nephrectomies). No patients required conversion to open procedure and there was a total of 8 complications among the 19 patients treated with 2 surgical reinterventions required in the radical prostatectomy patients [26].

Wristed Laparoscopic Instruments

Given the substantial financial costs and learning curves associated with robotic surgery, many have sought to develop laparoscopic instruments that employ wristed technology to attain the dexterity-related benefits of robotic instruments at lower cost.

Traditional laparoscopic instruments are straight with a fulcrum or pivot point of the instrument created by the port placed in the body wall. These instruments consist of a handle, rigid shaft, and an end effector that is operated by the user with the handle of the device. With the development of wristed laparoscopic instruments, surgeons have the benefit of tactile feel with a hand held and operated instrument as well as the added dexterity of an articulating instrument with a wrist like joint. Articulation of the instrument is beneficial to reduce instrument crowding and allow for proper instrument triangulation when working in confined spaces. This becomes particularly important when working with pediatric patients. Such instruments could also be used for single-port laparoscopic surgery with sufficient triangulation given end-effector articulation.

Wristed instruments have two types of wrist-like mechanisms when deflected: a either a zero- bend radius (jaws integrated into wrist mechanism) or a curved arc (jaws separate from and distal to the wristed movement) when deflected [32]. Handheld technology and interaction with the instrument to achieve wrist articulation varies from product to product. The three main types of handheld control mechanisms include handle control, thumb control, and mixed control [33]. Handle control instruments allow the handle to articulate relative to the instrument shaft and deflect the wrist. Thumb controlled instruments use a ball or joystick that is manipulated by the users thumb to allow for and control wrist articulation. Mixed control devices use elements of each of the prior two control methods and each degree of wrist freedom is controlled by a different lever located on the handle. Kinetic directional mapping is an important factor in instrument design. This refers to the direction of wrist movement when mapped to the direction of movement by the user. In parallel mapping, the control handle and end effector remain in parallel in relation to the central axis during articulation. In reverse mapping, the end effector and control handle move perpendicular in relation to the central axis of the instrument with articulation (handle deflection downward leads to downward deflection of end effector) [32].

In 2016, Anderson et al published a thorough review of the current available and in production technology in wristed laparoscopic instrumentation [32]. We offer a brief review of the major instrument types discussed in their publication with Table 5.2 as a summary of the devices discussed. The first design type is the pistol-grip handle controlled-devices with curved wrists. These instruments have reverse kinematic mapping with a handle that articulates relative to the instrument shaft for wrist control. The wrist itself is a curved device that is driven by tendons. Axial rotation of the end effector is achieved by manipulation of a knob on the handle of the instrument. Examples of this design of instrument include RealHand by Novare Surgical Systems Inc., the Autonomy Laparo-Angle articulating instruments by Cambridge Endoscopic Devices, Inc, and the Medtronic-Covidien SILS Hand

Table 5.2 Laparoscopic wristed instruments

Device	Kinetic mapping	Wrist type	Handle design	Reusable?	Entity producing or developing	Availability status
FlexDex	Parallel	Pinned	Forearm mounted	No – planned for future design	FlexDex Surgical	Commercially available in US with distribution via Olympus America, Inc
Radius Surgical System	Neither	Pinned	Lever/knob	Yes	Tuebingen Scientific, GmbH	Commercially available
SILS Hand Instruments	Reverse	Curved	Pistol	No	Medtronic (previously Covidien)	Commercially available (SILS™ Dissect, Clinch, Shears, Hook)
Intuitool	Reverse	Pinned	Pistol/trackball	Unknown	University of Nebraska	Seeking commercial partners
Maestro	Either	Pinned	Symmetric-reverse hemostat	Unknown	Vanderbilt University	Not commercially available
MiFlex	Reverse	Curved	Pistol/joystick	Handle: yes End effector: no	DEAM and Indes	Under development
Autonomy Laparo-angle	Reverse	Curved	Pistol	No	Cambridge Endoscopic Devices, Inc	Was commercially available – company out of business
RealHand	Reverse	Curved	Pistol	No	Novare Surgical System, Inc	Was commercially available – company out of business

Reprinted from Anderson et al. [32] with permission of Taylor & Francis, Ltd. (http://www.tandfonline.com)

Instruments. Only the SILS instruments are currently commercially available in the form of the SILS™ Dissect, SILS™ Clinch, SILS™ Shears and SILS™Hook. The former two companies filed bankruptcy and their products are not commercially available. These instruments are all disposable, single use, 5 mm diameter shaft devices. They also have the ability to be used without the articulating wrist as a standard laparoscopic instrument. The end effector of all of these instruments can be locked to improve ease of suturing. Such instruments however require a sweep motion of the user's hand over a large arc in order to deflect the wrist. This is problematic for learning as well as potentially prohibitive in confined working spaces in pediatric patients.

An example of a device that uses the mixed control mechanism is the Radius Surgical System by Tuebungen Scientific, GmbH. Wrist deflection occurs unidirectionally as the handle is deflected relative to the shaft of the device while axial rotation is controlled by a thumb knob. A multi-finger trigger on the device handle operates the jaws of the end effector. Gears, rather than cables are used to deflect and rotate the device. One major limitation of this device for the use in pediatric patients is the 10 mm shaft diameter (compared to 5 mm diameter of pistol-grip, handle devices). This device has been used in training model studies as well as in clinical practice for performance of a variety of laparoscopic procedures. Reports suggest improved ergonomics over conventional laparoscopic instruments [34–36]. The learning curve for this instrument however seems to be challenging given that the degrees of freedom are decoupled with a shaft rotation provided by thumb motions and unidirectional wrist articulation provided by movement of the handle. These instruments also rely on body wall reaction forces for stabilization of the shaft of the instrument. This may prove to be problematic if used in pediatric patients.

The Maestro, developed at Vanderbilt University, uses a handle-controlled mechanism with parallel and reverse kinetic mapping. The axes that articulate the handle are placed relative to the instrument shaft within the user's hand grasp. The device handle can be rotated within the user's hand to generate axial shaft rotation. Movements are similar to that of the da Vinci robotic system. The end of effector is tendon driven by steel cables, each anchored by a pulley. Large sweeping motions of the jaws are not required during articulation, making this device more favorable for smaller working spaces. A jaw locking mechanism is provided, allowing the end effector to be locked while allowing wrist articulation. There are currently no data on clinical use of this system.

FlexDex, has a unique design, and is currently distributed via Olympus America Inc. This instrument has an interface that connects to the user's forearm. The user's wrist deflections are mapped to the wrist deflections inside the patient with parallel mapping. The wrist articulation axes are located at the center of the surgeon's wrist. This allows decoupling of wrist movements from the traditional 4 degrees of freedom with laparoscopy. The surgeon is able to the control the standard degrees of freedom with her forearm and then add in wrist articulation as needed. The design is advantageous given direct wrist mapping. The forearm design however makes picking up and putting down the device challenging.

The last class of device is the thumb-controlled mechanism. Here, the handle is connected to the instrument shaft and wrist articulation is controlled by a thumb interface. The MiFlex and Intuitool devices both use a pistol-grip handle with thumb interface that controls instrument wrist movement within the patient. Both devices use reverse mapping. The MiFlex instrument was developed by DEAM B.V. with handle design by Indes B.V. This instrument is 5-mm in diameter and uses a rolling thumb joystick that is mounted on the device handle. The handle of the device is reusable while the end effector is single-use. The Intuitool device was designed at the University of Nebraska and similarly used a thumb trackball which allows transmission of the track-ball movements to rods within the shaft of the instrument. This leads to articulation of the wrist joint with ±60° wrist articulation. There is a knob for axial shaft rotation and the end effector jaws are operated by a trigger on the pistol-grip handle.

While numerous devices have been designed and are in development, many questions remain in regard to instrument design and use. For example, there is no clear consensus on which type of control is easiest to use, or which type of kinetic mapping is best. For those cases in which instrument triangulation is necessary, such as pediatric urologic intraabdominal surgery, reverse mapping may be superior for surgeon hand positioning and comfort. Widespread use of these instruments in the clinical setting remains insufficient to answer such technical questions. Various authors have assessed performance with articulating instruments for LESS with surgical simulator training. One study assessed surgeon kinematics and ergonomics with a particular articulating instrument and found that skilled minimally invasive surgeons were frustrated when using the instrument and developed upper back and extremity discomfort secondary to the increased range of motion of the wrists and abnormal joint posturing [37]. While such stress may not be as applicable to multiport surgery with articulating instruments, the authors suggest that continued ergonomic and kinematic improvements should be made in device design. A second simulation-based training study found that participants had the greatest success in task performance with LESS when using one straight laparoscopic instrument and one articulating instrument compared to using either two straight instruments or two articulating instruments [38]. No increased surgeon workload was appreciated when using the articulating instruments. This supports the continued use of articulating instruments in future human studies.

It also does not appear that any of these devices have been employed for use in pediatric patients to date. Regardless, such instruments do show promise in combining the benefits of wristed movement provided by robot assisted surgery at likely substantially lower costs.

Conclusion

We in pediatric urology have been the beneficiaries of dramatic improvements in surgical instrumentation. While not one of the instruments discussed above has been developed with the tiny pediatric urology market as its primary target, with our field's ingenuity we have adapted these tools to fit our needs. Our patient's lives have been improved. The previous decade has proven that a standard, adult-sized robot with three or more ports can accomplish a wide variety of pediatric urologic reconstructive procedures. The next decade may be more interesting still, as changes in port number, instrumentation, advanced laparoscopic instruments, and increasing competition between device manufacturers may be hold yet more advances.

References

1. Hagen ME, Stein H, Curet MJ. Introduction to the robotic system. In: Kim KC, editor. Robotics in general surgery. New York: Springer; 2014. p. 9–15.
2. Sung GT, Gill IS. Robotic laparoscopic surgery: a comparison of the DA Vinci and Zeus systems. Urology. 2001;58(6):893–8.
3. Yates DR, Vaessen C, Roupret M. From Leonardo to da Vinci: the history of robot-assisted surgery in urology. BJU Int. 2011;108(11):1708–13; discussion 14.
4. Rassweiler JJ, Autorino R, Klein J, Mottrie A, Goezen AS, Stolzenburg JU, et al. Future of robotic surgery in urology. BJU Int. 2017;120(6):822–41.
5. Gettman M, Rivera M. Innovations in robotic surgery. Curr Opin Urol. 2016;26(3):271–6.
6. Kallingal GJ, Swain S, Darwiche F, Punnen S, Manoharan M, Gonzalgo ML, et al. Robotic partial nephrectomy with the Da Vinci xi. Adv Urol. 2016;2016:9675095.
7. Berlinger NT. Robotic surgery--squeezing into tight places. N Engl J Med. 2006;354(20):2099–101.
8. Patel MN, Hemal AK. Does advancing technology improve outcomes? Comparison of the Da Vinci standard/S/Si to the Xi Robotic Platforms During Robotic Nephroureterectomy. J Endourol. 2018;32(2):133–8.
9. Meininger DD, Byhahn C, Heller K, Gutt CN, Westphal K. Totally endoscopic Nissen fundoplication with a robotic system in a child. Surg Endosc. 2001;15(11):1360.
10. Bruns NE, Soldes OS, Ponsky TA. Robotic surgery may not "make the cut" in pediatrics. Front Pediatr. 2015;3:10.
11. Chang C, Steinberg Z, Shah A, Gundeti MS. Patient positioning and port placement for robot-assisted surgery. J Endourol. 2014;28(6):631–8.
12. Howe A, Kozel Z, Palmer L. Robotic surgery in pediatric urology. Asian J Urol. 2017;4(1):55–67.
13. Finkelstein JB, Levy AC, Silva MV, Murray L, Delaney C, Casale P. How to decide which infant can have robotic surgery? Just do the math. J Pediatr Urol. 2015;11(4):170 e1–4.
14. Cundy TP, Marcus HJ, Hughes-Hallett A, MacKinnon T, Najmaldin AS, Yang GZ, et al. Robotic versus non-robotic instruments in spatially constrained operating workspaces: a preclinical randomized crossover study. BJU Int. 2015;116(3):415–22.
15. Meehan JJ, Sandler AD. Robotic resection of mediastinal masses in children. J Laparoendosc Adv Surg Tech A. 2008;18(1):114–9.
16. Thakre AA, Bailly Y, Sun LW, Van Meer F, Yeung CK. Is smaller workspace a limitation for robot performance in laparoscopy? J Urol. 2008;179(3):1138–42; discussion 42–3.
17. Ballouhey Q, Clermidi P, Cros J, Grosos C, Rosa-Arsene C, Bahans C, et al. Comparison of 8 and 5 mm robotic instruments in small cavities : 5 or 8 mm robotic instruments for small cavities? Surg Endosc. 2018;32(2):1027–34.
18. Baek M, Silay MS, Au JK, Huang GO, Elizondo RA, Puttmann KT, et al. Does the use of 5 mm instruments affect the outcomes of robot-assisted laparoscopic pyeloplasty in smaller working spaces? A comparative analysis of infants and older children. J Pediatr Urol. 2018;14:537–e1.
19. Stephan D, Salzer H, Willeke F. First experiences with the new Senhance(R) telerobotic system in visceral surgery. Visc Med. 2018;34(1):31–6.

20. Bozzini G, Gidaro S, Taverna G. Robot-assisted laparoscopic partial nephrectomy with the ALF-X robot on pig models. Eur Urol. 2016;69(2):376–7.
21. Fanfani F, Monterossi G, Fagotti A, Rossitto C, Gueli Alletti S, Costantini B, et al. The new robotic TELELAP ALF-X in gynecological surgery: single-center experience. Surg Endosc. 2016;30(1):215–21.
22. Gueli Alletti S, Perrone E, Cianci S, Rossitto C, Monterossi G, Bernardini F, et al. 3 mm Senhance robotic hysterectomy: a step towards future perspectives. J Robot Surg. 2018;12(3):575–7.
23. deBeche-Adams T, Eubanks WS, de la Fuente SG. Early experience with the Senhance(R)-laparoscopic/robotic platform in the US. J Robot Surg. 2018;13:357–9.
24. Rao PP. Robotic surgery: new robots and finally some real competition! World J Urol. 2018;36(4):537–41.
25. Chang KD, Abdel Raheem A, Choi YD, Chung BH, Rha KH. Retzius-sparing robot-assisted radical prostatectomy using the Revo-i robotic surgical system: surgical technique and results of the first human trial. BJU Int. 2018;122(3):441–8.
26. Kaouk JH, Haber GP, Autorino R, Crouzet S, Ouzzane A, Flamand V, et al. A novel robotic system for single-port urologic surgery: first clinical investigation. Eur Urol. 2014;66(6):1033–43.
27. Nelson RJ, Chavali JSS, Yerram N, Babbar P, Kaouk JH. Current status of robotic single-port surgery. Urol Ann. 2017;9(3):217–22.
28. Buffi NM, Lughezzani G, Fossati N, Lazzeri M, Guazzoni G, Lista G, et al. Robot-assisted, single-site, dismembered pyeloplasty for ureteropelvic junction obstruction with the new da Vinci platform: a stage 2a study. Eur Urol. 2015;67(1):151–6.
29. Schraibman V, Epstein MG, Maccapani GN, Macedo AL. Single-port robotic cholecystectomy. Initial and pioneer experience in Brazil. Einstein (Sao Paulo). 2015;13(4):607–10.
30. Gonzalez A, Murcia CH, Romero R, Escobar E, Garcia P, Walker G, et al. A multicenter study of initial experience with single-incision robotic cholecystectomies (SIRC) demonstrating a high success rate in 465 cases. Surg Endosc. 2016;30(7):2951–60.
31. Maurice MJ, Ramirez D, Kaouk JH. Robotic laparoendoscopic single-site retroperitoneal renal surgery: initial investigation of a purpose-built single-port surgical system. Eur Urol. 2017;71(4):643–7.
32. Anderson PL, Lathrop RA, Webster RJ III. Robot-like dexterity without computers and motors: a review of hand-held laparoscopic instruments with wrist-like tip articulation. Expert Rev Med Devices. 2016;13(7):661–72.
33. Fan C, Dodou D, Breedveld P. Review of manual control methods for handheld maneuverable instruments. Minim Invasive Ther Allied Technol. 2013;22(3):127–35.
34. Frede T, Hammady A, Klein J, Teber D, Inaki N, Waseda M, et al. The radius surgical system - a new device for complex minimally invasive procedures in urology? Eur Urol. 2007;51(4):1015–22; discussion 22.
35. Heemskerk J, Zandbergen R, Maessen JG, Greve JW, Bouvy ND. Advantages of advanced laparoscopic systems. Surg Endosc. 2006;20(5):730–3.
36. Shibao K, Higure A, Yamaguchi K. Laparoendoscopic single-site common bile duct exploration using the manual manipulator. Surg Endosc. 2013;27(8):3009–15.
37. Hallbeck MS, Lowndes BR, McCrory B, Morrow MM, Kaufman KR, LaGrange CA. Kinematic and ergonomic assessment of laparoendoscopic single-site surgical instruments during simulator training tasks. Appl Ergon. 2017;52:118–30.
38. Corker HP, Singh P, Sodergren MH, Balaji S, Kwasnicki RM, Darzi AW, et al. A randomized controlled study to establish the effect of articulating instruments on performance in single-incision laparoscopic surgery. J Surg Educ. 2015;72(1):1–7.

Chapter 6
Patient Positioning, Trocar Placement and Initial Access

Fadi Y. Zu'bi and Walid A. Farhat

Introduction

Robot oriented surgery (ROS) has gained popularity in both adult and pediatric urology. ROS has several advantages over conventional laparoscopic surgery, particularly in the improved exposure via magnified 3-dimensional view and simplification of suturing with the increased degree of freedom and movement of the robotic arm. Pediatric urologists have adopted robot oriented procedures in selected centers, performing procedures such as pyeloplasty for ureteropelvic junction obstruction, partial and complete nephrectomy, and ureteral reimplantation. In this chapter we describe logistical issues pertaining to patient positioning, trocar placement and initial access for the two quadrants of commonly performed urologic operations: those in the pelvis, or upper tract. Emphasis will be placed on patient safety issues, ergonomics, and optimizing surgical exposure.

Nuances of Minimal Invasive Surgery in Pediatrics

Minimal invasive surgery (MIS) in pediatric population is relatively challenging secondary to small size of the abdominal cavity. Desufflation and abdominal collapse may happen immediately as a result of any gas leak, which makes working in an already small workspace even more hazardous. Thus, port placement is of

---

F. Y. Zu'bi (✉)
Department of Urology, The Nazareth Hospital EMMS, Nazareth, Israel

Department of Urology, Rambam Health Care Campus, Haifa, Israel

W. A. Farhat
University of Wisconsin School of Medicine and Public Health, Department of Urology, Madison, WI, USA
e-mail: wfarhat@wisc.edu

© Springer Nature Switzerland AG 2020
P. C. Gargollo (ed.), *Minimally Invasive and Robotic-Assisted Surgery in Pediatric Urology*, https://doi.org/10.1007/978-3-030-57219-8_6

paramount importance with MIS in children. Due to the relatively restricted space, trocars must be placed carefully under direct sight to avoid bleeding, visceral injury and to allow optimal use of the available space [1]. The nuances of MIS in the pediatric population are further related to size of the patients, instruments, and more importantly the physiologic effects of pneumoperitoneum on the respiratory, cardiovascular, renal, and gastrointestinal tracts, particularly at higher pressures. Hence, surgeons embarking on incorporating MIS in their practice are advised to have a good understanding of the evolving technology and the physiology of children.

Positioning

Robotic surgery entails unique positioning requirements due to physical space restrictions and patient safety concerns [2, 3]. Conventional patient positioning on the operating room table and positioning devices, need to be appropriately tuned to meet the specific demands of robotic surgery [4]. Spatial position of the motorized operating room table, anaesthesia workstation, robotic console, robotic patient cart, drip stand and instruments trolley, must to be optimized relative to each other for each type of robotic surgery (Fig. 6.1). The robotic surgical team must be careful and work

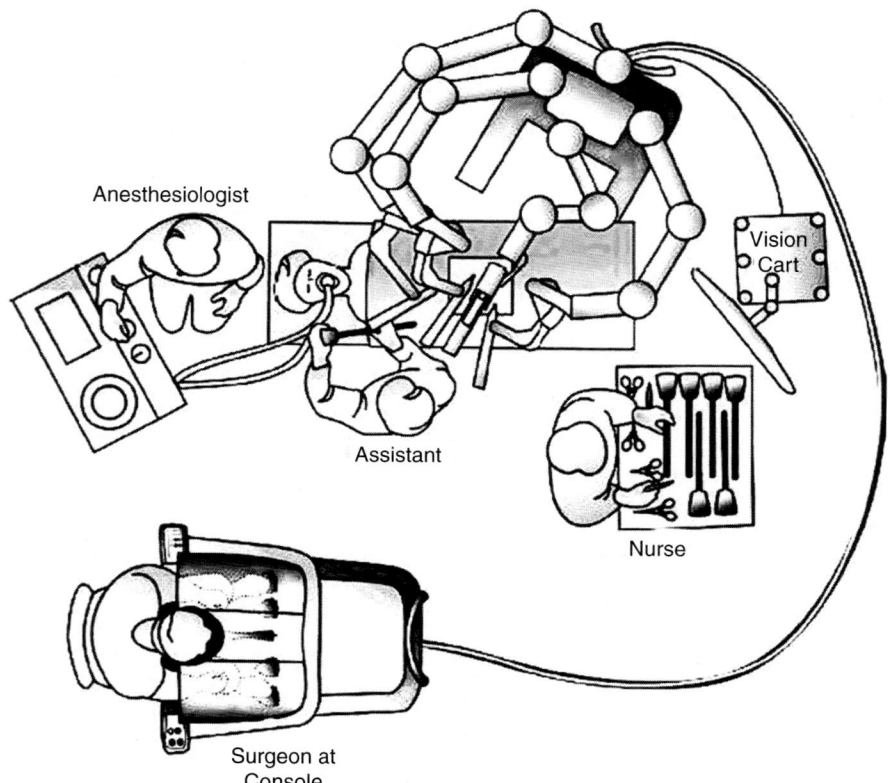

Fig. 6.1 Room setup for left sided procedures

together during positioning and setting up the device to avoid possible complications. Proper positioning of the patient during the operative period is important to optimize surgical exposure and to reduce the risk of positioning related injuries. Furthermore, understanding the pathophysiologic changes and special considerations associated with each position helps reduce positioning-related morbidity. For instance, a variety of positioning devices and accessories may be needed to aid in achieving the optimum surgical position and to provide safety and comfort for the patient (Fig. 6.2):

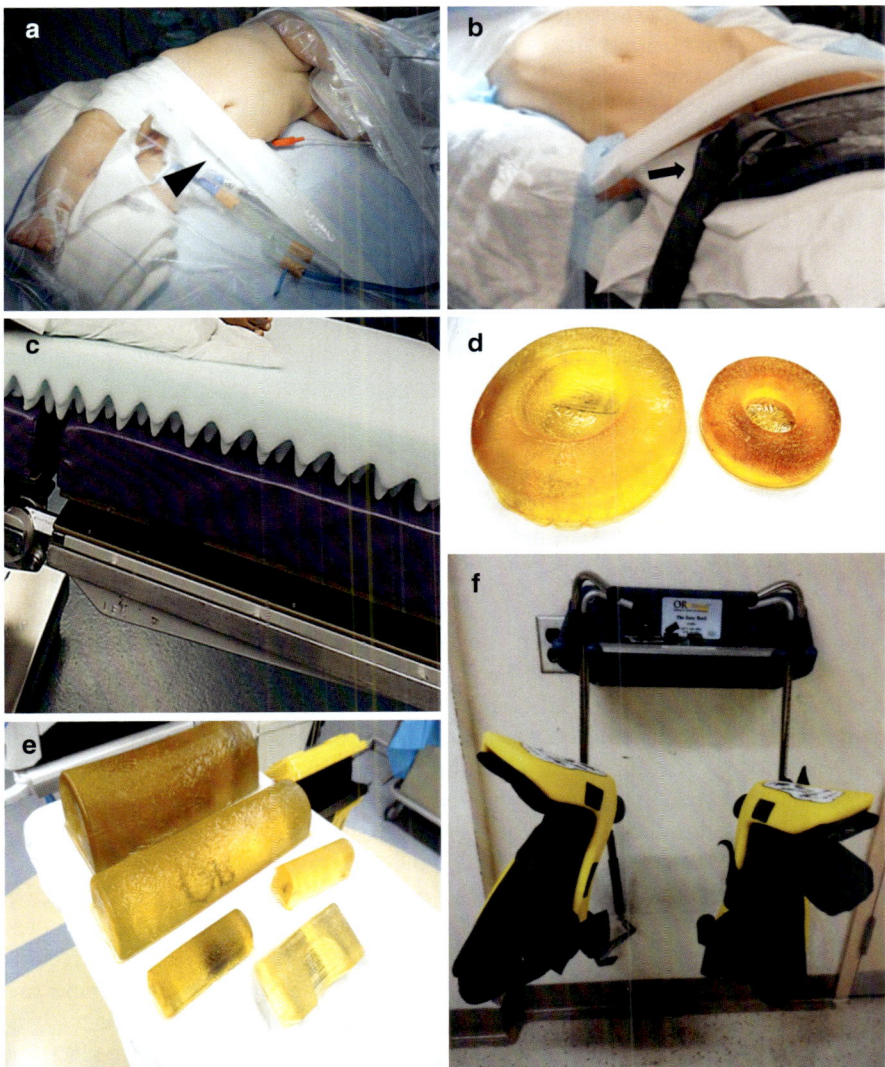

Fig. 6.2 (**a**) Silk tape to secure the patient (arrowhead) (**b**) Securing belt (arrow). Before prepping the patient, it is recommended to rotate carefully the operative table to confirm that the patient is well secured. (**c**) Honey Comb facing down to avoid skin marks (**d**) Head rest in different sizes (**e**) Gel bolsters. (**f**) Stirrups

- The procedure table itself, including general-purpose tables, and fixed-base systems with interchangeable tabletops. Occasionally, spinal tables are used for prone positioning.
- Procedure table mattresses include gel (standard/warming), foam (standard/alternating pressure), air operated warming, vacuum and static-air, viscoelastic (polyether/ polyurethane) honey comb, anti-decubitus mattresses.
- Equipment that attaches to the procedure table (e.g., headrests/holders, overhead arm supports, stirrups for pelvic procedure).
- Support devices for the head, arms, chest, iliac crests and lumbar areas.
- Gel bolsters in a variety of sizes and shapes to protect pressure points (e.g., the head, elbows, knees, ankles, heels).
- Securing devices (e.g., safety belts, tapes, vacuum beanbags).

Upper Urinary Tract Procedures

In the pediatric population, numerous upper urinary tract procedures may be performed robotically such as: dismembered pyeloplasty, nephrectomy /heminephrectomy, and upper ureteroureterostomy. Those procedures can be performed either through the transperitoneum or less commonly in retroperitoneal approach.

Transperitoneal Approach

Patient Positioning

After general anesthesia is induced, the patient is placed in a lateral decubitus position, rotated approximately 30–45° off the vertical plane (Fig. 6.3). The patient is positioned close to the edge of the table to allow for unhindered robotic arm movement. Once this is achieved, the bottom arm is placed on an arm board padded with egg crate foams. The upper arm is allowed to rest on the side of the patient. Additional foam padding is used to protect the face from unintentional injury. The patient is secured to the operating table at the level of the lower rib cage and hips using foam padding and silk tape. Finally, the table is flexed approximately 15° at the kidney rest. It is worth mentioning that elevating the kidney rest might decrease the distance from the great vessels, thus, increasing the risk of vascular injury during trocar placement. To decrease the risk of major vascular injury, it may be recommended to flex the table only when all trocars in place. Sometimes, clear drapes are used to cover the head of the patient, and all cables should be placed in such a way to avoid resting on the patient. A urethral catheter and orogastric tube are placed at the start of the procedure. At all times, timely and effective communication between the surgical and anesthesia teams, including read backs as necessary, may help avoid errors that could result from miscommunication.

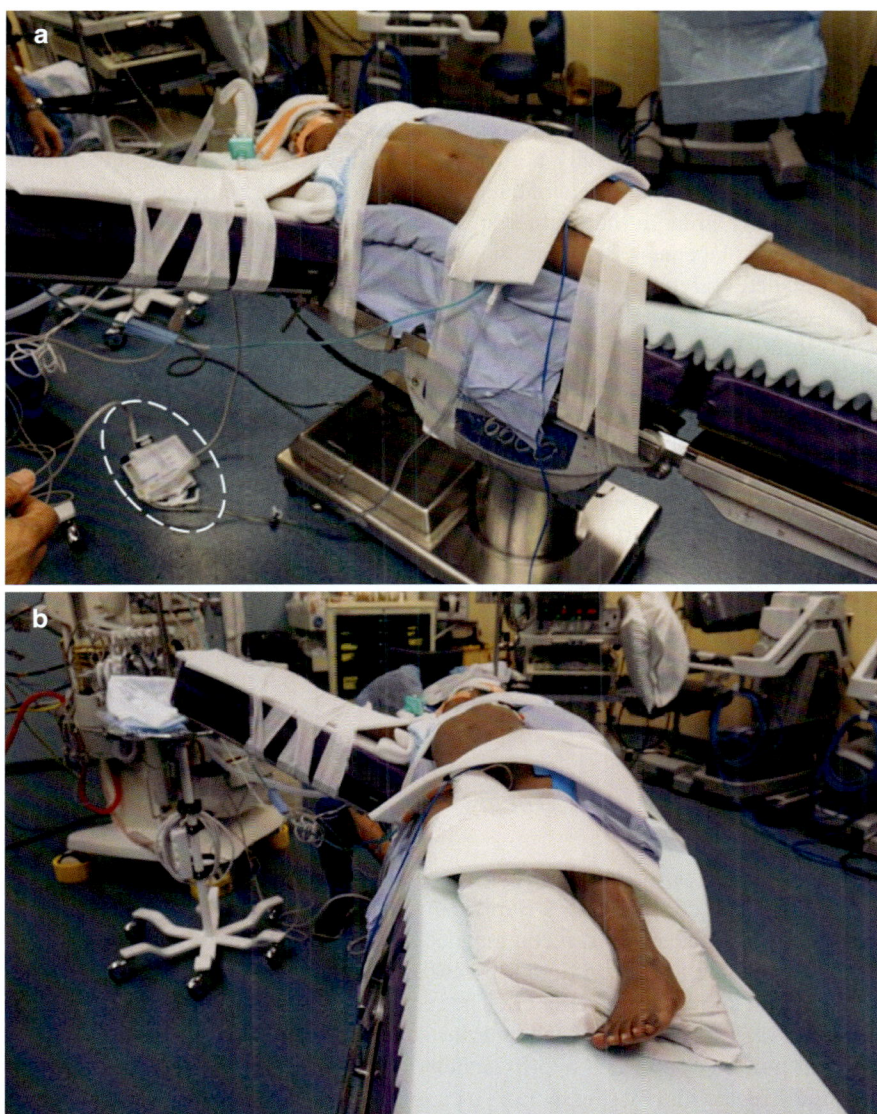

Fig. 6.3 (**a**) The patient is placed in a lateral decubitus position, rotated approximately 30–45° off the vertical plane. The urine bag (dotted ellipse) is accessible and close to the anesthesia team to monitor urine output. (**b**) Notice the foam padding protecting the face and extremities

Port Placement:

Typically, an open-access (Hasson) technique is used first to place the camera port. This technique involves opening the skin, fascia, and muscle until the peritoneum is exposed. The peritoneal cavity is then entered and the trocar placed under direct vision. The use of this open technique has been shown to decrease the risk of major vascular injury in large multicenter analyses [5, 6]. An alternate approach for the initial trocar placement is to use the Veress needle. The needle itself utilizes a spring-loaded "safety" insert that is designed to prevent iatrogenic visceral injury. The Veress needle is placed blindly into the abdominal cavity, and insufflation occurs through the needle. Proper placement is supported by placement of a saline-filled syringe on the needle. Aspiration should show gas in the syringe, and saline injected into the needle as the syringe is removed should quickly enter the abdomen (the so-called hanging saline drop test). When gas is insufflated via the Veress needle, one should see high flow rates at low pressure. If these findings are not observed, the needle should be withdrawn and placement reattempted before the trocar is inserted. The camera port is usually placed either in the umbilicus or in the inferior aspect of the umbilicus. We traditionally perform trans-umbilical access using the open "Hasson" technique (Fig. 6.4). Our current norms used for CO_2 working pressure and flow rate is summarized in Table 6.1 according to age. The abdomen is insufflated with CO_2 at the desired pressure, and the telescope is inserted to view the area of insertion for iatrogenic trauma.

Accessory and Assistant Trocars

The working trocars (often two separate 5-mm/8-mm trocars) are inserted under direct vision. Injection of 0.25% Bupivicaine (2.5 mg/mL) with 1:100000 epinephrine before port placement is recommended to provide preemptive analgesia and to minimize postoperative pain. In our practice, the first working port is placed in the midline 8 cm above the camera port. The second working port is placed in the midclavicular line at the level of the anterior superior iliac spine. If needed, a 5-mm assistant port can be placed approximately 6 cm lateral to the camera port, away from the affected kidney (Fig. 6.5a).

In infants, because of limited working space, we traditionally recommend to place working ports in the midline 4 cm from each other, with camera port by the umbilicus. As a general rule, port triangulation leads to excessive collision of the robotic arms. When placing ports suprapubically, caution must be taken to avoid iatrogenic injury, especially to the bladder.

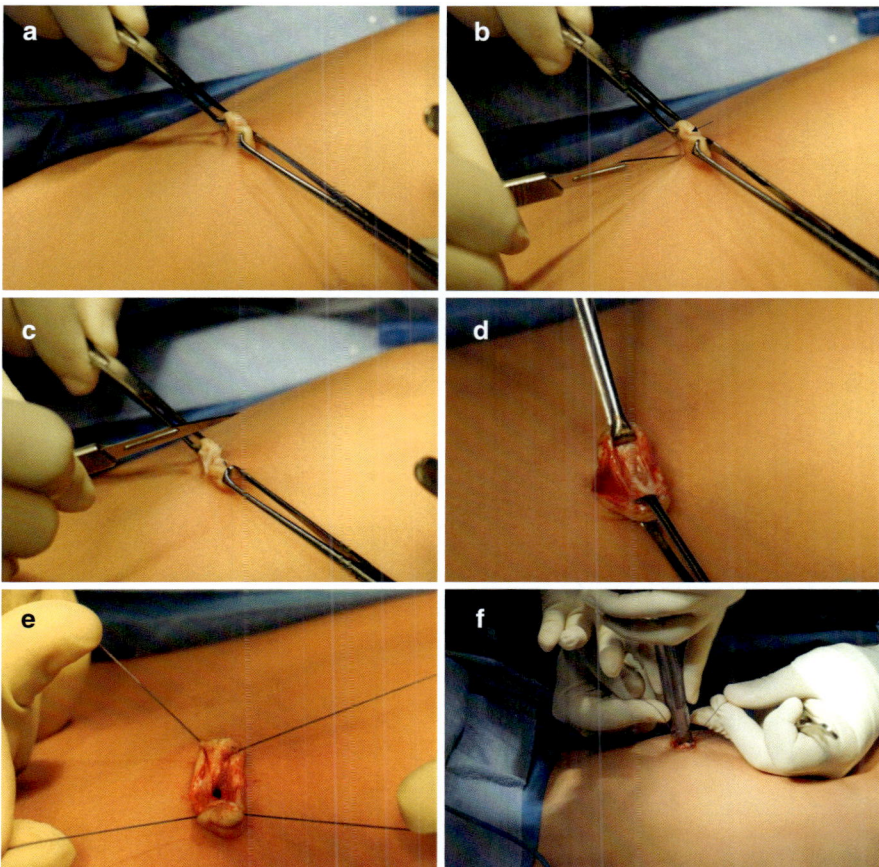

Fig. 6.4 The umbilical port insertion technique. (**a**) The umbilicus is everted and cleaned, with meticulous attention to hygiene (**b**) After identification of the central 'axle' of umbilicus (black arrow), to perform the incision (**c**) adherent to the midline (inside out fashion) (**d**) Fascial ring and the opening to the peritoneum identified (**e**) After widening the peritoneal opening to apply "U" stich on the fascial ring using 2-0 Vicryl suture (**f**) Camera port inserted according to "Hasson" technique while lifting the abdomen with the 2-0 Vicryl stay suture

Table 6.1 Recommended CO_2 working pressure and flow rate according to age

Age (year)	Flow rate (L/min)	Working pressure (mm Hg)
0–2	0.5	8–10
2–10	1	10–12
>10	2	12–15

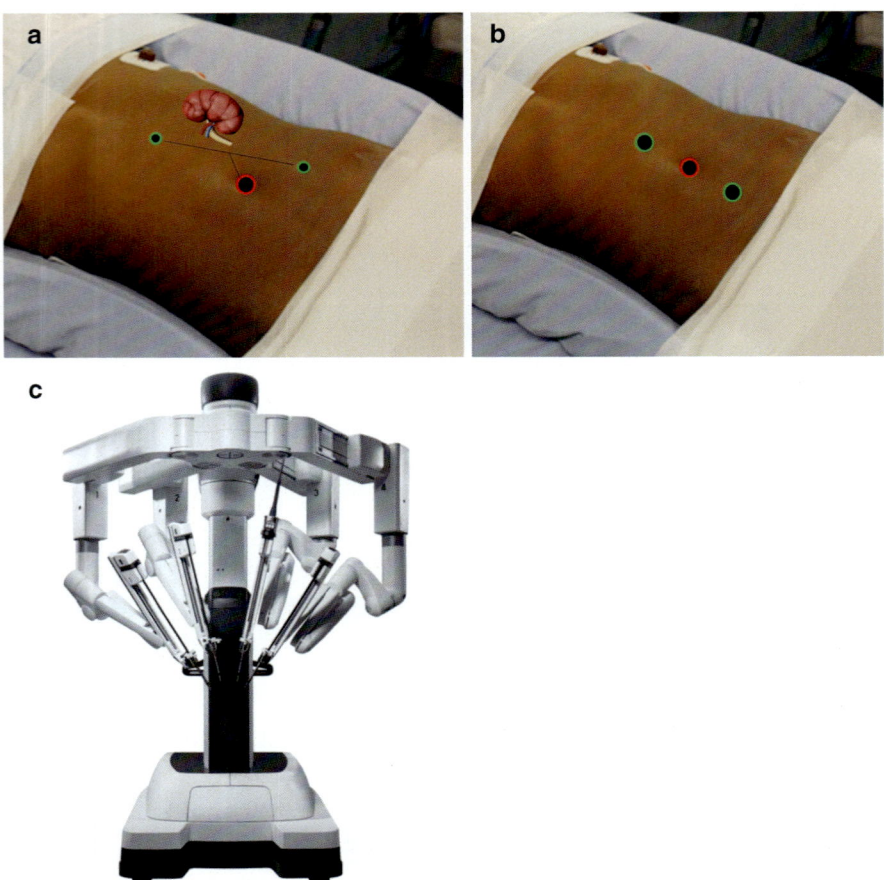

Fig. 6.5 (**a**) Port arrangement for renal surgery using the *Da Vinci Si* system. The arrangement of the arms and camera port is oriented symmetrically toward the area of surgery. Red – camera port, green – working robotic ports. (**b**) Straight line port position for most patients using the *Da Vinci Xi* system. The trocar should have at least 3 cm of separation in order to avoid robotic arms collision. Red – camera port, green – working robotic ports. (**c**) *Da Vinci Xi s*ystem with a horizontal FLEX joints

Docking

For upper urinary tract procedures, the ***Si*** robotic device is docked from the ipsilateral side. The *da Vinci **Xi*** model, on the other hand, with its rotating boom-mounted arms, could achieve a four-quadrant anatomical access while being docked from any position around the patient. The docking procedure is also facilitated by laser

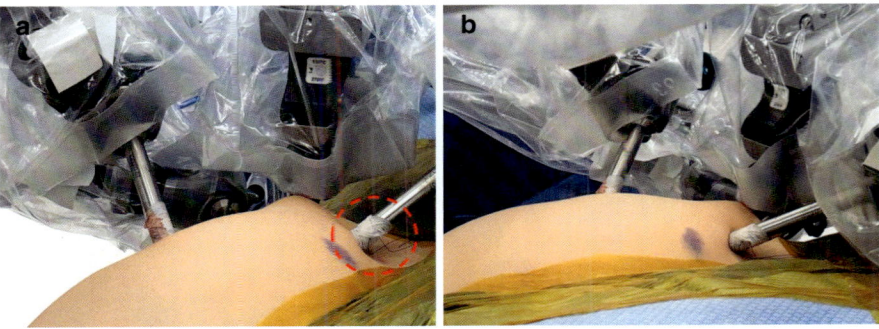

Fig. 6.6 The port is indenting the abdominal wall (**a**); the ports should be "burped" to allow sufficient intracorporeal working space (**b**). (*Courtesy of Daniel G. DaJusta, MD*)

targeting and improved cannula mounts. These features allow the use of a simplified "linear" port configuration and abbreviated docking time (Fig. 6.5b). Moreover, the new model has a horizontal FLEX joints that need to be compacted, leaving one-fist-width spacing between each arm. This configuration allows the arms to move in parallel with each other, avoiding collision between the instrument carriages and the adjacent arm during the procedure (Fig. 6.5c).

Once ports are placed, they should be pulled back (burped) to create more working space rather than indenting the abdominal wall. In order to do so, the arms should be clutched and the ports lifted away from the abdomen (Fig. 6.6).

Hidden Incision Endoscopic Surgery (HIdES)

This technique was first described by Gargollo [7], which allows all port sites to be hidden at the level of a Pfannenstiel incision and thus provide them nonvisible scars. For this technique, pneumoperitoneum is established using a Veress needle in an infraumbilical location. Initially a 5 mm trocar is used along with a 5 mm laparoscope to allow under direct vision insertion of an 8 or 5 mm robotic working port, 12 or 10 mm camera port and 5 mm assistant port below the line of a Pfannenstiel incision (Fig. 6.7). Once complete, the 5 mm infraumbilical port is exchanged for a robotic working port (5 or 8 mm). The robot is docked from the corner of the operating table for the camera arm to reach and stay within the operative sweet spot. The procedure is then carried out depending on the nature of the case. It is worthy to mention that using *HIdES* will provide a different intracorporeal view from the traditional access.

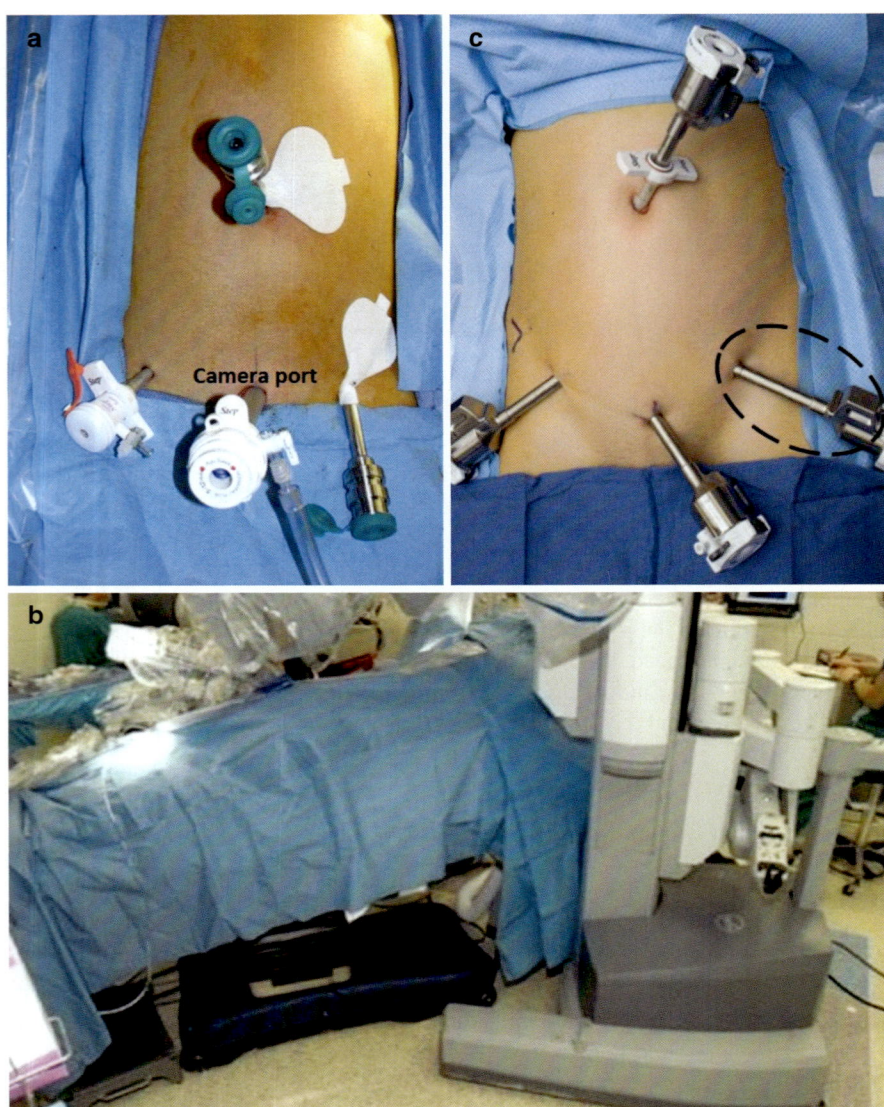

Fig. 6.7 (**a**) Trocar placement in HIdES procedure. Note how trocars (Si robotic device) are dropped below Pfannenstiel incision line (**b**) *Da Vinci Si* device feet have to straddle the top corner of the bed contralateral to the procedure side (**c**) *Da Vinci Xi* robotic device ports. Notice the 4th assisting arm (dotted ellipse) that can also be used for bilateral procedures. (**d**) The *Da Vinci Xi* model can be docked from any position around the patient. The main intraoperative change with HIdES from standard Laparoscopic port positioning is the view. The view changes from medial to lateral approach with standard port positioning (**e**) to a complete caudal to cranial approach (**f**). Healed scars with HIdES (**g**) versus standard Laparoscopic port positioning (**h**). (*Courtesy of Patricio C. Gargollo, MD*)

6 Patient Positioning, Trocar Placement and Initial Access

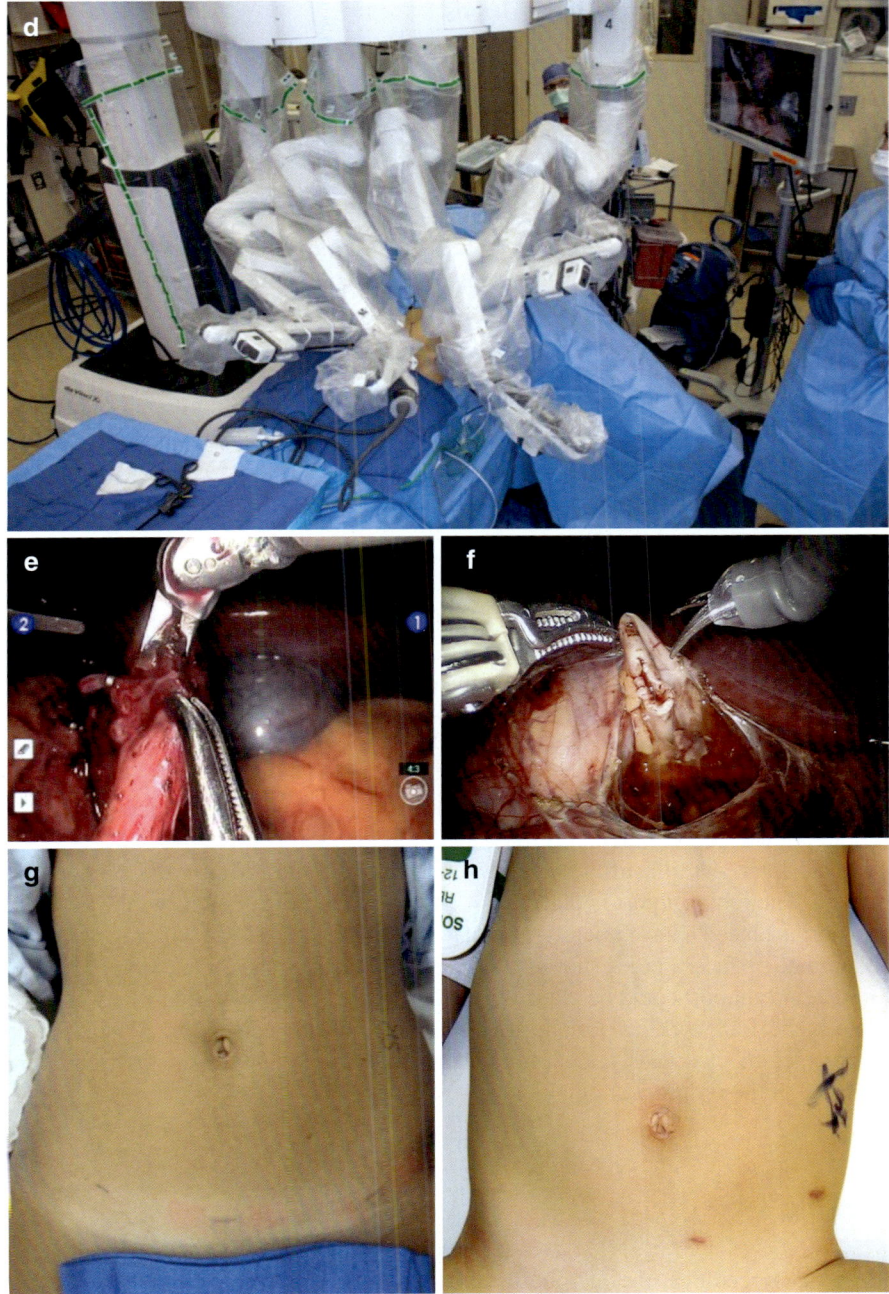

Fig. 6.7 (continued)

Lower Urinary Tract Procedures

Positioning

In pediatric urology, pelvic procedures that can be performed robotically include ureteral reimplantation, cystoplasty, creation of continent catheterizable channels and bladder neck reconstructive procedures. Depending on the robot platform to be used and the preference of the surgeon, patient is positioned in either supine or semilithotomy with both knees low lying to avoid collisions with the robotic arms. Feet and hands must be padded; arms are usually placed at the patient's side with palms up to prevent ulnar nerve damage. Wide egg crate pad can be used across the chest to secure the patient to the bed. Care should be taken to keep the padding infirm on the chest to allow adequate chest wall movement. Additional foam padding is used to protect the face from unintentional injury. The patient is placed in a Trendelenburg position approximately 25° from the horizon to encourage the bowel to fall out of the pelvis.

Accessory and Assistant Trocars

Camera port placement is achieved by measuring at least 10–12 cm from the pubic symphysis cranially and better be placed supraumbilically to increase the distance and space, especially in children with short puboumbilical distance like Kyphoscoliosis.

For *cystoplasty procedures*, it is recommended to place the camera port in a supraumbilical position. It is recommended to follow the same steps detailed earlier in this chapter. After insufflation of the abdomen, the sites of the working port are marked. The left arm port is placed 6–8 cm lateral to the umbilicus while the right arm port is placed approximately 9 cm lateral to the umbilicus. In children with less abdominal surface area, a shorter working distance of 4 to 5 cm is preferred. A 5-mm assistant port could be placed in the left upper quadrant, halfway between the camera and left working port. In a complex pelvic procedures eg. Bladder neck reconstruction, cystoplasty, a 12-mm port is used instead, and a 5-mm assistant port is placed in the right lower quadrant (Fig. 6.8).

Docking

In pelvic procedures, the **Si** robotic device is situated at the patient's feet in the midline when bilateral reimplantation or cystoplasty to be performed. However, for unilateral repairs the *Si* robotic device can be positioned at the ipsilateral foot. If *da Vinci Xi* model to be used, docking can be performed from any position around the patient.

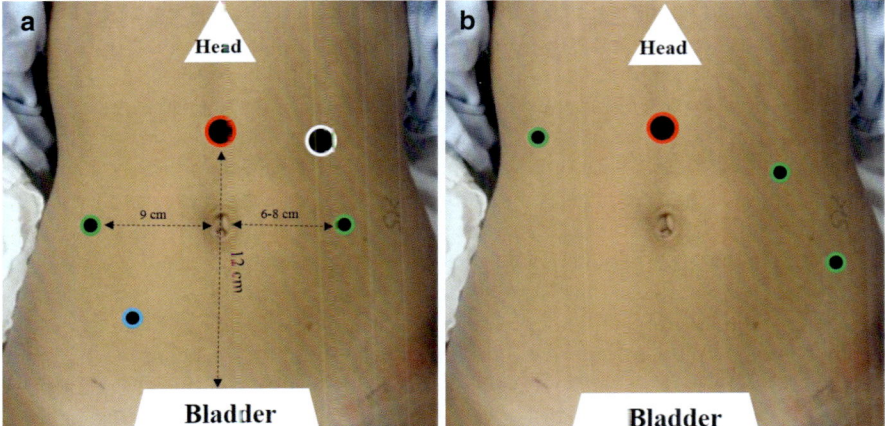

Fig. 6.8 (a) Port placement for pelvic procedures. Red – 12 mm camera port, green – 8 mm working robotic ports, white – 12 mm assistant port, blue – 5 mm assistant port. (b) Robotic port placement with 4th arm alternative for pelvic procedures. 5 mm assistant port placement is optional

Uncommon Approaches

Robotic Assisted Transvesical Antireflux Surgery

Peters in 2004 was the first to describe this technique, reporting that correction of reflux was achieved in 89% of refluxing units [8]. In his first published series [9], patients were positioned supine on the operative table, with the legs apart, and the feet were placed at the tip of the table. The urinary bladder was filled with saline using a urethral catheter. The initial 12 mm camera port was placed at the dome of the bladder by performing 12 mm transverse incision. A 12-mm VersaStep® sheath and cannula were placed and secured with 3-0 Vicryl box stitch. After inspection with the camera (using 0° telescope), another 8 mm working port were placed midway between the umbilicus and the pubis. Veress needle was used to place the VersaStep sheath, followed by the blunt-tip obturator of the 8 mm robotic cannulas. Similar to the initial access, all working ports were secured with purse string to avoid CO_2 loss and and can be used to close bladder punctures at the end. The normal saline in the bladder was evacuated by insufflating CO_2 with a pressure of 8–10 mm Hg. Lastly, the robotic device was situated at the patient's feet in the midline. The remaining steps of this procedure are similar to open technique.

Retroperitoneal Approach

Retroperitoneal access has some potential advantages with regard to urine leakage and avoiding lesions of the intra-abdominal organs such as adhesions. In children, retroperitoneal approach is considered a standard approach for open pyeloplasty. Based on this approach and on the original concept of retroperitoneoscopic pyeloplasty in children [10], Olsen et al. [11] reported in 2004 the first series involving 13 children, with ages ranging 3.5–16.2 years (median age of 6.7 years), who underwent 15 pyeloplasties with follow-up of 1–7 months with good outcomes. They later reported a larger series involving 67 pyeloplasties in 65 patients with 5-year follow-up, showing a complication rate of 17.9%, with only one patient requiring conversion to open surgery and with four patients requiring reoperation. In their experience, retroperitoneoscopic approach involved a shorter operative time and produced comparative results.

Despite the large experience in retroperitoneal laparoscopic procedures, we have not embarked on performing retroperitoneal approach using the robot device. According to the European experience [11], the primary access to the retroperitoneum is done with the patient placed in a 100° lateral semiprone position. A 15 mm incision 1–3 cm is done below the tip of the 12th rib, then the retroperitoneum is entered by blunt dissection, and the retroperitoneal space is developed by balloon dissection with 200–400 ml air. Two 8 mm Da Vinci ports are placed under direct guidance of a retroperitoneally placed finger of the surgeon to avoid damage to the edge of the peritoneum and colon. The first port to be placed anterior to the quadratus lumborum muscle close to the iliac crest, and the second to place in the anterior axillary line close to the costal curvature (Fig. 6.9). A 5 mm port for assistance with suction, sutures and cutting could be placed close to the anterior iliac spine. A 12 mm camera port to be placed in the primary incision and a zero telescope to be used during the procedure. Insufflation to be started with a pressure of 10–12 mm Hg CO_2. Da Vinci arms are docked from behind at an angle of 45–60° to the mid axillary line.

"Docking" Process with *da Vinci Si device*

After positioning the patient and all ports are placed, the robotic arms are attached in a process called docking. Camera arm should be docked first by using the clutch button to change the angle of camera arm to match the cannula so that it points to target anatomy. It is recommended to stabilize the cannula at the port site with one hand, and to bring the cannula into the cannula mount on the camera arm and clip both wings shut to hold the cannula in place.

Fig. 6.9 Port placement in robot oriented retroperitoneal pyeloplasty. Red – camera port, green – working robotic ports, blue – assistant 5 mm port

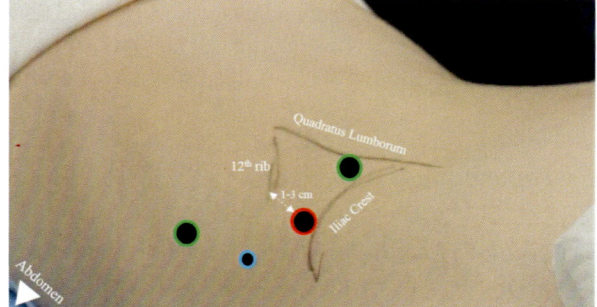

Camera arm setup joint #2 is placed opposite the instrument arm 3 (Fig. 6.10a). Setup joints are numbered starting from the joint closest to the center column. Setting the system in this position allows maximum range of motion for all

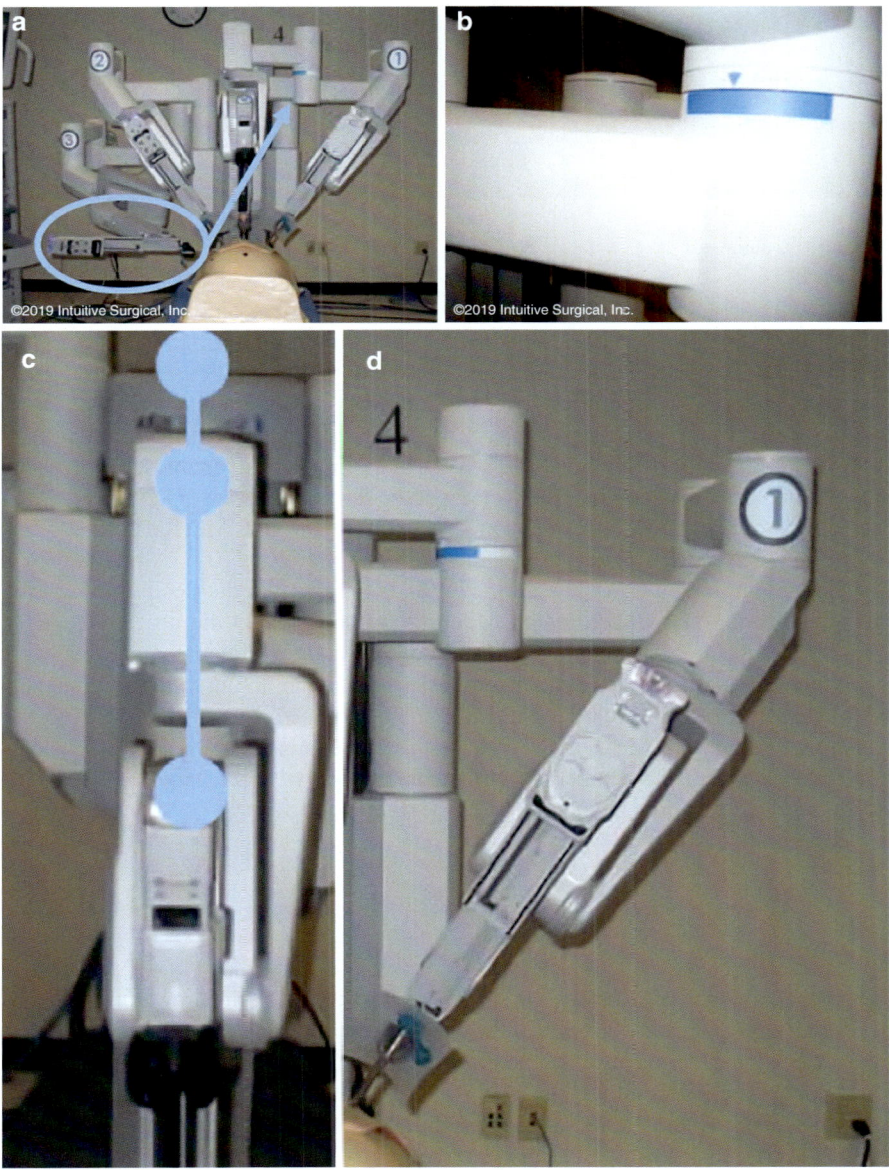

Fig. 6.10 (**a**) Setup Joint #2 opposite of 4th Arm. (**b**) Align Sweet Spot by lining up the blue arrow with the center of the thick blue line. (**c**) Align Camera Arm Clutch Button, 3rd setup Joint, and Center Column. (**d**) Position the arms so that the numbers on each instrument arm and the sterile adapter portion are facing forward. (**e**) 4th Arm positioning must be ~90° with arm horizontal to the floor and arm to arm angle must be ~45°. (**f**) Separate instrument arms and check setup joint angles to minimize potential collisions, and the angle at setup joint 2 must be ~90°. (*Copyright © 2019 Intuitive Surgical, Inc*)

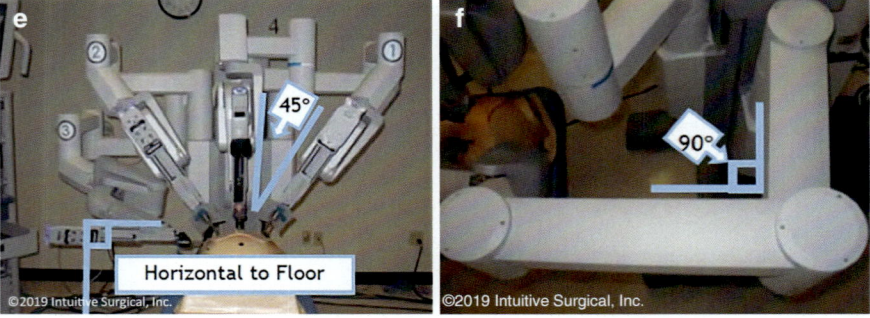

Fig. 6.10 (continued)

instrument arms. There is a thick blue line and a blue arrow on setup joint #2 indicating the sweet spot of the camera arm. Sweet spot should be aligned by lining up the blue arrow with the center of the blue line (Fig. 6.10b). Setting sweet spot gives the robotic arms maximum range of motion ensuring instrument and endoscope reach of all parts of target anatomy. Note that docking of the camera is done by using robotic arm port clutch buttons only. It is important to maintain the sweet spot and alignment of the camera arm throughout the docking process (Fig. 6.10c). After docking the camera arm, instrument arms must be positioned with the numbers and sterile adapter portion on each arm facing forward (Fig. 6.10d). Allow approximately 45° angle between each arm (Fig. 6.10e). Note that the position of instrument arm 3 can vary according to patient body habitus and the procedure. After positioning, ensure that the arms will not collide with the patient or interfere with each other. Bring the instrument arm by using the clutch button to the cannula and lock the wings of the quick click cannula mount on the arm to clip the arm to the cannula. Confirm that the remote center of the port is present at the desired place in the abdominal wall. Remember to stabilize the cannula with one hand at the port site while docking the instrument arm.

Checking System Setup

- After docking the instrument arms, it important to check the arm setup. Start by confirming that the sweet spot of the camera arm is in right position as mentioned earlier. If needed, the arm can be moved into position taking care to stabilize the cannula at the port site. Next step, to check the alignment of the camera port, target anatomy and the center column of the patient cart. Now separate the instrument arms to maximize the range of motion. Check the setup joint angles to minimize potential collisions. The angle at the setup joint 2 should be approximately 90° (Fig. 6.10f). Insert the endoscope into the cannula keeping the intuitive logo on the camera head facing the camera arm. Instrument insertion is done in the following steps:

- Straighten instrument wrist
- Close instrument tips
- Insert instrument tip into the cannula
- Attach instrument housing to the sterile adapter
- Press Instrument Arm clutch button and insert instrument under direct vision
- When instrument has reached desired location, press Instrument Arm clutch button to lock the instrument in place

Transition to Da Vinci Xi Model

The da Vinci Xi (Intuitive Surgical, Sunnyvale, CA, USA), launched in 2014, serves to address many of the limitations posed by the older da Vinci systems. The new system has overhead architecture, slimmer rotating boom-mounted arms, extended instrument reach, guided targeting, and integrated auxiliary technology. As mentioned earlier, the Xi surgical cart can achieve four-quadrant anatomical access while being docked from any position around the patient. The docking procedure is also facilitated by laser targeting and improved cannula mounts. These features allow the use of a simplified "linear" port configuration and an abbreviated docking time.

The external arms must be widely spaced in order to maximize the working field and to minimize collision, the opposite is true for the Xi – the horizontal FLEX joints need to be compacted, leaving one-fist-width spacing between each arm. The redesigned 8-mm Xi endoscope is able to be inserted through any of the 8-mm robotic ports – a feature known as "port hopping". Compared to the earlier da Vinci systems, the 30° endoscope can be inverted from the surgeon console. Table 6.2 summarizes the major differences between Si and the recent Xi system.

Table 6.2 Major differences between Da Vinci Si and Xi system

Si system	Xi system	Remarks
Single quadrant surgery	Multiquadrant surgery	Multiquadrant surgery is possible in Si system but would need redocking
4 arms: 3 instrument arms, 1 camera arm	4 similar arms	In Xi any arm can be camera
Endoscopes: 12 mm, 8.5 mm 0° and 30°	Only 8.5 mm endoscope 0° and 30°	–
Camera and instrument arm drape is required	No camera drape is required Arm drape is required	In the Xi endoscope is integrated with the camera with a chip on the tip
8 mm and 5 mm are available	Only 8 mm instruments, at present no 5 mm instruments	All Xi instruments are longer by 4.5 cm
Supports single site instruments	Does not support single site instruments	–
Arm clutch to be used for arm movement	"Grab and move" feature for arm movement	"Grab and move" feature is no longer available after docking the arm to cannula

Complications

Similar to other surgical approaches, minimizing morbidities and complications is a pivotal goal of robotic assisted procedure. Numerous reports of iatrogenic complications related to positioning, trocar placement, gas insufflation, and surgical technique have been published [3, 12–14]. Patient-related factors such as comorbidities may impact the incidence and severity of perioperative complications. Early recognition is essential to minimize the morbidity that may be endured by the patient. Complications related to patient positioning, and trocar placement along with preventive measures will be discussed in this chapter.

Patient Positioning

The risk for perioperative position related complications is increased by incorrect patient positioning, inadequate fixation or even a longtime in the proper patient positioning. Prolonged immobilization under general anesthesia is ideal for decubitus pressure skin lesions at various points. Inadequate padding and improper positioning might potentiate this type of complication. Once the patient is positioned and before docking the robot, a test roll should be conducted to confirm the patient is secured to the table with appropriate padding in areas that may experience increased pressures. Robotic arms can also be responsible for direct injury, primarily on the face especially in infants, thus face padding is useful to minimize unintentional injuries and the bedside assistant should be observant to prevent it.

Position related nerve injury risk may increase as much as 100- fold for each hour of surgery for both upper and lower limbs nerves [3, 12]. For instance, arm hyperabduction can cause brachial nerve plexus injury, thus it must be avoided by keeping the arms close to the body. In lateral decubitus position, an axillary roll should be placed to prevent contralateral brachial plexus compression and the ipsilateral arm can be positioned on the side to avoid trauma that can be caused by robotic arm collision. Based on the experience of adult practice, side docking has been proposed instead of standard low lithotomic position to overcome nerve injury of the lower limbs [15].

Port Placement and Access

As mentioned earlier, Veress needle access, Hasson open technique are the most common access techniques. A Veress needle is a sharp instrument placed blindly through the abdominal wall, thus safety checks, aspiration/injection and lifting the abdominal wall upwards help to minimize the risk of complications. If the Veress is in proper intraperitoneal position, it will flush easily with no return on aspiration.

Another indicator for improper Veress needle placement is high insufflation pressure with low volumes. As opposed to Veress needle access, the Hasson open technique allows direct view of abdominal and pelvic structures during access.

The open technique is thought to be safer although the Veress needle has also resulted in low complication rates [5, 6]. Passerotti et al. conducted a retrospective review which identified a complication rate of 2% with the Veress technique and 0.8% with the open technique, with no statistical difference.

Abdominal wall vessels can be injured during abdominal access, thus direct visualization and transillumination of the anterior abdominal wall is recommended to allow visualization and subsequent avoidance of vessels. If injury does occur, the vessel may be coagulated directly through another port. If the bleeding is significant and difficult to stop, fascial sutures may be placed in a figure of eight fashion to occlude the vessel. Other method was described [14] include placement of a foley catheter through the site, inflating the balloon and putting upward traction on the foley to tamponade the bleeding If the injury is severe in nature requiring immediate open exploration, the misplaced trocar should be left in position to potentially tamponade the injury as well to expedite identifying the location and guide the surgeon to the site of injury. If visceral injury does occur, the injury may be addressed laparoscopically or by a laparotomy depending on the extent of injury.

During CO_2 insufflation, communication with the anesthesia team is paramount. Although rare, insufflation complications take place when the Veress needle is accidentally placed into visceral structures or after rapid insufflation, CO_2 absorption might happen and lead to hypercarbia, acidosis, venous gas embolism. Surgeons should have a low threshold of suspicion for any of the above mentioned complications. The ideal way to manage complications is to prevent them. A dedicated pediatric robotic team is essential to reduce perioperative complications.

References

1. Passerotti C, Peters CA. Pediatric robotic-assisted laparoscopy: a description of the principle procedures. Sci World J. Hindawi. 2006;6:2581–8.
2. Sutton S, Link T, Makic MBF. A quality improvement project for safe and effective patient positioning during robot-assisted surgery. AORN J. John Wiley & Sons Ltd. 2013;97(4):448–56.
3. Shveiky D, Aseff JN, Iglesia CB. Brachial plexus injury after laparoscopic and robotic surgery. J Minim Invasive Gynecol. 2010;17(4):414–20.
4. Coppieters MW, Van De Velde M, Stappaerts KH. Positioning in anesthesiology. Anesthesiology. 2002;97(1):75–81.
5. Yanke BV, Horowitz M. Safety of the Veress needle in pediatric laparoscopy. J Endourol. Mary Ann Liebert, Inc. 2 Madison Avenue Larchmont, NY 10538 USA. 2007;21(7):695–7.
6. Passerotti CC, Nguyen HT, Retik AB, Peters CA. Patterns and predictors of laparoscopic complications in pediatric urology: the role of ongoing surgical volume and access techniques. J Urol. 2008;180(2):681–5
7. Gargollo PC. Hidden incision endoscopic surgery: description of technique, parental satisfaction and applications. J Urol. 2011;185(4):1425–31.
8. Peters CA. Robotically assisted surgery in pediatric urology. Urol Clin North Am. 2004;31(4):743–52.

9. Peters CA, Woo R. Intravesical robotically assisted bilateral ureteral Reimplantation. J Endourol. Mary Ann Liebert, Inc. 2 Madison Avenue Larchmont, NY 10538 USA. 2005;19(6):618–22.
10. Yeung CK, Tam YH, Sihoe JDY, Lee KH, Liu KW. Retroperitoneoscopic dismembered pyeloplasty for pelvi-ureteric junction obstruction in infants and children. BJU Int. John Wiley & Sons, Ltd. 2002;87(6):509–13.
11. Olsen LH, Rawashdeh YF, Jorgensen TM. Pediatric robot assisted retroperitoneoscopic pyeloplasty: a 5-year experience. J Urol. 2007;178(5):2137–41.
12. Barnett JC, Hurd WW, Rogers RM Jr, Williams NL, Shapiro SA. Laparoscopic positioning and nerve injuries. J Minim Invasive Gynecol. 2007;14(5):664–72.
13. Tomaszewski JJ, Casella DP, Turner RM, Casale P, Ost MC. Pediatric laparoscopic and robot-assisted laparoscopic surgery: technical considerations. J Endourol. Mary Ann Liebert, Inc. 140 Huguenot Street, 3rd Floor New Rochelle, NY 10801 USA. 2012;26(6):602–13.
14. Pemberton RJ, Tolley DA, van Velthoven RF. Prevention and management of complications in urological laparoscopic port site placement. Eur Urol. 2006;50(5):958–68.
15. Cestari A, Ferrari M, Zanoni M, Sangalli M, Ghezzi M, Fabbri F, et al. Side docking of the da Vinci robotic system for radical prostatectomy: advantages over traditional docking. J Robot Surg. Springer London. 2015;9(3):243–7.

Part II
Upper Tract Surgery

Chapter 7
Pyeloplasty

Chad Crigger, John Barnard, Daniel J. McClelland, and Michael Ost

Introduction and Background

Ureteropelvic junction obstruction (UPJO) represents a structural and/or functional impediment to the transit of urine from the renal pelvis to the proximal ureter [1]. UPJO can be further subdivided into congenital or acquired as well as intrinsic or extrinsic etiology for the obstruction [2, 3]. In the pediatric population and as a whole, congenital UPJO is far more common, and can be the result of numerous underlying pathologies including, but not limited to, an anterior crossing vessel, medial hyperplasia of the ureter, or an aperistaltic segment of the ureter. The incidence has been quoted at approximately 1 in every 2000 live births, with a male predominance [3, 4]. When left untreated, UPJO often leads to persistently elevated pressures in the pelvicalyceal system, hydronephrosis, and progressive deterioration of ipsilateral renal function. The likelihood of renal deterioration and surgery has been correlated with higher grades of hydronephrosis as well as when diagnosis is made by prenatal ultrasound, while mild hydronephrosis secondary to UPJO has been demonstrated to have a more benign course, often resolving spontaneously [4].

Treatment of ureteropelvic junction obstruction (UPJO) in the pediatric population has undergone evolution in the past several decades [5]. Historically, the gold standard for treatment was open dismembered pyeloplasty via a flank approach; however, with the widespread adoption and use of minimally invasive techniques there has been a transition favoring the robotic approach. Although laparoscopy preceded the implementation of robotics in pediatric urology, the technical

---

C. Crigger (✉) · M. Ost
West Virginia University School of Medicine, Department of Urology,
Morgantown, WV, USA
e-mail: chad.crigger@hsc.wvu.edu; michael.ost@hsc.wvu.edu

J. Barnard · D. J. McClelland
West Virginia University, Department of Urology, Morgantown, WV, USA
e-mail: jbarnard@hsc.wvu.edu

© Springer Nature Switzerland AG 2020
P. C. Gargollo (ed.), *Minimally Invasive and Robotic-Assisted Surgery in Pediatric Urology*, https://doi.org/10.1007/978-3-030-57219-8_7

difficulty and steep learning curve were barriers to its widespread use in the pediatric population [6]. The ergonomics of robotic surgery have been demonstrated in multi-institutional trials, and robotic pyeloplasty has now become the standard of care in the pediatric population across age groups with success rates of 96–100% [7]. It has been demonstrated that operative times and success rates approach those of an open approach after 15–20 cases, and complications tend to be technical in nature, and more common early in surgeons' experience with this approach [8]. Although robotic surgery has been demonstrated to have decreased length of stay, less post-operative pain, lower risk of wound infection, and lower risk of incisional hernia, opponents to its implementation cite increased operative times, high cost, no uniformity in training, and lack of haptic feedback [9, 10].

Patient Presentation and Diagnostic Evaluation

Historically, the classic presentation of UPJO was a neonate or infant with a palpable flank mass. However the widespread use of routine antenatal ultrasounds has drastically changed the clinical presentation of children with UPJO. Today, many children with this condition are identified prenatally or early in life while still asymptomatic, often incidentally as part evaluation for other clinical entities such as febrile urinary tract infections (UTIs).

Age at presentation can aid in diagnosis. Typically, newborns and infants presenting with UPJO have an obstruction caused by an intrinsic aperistaltic segment of the proximal ureter, characterized by an arrest in the development of circular muscular fibers resulting in a functional obstruction [11]. UPJO of childhood and adolescence is usually the result of an external compression by a crossing accessory vessel to the lower pole of the kidney resulting in a mechanical obstruction of the ureter that is often accompanied by nausea, vomiting and flank pain [11].

Other common presentations include recurrent infections and hematuria, either gross or microscopic. Some children may present with nephrolithiasis; a UPJO is associated with nephrolithiasis one-third of the time [12]. Urinary stasis promotes stone crystallization with subsequent development of calculi. Narrowing of the UPJ decreases the likelihood of spontaneous passage, propagating more crystal deposition. In those without symptoms, an elevated creatinine or hypertension may be clues to the diagnosis of UPJO.

Once UPJO is suspected on an Ultrasound or CT scan a functional study such as an IVP or renal scan may be obtained. Diuretic renography is a widely utilized, noninvasive technique that provides an estimate of split renal function. Using technetium-99m mercaptoacetyletriglycerine (^{99m}Tc-MAG3) as a tracer and correlation with the half-life (T1/2) washout curve, renal function is calculated. An ipsilateral split renal function <40%, is considered significant [13]. Furthermore (T1/2) > 20–25 min with a plateaued drainage curve is considered diagnostic. Magnetic resonance imaging (MRI) may be utilized in elucidating vascular anatomy in special circumstances of UPJO (such as horseshoe kidney, malrotated kidney, or cross-fused ectopia).

Indications for Surgery

Approximately one-third of children with UPJO ultimately undergo surgical intervention. Indications for surgery include worsening hydronephrosis under surveillance, symptoms (such as pain), persistent and/or poorly controlled hypertension, and low or decreasing differential renal function indicated by ipsilateral UPJO <40% on diuretic renography [14].

Surgical Considerations

Endoscopic Management

Minimally invasive techniques for treating UPJO started with ante- or retrograde endopyelotomy or balloon dilatation. While the success of this technique in treatment of strictures secondary to significant stone disease approached 94%, outcomes were less promising when treating congenital UPJO. In a series of 40 patients treated with balloon dilatation, those patients 18 or older and symptomatic had success rates of 57% while symptomatic patients presenting younger than 18 years had a 25% success rate [15]. The most robust review on endopyelotomy assessing the 25 year experience of one institution reported a primary endopyelotomy success rate of 65%, concluding that primary endopyelotomy was less successful than primary pyeloplasty. However, when considering secondary endopyelotomy with concomitant ureteral stenting after failed primary pyeloplasty, the success rate improved dramatically to 94% [16]. Given the success rate of primary pyeloplasty, we prefer this technique to initial endoscopic management.

Patient Positioning, Trocar Placement and Accessing the Abdomen

For laparoscopic or robotic-assisted pyeloplasty the patient is in a gentle or modified flank position, at approximately 45-degrees. We utilize gel rolls and foam padding to properly and safely position to the patient to avoid any peripheral nerve injuries from poor patient positioning. The patient is then secured with Velcro straps and the table is test-rolled to ensure the patient is immobile. This position also aids gravity to draw abdominal contents away from the retroperitoneal surgical site. This is most useful in the instance of UPJO in the morbidly obese child.

Pyeloplasty can be performed via a transperitoneal or retroperitoneal approach. The transperitoneal route has been employed more often due to familiarity and increased working space for suturing compared to the retroperitoneal approach. Due to patient positioning and the perceived decreased working space, the retroperitoneal approach has historically been favored at select centers which utilize this technique more commonly. Several reviews of reported series demonstrated that the two techniques were comparable in terms of operative time, blood loss, and rate of conversion to open surgery [17, 18]. It was not until 2015, however, that the first prospective, randomized head-to-head study comparing these two approaches was reported. Based on results of 38 children who were equally randomized, the authors demonstrated statistically significant shorter operative times, median hospital stays and time to oral feeding after surgery in the retroperitoneal group with comparable complication rates [19]. Though these results favor a retroperitoneal approach, the technique ultimately selected depends on surgeon comfort and familiarity.

We prefer gaining access in younger children utilizing the Bailez Technique, and reserve the Veress needle placement for adolescents [20]. Once access is obtained, insufflation is initiated to 8–10 mmHg through a 5 mm optical trocar that has been placed under direct vision at the infraumbilical position. Port placement using the Da Vinci Xi system (Intuitive Surgical, Sunnyvale, California) is in a linear fashion (Fig. 7.1), while placement is triangulated if utilizing the Da Vinci Si or a pure laparoscopic approach.

Internal Versus External Pyeloureteral Stenting

The use of pyeloureteral stents in pyeloplasty has traditionally been widespread amongst pediatric urologists. Transanastomotic standard double-J stents have historically been deployed to allow the anastomosis to heal, decompress the upper tract, and decrease risk of leakage. However, since the introduction of the percutaneous pyeloureteral stent, most commonly the Salle intraoperative pyeloureteral

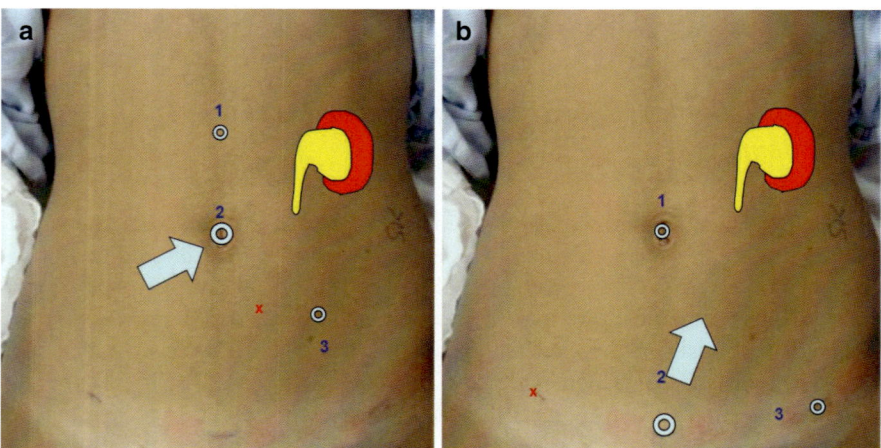

Fig. 7.1 Port placement for Robotic-assisted laparoscopic pyeloplasty showing the traditional (**a**) vs HIdES configurations (**b**). Light blue arrow is the camera port. Red x represents optional assist port. (*Courtesy of Patricio C. Gargollo, MD*)

stent (Cook Urological, Spencer, Indiana), much debate has ensued. In a head-to-head analysis reviewing outcomes and cost comparison, the two categories of stents were equivalent in terms of overall complication and success rates after pyeloplasty. When considering cost comparison the percutaneous pyeloplasty stent saved costs and, more importantly, prevented a second general anesthesia required for standard double-J placement [21–23].

More recently the dogma requiring ureteral drainage has been challenged and stentless pyeloplasty has entered the debate, further muddying the controversy. Recent trials have evaluated pyeloplasty outcomes comparing traditional double-J stents, external percutaneous stents and, finally no stent. When comparing quality adjusted life-years and costs, external percutaneous stenting emerged as a clear winner in terms of costs and reducing the morbidity and discomfort experienced with a standard double-J stent or potentially not leaving a stent. While external stenting distinguished itself over no stents or internal stents, no stents performed better than internal stents with regard to cost [24].

The debate and argument for stentless pyeloplasty continued with controversy citing the morbidity and bothersome lower urinary tract symptoms seen in stenting, in addition to the possible risk of stent migration [25]. While robotic stentless pyeloplasty appears feasible, pediatric urologists enjoy high success rates in pediatric robotic pyeloplasty regardless of technique and future research maximizing overall patient comfort will undoubtedly continue.

Technique

Dismembered Pyeloplasty Procedure Overview

While several techniques for minimally-invasive pyeloplasty exist, the Anderson-Hynes dismembered pyeloplasty has long been considered the standard in UPJO repair in large part due preserving a crossing vessel and also excising an aperistaltic segment. It is usually the most transferrable technique and hence most often used in robotics. They key steps of the procedure are the following:

After obtaining informed consent from the patient's guardian(s) and general anesthesia is induced, an age-appropriate Foley catheter is placed to decompress the bladder. The patient is then repositioned into a modified lateral decubitus position with the affected side up. Care is taken to properly pad all joints and secure the patient to the bed prior to test rolling the bed at maximum pitch positions to detect patient movement. After prepping and draping the patient in usual sterile fashion, intraperitoneal access is gained at the umbilicus using either the Bailez Technique or Veress needle placement. A sheath with trocar is then advanced without any resistance into the peritoneal cavity and the abdomen insufflated with careful consideration of initial abdominal pressures to a maximum insufflation pressure of 8–15 mmHg, depending on the child's age. A 5 mm laparoscopic camera is then used to inspect the abdominal cavity for any inadvertent injury.

Under direct visualization, 8 mm robotic trocars are then placed for the right and left robotic arms at the midline in the corresponding subxiphoid and suprapubic region. Under direct visualization, the initial 5 mm laparoscopic port is exchanged for an 8 mm robotic camera port. The robot is docked into place and all robotic instruments are advanced into the surgical field under direct visualization. Attention is first drawn to the white line of Toldt. This is incised from the level of the corresponding colic flexure to the level of the iliac vessels. The colorenal ligaments are then divided to reflect the bowel medially maximizing space within the surgical field and expose the anterior surface of the kidney within Gerota's fascia. At this point the kidney and ureter should be easily identified in addition to the level of the ureteropelvic junction obstruction. Care is taken to preserve any crossing vessel if present. A transmesenteric approach can be used for left sided UPJO in infants when the UPJO is readily seen. Port configurations can be a traditional port positioning or the hidden incision (HIdES) configuration described by Gargollo et al. [26] (Fig. 7.1a, b).

The proximal ureter and renal pelvis are then dissected free from all surrounding structures. Using a Keith needle, a stitch is placed through the anterior-medial portion of the renal pelvis and tension is applied percutaneously to properly tent this segment of interest. The UPJO is incised, disconnecting the proximal ureter from the ureteropelvic junction (if an inwelling stent was previously placed, the stent is preserved at this point). The ureter is then spatulated on its posterior-lateral aspect through any stenotic segment until normal caliber ureter is encountered. Once spatulation yields a sufficiently patent ureter, Anderson-Hynes dismembered pyeloplasty is performed (Fig. 7.2a, b) [27, 28]. Transposition of the proximal ureter and renal pelvis is performed over any crossing vessel if there is evidence of it causing extrinsic compression.

For the anastomosis 4-0 or 5-0 vicryl suture is used based on patient age and surgeon preference. In order to ensure a watertight anastomosis, two "marking sutures" are placed at the crotch of the spatulated ureter and dependent portion of the open renal pelvis. Typically, the anterior anastomosis is completed first followed by the posterior anastomosis; this minimizes the complexity of the repair and facilitates stent placement (if desired) or stent exchange once the anterior anastomosis is complete (Fig. 7.3a, b) [29, 30]. The anastomosis is inspected for any leak. The percutaneous Hitch stitch is released placing the ureter and ureteropelvic junction into proper orientation. The repair is once again inspected in its anatomic position to ensure a tension-free anastomosis and orthotopic lie. The surgical field is irrigated and suctioned and if desired, a percutaneous drain is placed posterior to the proximal ureter under direct visualization. At this point, the robotic instruments are removed under direct visualization and the robot undocked. The robotic arms are then removed and trocar sites are closed using 3-0 vicryl sutures.

Complications

Contemporary studies at academic institutions suggest that the overall complication rate is approximately 3% for robotic pyeloplasty which is similar to the open and laparoscopic approach [7]. As with any retroperitoneal surgery, vascular injury,

7 Pyeloplasty

Fig. 7.2 (**a**) Spatulation of proximal ureter after excising aperistaltic segment. (**b**) Posterior anastomosis of Anderson-Hynes pyeloplasty

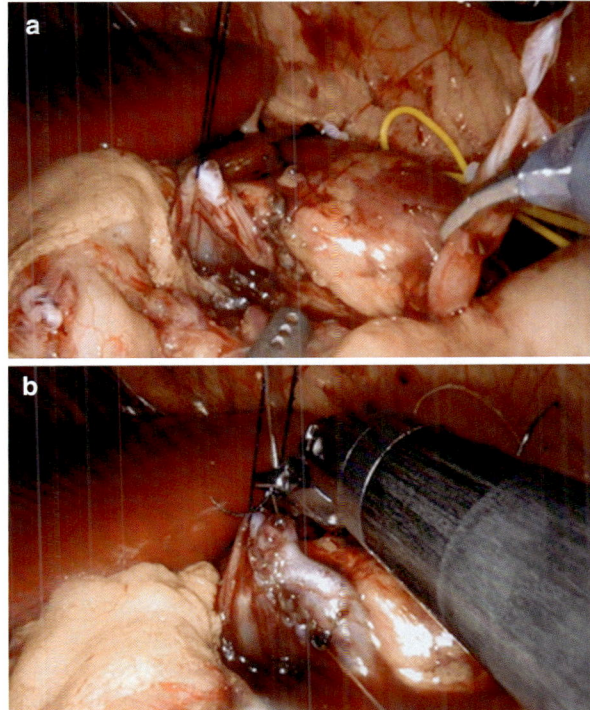

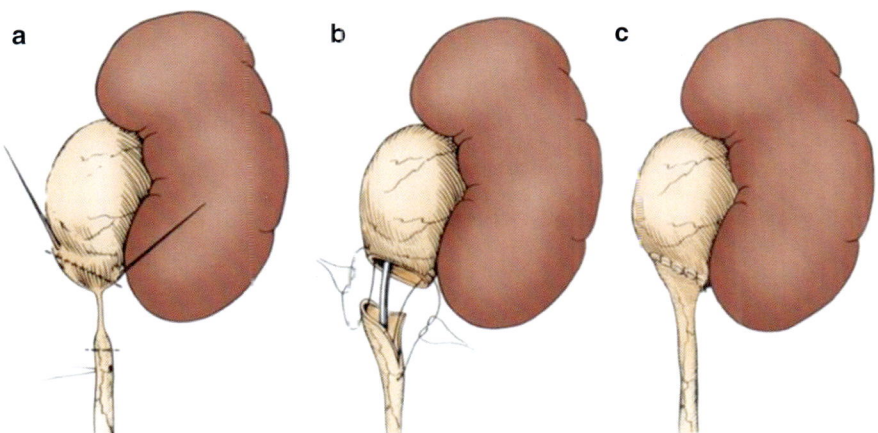

Fig. 7.3 (**a**) Stay sutures are placed at the medial and lateral aspects of the inferior portion of the renal pelvis. A third suture is placed on the lateral aspect of the proximal ureter below the level of the obstruction in preparation for the dismembered pyeloplasty to maintain proper orientation throughout the repair. (**b**) The obstructed segment is excised and the proximal ureter is spatulated on its lateral aspect. The anastomosis is then created as follows: the apex of the laterally spatulated ureter is joined to the inferior aspect of the pelvis while the medial side of the ureter is approximated to the superior border of the pelvis. (**c**) The anastomosis is completed with absorbable suture in a watertight fashion. (Adapted text [28, 29])

damage to adjacent viscera (bowel, spleen, liver), and failure to correct the underlying pathology are possible. Post-operative urine leak or urinoma formation is reported at approximately 1–2% across several series [31].

Despite success rates ranging from 90–100% across all surgical approaches, failure of initial pyeloplasty remains an issue of concern. One of the largest series published on re-operative robotic assisted laparoscopic pyeloplasty showed resolution or improvement of hydronephrosis in 91%, stability in 6%, and worsening hydronephrosis in 3% [32]. All children were symptom free and the sub-group who received preoperative and postoperative diuretic renography showed stable or improved renal function. This suggests failure of initial pyeloplasty can be reliably addressed by a re-operative robot assisted laparoscopic approach with similar success to a primary operation. Retrograde endopyelotomy is also a viable option; however, success rates are quoted at approximately 40–70% after failed pyeloplasty and decrease as the length of the stricture exceeds 1 cm and patient age less than 4 years [31, 33]. Balloon dilatation exhibits less desirable results with success rates around 10–20%.

Overall, robotic assisted laparoscopic pyeloplasty has a low complication rate and high success, even in the re-operative setting. Patients typically spend 1–2 days in the hospital post operatively, and the ICU admission rate is about 3% [10]. Surgeon volume has shown a trend toward decreasing complication rate, and underlying comorbidities have been shown to increase the risk of complications by up to threefold. This suggests better outcomes may be achieved at larger academic centers with higher surgical volumes and a full complement of pediatric subspecialties to optimize and manage comorbid conditions in the perioperative period.

References

1. Krajewski W, Wojciechowska J, Dembowski J, Zdrojowy R, Szydelko T. Hydronephrosis in the course of ureteropelvic junction obstruction: an underestimated problem? Current opinions on the pathogenesis, diagnosis and treatment. Adv Clin Exp Med. 2017;26(5):857–64.
2. Singh I, Strandhoy J, Assimos D. Chapter 40: pathophysiology of urinary tract obstruction. In: Campbell-Walsh urology. 10th ed. Philadelphia: Elsevier Saunders; 2012. p. 212–9.
3. VanDervoort K, Lasky S, Sethna C, Frank R, Vento S, Choi-Rosen J, et al. Hydronephrosis in infants and children: natural history and risk factors for persistence in children followed by a medical service. Clin Med Pediatr. 2009;3:63–70.
4. Lim D, Park J, Kim J, Paick S, Oh S, Choi H. Clinical characteristics and outcome of hydronephrosis detected by prenatal ultrasonography. J Korean Med Sci. 2003;18(6):859–62.
5. Satyanarayan A, Peters C. Advances in robotic surgery for pediatric ureteropelvic junction obstruction and vesicoureteral reflux: history, present, and future. World J Urol. 2020;38(8):1821–6.
6. Kassite I, Braik K, Villemagne T, Lardy H, Binet A. The learning curve of robot-assisted laparoscopic pyeloplasty in children: a multi-outcome approach. J Pediatr Urol. 2018;14(6):570.e1–570.
7. Howe A, Kozel Z, Palmer L. Robotic surgery in pediatric urology. Asian J Urol. 2017;4(1):55–67.
8. Ganpule A, Sripathi V. How small is small enough? Role of robotics in paediatric urology. J Minim Access Surg. 2015;11(1):45–9.
9. Andolfi C, Kumar R, Boysen W, Gundeti M. Current status of robotic surgery in pediatric urology. J Laparoendosc Adv Surg Tech A. 2019;29(2):159–66.

10. Chan Y, Durbin-Johnson B, Sturm R, Kurzrock E. Outcomes after pediatric open, laparoscopic, and robotic pyeloplasty at academic institutions. J Pediatr Urol. 2017;13(1):49.e1–6.
11. Gonzalez R, Schimke C. Ureteropelvic junction obstruction in infants and children. Pediatr Clin N Am. 2001;48(6):1505–18.
12. Leavitt DA, Rosette J, Hoenig DM. Chapter 53: strategies for nonmedical management of upper urinary tract calculi. In: Campbell-Walsh urology. 10th ed. Philadelphia: Elsevier Saunders; 2012. p. 1235–59.
13. Morales-Lopez RA, Perez-Marchan M, Brayfield MP. Current concepts in pediatric robotic assisted pyeloplasty. Front Pediatr. 2019;7(4):1–7.
14. Gordon I, Dhillon HK, Gatanash H, Peters AM. Antenatal diagnosis of pelvic hydronephrosis: assessment of renal function and drainage as a guide to management. J Nucl Med. 1991;32(9):1649–54.
15. Osther P, Geersten U, Nielsen H. Ureteropelvic junction obstruction and ureteral strictures treated by simple high-pressure balloon dilation. J Endourol. 1998;12(5):429–31.
16. Kim E, Tanagho Y, Traxel E, Austin P, Figenshau R, Coplen D. Endopyelotomy for pediatric ureteropelvic junction obstruction: a review of our 25-year experience. J Urol. 2012;188(4):1628–33.
17. Turra F, Escolino M, Farina A, Settimi A, Esposito C, Varlet F. Pyeloplasty techniques using minimally invasive surgery (MIS) in pediatric patients. Transl Pediatr. 2016;5(4):251–5.
18. Antoniou D, Karetsos C. Laparoscopy or retroperitoneoscopy: which is the best approach in pediatric urology? Transl Pediatr. 2016;5(4):205–13.
19. Badawy H, Zoaier A, Ghoneim T, Hanno A. Transperitoneal versus retroperitoneal laparoscopic pyeloplasty in children: randomized clinical trial. J Pediatr Urol. 2015;11(3):122.e1–6.
20. Franc-Guimond J, Kryger J, Gonzalez R. Experience with the Bailez technique for laparoscopic access in children. J Urol. 2003;170(3):936–8.
21. Braga L, Armando J, Farhat W, Bagli D, Koury A, Salle J. Outcome analysis and cost comparison between externalized pyeloureteral and standard stents in 470 consecutive open pyeloplasties. J Urol. 2008;180:1593–9.
22. Helmy T, Blanc T, Paye-Jaouen A, El-Ghoneimi A. Preliminary experience with external ureteropelvic stent: alternative to double-j stent in laparoscopic pyeloplasty in children. J Urol. 2011;185:1065–70.
23. Dangle P, Shah A, Gunceti M. Cutaneous pyeloureteral stent for laparoscopic (robot)-assisted pyeloplasty. J Endourol. 2014;28(10):1168–71.
24. Yiee J, Baskin L. Use of internal stent, external transanastomotic stent or no stent during pediatric pyeloplasty: a decision tree cost-effectiveness analysis. J Urol 2011;185:673–81.
25. Silva M, Levy A, Finkelstein J, Van Batavia J, Casale P. Is peri-operative urethral catheter drainage enough? The case for stentless pediatric robotic pyeloplasty. J Pediatr Urol. 2015;11:175.e1–5.
26. Gargollo PC. Hidden incision endoscopic surgery: description of technique, parental satisfaction and applications. J Urol. 2011;185(4):1425–31.
27. Anderson J, Hynes W. Retrocaval ureter: a case diagnosed pre-operatively and treated successfully by a plastic operation. Br J Urol. 1949;21(3):209–14.
28. Peters C, Schlussel R, Retik A. Pediatric laparoscopic dismembered pyeloplasty. J Urol. 1995;153(6):1962–5.
29. Henning O, Rawashdeh Y. Chapter 133: surgery of the ureter in children. In: Campbell-Walsh urology. 10th ed. Philadelphia: Elsevier Saunders; 2012. p. 3057–74.
30. Bergesen A, Thomas R, Lee B. Robotic pyeloplasty. J Endourol. 2018;32(1):S68–72.
31. Samarasekera D, Stein R. Robotic-assisted laparoscopic approaches to the ureter: pyeloplasty and ureteral implantation. Indian J Urol. 2014;30(3):293–9.
32. Jacobson D, Shannon R, Johnson E, Gong E, Liu D, Flink C, et al. Robot-assisted laparoscopic reoperative repair for failed pyeloplasty in children: an updated series. J Urol. 2019;201(5):1005–11.
33. Braga L, Lorenzo A, Skeldon S, Dave S, Bagli D, Khoury A, et al. Failed pyeloplasty in children: comparative analysis of retrograde endopyelotomy versus redo pyeloplasty. J Urol. 2007;178(6):2571–5.

Chapter 8
Robot Assisted Laparoscopic Heminephrectomy

Geeta Kekre, Arun Srinivasan, and Aseem R. Shukla

Introduction

A heminephrectomy is the most common operation performed in the setting of a duplication anomaly. Advancement in laparoscopic techniques has made it possible to safely perform surgery for this complex anomaly through tiny incisions resulting in lesser post operative pain and faster recovery. The robot, with its enhanced 3-dimensional magnified vision, greater degrees of freedom of movement, and superior ergonomics, has only raised the bar for minimal access surgery. The ability to visualise the ureters in their entirety is a strong argument in favour of a laparoscopic approach in the surgery for duplication anomalies.

The indications for performing a robot-assisted laparoscopic heminephrectomy are the same as for performing an open heminephrectomy. Although upper pole nephrectomies are more common, many cases require the lower pole to be removed. Incontinence from an ectopic ureter, recurrent infections in a refluxing or obstructed moiety and a non-functioning moiety are some of the situations in which a heminephrectomy may be considered. The surgery can be performed transperitoneally or retroperitoneoscopically. In this chapter, we describe both the techniques.

G. Kekre
Children's Hospital of Philadelphia, Philadelphia, PA, USA

Lokmanya Tilak Municipal Medical College and General Hospital, The Department of Paediatric Surgery, Mumbai, India

A. Srinivasan · A. R. Shukla (✉)
Children's Hospital of Philadelphia, Perelman School of Medicine at the University of Pennsylvania, Division of Urology, Philadelphia, PA, USA
e-mail: srinivasana@email.chop.edu; shuklaa@email.chop.edu

Anatomical Considerations

It is critical to know the anatomy of the duplicated ureters in relation to each other to safely perform a heminephro-ureterectomy. Often times, these ureters are surrounded by a common sheath, sharing much of their blood supply. Overzealous dissection of the affected ureter may result in devascularisation of the unaffected one, with disastrous consequences. An MR Urogram usually provides the necessary information. Many surgeons will perform a cystoscopy with a retrograde pyeloureterogram to delineate the anatomy of the ureters before they begin the heminephrectomy. A stent can be placed at this time in the healthy ureter, so as to facilitate identification. The pelvis of the moiety to be excised is usually dilated and enlarged, but the parenchyma itself is usually small. The affected upper pole parenchyma may be hidden from view by the liver or spleen in a transperitoneal approach. An upper pole ureter will pass posterior to the renal pedicle, making it necessary to dissect near the hilar structures. This is of note in robotic surgery because there is no haptic feedback, and hence the surgeon must be familiar with the visual cues that enable one to gauge the tension being applied to these vessels by the robotic arm.

Equipment

The da Vinci surgical robot currently uses 5 mm and 8 mm instruments. While the 8 mm instruments have increased manoeuvrability, the 5 mm instruments are still popular among many paediatric urologists operating on small children. The robotic instruments currently available include a hook cautery, needle drivers, scissors, Debakey forceps and grasping forceps. An 8 mm suction- irrigation device is also available. Conventional laparoscopic instruments may be used through a separate port for liver retraction. Some surgeons may prefer to use a Ligasure or Harmonic device as well. 5 mm clips may be used if necessary.

The Transperitoneal Approach

Patient Position

A supine or a partial flank position is best for a transperitoneal minimal access heminephrectomy. For a partial flank position, a sand bag or a bolster is placed under the ipsilateral flank to give a 45° rotation. Another bolster or bean bag is used to support the child and keep him/her in place. The child must be secured to the table with cotton tape or similar because it is often necessary to rotate the table during the surgery. Attention must be paid to the pressure points. These must be padded to avoid sores and injuries. Some surgeons use inflatable pressure bags, especially in bilateral cases, to raise the ipsilateral flank as needed. Once the patient is positioned and secured, the table can be rotated so that the patient is effectively supine during port insertion and closure.

Trocar Placement

Typically, one camera port and two working ports are necessary to perform a heminephrectomy. A fourth port is required more often than not for retraction of the liver or spleen. The camera port is usually placed at the umbilicus. The working ports are placed so as to achieve maximum triangulation as well as maximum working space, which can be a challenge in smaller children. The second generation da Vinci systems have an auto targeting feature that enables the robotic arms to rotate away from each other and the patient so that working space can be optimised.

The camera port is placed at the umbilicus by the open Hassan technique, which has a lower risk of injury than the Veress technique [1].

The umbilicus is grasped with an Allis forceps and everted. A vertical or a "smiling" incision is made within the umbilicus and is dissected with an artery forceps to reach the junction of the umbilical tube with the rectus fascia. Two stay sutures of 2-0 vicryl may be placed on the fascia. Using a No.11 blade, the umbilical tube is gently incised between the stays, breaching the peritoneum. It is important to communicate with the anaesthesiologist at this point, who will then momentarily hold ventilation to minimise visceral excursion and prevent bowel injury. An artery forceps is then introduced and this incision is widened. A 10 mm robotic trocar and cannula is placed through the incision and pneumoperitoneum is created.

Insufflation is usually done at not more than 2 L/min, and a pressure of 10–12 mm of Hg is maintained. In smaller children and infants, it is usually necessary to create a pressure of no more than 8 mm of Hg.

The telescope is introduced and the abdominal cavity is inspected for any injuries. The two working ports are introduced under vision. One port is placed in the epigastric region under the ribs, just off the midline on the ipsilateral side and the other is placed in the ipsilateral iliac region between the umbilicus and the iliac crest at the midclavicular line. In smaller patients, it may be helpful to place this port closer to the midline or even on the opposite side of the midline (Fig. 8.1). While this does not allow for triangulation, it does provide more working space. The fourth port for retraction of the liver or the spleen can be placed in the midclavicular line at the level of the umbilicus. In fact, this need not a be a port at all- a 3 mm instrument can be inserted directly through the abdominal wall, leaving behind a very tiny wound. Alternatively, the robotic elbow can be used for retraction, eliminating the need for an additional port. When a clip applier or suture is to be passed, a robotic arm is removed and the assistant uses the same port [2].

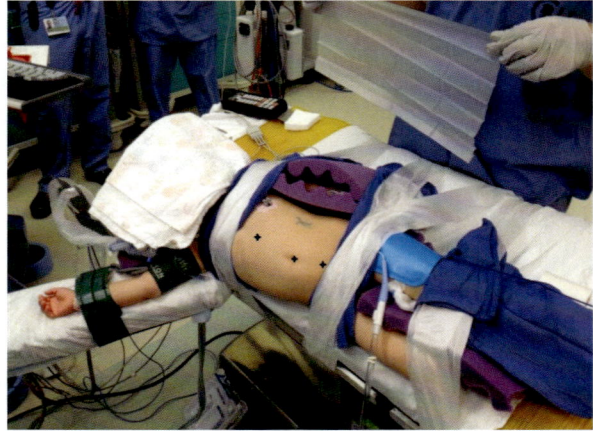

Fig. 8.1 Patient position and trocar placement for a transperitoneal robot assisted heminephrectomy. Note that the patient is secured to the table in a lateral position, but the table can be rotated during insertion of the umbilical port so that the patient is effectively supine. A fourth port can be placed for liver retraction

Placement of the Robot

The robot is angled over the ipsilateral shoulder of the patient, so that the entire patient cart stands on the ipsilateral side of the patient. Alternatively, we bring the robot perpendicular to the table and then rotate the foot end of the table away. Three robotic arms are engaged with the laparoscopic ports. The 30° lens is used at the umbilical port (Fig. 8.2.)

Dissection

We generally begin dissection with an atraumatic grasper in the left hand and a monopolar cautery hook or scissors in the right hand. The peritoneum is incised at the white line of Toldt and the colon is reflected medially to expose Gerota's fascia. It is necessary to take down the splenic flexure on the left side and the hepatic flexure on the right when performing an upper pole nephrectomy. Care must be taken to identify and preserve the mesocolon and its vessels during this dissection. The Gerota's fascia is opened to expose the renal moieties and pelves. The distal ureters can easily be identified as they course over the psoas and are traced upwards toward the renal pelves. It is important not to loop up the ureter until both the ureters have been identified.

The liver or spleen can be retracted using an S retractor. Alternatively, an atraumatic grasper or a suction canula can be used for this purpose. The ureter of the upper moiety passes posterior to the main renal pedicle. A plane is created between the upper moiety ureter and main the renal vessels using gentle blunt dissection (Fig. 8.3). Attention must be paid to the amount of tension being applied to the vessels during this dissection. Once the upper moiety ureter is clearly identified, it is

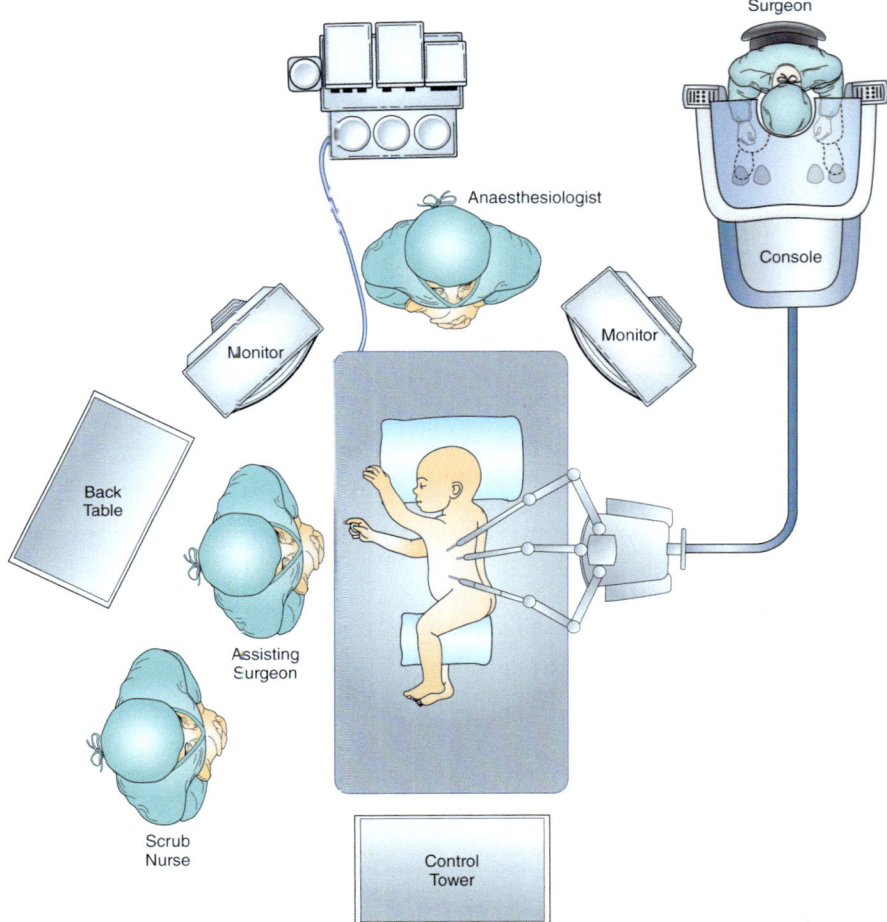

Fig. 8.2 Position of the robot and operating room set up

looped up as distally as possible where a window can be created between it and the lower moiety ureter. The upper moiety ureter is then divided closer to the renal pelvis using robotic scissors at the distal working port. The distal stump is ligated with a 3-0 vicryl suture square knot tied with the use of the robotic needle driver and the grasper. The proximal stump of ureter is then passed posterior to the renal pedicle and brought superiorly. Traction can be given to this proximal ureteral stump now, and using diathermy, the upper moiety pelvis is dissected from the surrounding tissue. The upper moiety vessels are identified during this dissection. These are usually small vessels that arise from the main renal vessels. There may be more than one artery and vein supplying the upper moiety. In many cases, the main renal artery may branch early to give rise to vessels supplying both moieties. These vessels are

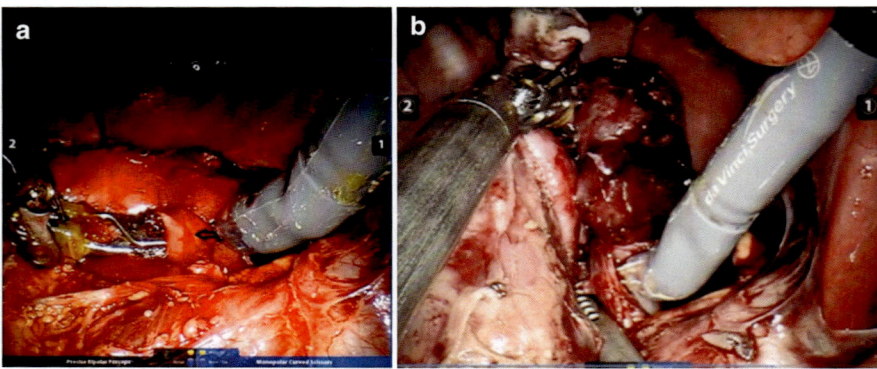

Fig. 8.3 Dissection of the lower pole hilum. (**a**) A plane is created posterior to the lower pole vessels (arrow) by blunt dissection. (**b**) The divided upper pole ureter being passed under the lower pole pedicle. (*Photographs courtesy Dr. Mohan. S. Gundeti, Comer Children's Hospital, The University of Chicago Medicine and Biological Sciences*)

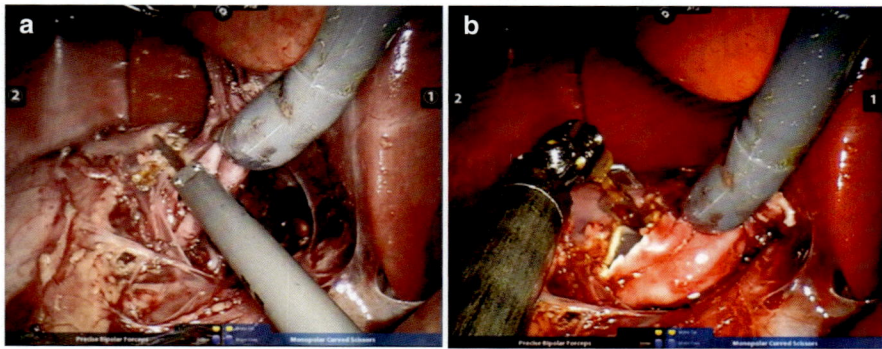

Fig. 8.4 (**a, b**) Separation of the upper pole from the lower pole. The upper pole has been incised, leaving sufficient capsule on the remnant pole to allow closure. (*Photographs courtesy Dr. Mohan. S. Gundeti, Comer Children's Hospital, The University of Chicago Medicine and Biological Sciences*)

often splayed over a hydronephrotic pelvis making them difficult to identify and dissect. Therefore, it is necessary to clearly identify a vessel as supplying the upper pole before ligating it.

The vessels may be ligated using a 5 mm clip and applier, a Ligasure device, a vessel sealer or a ligature. The moiety will change colour when its blood supply is eliminated, but this may not be clearly appreciated in a thinned out, non-functioning, pale moiety. It is important to note that the healthy moiety remains unchanged. A clear demarcation between the two moieties can easily be appreciated. Using the robotic diathermy hook and grasper, the upper moiety is separated from the lower pole. The Harmonic or Ligasure devices may also be used for this purpose. As much of the renal capsule as possible is spared while excising the parenchyma of the moiety, so that this capsule can be sewn over (Fig. 8.4). A small, non functioning upper pole can often be removed without much bleeding. If bleeding does occur, haemostatic mattress sutures must be placed. A careful inspection must be done to identify any breach in the lower pole parenchyma or pelvicalyceal system. Such a breach needs to be sutured with absorbable sutures, and a stent must be placed in the ureter. A haemostatic material such as Floseal® or Surgicel® can be placed over the cut surface. Masson et al., found that suturing the cut surface over a fat pad reduced the incidence of urinoma formation [2] The distal ureter is then dissected down to the uretero-vesical junction where it is ligated with an absorbable suture, divided and excised. Utmost care must be taken to preserve the vascularity of the healthy ureter. When the ureters run through a common sheath, it may be impossible to dissect one ureter without injuring the other and in such cases it becomes advisable to leave behind the distal ureteral stump. This becomes particularly significant in patients with sympotomatic reflux, and a secondary ureterectomy may be required later [3]. The specimen is usually retrieved via the umbilical incision. For this purpose, the 10 mm telescope is replaced with a 5 mm one placed at the distal port. A retrieval bag is usually not necessary unless the specimen contains a tumour. The incision on the fascia may be extended to deliver the specimen. It is useful to suction any liquid content out of the specimen. In case of a large specimen, such as a tumour, a separate Pfannensteil incision can be made for delivery of the specimen. Placement of a drain in the renal fossa is at the discretion of the surgeon.

A lower pole nephrectomy is performed in much the same way. The line of demarcation between a hydronephrotic lower pole and the upper pole is often difficult to identify and dissection may take some effort. The dissection is usually inferior to the renal pedicle, and perihilar dissection is not needed. While separating the lower pole parenchyma from the upper pole, it is important to bear in mind that the dilated lower pole pelvicalyceal system often projects into the upper pole and the cut surface must be carefully examined before closure.

The Retroperitoneal Approach

Retroperitoneoscopic paediatric heminephrectomy was first reported by Diamond et al. in 1995. More recently, the robot has been used to perform this procedure. While less popular than the transperitoneal approach, the retroperitoneoscopic approach is anatomically feasible in children because of less perinephric fat and less muscle bulk than adults. This approach offers direct access to the kidney and pelvis, and obviates the need for perihilar dissection in an upper pole nephrectomy [4, 5]. However, visualisation and dissection of the distal ureter close to the vesicoureteral junction is challenging, and working space is limited. Retroperitoneoscopy may be performed with the patient in flank position or prone.

Equipment

The equipment required is the same as that for transperitoneal heminephrectomy. In addition, a laparoscopic balloon trocar is required to create the retroperitoneal working space. Alternatively, surgeons have used soaked sponges, gloves and condoms to create the retroperitoneal space in children. As in the transperitoneal approach a cystoscopic stenting of the ureter to be preserved may be performed.

The Flank Approach

The patient is placed with the back flush to the edge of the table. A roll or bolster is placed under the contralateral side to support the torso and to raise the ipsilateral flank. The patient must be supported and secured to the table. A 1 cm incision is made about a centimetre lateral to the tip of the 12th rib and is deepened by splitting the muscle fibres with the tips of a pair of dissecting scissors. Once the retroperitoneum is reached, a fine right angle or "S" retractor is inserted into the incision and a careful inspection is made to ensure that the peritoneum has not been breached. The balloon trocar is inserted through this incision and inflated to create the retroperitoneal working space. Alternatively, a soaked sponge is gently pushed into the retroperitoneum to create space. The balloon trocar (or sponge) is withdrawn and a 2-0 Vicryl U-stitch is placed on the fascia. A 10 mm port is then inserted through the incision and a 30° telescope is introduced. The trocar can be used to further sweep away the peritoneum and enlarge the retroperitoneal space. Insufflation is begun only after the integrity of the peritoneum has been confirmed. A gas flow rate of 1 L/min gradually raised to a maximum of 3 L/min is used to obtain a pressure of not more than 12 mm of Hg. The U-stitch is used to secure the fascia around the trocar and prevent any gas leaks. The Two 5 mm working ports are inserted – one anterior to the sacrospinalis muscle and the other about a centimetre and a half superior to the iliac crest in the mid axillary line (Fig. 8.5). It is imperative to ensure that the peritoneum has been reflected medially adequately before insertion of these ports, lest the trocar should penetrate the peritoneum and cause visceral injury.

The robot is brought perpendicular to the table and angled over the patient's shoulder to engage at the three ports. Dissection is typically begun with atraumatic robotic graspers and robotic scissors.

The psoas muscle forms an important landmark in the retroperitoneal approach. An additional instrument may be required to retract the kidney off the psoas to approach the renal hilum. The ureters are identified and are traced to their respective moieties. The upper moiety ureter is ligated and disconnected at a suitable site and its proximal stump is used to apply gentle traction on the upper moiety. The upper moiety is bluntly separated from the surrounding tissue. However, the kidney remains attached to the peritoneum anteriorly. Reflecting the moiety off the psoas, the renal hilum is dissected. Vessels supplying the upper moiety are identified,

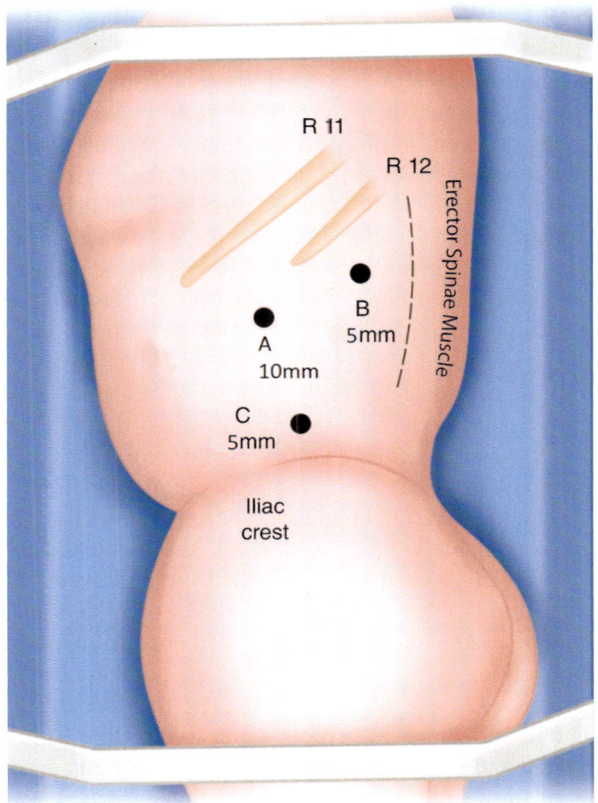

Fig. 8.5 Trocar placement for retroperitoneoscopic robot assisted heminephrectomy in the flank position

clipped and divided. The parenchyma of the moiety is excised sparing as much capsule as possible. This capsule is sewn over the cut surface. Care must be taken to identify any breach in the lower pole pelvicalyceal system. Such a breach must be repaired. The ureter is dissected as far distally as possible and excised. In the retroperitoneoscopic approach, extensive dissection of the ureter is challenging.

The specimen is usually delivered through the 1 cm incision at the tip of the 12th rib. A 5 mm laparoscope is introduced through the inferior port and the specimen is extracted through the 10 mm port. This incision can be extended as needed. A drain may be kept in the renal fossa before closure. The U stitch placed on the fascia at the time of port insertion assists in closing the fascia.

A lower pole nephrectomy is performed in a similar manner, although delineating the lower pole pelvis may be more difficult as its line of demarcation is less clear. Also, the pelvicalyceal system of the hydronephrotic lower pole may project into the upper pole parenchyma, a detail to which attention must be paid during excision.

The Prone Approach

While the retroperitoneal flank approach offers direct access to the kidney and its hilum, the prone approach has become popular among some surgeons operating on young children. In this position, the kidney falls away from the psoas muscle, and retraction is not needed. The patient is placed prone with supports under the chest and the hips [6]. The abdomen is freely suspended over the surface of the table, but supports are placed such that the space between the iliac crest and the 12th rib is maximised. The ipsilateral side is brought close to the edge of the table. All pressure points must be padded. Close coordination between the surgeon, the anaesthesiologist and the nursing team is essential during positioning of the patient.

Access is gained through a 1 cm incision in the costovertebral angle lateral to the erector spinae muscles. The muscles are split with the tips of a pair of dissecting scissors to enter the retroperitoneum through the dorsolumbar fascia at the anterior margin of the quadratus lumborum. The psoas does not form an anatomic landmark in this approach hence orientation is difficult. The retroperitoneal space is created using a balloon trocar or a sponge as described in the flank approach. A 2-0 absorbable U stitch is placed in the fascia and a 10 mm port with a 30° telescope is introduced to confirm that the peritoneum is intact. Insufflation is then carried out at 1–3 L/min to a pressure of 12 mm of Hg. The telescope and port may be used as a unit to sweep the peritoneum medially, away from the sites of the working ports. Two 5 mm working ports are inserted, one a centimetre off the tip of the 12th rib, and the other above the iliac crest in the posterior axillary line. The robot is brought perpendicular to the table from the contralateral side of the patient and docked to the three ports. Dissection proceeds in much the same way as in the flank approach, although hilar dissection is easier as the kidney falls away from the psoas. The specimen is delivered at the costo-vertebral angle, where the incision may be extended if needed. The U stitch helps secure closure of the fascia.

Transperitoneal Versus Retroperitoneal Approach

Studies comparing the retroperitoneal approach and the transperitoneal approach have demonstrated no significant advantage of the former over the latter [7, 8]. The retroperitoneal approach demands greater dexterity in a limited working space. The transperitoneal approach is decidedly advantageous when combined upper and lower tract procedures are to be done [9].

However, while the transperitoneal approach remains more popular, there are some situations where the retroperitoneal approach is more desirable. This includes patients who have had multiple abdominal surgery, where entering the peritoneal cavity entails a high risk of organ injury, need for more extensive dissection and possibility of greater blood loss.

Borzi [8] compared the flank and the prone retroperitoneal approach in his series of 36 complete and 19 partial nephroureterectomies. While he found no statistically significant difference in the mean operating time for the two approaches, he found better access to the distal ureter in the flank approach. He recommend the flank approach where complete ureterectomy is needed in a child older than 5 years or in a case of renal ectopia or fusion [8].

Post Operative Care and Pain Relief

Post operative pain can usually be managed with scheduled acetaminophen or ibuprofen, although opiates have been used in early series [6]. Port site infiltration with local anaesthetic such as lidocaine or bupivacaine, either at the time of insertion of the port or at the time of closure, also contributes to pain relief.

Patients can usually be discharged from hospital the same day or the next morning. A ureteral stent, if placed, is removed 4–6 weeks later. The length of post surgical hospital stay depends on any concurrent procedures performed on the patient and any medical co morbidities.

Complications and Outcomes

The complication profile of robotic heminephrectomy includes those risks associated with any minimal access urologic surgery. That includes complications of access such as trocar puncture trauma to organs or vessels and development of hernias at the trocar site. The OR team must always be prepared for the possibility of robotic malfunction and the failure to complete the procedure robotically.

During a heminephrectomy, injuries are possible to the bowel, liver and spleen. The duodenum can be injured while exposing the right upper pole. Vascular injuries are possible if the camera isn't oriented properly- it is possible to mistake the inferior vena cava for the right renal vein in small children. Ischaemic injury to the lower pole can result from arterial spasm caused by too much tension on the pedicle during dissection [10]. Urinoma formation, nephrectomy bed fluid collections and abscesses are also known to occur (Table 8.1). The rate of occurrence of complications seems to be associated with the age of the patient rather than the technique used. Interestingly, in a single institute study by Varda et al. that showed a 12% complication rate, all complications were found to occur in cases with lower pole pathology [11].

"Cyst formation" or benign fluid collections in the nephrectomy bed have been found on follow up ultrasounds of patients of heminephrectomy, irrespective of the approach. These probably arise from unrecognized collecting system injuries or partial transection of the diseased moiety that leaves exposed urothelium [11]. Mason et al. found a collection in 29% of their 21 patients undergoing robot assisted

Table 8.1 Outcomes of robot-assisted heminephrectomy

Author	Approach	Number	Mean age (months)	OR time (min)	Upper poles/lower poles	LOS (days)	Reoperation rate	Urinoma formation	Cyst formation/contained fluid collections	Perinephric abscess	Mean change in renal function	Urine leak	Overall complication rate
Varda, Rajender, Yu, Lee (2018)	Transperitoneal robotic	27	3.6 y	206	27/16	1		1	5	1	NR	NR	11%
Esposito, Escolino, Castagnetti et al. (2016)	Transperitoneal laparoscopic	52	50 m	NR	42/10	NR	0	4	NR	NR	NR	4	30.0%
Malik, Pariser, Gundeti (2015)	Retroperitoneoscopic	50	50 m	NR	41/9	NR	2	6	NR			1	19%
	Transperitoneal robotic	16	37 m 30 s	135	NR	2	2	2	4	0	−2.7% decreased function in 6 patients	NR	NR
Marte, Paparella, Pintozzi (2015)	Laparoscopic	22	3.9 y	154	NR	2–4	0	NR	5	0	NR	1	NR
Herz, Smith, et al. (2015)	Transperitoneal robotic	20	3.1 y	209	17/3	NR	NR	NR	NR	NR	NR	NR	5%
Mason, Henderson, et al. (2014)	Transperitoneal robotic	21	4.1 y	301	17/4	1.583	NR	NR	6	NR	NR	NR	NR
Jayram, Roberts, et al. (2011)	Retroperitoneoscopic	142	11.4	120	NR	2	1	7	38	0	Loss of function in 7	NR	
Garcia-Aparicio, et al. (2009)	Transperitoneal laparoscopic	9	14 m	182	NR	2.44	NR	NR	NR	NR	NR	NR	0
Leclair, Vidal, Suply, et al. (2009)	Retroperitoneoscopic	48* (10 converted)	8 m 36 s	120	36/12	3	1	1	NR	NR	Complete loss of function in 1 patient	NR	2/48

LOS length of stay in hospital, *NR* not reported. *This series included retroperitoneal laparoscopic operations.

heminephrectomy [2]. These fluid collections are usually asymptomatic, and all resolve spontaneously over a period of months to years. In a series by Lee et al., one patient required drainage of a urinoma [12]. Mason et al. proposed that the rate of urinoma formation is lower for surgeons who use a fat bolster to close the cut surface of the kidney, although the difference in their series did not reach statistical significance [2]. They reported a collection arising out of a forniceal rupture of the healthy moiety during a retrograde pyelogram at the start of the procedure, which was managed by stent placement for 17 days. They also reported an incarcerated port site hernia in one patient.

Loss of function of the ipsilateral remnant moiety after a minimal access heminephrectomy has been reported in multiple series, with an incidence ranging from 0 to 7% [13]. While Malik et al. have reported a decrease in function up to 10% [3], Strine et al. found that post operative renal scintigraphy usually demonstrates an average decrease in function of 3.6%. It was proposed that this decrease in renal function could be because the preoperative scintigraphy included the poorly functioning moiety, which would contribute to some uptake [13]. Wallis attributed the loss of function in the remnant moiety in 2 of their 26 patients to smaller size and younger age [14], but Jayaram et al. in their multicentre review found an increased risk of function loss in children undergoing upper pole nephrectomy (83% vs 13%) [10]. They proposed that the hilar dissection during upper pole nephrectomy could result in ischaemic damage to the lower pole, irrespective of the age of the patient, or the approach used. That said, it is not mandatory to perform a scintigraphy in the follow up of a heminephrectomy. A renal Doppler ultrasound can also assess the function of the remnant moiety [13].

The incidence of delayed infection in the ureteral stump requiring a completion ureterectomy varies. In Ade-Ajaye's series of 58 patients, 8 required completion ureterectomy for recurrent infections [15]. Mushtaq's series of 54 patients demonstrated visible stumps on ultrasound in 12%, but none required ureterectomy [6]. However, VUR induced infection does occur in 10–25% of ureteral stumps, necessitating completion ureterectomy [16].

At the time of surgery, it is necessary to weigh the risks of injury to the healthy ureter versus the need for a second surgery to complete the ureterectomy.

Conclusion

Minimal access techniques are the preferred method of treating duplex anomalies in children. The robot is slowly establishing its utility and safety in tackling these complex cases in younger patients.

References

1. Passerotti CC, Nguyen HT, Retik AB, et al. Patterns and predictors of laparoscopic complications in paediatric urology: the role of ongoing surgical volume and access techniques. J Urol. 2008;180:681.

2. Mason MD, Anthony Herndon CD, Smith-Harrison LI, Peters CA, Corbett ST. Robotic-assisted partial nephrectomy in duplicated collecting systems in the pediatric population: techniques and outcomes. J Pediatr Urol. 2014;10(2):374–9.
3. Malik RD, Pariser JJ, Gundeti MS. Outcomes in pediatric robot-assisted laparoscopic heminephrectomy compared with contemporary open and laparoscopic series. J Endourol. 2015;29(12):1346–52.
4. El-Ghoneimi A, Farhat W, Bolduc S, et al. Retroperitoneal laparoscopic vs open partial nephroureterectomy in children. BJU Int. 2003;91:532–5.
5. Traxel EJ, Minevich EA, Noh PH. A review: the application of minimally invasive surgery to pediatric urology: upper urinary tract procedures. Urology. 2010;76:122–33.
6. Mushtaq I, Haleblian G. Laparoscopic heminephrectomy in infants and children: first 54 cases. J Pediatr Urol. 2007;3(2):100–3.
7. Garcia-Aparicio L, Krauel L, Tarrado X, Olivares M, Garcia-Nunez B, Lerena J, et al. Heminephrectomy for duplex kidney: laparoscopic versus open surgery. J Pediatr Urol. 2010;6(2):157–60.
8. Borzi PA. A comparison of the lateral and posterior retroperitoneoscopic approach for complete and partial nephroureterectomy in children. BJU Int. 2001;87:517–20.
9. Harrell WB, Snow BW. Minimally invasive pediatric nephrectomy. Curr Opin Urol. 2005;15:277–81.
10. Jayram G, Roberts J, Hernandez A, Heloury Y, Manoharan S, Godbole P, Leclair M, Mushtaq I, Gundeti MSL. Outcomes and fate of the remnant moiety following laparoscopic heminephrectomy for duplex kidney: a multicenter review. J Pediatr Urol. 2011;7:272–5.
11. Varda BK, Rajender A, Yu RN, Lee RS. A contemporary single-institution retrospective cohort study comparing perioperative outcomes between robotic and open partial nephrectomy for poorly functioning renal moieties in children with duplex collecting systems. J Pediatr Urol. 2018;14(6):549e1–8.
12. Lee RS, Sethi AS, Passerotti CC, et al. Robot assisted laparoscopic partial nephrectomy in children: a viable and safe option in children. J Urol. 2009;181(2):823–8.
13. Strine AC, Whittam BM, Misseri R, Kaefer M, Rink RC, Karmazyn B, Cain MP. Is renal scintigraphy necessary after heminephrectomy in children? J Pediatr Urol. 2016;12(1):38.e1–4.
14. Wallis MC, Khoury AE, Lorenzo AJ, Pippi-Salle JL, Bägli DJ, Farhat WA. Outcome analysis of retroperitoneal laparoscopic heminephrectomy in children. J Urol. 2006;175:2277–82.
15. Ade-Ajayi N, Wilcox DT, Duffy PG, Ransley PG. Upper pole heminephrectomy: is complete ureterectomy necessary? BJU Int. 2001;88(1):77–9.
16. Caluwé D, Chertin B, Puri P. Long-term outcome of the retained ureteral stump after lower pole heminephrectomy in duplex kidneys. Eur Urol. 2002;42:63–6.

Chapter 9
Nephrectomy: Minimally Invasive Surgery

Benjamin Whittam, Kahlil Saad, and Matthieu Peycelon

Introduction

For decades pediatric urologists have been performing laparoscopy for non-palpable testis. The passage from diagnostic to therapeutic indications has been a long and hesitating course for pediatric urologists. During the 1990s minimally invasive renal surgery was limited to ablative indications and used only in a limited number of centers, with the first laparoscopic pediatric nephrectomy performed in 1992. In the early experience, the indications for laparoscopy in pediatric urology were unclear and unproven compared to the advantages of open procedures. It is only in the last several years that minimally invasive surgery has taken a foothold in practice and research in pediatric urology. Since that time, laparoscopic and robotic approaches to pediatric nephrectomy have become an essential part of the pediatric urologist's armamentarium.

This chapter will address first the established technique of laparoscopic nephrectomy and second the development of robotic-assisted laparoscopic nephrectomy including particular applications, complications and outcomes.

Surgical Technique

Patient Preparation

Patient preparation is not different from the conventional pediatric urology preparation. Usually, no specific diet measures are prescribed before surgery. Usual

---

B. Whittam (✉) · K. Saad M. Peycelon
Riley Hospital for Children at Indiana University, Division of Pediatric Urology,
Indianapolis, IN, USA
e-mail: bwhittam@iupui.edu

© Springer Nature Switzerland AG 2020
P. C. Gargollo (ed.), *Minimally Invasive and Robotic-Assisted Surgery in Pediatric Urology*, https://doi.org/10.1007/978-3-030-57219-8_9

recommendations for general anesthesia preparations are followed. All patients are screened for blood type. Serum electrolytes, creatinine, and coagulation studies should be performed, and all patients should have preoperative sterile urine cultures, as indicated. The child is on strict NPO diet for a period between 4 and 8 hours depending on his/her age, and premedicated before going to the operating theatre. Some surgeons recommend fluid diet and enema on the night preceding surgery [1]. A nasogastric tube may be placed after the endotracheal general anesthesia. Noninvasive hemodynamic and ventilatory monitoring is needed during laparoscopic nephrectomy in either trans- or retroperitoneal approach. Cephalosporin is often administered intravenously in the operating room.

Renal Access

The kidney can be safely accessed by during laparoscopy by either a retroperitoneal or a transabdominal transperitoneal approach. Additionally, there are several patient positioning options and newer approaches utilizing a single surgical site.

Retroperitoneal

Lateral

The patient is placed lateral, with enough flexion of the operating table to expose the area of trocar placement, between the last rib and the iliac crest. In infants and young children (under 6 years), the use of a lumbar padding to laterally flex the patient without flexing the operating table may be needed. Retroperitoneal access is achieved through the first incision, 15 mm in length, and one finger width from the lower border of the tip of the 12th rib. The use of narrow retractors with long blades allows a deep dissection despite a short incision. Gerota's fascia is approached by a muscle splitting blunt dissection, then it is opened under direct vision and the first blunt trocar (5 mm, 0° lens) is introduced directly inside the opened Gerota's fascia. A working space is created by gas insufflation's dissection, and the first trocar is fixed with a purse-string suture that is applied around the deep fascia to ensure an airtight seal and to allow traction on the main trocar if needed to increase the working space. This suture is preferably done before putting the trocar as the small incision is too tight around the trocar. A second trocar (5 mm) is inserted posteriorly in the costovertebral angle, in front of the lumbosacral muscle. A third 5-mm trocar is inserted, in the anterior axillary line, a finger width from the top of the iliac crest. To avoid transperitoneal insertion of this trocar, the working space is fully developed, and the deep surface of the anterior wall muscles is identified before trocar insertion. Insufflation pressure should not exceed 12 mm Hg, and the CO_2 flow rate is progressively increased from 1L to 3L/min. Access to the retroperitoneum and creation of the working space are the keys to success in retroperitoneal renal surgery.

Age is not a limiting factor for this approach [2]. Young children have less fat and the access is even easier.

Prone Posterior

The access begins with an incision in the costovertebral angle at the edge of the paraspinous muscles The secondary trocars are placed just above the iliac crest, one medially at the edge of the paraspinous muscles, and one laterally at the posterior clavicular line [1, 3, 4]. This approach gives the advantage of excellent exposure of the pedicle with spontaneous traction on the pedicle by the gravity. The difficulty in this approach is to go to the distal part of the ureter. Borzi et al. compared in a randomized prospective study the lateral to the posterior retroperitoneal approach in children undergoing laparoscopic nephrectomy and found no significant difference in the operative time [5].

Other Tips for Access

Since the description by Gaur et al., balloon dissection has been the method applied by most urologists [6]. Disadvantages of the balloon are the cost of the disposable material and the possible complications related to rupture of the balloon [7]. On the other hand, balloon dissection allows creating a working space without opening Gerota's fascia, which is important for radical removal of malignant tumors in adults. Capolicchio et al. [8] described a modification of lateral access [8]. They recommend the insertion of the first trocar through the costovertebral angle. This modification helped them to avoid an accidental peritoneal tear during access through the first lateral incision and allowed a smaller incision for the laparoscope. One of the possible disadvantages of the use of this device is that the placement of the device can be incorrectly inserted and the Gerota's fascia would be approached more anteriorly. This common mistake may lead to downward release of the kidney and makes the retroperitoneal approach more difficult with the need to retract the kidney upwards. Micali et al. reported the use of the VisiPort© (Medtronic, Minneapolis, MN, USA) visual trocar to access directly to the retroperitoneal space, which was originally described by Cadeddu et al. [9, 10]. The advantage of this method is the possibility to use a small incision for the first trocar, which is helpful in reconstructive surgery but not in ablative surgery as the first incision is needed for organ retrieval.

Transperitoneal

Several options exist in terms of patient positioning. The most frequently described is the flank position [1]. The pneumoperitoneum is created through an open umbilical approach. The child is positioned with the surgeon standing in front of the abdomen (opposite side of the kidney). The most frequent configuration has been with the umbilical port and two operating ports in the midline above and below the umbilicus. A fourth trocar may be placed in the mid-clavicular line if needed for exposure. The kidney is exposed by medial mobilization of the colon. One significant advantage of a transperitoneal approach is clear identification and dissection of the distal part of the ureter as well as navigation by familiar intraabdominal landmarks.

Single-Site Access

Johnson et al. published in 2009 the first pediatric single-port-access nephrectomy for a multicystic, dysplastic kidney [11]. With the patient in a right lateral decubitus position, a semicircular infra-umbilical incision was made. A R-port was utilized to establish laparoscopic access. It is a unique single-access port consisting of two components: a fascial retractor containing an inner and an outer ring with an intervening plastic sleeve and a multichannel valve. Each component is covered with a thermoplastic elastomer that maintains pneumoperitoneum while allowing the introduction of flexible or rigid instruments. A 2-cm rectus fasciotomy was made, and the R-port was secured. Mobilization of the spleen and left colon allowed identification of the left kidney and ureter. A harmonic scalpel can be used to take the renal artery, renal vein and ureter. After complete mobilization, the kidney is secured in an entrapment bag, morcellated and removed through the single infra-umbilical incision. Beyond the initial hurdles and learning curve, this technique is promising and has the potential to be extended to other procedures in pediatric urology [12–16]. The use of adjacent fascial puncture sites for instrumentation can obviate the need for a commercial port or multiple trocars [17].

Technique of Laparoscopic Nephrectomy

Laparoscopic Retroperitoneal Approach

First described by Diamond et al. and Valla et al. in 1995 [18–20], patients are placed in a modified lateral decubitus position with table flexion and kidney rest elevation and the procedure is performed via the lateral retroperitoneal approach [21–23]. The retroperitoneal access is achieved via the first incision, 15–20 mm in length, and one finger width from the lower border of the tip of the 12th rib. The Gerota's fascia is approached by a muscle-splitting blunt dissection and is then opened under direct vision. The first blunt trocar (5 or 10 mm) is introduced directly inside the opened Gerota's fascia. A working space is created by gas insufflation dissection. A second trocar (5 mm) is inserted posteriorly in the costovertebral angle and a third trocar (5 mm) is inserted, in the anterior axillary line, a finger width from the top of the iliac crest. The renal pedicle is identified and approached posteriorly and dissected close to the junction with the aorta and vena cava. On the left side the vein is ligated distal to the genital and adrenal branches. After dissecting the renal artery then the vein, the vessels are clipped, ligated or coagulated. The choice of method depends on the vessel diameter. In general, small arteries of MCDK can be coagulated by bipolar cautery or harmonic scalpel, while the most common method is to double ligate the artery proximally by two clips and distally by one. The vein is generally clipped in the same way, if the diameter is bigger than the length of the clip, the vein is first ligated by a resorbable intracorporeal knot; the diameter is thus reduced, and the ligature is secured by juxtaposed clips. The ureter is then identified and dissected as far as necessary. In the absence of reflux, the ureter is coagulated and sectioned at the level of the lumbar ureter (especially in pretransplant nephrectomy, the native ureter might be used for the transplantation). In the presence of reflux, the dissection is distally followed, the vas deferens is identified in males, and the ureter is ligated as close as possible to the ureterovesical junction. The last part of dissection is the anterior surface of the kidney. The kidney is dissected from the peritoneum very close to its capsule in the cleavage plan of areolar tissue. Usually no hemostasis is necessary in this plane, but in inflammatory adherent kidneys a sharp dissection with bipolar coagulation may be necessary. The kidney is usually retrieved through the main incision at the tip of the 12th rib. A 5-mm telescope is inserted through the accessory port, and a toothed grasping forceps is introduced through the first port to extract the kidney. The kidney is grasped at one of the poles, and pulled in this axis, to pull on the smallest diameter of the kidney. In most cases, the kidney can be divided under vision during extraction through the muscle wall. In cases of severe pyelocaliceal dilation or MCDK, direct evacuation by puncture helps in organ retrieval. An extraction bag is used for infected or large kidneys, and the kidney is morcellated inside the bag.

Laparoscopic Transperitoneal Approach

The child is placed, supported, and strapped in the semilateral position with a degree of contralateral flexion of the spine to open the renal angle. This position allows the intestine to fall medially by gravity. The surgeon stands in front of the patient. In the traditional kidney position three trocars are inserted after creation of a pneumoperitoneum: 10 mm periumbilical (port I), 10/12 mm subcostal (port II) and 12/10 mm above the iliac spine (port III) in the mamillary line [24, 25]. Although a 0° laparoscope may be used successfully in some cases, a 30° laparoscope gives better visibility and versatility. After laterocolic incision the colon is reflected away from the lateral wall. Thereafter two 5-mm trocars (ports IV, V) are inserted into the lateral abdominal wall parallel to ports II and III. Following clipping and dissection of the gonadal vein, the ureter is isolated and divided. Then the cranial part of the ureter is used as a retractor exposing the renal hilum for dissection of the renal vessels. The main renal artery and vein are dissected separately by use of an endoscopic stapling device. Finally, the kidney including Gerota's fascia is isolated from the adrenal and the upper peritoneum. Entrapment of the organ is performed with a specially designed bag. The neck of the bag is brought out onto the surface of the abdomen (via port II/III) allowing digital morcellation with index finger inside the bag and removal of the organ in several pieces can be performed if necessary [26]. After a final inspection of the operative field and evacuation of the pneumoperitoneum, incisions >3.5 mm are closed using absorbable sutures. The cannula sites are infiltrated with local anesthetic agents.

Technique of Robot-Assisted Nephrectomy

Nephrectomy is a valuable tool in the armamentarium of the pediatric urologist to treat a wide variety of conditions. While robotic procedures have increased dramatically recently, most focus by pediatric urologists on the upper tracts has been on reconstructive or minimally ablative procedures such as pyeloplasty, ureteroureterostmy and partial nephrectomy [27]. A robotic approach to nephrectomy will replicate similar approaches used in reconstruction applied to a purely extirpative procedure. The surgeon must select the appropriate approach for the patient based on the case particulars, even with acknowledgement of higher reported total costs, but shorter hospitalization [28]. Additionally, a robotic approach may be advantageous such as in bilateral procedures, where a nephrectomy/nephroureterectomy may combined with a contralateral procedure such as a ureteral reimplant as Lee et al. reported in four patients with concurrent contralateral extravesical ureteral reimplantation [29, 30]. A mixed pure-laparoscopic and robotic approach for bilateral upper pole heminephrectomies has also been reported for non-functional moieties [31]. Lastly, while current robotic ports are 8 mm in size, they offer not only articulated instruments, but a wide variety of instruments that the surgeon may find useful. Smaller sized ports and instruments exist, but their adoption is not as widespread.

Patient preparation is similar for a robotic assisted approach. Appropriate blood work, including type and screen, CBC, and BMP should be considered. Should entry into the urinary tract other than ligation of the ureter be anticipated, or in cases or recurrent infections, obtain a urine culture and treat prior to proceeding. Besides a standard NPO period prior to surgery, a bowel preparation is not necessary, unless the surgeon expects significant constipation that may hinder dissection. Antibiotic prophylaxis should be guided by best-practices including any expected entry into the urinary system or the presence of long-standing infection. In the absence of this, the procedure may be treated as a clean procedure with common antibiotic prophylaxis choice such as cefazolin. The surgeon may consider a neuraxial block or regional block to be performed by the anesthesiologist (such as a transversus abdominis plane, i.e., TAP block) versus local anesthetic infiltration into the port sites, with reported similar pain control [32].

Patient positioning is surgeon-dependent, however should at least initially be undertaken with the anesthesiologist to ensure careful padding and avoid compression or hyperextension that may lead to neuropraxia. Patients should be secured a multiple points, and the bed rotation tested for stability. As with a pure laparoscopic approach, renal access may proceed in a retroperitoneal or transperitoneal fashion. A retroperitoneal approach is taken with similar position to an open surgery with the patient in the lateral decubitus position, with the head well-supported and the arms either both forward in a neutral position, or with the ipsilateral arm tucked to the side if space permits. The legs are placed in a neutral, well-padded position and the table may be slightly flexed, either with or without the kidney rest deployed, just enough to open the space between the iliac crest and the inferior border of the ribs.

For a transabdominal approach, the patient may be placed in one of three different positions: pure flank, modified flank or supine. Flank position is similar as described above for a retroperitoneal approach. In a modified flank approach the patient is placed with approximately 45 degrees of lift of the operative side via the use of gel rolls and gentle padding. The ipsilateral hip and back are bumped in the fashion with the legs slightly flexed. In this position the ipsilateral arm is most easily tucked at the side. In a supine position, arms may be tucked or folded over the chest, and a X-pattern of tape over the chest often works well the secure the arms at the side. We favor the supine in older children for its ease of position with the ability to replicate a modified flank position internally simply tilting the operative table.

With a retroperitoneal approach, ports may be placed in a fashion similar to a pure laparoscopic depending on a prone posterior versus flank approach and dilation of the potential retroperitoneal space. The first port may either be placed at the tip of the 12th rib, or in the costovertebral angle at the lateral boarder of the paraspinous muscles. The potential space is developed, and two more working ports placed as above. Rarely are more than three ports necessary with a robotic setup, although placement of a fourth arm or an assistant port is possible, usually inferior to the camera, though a superior placement may be done if needed for creating space under the liver.

Port placement for a transabdominal approach may depend on the robotic platform being used (Fig. 9.1). With the Si series of Da Vinci robots, side docking was necessary which required certain port placement with triangulation of the operative field. Currently, with the Xi series, port placement may proceed in standard triangulation or in a straight line in the midline using the umbilicus for the camera port. This has been reported for use in bilateral procedures where midline placement obviates the need for replacing or adding new trocar sites [33]. This approach easily allowed for five midline ports in a 14 kg child as reported by Sala et al. for a bilateral Wilms nephrectomy. Three port placement may be accomplished with an umbilical camera port and ipsilateral ASIS and infracoastal ports to triangulate the kidney. If needed, a fourth port for either the third robotic arm or an assistant port may be added at a suprapubic location or midway between the superior ports at the lateral edge of the rectus muscle. Recently popularized, the HiDES technique can be used to place two of the ports other than the umbilical incision below the waistline [34]. After standard access through the umbilicus, ports can be placed just medial the ipsilateral ASIS and at the midline suprapubic, both with a transverse incision. The skin and facial ports entry sites may be slid along each other to allow for a lower skin incision while still maintaining reasonable access and working room. Using an

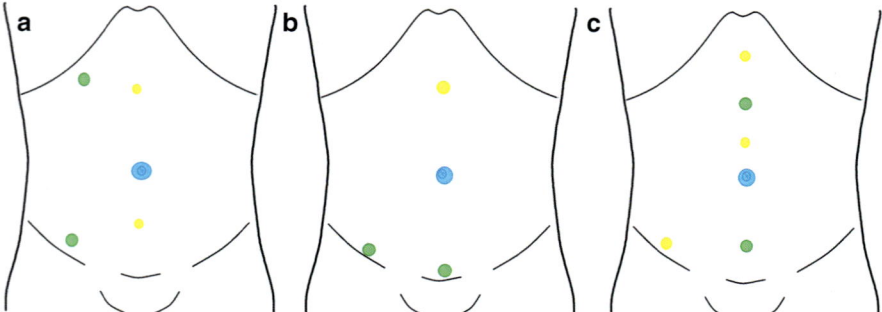

Fig. 9.1 Port placement for a robotic setup will depend on platform and number of ports needed. (**a**) Standard three-port triangulation with the camera (blue) in the umbilicus and working ports (green) in a sub-costal location and off of ASIS. Additional ports (yellow) may be placed as need for retraction, dissection or for an assistant. (**b**) Three-port placement for a HiDES approach to the kidney. (**c**) Midline port placement possible with the Xi DaVinci system. The inferior working port may be placed in a HiDES position

Si platform, the robot is brought over the patient's should at approximately 45 degrees to allow for the instruments to triangulate on the kidney. With standard or inline placement using the Xi system the boom may be rotated to the correct orientation. Multiple instruments are available, with robotic hem-o-lock appliers, and robotic articulating stapling instruments now available on standard 8 mm sizes [35].

Dissection of the kidney may then proceed from several approaches. Via a retroperitoneal approach the space has already been created and careful dissection around the kidney will allow access to the vessels at the hilum. In a transabdominal approach, obtain access to the retroperitoneum by reflecting the colon along the white line of Toldt on the operative side. If bleeding is a concern early vascular control may first be obtained with dissection and vascular control of the hilum. The kidney may be dissected away from surrounding tissues with a bottom-to-top approach utilizing the ureter as the initial landmark and lifting the kidney away from the psoas muscle. Release of the kidney from the lateral attachments may be delayed as needed or order to perform the medial dissection including hilar control. Often the superior dissection is performed at last, usually leaving the adrenal unless dictated by oncologic concerns.

Special Situations

Non-orthotopic kidneys, such as pelvic kidneys, horseshoe kidneys and those with expected deviations in anatomy, especially vascular, require careful workup prior to extirpation.

Horseshoe kidney occurs in approximately 1 of every 400 individuals. Cross-sectional imaging should identify relevant vasculature. Previously reported case series in laparoscopy are immediately applicable to a robotic approach, with the added ease of a third robotic arm being able to substitute for an assistant to provide traction and positioning in the peritoneum. Agrawal reported three cases of laparoscopic nephrectomy for non-functioning moieties in two and a renal mass requiring radical right nephrectomy [36]. The small vessels and isthmus were taken with a hook cautery, 10 mm Ligasure™, or using hem-o-lock clips for hemostasis. Recently, Lottman reported a left retroperitoneoscopic nephrectomy for nephrotic syndrome [37]. Care should be taken to identify the true line of fusion, as complications from incomplete resection have been reported as up to 60% of lower pole fusion may be lateral and not midline [38]. Kumar reported a case of robot-assisted heminephrectomy for chromophobe renal cell carcinoma in a case of fused ectopic kidneys [39]. Indocyanine green (ICG)-aided near infrared fluorescence has been reported for selective atrial mapping during heminephrectomy to prevent inadvertent injury to non-operative moiety, and may be useful for determining isthmus blood supply during dissection of a horseshoe kidney [40].

Pelvic kidneys offer a unique challenge given location with the pelvis and aberrant arising vessels that may descend directly from the aorta or lateraling from the iliac arteries. Oyinloye reported a Wilms tumor a of a left pelvic kidney in a 10-year old girl, treated with open nephrectomy [41]. As to date there are no reports of robotic removal of a pelvic kidney, although we would expect case series soon.

Tips and Tricks

Ligation of the Ureter

As previously described, ureteral ligation may be accomplished using a number of tools but will depend on the reason for removal. Simple transection with cautery may be acceptable for non-refluxing units, but refluxing units may require further ureteral dissection and transection of the ureter at the ureterovesical junction with further plication of the ureter to prevent urine leak. The ureteral stump may ligated with a hem-o-lock clip, and may be over sewn robotically if large and a concern for reflux. Care should be taken to dissect as close as possible to the ureterovesical junction if excision for reflux, without injury to the vas deferens in a male or uterine vessels in a female.

Kidney Retrieval

Retrieval of the kidney will depend on any oncologic concerns and size of the organ. A multicystic kidney or large hydronephrotic kidney may be decompressed prior to removal to facilitate removal without much need to enlarge ports. The robot is well-suite toward removal of a MCDK, and increased use of the robot for this despite a decrease in overall nephrectomies has been reported [42]. Numerous commercial laparoscopic retrieval bag systems exist, with various port sizes (5–25 mm) and bag volumes (150–4000 mL). Previous laparoscopists have reported no increased risk of surgicalsite infection and a 1% rate of retrieval site hernias among 373 elective cholecystectomies without the use of a bag for organ retrieval [43]. Surgeons have also devised homemade retrieval systems at the bedside in order to reduce cost and facilitate removal. The finger of a sterile glove may be used for small dysplastic kidneys, with a hem-o-lock clip on a string used to close the finger bag and retrieve the specimen. Kao et al. reported on 135 patients undergoing laparoscopic adrenalectomy or prostatectomy using the palmer portion of a sterile glove, 2-0 nylon for a drawstring and 1-0 Vicryl to secure the bottom of the bag, with no reported perioperative complications or evidence of leak in the form of wound metastases [44]. A further retrieval system, the Nadiad bag, constructed from a plastic sheet, nylon thread and a 5-Fr ureteral catheter has been reported [45] with a 4-min retrieval time in 100 nephrectomies [46] and no saline leak. In-bag morcellation systems are available, but should only be considered for extremely large, non-malignant kidneys that cannot be decompressed with any of the above techniques.

Role of Prophylactic Antibiotics

According to the WHO and the EAU, surgical antibiotic prophylaxis is not recommended for laparoscopic nephrectomy in children. However, AUA guidelines recommend the use of a single use of cefazolin or TMP-SMX injection after induction [47].

Lymph Node Dissection

In an oncologic setting, the lymph node samples can be picked up along the aorta above the level of the mesenteric artery and this sampling is very important for accurate staging, and decreases the risk of undertreating the child in case of malignant renal tumors [48]. There has been controversy regarding the impact on survival of the number of lymph nodes examined in. Among 1340 Wilms' tumors reported by Zhuge et al. with lymph node data available following surgery, the 5-year survival was significantly lower for patients with no lymph nodes sampled (87%) or one to five lymph nodes sampled (91%), versus 6–10 lymph nodes (93%) or more than 10 lymph nodes (95%) [49]. However, Kieran et al. demonstrated recently that the number of lymph nodes sampled did not predict 5-year event-free survival variations from 3409 patients; the effect of lymph node positivity was greater only for patients with anaplastic tumors [48]. Nevertheless, although this study confirmed the great importance of sampling at least some lymph nodes, allowing an accurate staging, extensive lymph node dissection seems unnecessary as no patient had positive distant lymph nodes in the setting of negative hilar lymph nodes. Thus, radical nephrectomy with lymph node sampling can be performed under laparoscopy as in open surgery. Bouty et al. published in 2020 a large study including 50 transperitoneal laparoscopic total nephrectomies [50]: lymph node sampling is recommended for all patients, with an ideal number of seven nodes sampled [51, 52]. It is often reported that MIS does not allow for as good a lymph node picking as open surgery [53]. However, Bouty et al. demonstrated the contrary [50, 54].

Indication and Outcome

Laparoscopy

Renal Cancer

In the International Society of Pediatric Oncology (SIOP) protocol, the old standard for therapy is open total nephrectomy, preceded by neoadjuvant chemotherapy [55]. However, increased morbidity, such as the risk of adhesion-related complications and the presence of scars altering the quality of life of long-term survivors, is not uncommon [56, 57]. It is now well established that these risks are lower with minimally invasive surgery (MIS) [56]. Therefore, modern protocols now focus on reducing these risks, while maintaining excellent oncological outcomes. First described in 2004 by Duarte et al., the use of MIS for WT has been reported in the literature in approximately 100 cases [58, 59]. The first series of minimally invasive surgery for unilateral WT by laparoscopy in children was reported by Duarte et al. in 2006 in eight cases with good results [60]. They showed that LRN was feasible after preoperative chemotherapy, including for rather large tumors, even if the follow-up was short. Local control was achieved, as only a 1/8 tumor had microscopic residual disease and required flank radiotherapy. Varlet et al. first reported five cases (mean age: 4 years; mean renal tumor diameter: 50 mm) in 2009 [61]. All tumors and lymph node samples were removed completely by laparoscopy without rupture. No conversion to laparotomy was necessary and there was neither intraoperative bleeding nor complications. The mean operative time was 90 min (60–117). No recurrence was reported after a mean follow-up of 18 months. Varlet et al. concluded that LRN in children for renal cancer was feasible after preopretavive chemotherapy by experiment surgeons in oncology and laparoscopic procedures, with the same oncologic strategies as open surgery, giving the advantage that the tumor needs less mobilization before vessel coagulation, and leads to less blood loss [61]. The laparoscopic approach not only improves the convalescence, the pain, the hospital stay, and the cosmetic outcome in these patients, but also allows planned postoperative chemotherapy or radiation therapy to proceed at an earlier date than open procedure.

The criteria for selection to allow performed LRN in unilateral renal tumors include unilaterality, size of tumors post chemotherapy without crossing the midline, and absence of the thrombus in the renal or cava vein. The tumors beyond the midline after chemotherapy, thrombus of the renal and cava vein, and primary tumors not treated with preoperative chemotherapy should serve as contraindications, as the open surgical procedure is still the standard care. The size of the tumor may also be a contraindication but depending on the size and age of the child, if a large tumor can be extracted by a suprapubic incision without rupture, the size is not a problem; however this incision must be large enough to avoid this complication. It seems reasonable that a low suprapubic incision for removal of the tumor is not only more cosmetic than flank incision but probably better tolerated by patients.

A retrospective multicentric study of children having undergone laparoscopic radical nephrectomy for a malignant renal tumor in the pediatric surgery institutions of the French Society of Pediatric Oncology was published in 2014, including 17 patients with unilateral small malignant tumors at the time of surgery, with or without neoadjuvant chemotherapy, whose medial edge did not cross the lateral edge of the vertebra, allowing an easy approach to the renal pedicle [62]. None of these tumors had preoperative suspicion of extrarenal extension, vena cava thrombosis, preoperative rupture, or large lymph node involvement around the vena cava and the aorta. Median age at surgery was 26 months (5 months–11 years). After chemotherapy, only three tumors were more than 51 mm and 14 were less than 50 mm. The tumor did not cross the lateral edge of the vertebra in 16 but crossed it in one case (the largest one was 8 cm in diameter), the medial edge of the tumor being on the midline. Tumors were located as follows: seven in the upper pole, three in the lower pole, and seven in the medial part of the kidney. Two conversions were necessary for difficult dissection of the renal artery, especially for the largest tumor (8 cm) crossing the lateral edge of the vertebra. No tumoral rupture occurred and the median operative time was 124 min (70–210). The immediate follow-up was uneventful for 16 children. Local staging was stage I in eight patients, stage II in six, and stage III in one. This stage III right WT was not related to spillage or incomplete resection, but to the presence of a vascular tumoral thrombus on the margins of the renal vein division. With a median follow-up of 42 months [12–77], 88.2% children were in complete remission without evidence of disease. None of them had oncological complications (port site or retroperitoneal recurrence, secondary pulmonary metastasis) and no small bowel obstruction occurred. One stage I intermediate-risk left upper pole nephroblastoma relapsed locally 9 months after surgery in the kidney area and was treated by second-line chemotherapy and open surgery; he was in second complete remission at 6 months. The child with the *TFE3* renal cell carcinoma had a local needle biopsy site recurrence 13 months after the biopsy, treated by a parietectomy, but she died 4 years and 2 months after laparoscopic nephrectomy because of pulmonary and cerebral metastases; she had no evidence of port site or retroperitoneal or parietal recurrence.

The indications of laparoscopic radical nephrectomy in children can be summarized, for trained laparoscopic surgeons, as small tumors that do not cross the lateral edge of the vertebra at the time of surgery (Fig. 9.2). Thus, the indications will be probably more frequent in the SIOP protocol with preoperative chemotherapy than in COG protocols without adjuvant chemotherapy [63]. Contraindications include cava or renal thrombosis at time of surgery, adhesions to other organs and initial tumoral rupture to avoid peritoneal spillage, and diffusion by the pneumoperitoneum, even if peritoneal metastases could be removed under laparoscopy, as in one case disease-free at 19 months after surgery [64]. A difficult question remains

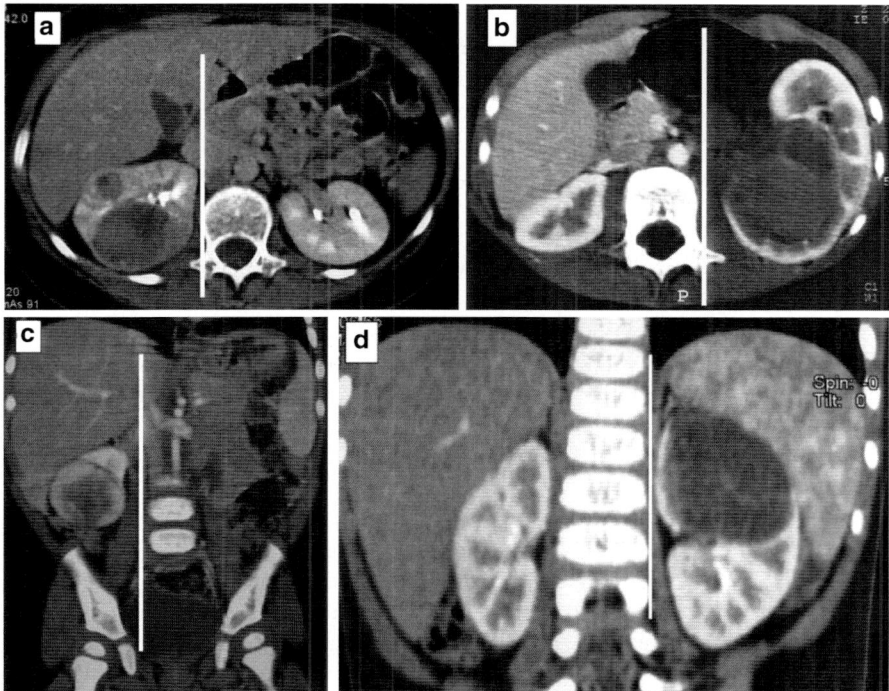

Fig. 9.2 The medial edge of the tumor does not cross the lateral edge of the vertebra (white line). (**a**) TFE3 renal cell carcinoma. (**b**) Wilms' tumor after chemotherapy. (**c**) Clear cell sarcoma. (**d**) Cystic Wilms' tumor (from Varlet et al.) [62]. (*Reprinted with permission from Elsevier*)

concerning the choice between laparoscopic radical nephrectomy and partial open nephrectomy for small polar tumors, that is the choice between the risk of possible renal failure in the long term, about 1% with radical nephrectomy in non-syndromic patients, versus the risk of local recurrence with partial nephrectomy, increased from 3% with radical nephrectomy up to 7–8% in unilateral Wilms' tumor with a poor prognosis in spite of intensive chemotherapy [49, 65–67].

If the surgeon has appropriate training in both endosurgery (nephrectomy, pyeloplasty, or other complex abdominal and thoracic procedures) and surgical oncology, we believe the risk of rupture is similar to open radical nephrectomy in carefully selected cases of renal tumor. Imaging magnification and modern coagulating devices allow safe dissection and little movement of the instruments in the abdominal cavity, avoiding any damage to the tumor [62].

Other articles have been published on the feasibility and satisfactory oncological outcomes for malignant renal tumors:

- Romao et al. in 2014 compared the outcomes of laparoscopic nephrectomy (LN) with open radical nephrectomy (ORN) in the management of consecutive pediatric neoplasms [68]. Demographics from the 45 patients (13 LN, 32 ORN) were similar, and tumors in the LN group were significantly smaller (6.6 ± 1.8 cm *vs.* 11 ± 3 cm ORN). No tumor ruptures occurred with either technique. Wilms tumor (seven LN, 24 ORN) was the most common diagnosis, followed by renal cell carcinoma (four LN, four ORN). Mean length of stay was significantly shorter for LN (3 vs. 6 days). Postoperative narcotic requirements and use of nasogastric tube were higher in the ORN group. After a median follow-up of 18 (LN) and 33 months (ORN), 1 and 4 recurrences occurred, respectively.

- Warmann et al. in 2014 included 24 children undergoing MIS for tumor nephrectomy in the SIOP 2001 trial [52]. Median age at operation was 40 months [14–65]. All patients received preoperative chemotherapy. Median tumor volume was 178 mL at diagnosis (47–958) and 73 mL at surgery (4–776). There was one surgical complication (splenic injury), no intraoperative tumor rupture occurred. Abdominal stage was I in 14, II in 7, and III in 3 patients. Adequate lymph node sampling was performed in only 2 patients. One local relapse occurred. Event-free survival was 23/24, overall survival was 24/24, median follow up was 47 months (2–114).
- Bouty et al. in 2018 analyzed the risk of local recurrence [59]. One hundred and four LTRNs have been performed for WT with neoadjuvant chemotherapy in 93 cases. Tumor was ruptured preoperatively in three cases but never intraoperatively. The median volume of the tumor was 229 mL (4–776 mL). Local stage was specified in 86 cases: 49 stage I, 28 stage II, and nine stage III. Lymph nodes were sampled in 48 patients (median 2.3 [0–14] nodes). Three tumors were initial local stage I (2 intermediate and 1 high risk) and one stage III. With a median follow-up of 20.5 months (1–114), there were four local recurrences (3.8%) at a median of 8.5 [7–9] months after surgery. This local recurrence incidence is lower than previously reported after open resection. However, tumors amenable to minimally invasive surgery are smaller, with higher numbers of low stage and standard histology. Additionally, the quality of the reports is suboptimal, and follow-up is relatively short. However, LTRN does not seem to increase the incidence of local recurrence in WT.
- Harris et al. in 2018 focused on the size of the tumor. Tumors in the laparoscopic group were significantly smaller, but it was possible to excise tumors more than 300 mL. A ratio of tumor to contralateral kidney may be a better guide to safe excision than an overall volume cutoff [69].
- Flores et al. in 2018 described preliminary results of laparoscopic nephrectomies (LN) for the treatment of unilateral Wilms tumors (WT) [70]. Among 105 patients with WT, 14 underwent LN. Median tumor volume for the patients undergoing LN was 72 mL (7–169). Estimated 5-year overall survival for all patients with WT during this period was 88.7%. Two patients underwent conversion. No recurrence or related death was found at a mean 32-month follow-up period.
- Schmidt et al. in 2019 presented their experience (N = 9) with special regard to patient selection and technical aspects [71]. Median tumor volume at surgery, maximal diameter, and specimen weight was 74 mL (15–207), 6.5 cm (3.5–9.3), and 125 g (63–310), respectively. No intra- or postoperative complications

occurred. Overall survival and event-free survival was 9/9, median follow up was 48 months [24–78]. These data were used to propose a patient selection algorithm. Technical aspects derived from our experience include usage of the ureter as leading structure, usage of a transabdominal traction suture around the ureter, and lymph node sampling before tumor nephrectomy.
- Bouty et al. in 2020 underlined the concerns with this approach, in particular with regard to the difficulty of lymph node sampling and the risk of local recurrence [50, 59]. Hence, the UMBRELLA SIOP – RTSG 2016 Wilms tumor protocol has defined criteria for the use and contraindications of MIS in WT [51]. Contraindications include infiltration of extrarenal structures, extension beyond the lateral border of the spinal column, presence of a venous thrombus, and little experience in laparoscopic nephrectomy. During the study period, 50 patients underwent transperitoneal MIS total nephrectomies. The median age at diagnosis was 38 months (6–181). All tumors were unilateral. Renal vein thrombus and preoperative rupture was present in three cases each (6%). Seven patients (14%) presented with lung metastases at diagnosis (stage IV). Twenty-one patients (42%) underwent a percutaneous biopsy prior to initiating treatment. The median volume of the tumors at diagnosis was 2336 mL (66–12,811). Neoadjuvant chemotherapy was vincristine – actinomycin D in 43 cases (86%) with localized disease, vincristine – actinomycinD – doxorubicin in six patients with stage IV WT and a combination of etoposide – carboplatin – cyclophosphamide and doxorubicin in the remaining patient, where WT developed on a previously treated nephroblastomatosis. Lymph node sampling was performed in 42 cases (84%), with a median of four lymph nodes [1–11] present on the pathology report. There were three perioperative complications (6%): one bowel, one splenic vein, and one renal vein injury. There were four diaphragmatic resections, of which two were repaired laparoscopically. Six (12%) patients were converted to an open approach: two for diaphragmatic tears with patients not tolerating insufflation, one for the splenic vein injury, one for the renal vein injury, one due to difficulty in dissecting the renal artery, and one because of an inability to perform the thrombectomy of the vena cava robotically for a thrombus not visible on preoperative CT. Conversions occurred more frequently at the beginning of the experience. There were no intraoperative tumor ruptures. After a median follow-up of 34 months (2–138), 47 patients (94%) were in complete remission, two (4%) presented with local relapse at 7 and 9 months after surgery (both stage I, intermediate risk) and one presented with metastatic relapse to the lungs 4 months after surgery (stage III, high risk). In conclusion, MIS can be used safely in about 20% of cases of WT, with no intraoperative rupture and a 3-year EFS of 94%. Although these tumors are smaller and of lower stages than usually reported, there was only 4% local relapse.

In conclusion, data suggest that laparoscopic nephrectomy for WT is feasible and has promising results in terms of event-free and overall survival [70]. In patients undergoing pre-operative chemotherapy the correct selection for LN is crucial. Following the basic oncological precepts and in experienced centers, LN represents a plausible modality in the care of these patients. One of the major advantage of MIS in WT are lower morbidity especially intestinal obstruction. Even though it is difficult to properly evaluate, the other benefits of laparoscopy likely include a more comfortable postoperative course, quick discharge at day 2 or 3 and a better cosmetic result on the abdominal wall, with three or four small scars on the abdomen and one suprapubic scar instead of a large abdominal scar [14]. This last point was discussed in a recent report providing prevalence data relating to scarring, disfigurement, and persistent hair loss in adult survivors of childhood cancer; they can affect psychological function and quality of life, especially chest or abdominal scars [57]. Minimal invasive surgery should also result in more rapid recovery of patients and immune function [72].

Finally, the risk-benefit balance for laparoscopic radical nephrectomy for Wilms' tumor when feasible seems favorable: the theoretical risks of tumoral rupture, peritoneal diffusion, and port site metastasis, not uncommon in open surgery, remain present with laparoscopy, but do not seem to be significantly increased in carefully selected indications. The benefits are more comfortable postoperative course, decreased hospital stay, improved hospital cost saving, better cosmetic results, and probably a decrease in the incidence of small bowel obstructions.

A prospective registration of performed cases seems mandatory to allow evaluation of the technique and its indications and longer follow-up is mandatory to confirm comparable oncological outcomes to ORN. Multicenter prospective studies are necessary to evaluate and compare the results of the laparoscopic approach with open surgery.

Benign Conditions: Nonfunctioning Kidney and End Stage Renal Disease (ESRD)

The majority of benign indications, e.g., renal dysplasia, non-functioning kidneys secondary to obstructive or refluxing uropathy, or ectopic ureter, or UPJO or MCDK, pretransplant nephrectomy for arterial hypertension, nephrotic syndrome or uremic hemolytic syndrome and nephrolithiasis is suitable for laparoscopic nephrectomy [19, 20, 23, 73, 74]. Same-day discharge after surgery is even feasible and safe for laparoscopic nephrectomy in children [75]. Several studies even indicate that laparoscopic nephrectomy for congenital benign disease in children is achieved safely and that the modality offers additional advantages in children as compared to adults in terms of blood loss, transfusion and perioperative complication [76]. Nonfunctioning kidneys are generally of small size, so they can be extracted via a 10- or 12-mm cannula site without morcellation [20].

The first article comparing open, transperitoneal and retroperitoneal laparoscopic nephrectomy in children for benign renal diseases was published in 1998 by Rassweiler et al. [24]. Analgesic medication requirement per patient and length of hospital stay were lower in case of MIS. They were the first team to conclude that their results demonstrated an overall clear advantage of a laparoscopic approach when compared to open surgery. The literature provides crystal-clear data: very low complications or conversions in well-trained hands are reported [20].

Furthermore, nephrectomy may be indicated in children with ESRD before transplantation. This procedure through a retroperitoneal laparoscopic approach is feasible in this high-risk group of pediatric patients. El Ghoneimi et al. in 2000 reported his series of 12 nephrectomies in nine children with ESRD performed at a mean age of 7 years (7 months–13 years) through three trocars [22]. Cases were classified as American Society of Anesthesiologists grade III and presented with ESRD, hypertension, thrombocytopenia and/or nephrotic syndrome. The renal artery and vein were ligated separately with endocorporeal knots and clips. No conversion nor intraoperative complications were recorded. The same conclusion was reported by Szymanski et al. in 2010 stating that retroperitoneoscopic nephrectomy for ESRD is a safe and effective technique that preserves peritoneal integrity in children who require immediate postoperative peritoneal dialysis [77]. Avoiding post-nephrectomy hemodialysis decreases patient morbidity, preserving vessels for future vascular access. Moreover, en-bloc removal of horseshoe kidney for ESRD is feasible through retroperitoneoscopy with early postoperative reinitiating peritoneal dialysis [78].

The introduction of laparoscopic procedures has allowed the development of techniques that reduce patient morbidity, hospital stay, and analgesia requirement. Steven et al. also reported a series of 13 children who underwent elective laparoscopic nephrectomy for unilateral multicystic dysplastic kidney and emphasized the advantages this procedure has to offer for their management [79].

Severe Urinary Tract Infections

A total of 23 successful retroperitoneoscopic nephrectomies for pyonephrosis were first performed by Lucan et al. and published in 2004 [80]. Although technically difficult, retroperitoneoscopic nephrectomy for pyonephrosis is feasible. The extraperitoneal approach allows direct access to the renal hilum and helps avoid spillage of pus into the peritoneum. Even if the operative time is longer than in classic lumbotomy, blood loss, hospital stay, wound complications and time of return to school are significantly in favor of laparoscopy.

Nephrectomy for xanthogranulomatous pyelonephritis (XGP) can be extremely challenging. Josh et al. published three laparoscopic nephrectomies performed at 1, 5 and 9 years for this severe and chronic infection [81]. Creation of retroperitoneal space was easier than anticipated despite the perinephric inflammation. Excellent visualization of renal pedicle was obtained. The renal vessels were divided using the ultrasonic dissector. Postoperative pain and morbidity were greatly reduced. However, in case of XGP, retroperitoneoscopy may be contraindicated according to Esposito et al. [74].

In conclusion, there is no data showing any superiority of retroperitoneal (RP) to transperitoneal (TP) and to posterior prone retroperitoneoscopic (PRP) approach for laparoscopic nephrectomy in children. Kim et al. published in 2009 a systematic review including 51 articles that reported the outcomes of 689 pediatric nephrectomies [82]. Of these, 401 were RP and 288 were TP laparoscopic renal surgeries in children. The mean patient age for RP and TP was 5.4 years and 4.8 years, respectively. The mean operative time was 129 min for RP and 154 min for TP. The hospital stay was 2.5 days for RP and 2.3 days for TP. The overall complication rate for RP was 4.3% and for TP was 3.5% ($p > 0.05$). The number of vascular injuries for RP was 2 and for TP was 0 ($p > 0.05$). The number of bowel injuries for RP was 2 and for TP was 1 ($p > 0.05$). Gundetti et al. also concluded in his series of 100 consecutive nephrectomies performed by MIS that both the TP and PRP approaches for nephrectomy are equally applicable in children [83]. It is also safe and feasible in infants younger than 12 months and weighing 10 kg or less [84].

Moreover, nephrectomy via laparo-endoscopic single site (LESS) surgery (also known as single incision laparoscopic surgery or SILS) is associated with shorter lengths of hospital stay and decreased postoperative pain medication use when compared with open surgery [14]. LESS nephrectomy in children is associated with similar surgical times, lengths of hospital stay and postoperative pain medication use as the other minimally invasive modalities (TP and RA) [16].

Complication rate is relatively low. Nephrectomy had a significantly lower frequency of grade III complications (1.2%) compared to pyeloplasty (3.6%), ureteral reimplantation (6.7%) and complex reconstruction (11.8%) ($p < 0.05$) in the largest systematic review of 5864 pediatric patients who had minimally invasive surgery [85]. Conversion rate is globally low too [85, 86]. Need for reoperation is often associated with the underlying diagnosis and the natural sequelae of the disease process.

Only Baez et al. reported the operating time may be slightly shorter and postoperative recovery significantly longer for transperitoneal nephrectomy (TP) in comparison to retroperitoneal nephrectomy (RP) [87]. TP may be associated with minimal paralytic ileus within the first 24 h, meanwhile RP requires a different surgical skillset, but the patient may have a postoperative tolerance. Esposito et al. in 2016 concluded that LN ($N = 101$) is easier and faster to perform compared to RN ($N = 48$) and complication rate was higher after RN compared to LN [74]. Eight complications (5.3%) were recorded: 3 small bleedings (2 RN, 1 LN) during dissection, 2 peritoneal perforations during RN requiring conversion in LN, 1 abdominal abscess in case of XGP after LN requiring a redo surgery to drain the abscess, 1 instrumentation failure (LN) and 1 refluxing ureteral stump after RN requiring a redo surgery to remove it. Moreover, they concluded that LN is better in case of nephroureterectomy for VUR as the symptoms related to a refluxing distal ureteral stump (DUS) occurred only in patients undergoing retroperitoneoscopic nephroureterectomy, where the DUS was longer than the DUS detected in laparoscopic patients [88].

In conclusion, retroperitoneal, prone posterior and transperitoneal have no clear sono significant advantage is gained by a RP, PPR or TP approach for laparoscopic nephrectomy. MIS is associated with a lower postoperative complication rate than for open procedures [89]. The management of renal pathologies using laparoscopy is now currently the approach of choice for most pediatric renal diseases [90]. The incidence of vascular and bowel injuries is rare for all approaches. Therefore, the choice of approach should be determined by surgeon preference, patient anatomy, or the procedure to be performed. Higher-volume MIS centers also reach a lower complication rate than lower-volume centers [89].

Robot-Assisted

As robotics continue to grow in use and applications we expect to see further reports of successful adoption of above laparoscopic success now applied with robotic assistance. This follows lateral spread of skills from existing laparoscopy in pediatric urology and surgery as well as transfer of techniques first implemented in adult robotic surgery. In this vein, Varda and colleagues reports on a series of eight pediatric urologic oncology cases done in collaboration with their adult colleagues, including one nephrectomy with pericaval lymph node dissection [91]. In the field of renal transplantation, successful donor nephrectomies have been reported in a small series [92]. A meta-analysis of adult patients comparing robotic and laparoscopic partial nephrectomy found similar operative time and EBL. Patients treated with robotic partial nephrectomy has larger tumors with higher mean R.E.N.A.L. nephrometry scores and had a decreased likelihood of conversion to open surgery, lower any and major (Clavien 1 or greater and Clavian 3 or greater) complications with shorter warm ischemia time [93]. Partial nephrectomies of both upper and lower pole non-functional moieties have been reported. Bansal et al. reported on 24 patients undergoing pediatric robotic-assisted laparoscopic nephro-ureterectomy versus a laparoendoscopic single-site approach [94]. There was no difference in age, weight, hospital stay and pain medication use. There was a longer operative time with a robotic approach (mean 227 min versus 174 min). In the question of robotic versus open surgical approaches, a comparison by Ballouhey of 28 pediatric patients undergoing heminephrectomy for duplex kidney found lower length of stay and total narcotic use, but similar operative time, renal outcomes and complication rate (drain-site omental hernia and an asymptomatic fluid collection in the robotic group) [95]. While further literature examining only pediatric robotic-assisted laparoscopic nephrectomies are fewer in the literature, this is likely due to the well-established role that laparoscopic nephrectomies have already been shown, with practice following and adopting robotics. Newer literature now focuses on complex reconstruction and partial nephrectomies in the pediatric urologic literature.

Conclusion

Indications for minimally invasive surgery in pediatric urology are expanding, with more centers being involved in the evolution of various procedures. To avoid a discouraging learning curve, we recommend that pediatric urologists acquire their experience in a progressive pattern. Nephrectomy for multicystic dysplastic kidney or hydronephrosis is a relatively safe and easy procedure which acquaints the surgeon with laparoscopic exposure to the upper tract. When the surgeon is familiar with this exposure, he/she can proceed to more difficult nephrectomies (pretransplant, partial nephrectomy). Time can only be limited by training. Today, training is easily available in many centers of adult and pediatric surgery. Experienced peers are also available to accompany the surgeon during the initial experience, especially in the era of robotic surgery. This might improve the results during the initial experience with laparoscopy and encourage its development among larger number of pediatric urologists. Minimal access procedures emphasize our goals of improving patient comfort and safety while adapting the laparoscopic procedures as closely as possible to conventional surgical techniques with respect to the operative time, cost, and surgical principles.

References

1. Peters CA. Laparoendoscopic renal surgery in children. J Endourol. 2000;14(10):841–7; discussion 847–848.
2. Joyeux L, Lacreuse I, Schneider A, Moog R, Borgnon J, Lopez M, et al. Long-term functional renal outcomes after retroperitoneoscopic upper pole heminephrectomy for duplex kidney in children: a multicenter cohort study. Surg Endosc. 2017;31(3):1241–9.
3. Heloury Y, Muthucumaru M, Panabokke G, Cheng W, Kimber C, Leclair MD. Minimally invasive adrenalectomy in children. J Pediatr Surg. 2012;47(2):415–21.
4. Jayram G, Roberts J, Hernandez A, Heloury Y, Manoharan S, Godbole P, et al. Outcomes and fate of the remnant moiety following laparoscopic heminephrectomy for duplex kidney: a multicenter review. J Pediatr Urol. 2011;7(3):272–5.
5. Borzi PA. A comparison of the lateral and posterior retroperitoneoscopic approach for complete and partial nephroureterectomy in children. BJU Int. 2001;87(6):517–20.
6. Gaur DD. Laparoscopic operative retroperitoneoscopy: use of a new device. J Urol. 1992;148(4):1137–9.
7. Adams JB, Micali S, Moore RG, Babayan RK, Kavoussi LR. Complications of extraperitoneal balloon dilation. J Endourol. 1996;10(4):375–8.
8. Capolicchio J-P, Jednak R, Anidjar M, Pippi-Salle JL. A modified access technique for retroperitoneoscopic renal surgery in children. J Urol. 2003;170(1):204–6.
9. Micali S, Caione P, Virgili G, Capozza N, Scarfini M, Micali F. Retroperitoneal laparoscopic access in children using a direct vision technique. J Urol. 2001;165(4):1229–32.
10. Cadeddu JA, Chan DY, Hedican SP, Lee BR, Moore RG, Kavoussi LR, et al. Retroperitoneal access for transperitoneal laparoscopy in patients at high risk for intra-abdominal scarring. J Endourol. 1999;13(8):567–70.
11. Johnson KC, Cha DY, DaJusta DG, Barone JG, Ankem MK. Pediatric single-port-access nephrectomy for a multicystic, dysplastic kidney. J Pediatr Urol. 2009;5(5):402–4.
12. Kocherov S, Lev G, Shenfeld OZ, Chertin B. Laparoscopic single site surgery: initial experience and description of techniques in the pediatric population. J Urol. 2011;186(4 Suppl):1653–7.
13. Liem NT, Dung LA, Viet ND. Single trocar retroperitoneoscopic nephrectomy for unilateral multicystic dysplastic kidney in children. Pediatr Surg Int. 2012;28(6):641–3.
14. Kim PH, Patil MB, Kim SS, Dorey F, De Filippo RE, Chang AY, et al. Early comparison of nephrectomy options in children (open, transperitoneal laparoscopic, laparo-endoscopic single site (LESS), and robotic surgery). BJU Int. 2012;109(6):910–5.
15. Cherian A, De Win G. Single incision retro-peritoneoscopic paediatric nephrectomy: early experience. J Pediatr Urol. 2014;10(3):564–6.

16. Aneiros Castro B, Cabezalí Barbancho D, Tordable Ojeda C, Carrillo Arroyo I, Redondo Sedano J, Gómez FA. Laparoendoscopic single-site nephrectomy in children: is it a good alternative to conventional laparoscopic approach? J Pediatr Urol. 2018;14(1):49.e1–4.
17. Patel N, Santomauro M, Marietti S, Chiang G. Laparoendoscopic single site surgery in pediatric urology: does it require specialized tools? Int Braz J Urol. 2016;42(2):277–83.
18. Diamond DA, Price HM, McDougall EM, Bloom DA. Retroperitoneal laparoscopic nephrectomy in children. J Urol. 1995 153(6):1966–8.
19. Valla JS, Guilloneau B, Montupet P, Geiss S, Steyaert H, el Ghoneimi A, et al. Retroperitoneal laparoscopic nephrectomy in children. Preliminary report of 18 cases. Eur Urol. 1996;30(4):490–3.
20. Valla JS, Guilloneau B, Mortupet P, Geiss S, Steyaert H, Leculee R, et al. Retroperitoneal laparoscopic nephrectomy in children: preliminary report of six cases. J Laparoendosc Surg. 1996;6(Suppl 1):S55–9.
21. El-Ghoneimi A, Valla JS, Steyaert H, Aigrain Y. Laparoscopic renal surgery via a retroperitoneal approach in children. J Urol. 1998;160(3 Pt 2):1138–41.
22. El-Ghoneimi A, Sauty L, Maintenant J, Macher MA, Lottmann H, Aigrain Y. Laparoscopic retroperitoneal nephrectomy in high risk children. J Urol. 2000;164(3 Pt 2):1076–9.
23. El-Ghoneimi A, Abou-Hashim H, Bonnard A, Verkauskas G, Macher M-A, Huot O, et al. Retroperitoneal laparoscopic nephrectomy in children: at last the gold standard? J Pediatr Urol. 2006;2(4):357–63.
24. Rassweiler J, Frede T, Henkel TO, Stock C, Alken P. Nephrectomy: a comparative study between the transperitoneal and retroperitoneal laparoscopic versus the open approach. Eur Urol. 1998;33(5):489–96.
25. Davies BW, Najmaldin AS. Transperitoneal laparoscopic nephrectomy in children. J Endourol. 1998;12(5):437–40.
26. Rassweiler J, Fornara P, Weber M, Janetschek G, Fahlenkamp D, Henkel T, et al. Laparoscopic nephrectomy: the experience of the laparoscopy working group of the German Urologic Association. J Urol. 1998;160(1):18–21.
27. Spinoit A-F, Nguyen H, Subramaniam R. Role of robotics in children: a brave new world! Eur Urol Focus. 2017;3(2–3):172–80.
28. Mahida JB, Cooper JN, Herz D, Diefenbach KA, Deans KJ, Minneci PC, et al. Utilization and costs associated with robotic surgery in children. J Surg Res. 2015;199(1):169–76.
29. Andolfi C, Kumar R, Boysen WR, Gundeti MS. Current status of robotic surgery in pediatric urology. J Laparoendosc Adv Surg Tech A. 2019;29(2):159–66.
30. Lee DI, Schwab CW, Harris A. Robot-assisted ureteroureterostomy in the adult: initial clinical series. Urology. 2010;75(3):570–3.
31. Pedraza R, Palmer L, Moss V, Franco I. Bilateral robotic assisted laparoscopic heminephroureterectomy. J Urol 2004;171(6 Pt 1):2394–5.
32. Srinivasan AK, Shrivastava D, Kurzweil RE, Weiss DA, Long CJ, Shukla AR. Port site local anesthetic infiltration vs single-dose intrathecal opioid injection to control perioperative pain in children undergoing minimal invasive surgery: a comparative analysis. Urology. 2016;97:179–83.
33. Sala LFM, Guglielmetti GE, Coelho RF. Bilateral nephrectomy robotic-assisted laparoscopic in children with bilateral Wilms' tumor. Urol Case Rep. 2020;31:101146.
34. Gargollo PC. Hidden incision endoscopic surgery: description of technique, parental satisfaction and applications. J Urol 2011;185(4):1425–31.
35. Chang C, Steinberg Z, Shah A, Gundeti MS. Patient positioning and port placement for robot-assisted surgery. J Endourol. 2014;28(6):631–8.
36. Agrawal S, Kalathia J, Chipde SS, Mishra U, Tyagi A, Parashar S. Laparoscopic heminephrectomy in horseshoe kidneys: a single center experience. Urol Ann. 2017;9(4):357–61.
37. Lottmann H, Pio L, Heloury Y, Boyer O, Aigrain Y, Blanc T. Left lateral retroperitoneoscopic total nephrectomy of a horseshoe kidney in a 3-year-old boy. J Pediatr Urol. 2019;15(5):574–5.

38. Venkat Ramanan S, Velmurugan P, Bhaskar Prakash AR, Arora A, Karri L. A case of incomplete removal of horseshoe kidney by laparoscopic nephrectomy in an adult leading to urinary leak: an eye opener. Case Rep Urol. 2019;2019:4132521.
39. Kumar S, Singh S, Jain S, Bora GS, Singh SK. Robot-assisted heminephrectomy for chromophobe renal cell carcinoma in L-shaped fused crossed ectopia: surgical challenge. Korean J Urol. 2015;56(10):729–32.
40. Herz D, DaJusta D, Ching C, McLeod D. Segmental arterial mapping during pediatric robot-assisted laparoscopic heminephrectomy: a descriptive series. J Pediatr Urol. 2016;12(4):266.e1–6.
41. Oyinloye AO, Wabada S, Abubakar AM, Oyebanji LO, Rikin CU. Wilms tumor in a left pelvic kidney: a case report. Int J Surg Case Rep. 2019;66:115–7.
42. Brown CT, Sebastião YV, McLeod DJ. Trends in surgical management of multicystic dysplastic kidney at USA children's hospitals. J Pediatr Urol. 2019;15(4):368–73.
43. Majid MH, Meshkat B, Kohar H, El Masry S. Specimen retrieval during elective laparoscopic cholecystectomy: is it safe not to use a retrieval bag? BMC Surg. 2016;16(1):64.
44. Kao C-C, Cha T-L, Sun G-H, et al. Cost-effective homemade specimen retrieval bag for use in laparoscopic surgery: experience at a single center. Asian J Surg. 2012;35(4):140–3.
45. Ganpule AP, Gotov E, Mishra S, Muthu V, Sabnis R, Desai M. Novel Cost-effective specimen retrieval bag in laparoscopy: Nadiad bag. Urology. 2010;75(5):1213–6.
46. Deshmukh CS, Ganpule AP, Islam MR, Sabnis RB, Desai MR. Laparoscopic and robotic specimen retrieval system (Modified Nadiad Bag): validation and cost-effectiveness study model. J Minim Access Surg. 2019;15(4):305–10.
47. Urologic Procedures and Antimicrobial Prophylaxis. American Urological Association [Internet]. 2019. [cited 2020 Apr 19]. Available from: https://www.auanet.org/guidelines/urologic-procedures-and-antimicrobial-prophylaxis-(2019).
48. Kieran K, Anderson JR, Dome JS, Ehrlich PF, Ritchey ML, Shamberger RC, et al. Lymph node involvement in Wilms tumor: results from National Wilms Tumor Studies 4 and 5. J Pediatr Surg. 2012;47(4):700–6.
49. Zhuge Y, Cheung MC, Yang R, Koniaris LG, Neville HL, Sola JE. Improved survival with lymph node sampling in Wilms tumor. J Surg Res. 2011;167(2):e199–203.
50. Bouty A, Blanc T, Leclair MD, Lavrand F, Faure A, Binet A, et al. Minimally invasive surgery for unilateral Wilms tumors: multicenter retrospective analysis of 50 transperitoneal laparoscopic total nephrectomies. Pediatr Blood Cancer. 2020;67(5):e28212.
51. van den Heuvel-Eibrink MM, Hol JA, Pritchard-Jones K, van Tinteren H, Furtwängler R, Verschuur AC, et al. Position paper: rationale for the treatment of Wilms tumour in the UMBRELLA SIOP-RTSG 2016 protocol. Nat Rev Urol. 2017;14(12):743–52.
52. Warmann SW, Godzinski J, van Tinteren H, Heij H, Powis M, Sandstedt B, et al. Minimally invasive nephrectomy for Wilms tumors in children - data from SIOP 2001. J Pediatr Surg. 2014;49(11):1544–8.
53. Burnand K, Roberts A, Bouty A, Nightingale M, Campbell M, Heloury Y. Laparoscopic nephrectomy for Wilms' tumor: can we expand on the current SIOP criteria? J Pediatr Urol. 2018;14(3):253.e1–8.
54. Stewart CL, Bruny JL. Maximizing lymph node retrieval during surgical resection of Wilms tumor. Eur J Pediatr Surg. 2015;25(1):109–12.
55. Pritchard-Jones K, Bergeron C, de Camargo B, van den Heuvel-Eibrink MM, Acha T, Godzinski J, et al. Omission of doxorubicin from the treatment of stage II-III, intermediate-risk Wilms' tumour (SIOP WT 2001): an open-label, non-inferiority, randomised controlled trial. Lancet Lond Engl. 2015;386(9999):1156–64.
56. Aguayo P, Ho B, Fraser JD, Gamis A, St Peter SD, Snyder CL. Bowel obstruction after treatment of intra-abdominal tumors. Eur J Pediatr Surg. 2010;20(4):234–6.
57. Kinahan KE, Sharp LK, Seidel K, Leisenring W, Didwania A, Lacouture ME, et al. Scarring, disfigurement, and quality of life in long-term survivors of childhood cancer: a report from the Childhood Cancer Survivor study. J Clin Oncol Off J Am Soc Clin Oncol. 2012;30(20):2466–74.

58. Duarte RJ, Dénes FT, Cristofari LM, Giron AM, Filho VO, Arap S. Laparoscopic nephrectomy for wilms tumor after chemotherapy: initial experience. J Urol. 2004;172(4 Pt 1):1438–40.
59. Bouty A, Burnand K, Nightingale M, Roberts A, Campbell M, O'Brien M, et al. What is the risk of local recurrence after laparoscopic transperitoneal radical nephrectomy in children with Wilms tumours? Analysis of a local series and review of the literature. J Pediatr Urol. 2018;14(4):327.e1–7.
60. Duarte RJ, Dénes FT, Cristofani LM, Odone-Filho V, Srougi M. Further experience with laparoscopic nephrectomy for Wilms' tumour after chemotherapy BJU Int. 2006;98(1):155–9.
61. Varlet F, Stephan JL, Guye E, Allary R, Berger C, Lopez M. Laparoscopic radical nephrectomy for unilateral renal cancer in children. Surg Laparosc Endosc Percutan Tech. 2009;19(2):148–52.
62. Varlet F, Petit T, Leclair M-D, Lardy H, Geiss S, Becmeur F, et al. Laparoscopic treatment of renal cancer in children: a multicentric study and review of oncologic and surgical complications. J Pediatr Urol. 2014;10(3):500–5.
63. Barber TD, Wickiser JE, Wilcox DT, Baker LA. Prechemotherapy laparoscopic nephrectomy for Wilms' tumor. J Pediatr Urol. 2009;5(5):416–9.
64. Javid PJ, Lendvay TS, Acierno S, Gow KW. Laparoscopic nephroureterectomy for Wilms' tumor: oncologic considerations. J Pediatr Surg. 2011;46(5):978–82.
65. Cost NG, Lubahn JD, Granberg CF, Schlomer BJ, Wickiser JE, Rakheja D, et al. Oncologic outcomes of partial versus radical nephrectomy for unilateral Wilms tumor. Pediatr Blood Cancer. 2012;58(6):898–904.
66. Godzinski J, Tournade MF, deKraker J, Lemerle J, Voute PA, Weirich A, et al. Rarity of surgical complications after postchemotherapy nephrectomy for nephroblastoma. Experience of the International Society of Paediatric Oncology-Trial and Study "SIOP-9". International Society of Paediatric Oncology Nephroblastoma Trial and Study Committee. Eur J Pediatr Surg. 1998;8(2):83–6.
67. Shamberger RC, Guthrie KA, Ritchey ML, Haase GM, Takashima J, Beckwith JB, et al. Surgery-related factors and local recurrence of Wilms tumor in National Wilms Tumor Study 4. Ann Surg. 1999;229(2):292–7.
68. Romao RLP, Weber B, Gerstle JT, Grant R, Pippi Salle JL, Bägli DJ, et al. Comparison between laparoscopic and open radical nephrectomy for the treatment of primary renal tumors in children: single-center experience over a 5-year period. J Pediatr Urol. 2014;10(3):488–94.
69. Harris AC, Brownlee EM, Ramaesh R, Jackson M, Munro FD, MacKinlay GA. Feasibility of laparoscopic tumour nephrectomy in children. J Pediatr Surg. 2018;53(2):302–5.
70. Flores P, Cadario M, Lenz Y, Cacciavillano W, Galluzzo L, Nestor Paz EG, et al. Laparoscopic total nephrectomy for Wilms tumor: towards new standards of care. J Pediatr Urol. 2018;14(5):388–93.
71. Schmidt A, Warmann SW, Urla C, Schaefer J, Fideler F, Fuchs J. Patient selection and technical aspects for laparoscopic nephrectomy in Wilms tumor. Surg Oncol. 2019;29:14–9.
72. Cribbs RK, Wulkan ML, Heiss KF, Gow KW. Minimally invasive surgery and childhood cancer. Surg Oncol. 2007;16(3):221–8.
73. Suzuki K, Ihara H, Kurita Y, Kageyama S, Ueda D, Ushiyama T, et al. Laparoscopic nephrectomy for atrophic kidney associated with ectopic ureter in a child. Eur Urol. 1993;23(4):463–5.
74. Esposito C, Escolino M, Corcione F, Draghici IM, Savanelli A, Castagnetti M, et al. Twenty-year experience with laparoscopic and retroperitoneoscopic nephrectomy in children: considerations and details of technique. Surg Endosc. 2016;30(5) 2114–8.
75. Ilie CP, Luscombe CJ, Smith I, Boddy J, Mischianu D, Golash A. Day case laparoscopic nephrectomy. J Endourol. 2011;25(4):631–4.
76. Ku JH, Byun S-S, Choi H, Kim HH. Laparoscopic nephrectomy for congenital benign renal diseases in children: comparison with adults. Acta Paediatr. 2005;94(12):1752–5.
77. Szymanski KM, Bitzan M, Capolicchio J-P. Is retroperitoneoscopy the gold standard for endoscopic nephrectomy in children on peritoneal dialysis? J Urol. 2010;184(4 Suppl):1631–7.

78. Weatherly D, Budzyn B, Steinhardt GF, Barber TD. En bloc retroperitoneoscopic removal of horseshoe kidney for end-stage renal disease. Urology. 2015;86(4):814–6.
79. Steven LC, Li AGK, Driver CP, Mahomed AA. Laparoscopic nephrectomy for unilateral multicystic dysplastic kidney in children. Surg Endosc. 2005;19(8):1135–8.
80. Lucan M, Iacob G, Lucan C, Yohannes P, Rotariu P. Retroperitoneoscopic nephrectomy v classic lumbotomy for pyonephrosis. J Endourol. 2004;18(3):215–9.
81. Joshi AA, Parashar K, Chandran H. Laparoscopic nephrectomy for xanthogranulomatous pyelonephritis in childhood: the way forward. J Pediatr Urol. 2008;4(3):203–5.
82. Kim C, McKay K, Docimo SG. Laparoscopic nephrectomy in children: systematic review of transperitoneal and retroperitoneal approaches. Urology. 2009;73(2):280–4.
83. Gundeti MS, Patel Y, Duffy PG, Cuckow PM, Wilcox DT, Mushtaq I. An initial experience of 100 paediatric laparoscopic nephrectomies with transperitoneal or posterior prone retroperitoneoscopic approach. Pediatr Surg Int. 2007;23(8):795–9.
84. You D, Hong S, Lee C, Kim KS. Feasibility and safety of laparoscopic ablative renal surgery in infants: comparative study with children. J Urol. 2012;188(4):1330–4.
85. Aksenov LI, Granberg CF, Gargollo PC. A systematic review of complications of minimally invasive surgery in the pediatric urological literature. J Urol. 2020;203(5):1010–6.
86. MacDonald C, Small R, Flett M, Cascio S, O'Toole S. Predictors of complications following retroperitoneoscopic total and partial nephrectomy. J Pediatr Surg. 2019;54(2):331–4.
87. Baez JJN, Luna CM, Mesples GF, Arias AJ, Courel JM. Laparoscopic transperitoneal and retroperitoneal nephrectomies in children: a change of practice. J Laparoendosc Adv Surg Tech A. 2010;20(1):81–5.
88. Escolino M, Farina A, Turrà F, Cerulo M, Esposito R, Savanelli A, et al. Evaluation and outcome of the distal ureteral stump after nephro-ureterectomy in children. A comparison between laparoscopy and retroperitoneoscopy. J Pediatr Urol. 2016;12(2):119.e1–8.
89. Tejwani R, Young BJ, Wang H-HS, Wolf S, Purves JT, Wiener JS, et al. Open versus minimally invasive surgical approaches in pediatric urology: trends in utilization and complications. J Pediatr Urol. 2017;13(3):283.e1–9.
90. Bowlin PR, Farhat WA. Laparoscopic nephrectomy and partial nephrectomy: intraperitoneal, retroperitoneal, single site. Urol Clin North Am. 2015;42(1):31–42.
91. Varda BK, Cho P, Wagner AA, Lee RS. Collaborating with our adult colleagues: a case series of robotic surgery for suspicious and cancerous lesions in children and young adults performed in a free-standing children's hospital. J Pediatr Urol. 2018;14(2):182.e1–8.
92. Akin EB, Aydogdu I, Barlas IS. Introducing robot-assisted laparoscopic donor nephrectomy after experience in hand-assisted retroperitoneoscopic approach. Transplant Proc. 2019;51(7):2221–4.
93. Leow JJ, Heah NH, Chang SL, et al. Outcomes of robotic versus laparoscopic partial nephrectomy: an updated meta-analysis of 4,919 patients. J Urol. 2016;196(5):1371–7.
94. Bansal D, Cost NG, Bean CM, Riachy E, Defoor WR, Reddy PP, et al. Comparison of pediatric robotic-assisted laparoscopic nephroureterectomy and laparoendoscopic single-site nephroureterectomy. Urology. 2014;83(2):438–42.
95. Ballouhey Q, Binet A, Clermidi P, Braik K, Villemagne T, Cros J, et al. Partial nephrectomy for small children: robot-assisted versus open surgery. Int J Urol. 2017;24(12):855–60.

Chapter 10
Complex Upper Tract Reconstruction

Angela M. Arlen, Karmon M. Janssen, and Andrew J. Kirsch

Introduction

The use of minimally invasive surgery (MIS) has gained widespread acceptance in the pediatric population, due to advantages including quicker postoperative recovery, fewer analgesic requirements, shorter length of hospital stay, and superior cosmetic outcomes [1]. Robotic technology has bridged the gap between open and laparoscopic surgery with magnified three-dimensionality, superior stereoscopic visualization and enhanced precision of movement that allows 90 degrees of articulation and 7 degrees of freedom, in addition to tremor filtration and ergonomic comfort [2]. These advantages make robot-assisted surgery (RAS) an ideal approach for complex upper tract reconstruction.

Ureterocalicostomy is a potential option for children with ureteropelvic junction obstruction associated with significant lower pole calicectasis; it is typically utilized in patients with a prior failed pyeloplasty and intrarenal pelvis. Horseshoe kidney is the most common renal fusion anomaly, and is associated with duplication, vesicoureteral reflux and ureteropelvic junction obstruction (UPJO). Because the joined kidneys fail to rotate, the pelvis and ureters are atypical in orientation, with an anterior position. Horseshoe kidneys have an increased risk of UPJO secondary to high ureteral insertion, aberrant crossing vessels and abnormal ureteral course anterior to the isthmus [3]. As pediatric surgeons expertise has grown, the indications for

A. M. Arlen
Yale University School of Medicine, Department of Urology, New Haven, CT, USA
e-mail: angela.arler@yale.edu

K. M. Janssen
Emory University, Children's Healthcare of Atlanta, Department of Pediatric Urology, Atlanta, GA, USA

A. J. Kirsch (✉)
Emory University, Children's Healthcare of Atlanta, Atlanta, GA, USA

robot-assisted laparoscopic surgery have expanded to include more anatomically challenging cases such as ureterocalicostomy and pyeloplasty in horseshoe kidney.

Indications

Options for definitive surgical intervention of complicated upper tract obstruction may include both reconstructive and extirpative procedures, depending upon function of the affected moiety. Persistent, symptomatic ureteropelvic junction obstruction after failed pyeloplasty represents a challenging clinical scenario. Ureterocalicostomy involves excision of hydronephrotic lower pole with anastomosis of the dismembered ureter directly to the lower pole calyx [4]. Indication for ureterocalicostomy are relative as it is a potential salvage option in children with ureteropelvic junction obstruction and significant lower pole calicectasis. It is often reserved for those patients with a prior failed pyeloplasty and a minimal pelvis, or patients with an exaggerated intrarenal pelvis [5, 6].

Surgical indications for UPJO in children with horseshoe kidney are the same as those with normal kidneys – symptomatic patients recurrent flank pain, poor drainage and declining renal function [7]. Traditionally, management included open dismembered pyeloplasty, with laparoscopic and robot-assisted laparoscopic pyeloplasty gaining increasing popularity and more widespread acceptance. The primary technical challenges of pyeloplasty in this population relate to aberrant lower pole vessels, unfamiliar caudal position with malrotation of the kidney, and the renal isthmus [8, 9]. While renal scintigraphy is often used to confirm obstruction, in cases of complex upper tract reconstruction such as fusion anomaly or secondary UPJO, the authors prefer magnetic resonance urography (MRU), as it has the unique advantage of providing both functional *and* anatomic details of the urinary tract [10].

General Surgical Principles

- Typical patient positioning is the modified flank/lateral decubitus position with arms at the sides and the affected side elevated approximately 45 degrees; the surgeon must ensure all pressure points are adequately padded and the child is appropriately secured to the table. Rotation thereafter places the patient in a more lateral position providing excellent exposure and avoiding the need for a traditional lateral decubitus position and the need for axillary role.
- Monofilament hitch stitch in renal pelvis is routinely used for traction to facilitate dissection.
- Limited direct handling of ureter with care taken to preserve ureteral blood supply.
- Anastomosis may be performed in a running or interrupted fashion; the authors prefer a small absorbable braided suture with knots placed extraluminally.

- After the posterior anastomosis is complete, a double J stent is placed if not previously done, followed by completion of the anterior anastomosis; the authors leave an indwelling stent for 4–6 weeks postoperatively. Anastomosis should be tension free and watertight. Pre-stenting may decompress the renal pelvis and make anatomy awkward and more difficult to discern tissue planes.
- Placement of a closed suction or penrose drain is at the surgeon's discretion; the authors do not routinely leave a drain.
- Renal-bladder ultrasound is obtained approximately 4–6 weeks after stent removal, with additional imaging obtained as clinically indicated

Robot-assisted Laparoscopic Ureterocalicostomy

Many factors are considered when determining the optimal surgical approach for a given child. Minimally invasive surgical techniques are increasingly utilized in the pediatric population for complex reconstruction, and pure laparoscopic ureterocalicostomy has been described in an adult patient cohort [11]. However, given the need for delicate intracorporeal suturing, robotic surgery is particularly advantageous for these reconstructive procedures [5, 12, 13]. In comparison to open surgery, robotic surgery has been associated with decreased morbidity, less postoperative pain, lower analgesic requirements, quicker postoperative recovery, and shorter hospital stays. While improved cosmesis is often considered a benefit over open surgery, the location in addition to scar size, impacts patient satisfaction [14].

Robotic ureterocalicostomy is considered when anatomy is not amendable to standard dismembered pyeloplasty but renal function warrants reconstruction rather than excision. A transperitoneal approach is taken, with port placement similar to pyeloplasty. After reflection of the colon and adequate dissection, the ureter is sharply transected and spatulated. The hilum is mobilized to allow for rapid vascular control if necessary. The most dependent lower pole calix is then amputated with a hot shears, and any bleeding controlled with electrocautery. The posterior anastomosis is performed with 5–0 absorbable sutures in a running fashion. A double J ureteral stent is then placed in an antegrade fashion. The anterior anastomosis is performed in an interrupted manner, allowing for visualization and approximation of the renal collecting system to the ureteral mucosa without placing tension on the renal parenchyma (Fig. 10.1).

Robot-assisted Laparoscopic Pyeloplasty in Horseshoe Kidney

Horseshoe kidney occurs in 1 in 400–600 individuals and affects males twice as often as females. The lower renal poles are fused by a fibrous or parenchymal isthmus over the spine across the midline (Fig. 10.2). As the kidneys fail to rotate, the pelvis and ureters are atypical in orientation, which may result in high ureteral

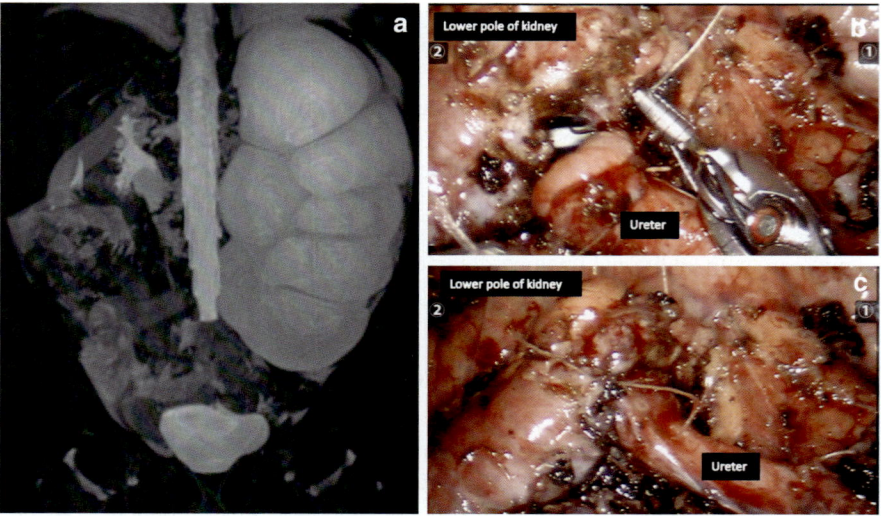

Fig. 10.1 Preop imaging of child with massively dilated left collecting system (**a**). After exposure of the lower pole and identification/mobilization of the ureter, the proximal ureter is transected distal to the level of obstruction. The ureter is then spatulated. The hydronephrotic lower pole is amputated and any bleeding controlled with electrocautery. The posterior anastomosis is performed in a running fashion with 5-0 Vicryl. After placement of a double J stent (**b**), the anterior anastomosis is performed in an interrupted fashion allowing for optimal visualization and approximation of the renal collecting system to the ureteral mucosa without placing tension on the renal parenchyma (**c**)

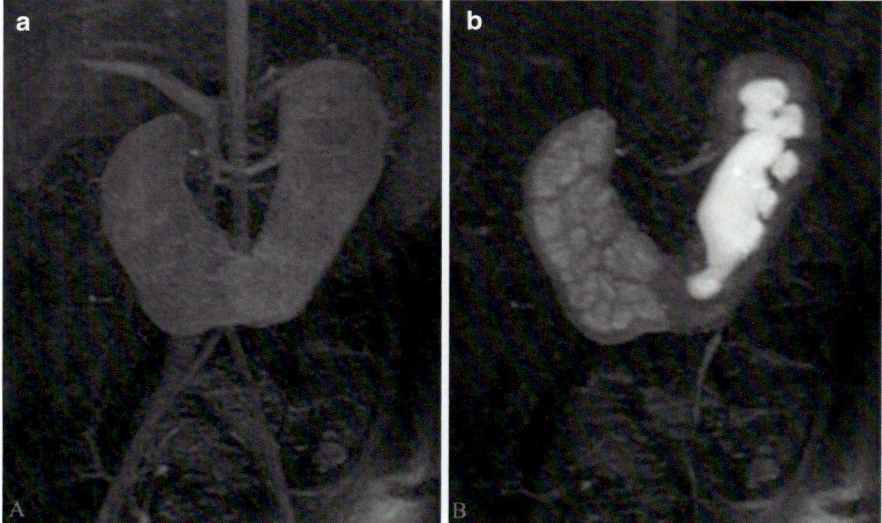

Fig. 10.2 Magnetic resonance urogram demonstrating the vasculature as well as the isthmus associated with a horseshoe kidney (**a**) and delayed cortical transit time with dense nephrogram of the right renal moiety suggesting obstruction (**b**)

insertion, abnormal ureteral course and/or anomalous vasculature contributing to UPJO [15]. Laparoscopic pyeloplasty in a patient with horseshoe kidney was initially described in 1995, and several pediatric series have since been published [16–18]. As with other reconstructive procedures, the robotic platform confers marked technical advantages over pure laparoscopy.

As for a standard pyeloplasty, the child is secured in a modified flank position with all pressure points appropriately padded. The camera port is placed just inferior to the umbilicus, with two operative 8 mm robotic ports placed after survey of the anatomy – these ports are typically placed in the midline 5–7 cm cephalad to the camera port and either 30 degrees rotated from the midline toward the kidney of interest or midline. The authors to do not use the robotic fourth arm or routinely use an assistant port. While the port sites are marked prior to placing the camera, it is prudent to ensure ports allow adequate visualization and working space. The remaining steps for anastomosis are the same for a standard pyelopasty.

Outcomes/Complications

Robotic upper tract reconstruction confers several advantages, with decreased morbidity and quicker postoperative recovery. In five studies evaluating pediatric robotic pyeloplasty, the combined complication rate was 7.2% [19]. The vast majority of complications were Clavien–Dindo grades I–III, and included post-operative urinary tract infection (UTI), ureteral stent or nephrostomy tube dislodgement, ileus, urine leak, hematuria, bleeding, and visceral organ injury. A recent systematic review of complications of pediatric minimally invasive surgery reported a 3.64% rate of Clavien-Dindo grade III complications, with no significant difference between laparoscopic and robotic approaches [20]. It stands to reason that given the challenging nature of ureterocalicostomy or pyeloplasty with aberrant anatomy such as horseshoe kidney, the complication rates may be higher. In a series including 14 children, complications included UTI in 1 (7.1%) and a ureteral stricture in 1 patient necessitating a secondary procedure (7.1%).

Ureterocalicostomy is often considered a last resort for renal preservation, and therefore is typically only considered in very challenging or redo cases. Recurrent obstruction is thought to be secondary to ischemia. Casale et al. reported the outcomes of 9 children undergoing robotic ureterocalicostomy for either failed prior pyeloplasty or exaggerated intrarenal collecting system – with no evidence of recurrent obstruction on diuretic renal scan performed 12 months postoperatively [5]. In our unpublished series of four patients who underwent robotic ureterocalicostomy, two (50%) patients had improvement where two patients had stability of hydronephrosis. Of those who had postoperative functional scans, all had improvement in kidney function, and there were no reported early or late complications. Success rates for robotic pyeloplasty in children with horseshoe kidney is similar to standard pyeloplasty, with Esposito reporting a 92.8% success rate in a series of 14 children [7].

Conclusions

As pediatric robotic urology continues to evolve, the indications for its role in complex upper tract reconstruction have broaden. Robotic ureterocalicostomy is an option for renal salvage when pyeloplasty is not feasible, most often in cases of failed pyeloplasty with an intrarenal pelvis. Robotic pyeloplasty in cases with renal fusion anomalies such as horseshoe kidney have success and complication rates similar to standard pyeloplasty.

References

1. Chen CJ, Peters CA. Robotic assisted surgery in pediatric urology: current status and future directions. Front Pediatr. 2019;7:90.
2. Camarillo DB, Krummel TM, Salisbury JK. Robotic technology in surgery: past, present, and future. Am J Surg. 2004;188:2S–15S.
3. Yohannes P, Smith AD. The endourological management of complications associated with horseshoe kidney. J Urol. 2002;168:5.
4. Ross JH, Streem SB, Novick AC, Kay R, Montie J. Ureterocalicostomy for reconstruction of complicated pelviureteric junction obstruction. Br J Urol. 1990;65:322.
5. Casale P, Muchsavage P, Resnick M, Kim SS. Robotic ureterocalicostomy in the pediatric population. J Urol. 2008;180:2643.
6. Jacobson DL, Shannon R, Johnson EK, Gong EM, Liu DB, Flink CC, et al. Robot-assisted laparoscopic reoperative repair for failed pyeloplasty in children: an updated series. J Urol. 2019;201(5):1005.
7. Esposito C, Masieri L, Blanc T, Manzoni G, Silay S, Escolino M. Robot-assisted laparoscopic pyeloplasty (RALP) in children with horseshoe kidney: results of a multicentric study. World J Urol. 2019;37(10):2257.
8. Chammas M, Feuillu B, Coissard A, Hubert J. Laparoscopic robotic-assisted management of pelvi–ureteric junction obstruction in patients with horseshoe kidneys: technique and 1-year follow-up. BJU Int. 2006;97(3):579.
9. Khoder WY, Alghamdi A, Schulz T, Becker AJ, Schlenker B, Stief CG. An innovative technique of robotic-assisted/laparoscopic re-pyeloplasty in horseshoe kidney in patients with failed previous pyeloplasty for ureteropelvic junction obstruction. Surg Endosc. 2016;30(9):4124.
10. Grattan-Smith JD, Little SB, Jones RA. MR urography evaluation of obstructive uropathy. Pediatr Radiol. 2008;38:S549.
11. Gill IS, Cherullo EE, Steinburg AL, Desai MM, Abreu SC, Ng C, et al. Laparoscopic ureterocalicostomy: initial experience. J Urol. 2004;171:1227.
12. Van Batavia JP, Casale P. Robotic surgery in pediatric urology. Curr Urol Rep. 2014;15:402.
13. Bilgutay AN, Kirsch AJ. Robotic ureteral reconstruction in the pediatric population. Front Pediatr. 2019;22(7):85.
14. Garcia-Roig ML, Travers C, McCracken C, Cerwinka W, Kirsch JM, Kirsch AJ. Surgical scar location preference for pediatric kidney and pelvic surgery: a crowdsourced survey. J Urol. 2017;197(3 Pt 2):911.
15. Natsis K, Piagkou M, Skotsimara A, Protogeroi V, Tsitouridis I, Skandalakis P. Horseshoe kidney: a review of anatomy and pathology. Surg Radiol Anat. 2014;36(6):517.
16. Janetschek G, Peschel R, Altarac S, Bartsch G. Laparoscopic and retroperitoneoscopic repair of ureteropelvic junction obstruction. Urology. 1996;47(3):311.

17. Blanc T, Koulouris E. Botto N, Paye-Jaouen A, El-Ghoneimi A. Laparoscopic pyeloplasty in children with horseshoe kidney. J Urol. 2014;191(4):1097.
18. Kawauchi A, Fujito A, Yoneda K, Soh J, Naitoh Y, Mizutani Y, et al. Laparoscopic pyeloplasty and isthmectomy for hydronephrosis of horseshoe kidney: a pediatric case. J Endourol. 2005;19(8):984.
19. Andolfi C, Adamic B, Oommen J, Gundeti MS. Robot-assisted laparoscopic pyeloplasty in infants and children: is it superior to conventional laparoscopy? World J Urol. 2020;38(8):1827–33.
20. Aksenov LI, Granberg CF, Gargollo PC. A systematic review of complications of minimally invasive surgery in the pediatric urological literature. J Urol. 2020;203(5):1010.

Part III
Lower Tract Surgery

Chapter 11
Ureteral Reimplantation

Jeffrey Villanueva, Janelle Fox, and Glenn Cannon

Abbreviation

RALUR   Robotic Assisted Ureteral Reimplant

Introduction

Anti-reflux surgery has evolved considerably from necessity at the time of bladder neck reconstruction to widespread adoption for correction of simple vesicoureteral reflux [1]. The intervention for vesicoureteral reflux (VUR) underwent a paradigm shift in the 1970s where spontaneous resolution of VUR was found to occur in the majority [2]. Numerous investigations confirmed the role of antibiotic prophylaxis in VUR management, contributing to a marked decrease in procedures to diagnose and treat VUR in the United States [3]. Overall, the utilization of surgical treatment has decreased with time, in favor of a more conservative approach toward expectant management [4–6]. This means the end-point for intervention in modern-day treatment of VUR has changed. It is no longer a child's likelihood of VUR resolution, rather the occurrence of breakthrough febrile urinary tract infections failing both antibiotic prophylaxis and adequate management of bowel and bladder dysfunction. Abdelhalim and Khoury have noted limitations to a top-down approach, which has attempted to minimize VCUG morbidity as well as unnecessary imaging and intervention. However, limited availability of DMSA, variable interpretation of DMSA scans, cost of nuclear medicine scans, increased ionizing radiation doses, and lack of distinction between congenital renal dysplasia and infection-related scarring have limited adoption of the top-down approach. In the end, a patient-centered approach to VUR has been suggested, given lack of clear outcomes benefit from either AAP, NICE or TDA guidelines [7].

Some have argued the knowledge of vesicoureteral reflux status may not change the clinical approach to a child with less than three UTIs [8]. Bandari and Docimo

---

J. Villanueva · J. Fox · G. Cannon (✉)
UPMC Children's Hospital of Pittsburgh, Division of Pediatric Urology, Pittsburgh, PA, USA
e-mail: Cannongm2@upmc.edu

© Springer Nature Switzerland AG 2020
P. C. Gargollo (ed.), *Minimally Invasive and Robotic-Assisted Surgery in Pediatric Urology*, https://doi.org/10.1007/978-3-030-57219-8_11

in 2019 additionally asserted that diagnosis and treatment of VUR has been most commonly performed in precisely the population for whom it may have the least long-term benefit: females with normal renal reserve and febrile UTIs. Our understanding of VUR has evolved from a simple and surgically curable disease to that of a symptom of less clear significance. To date, the field of Pediatric Urology has not been able to demonstrate that surgical correction of VUR definitively reduces progression to end stage renal disease, hypertension or proteinuria. The long-term impact of antibiotic prophylaxis on renal function has also been questioned. The multicenter, randomized controlled RIVUR and CUTIE trials comparing contemporaneous pediatric populations with and without Grades I-IV VUR failed to show differences in renal scarring [6, 9]. Instead, the preponderance of ESRD patients with VUR have been male or possessed congenital anomalies of the kidney and urinary tract (CAKUT). Aptly stated, "[t]aken together, diagnosing VUR would not provide prognostic or therapeutic value in preventing ESRD in a population of children with UTIs so long as UTI is promptly diagnosed and treated" [8]. So, when it is time to surgically intervene on the refluxing child with breakthrough UTIs in whom bowel and bladder dysfunction have been optimized, the Pediatric Urologist must offer treatments which are safe, effective, and certainly 'non-inferior' in his or her hands.

Incidentally, the use of robotic assisted laparoscopic ureteral reimplantation (RALUR) increased from 0.3% to 6.3% of ureteral reimplantations between 2009 and 2012, presumably due to a shorter learning curve compared with pure laparoscopic ureteral reimplantation [5]. Factors which may contribute are the platform's 3D vision, articulation of the laparoscopic instruments which facilitate suturing, and improved surgeon ergonomics [10]. While RALUR and LUR have been described transvesically, they have not been widely adopted due to suboptimal working space and difficulties with insufflation [11–14]. Similarly, while extravesical LUR has been described with good results, its limitation is mainly the use of challenging intracorporeal knot tying [15, 16]. Therefore, due to the simplification of laparoscopic suturing, most surgeons have adopted the extravesical RALUR approach [14].

Bilateral RALUR has been performed transvesically and extravesically [13, 17] Some reports have identified transvesical RALUR to have decreased ureteral drainage, hospital stays, and bladder spasms [18]. Although the transvesical RALUR was initially purported to have possibly decreased rates of urinary retention, extravesical RALUR can be used to spare the pelvic plexus by the ureter with a decreased concern for urinary retention [17]. Furthermore, RALUR has been safely performed in more complex cases as part of ureteral tapering, common sheath reimplantation, and periureteral diverticulectomy [19], though the technique is still considered experimental for complicated anatomy. Beyond anatomic abnormalities, the importance of assessment and aggressive treatment of bladder bowel dysfunction is central to both the workup and success of surgery [6, 20]. Furthermore, dysfunctional voiding has been thought to increase the failure rate of surgically corrected reflux, making the recognition of bladder bowel dysfunction important no matter how reflux is surgically corrected [21, 22]. Specifically for RALUR, preoperative bladder bowel dysfunction has been shown to be a risk factor for surgical failure [23].

There have been numerous investigations into the use of RALUR to treat vesicoureteral reflux. Initially, these reports were limited to a select number of Children's Hospitals that had access to the robotic platform. These early reports on RALUR appeared to have excellent results with success above 90%, [24–26] but were not consistently replicated in other centers as the procedure was more widely adopted by surgeons in their early learning curves [16, 23, 27]. Radiographic success ranged from 72% to 87.9% with Clavien 3 complication rates of 3–8% [16, 28]. Recent large multi-center clinical trials report success rates of 93.8% [26] and have been unable to identify factors responsible for failure of this technique compared with 'gold standard' open ureteral reimplantation surgery. While recent data on improved outcomes are encouraging, it is a cautionary tale that we do not yet know how we have achieved these improvements nor the patient population in whom RALUR is most beneficial.

Pain Control

The minimally invasive approach with RALUR has led some investigators to compare postoperative pain with the traditional open approach. In one study where anesthetic regimens were not standardized, intravesical RALUR had decreased bladder spasms compared to open ureteral reimplant. However, this group found no difference in pain scores between either approach (intravesical or extravesical) in open and RALUR [18]. Another retrospective study found that while narcotic use was decreased in bilateral extravesical RALUR compared to the open approach, this was not found in the comparison within the unilateral extravesical group [29]. Importantly, this group did not report the use of non-narcotic medications. Another group demonstrated that while children who undergo RALUR had decreased narcotic use on the first postoperative day compared to open reimplants, standardized post-operative pain scores, a more accurate assessment of pain, were not different between children [30]. A study using the PHIS (Pediatric Health Information System) which reviewed more than 6000 open and RALUR procedures showed that while RALUR used less opioids postoperatively, they also used ketorolac more frequently. It is unknown if this difference is independent of ketorolac use, or if the more recently trained urologists simply use fewer narcotic prescriptions [31].

Length of Stay

Decreased length of stay is a potential benefit to RALUR over the open approach, though in the authors' experience this is limited to older children and adolescents. In the early learning curve, the aforementioned 2014 study reported a 7–9 day postoperative stay for RALUR [32]. A More recent data suggest lengths of stay similar to or slightly lower than open ureteral reimplantation [30]. A recent paper looked at the discharge of unilateral, extravesical RALUR patients as a same day procedure where the patient is discharged from the Post-Anesthesia Care Unit (PACU). In this series, while all 27 patients were discharged from the PACU, one required readmission for constipation, one was diagnosed with a pneumonia, and one with bacterial cystitis. However, this study excluded those with grade V VUR which excluded grade V VUR and more than 80% of patients had grade II or III VUR [33]. Conversely, studies which successfully described outpatient and open extravesical ureteral reimplants have been performed, but also included grade V VUR, bilateral procedures, and complex reconstruction such as ureteral tapering [34].

Cost

One institutional series has reported that RALUR is cost effective compared with open ureteral reimplantation [35, 36]; however, all others have found RALUR costs to exceed OUR [37, 38]. This preliminary study found that higher robotic surgical charges were offset by shorter lengths of postoperative hospitalization. This analysis was limited in its use of hospital charges to define healthcare cost and also its limited population. It should be noted the open ureteral reimplantation group included analysis of patients hospitalized up to 5 days, rather than a more typical 1–2 day postoperative stay. From a nationwide sample, Kurtz et al. demonstrated that RALUR had about 18% higher direct costs than the open procedure, a difference which was partially comprised of the increased surgical complications and complication charges in the RALUR group [38]. In studies of other robotic pediatric urologic procedures, such a robotic pyeloplasty, patients identified via the PHIS database from 18 United States Childrens' hospitals still incurred higher costs of care compared with matched, open surgical counterparts. The majority of increased costs arose from operating room and anesthesia time, which is typically "costed" on a per-minute basis [39].

Cosmesis

The use of the robotic approach is typically seen as a procedure with more appealing surgical incisions. One large incision may have more wound tension and scarring compared to multiple smaller incisions [40]. However, a crowdsourced survey had shown that a Pfannenstiel incision was preferred over conventionally placed laparoscopic port incisions, especially when depicted in relation to undergarments [41]. This did not factor in "hidden incision endoscopic surgery" (HidES) incisions for port placement [42]. Alternatively, Barbosa et al. found that patients and parents who were considering surgery strongly preferred robotic incisions [43]. However, this paper's methodology has been criticized for the images the authors chose to represent scars after various surgeries [41]. Regardless of the surgical approach, Barbosa et al. found that parents preferred the technique with superior outcomes.

Complications

Cost and colleagues report port site hernias following pediatric abdominal laparoscopy of 3.2%, preferentially occurring in infants [44]. Among RALUR papers with a reported postoperative hernia, port site hernia accounted for 50% of Clavien 3 complications, hence the risk of port site hernia is far higher in the younger patient population who typically recovers better from an open Pfannensteil incision. Such preventable complications will be low in number amongst single institutional series and payer or registry database studies are needed. In addition, it cannot be overstated that port site herniation in children is different than in adults. Port site hernias can occur even through 3 mm port sites [45]; hence, every port site in a child should be closed and surgeons should avoid placement of drains through port sites if possible.

Due to both increased procedural cost and 90-day complications (13% vs 4.5% with open surgery), Kurtz and colleagues caution implementation of robotic ureteral reimplantation in centers with limited volume and experience, as well as systematic tracking of outcomes [38]. It is worth reminding ourselves that we all can improve upon our outcomes with systematic and objective tracking of not just institutional, but also personal surgical outcomes. It is not comfortable to do so, nor was it for Ernest Codman, who developed the concept of outcomes evaluation in his End-result System in 1918. However, "the ego of the surgeon must always be subservient to the patient's welfare" [46].

The apparent increased complication rate compared to CUR as well as notable Clavien 3 complications serve as a caution to any surgeon looking to incorporate RALUR into their repertoire [38]. Table 11.1 depicts the major RALUR studies with their success and classified Clavien complication. Despite more than 15 years of innovation in divisions well known for achievement in minimally invasive surgery, modest success and complication rates persist.

Operative Success

The first reports by Peters demonstrated the feasibility of RALUR, with radiographic VUR resolution of up to 88% [25]. As these results were encouraging despite early innovation of a novel procedure, several other groups replicated the results and improved overall reported success rate [24, 32, 47–52]. Kasturi et al. in 2012 described near universal radiographic resolution after intervention. This study included only toilet trained children who were evaluated for and treated for bladder bowel dysfunction prior to surgery. Despite bilateral extravesical dissection, there

Table 11.1 Reported outcomes and surgical complications of robotic ureteral reimplantation

Study	Year of publication	Number of ureters	Number of patients	Mean age (years)	Intravesical/ extravesical approach	Average follow up (months)	Average preoperative VUR grade from presented data	Clinical success rate	Radiographic VUR resolution	Complication rate (%)	Reported complication (%)	Clavien-Dindo score
Peters [25]	2004	27	24	5.8	0/24	6	2.8		88	13	Bladder leak (8)	1
											Ureteral obstruction (4)	3
Peters [13]	2005	12	6	5–15 (range)	6/0	NA	NA	NA	83	17	Urine leak (17)	3
Casale [24]	2008	82	41	3.2	0/42	At least 6	3.9	98	98	2	Febrile UTI (2)	1
Lee [47]	2010	4	4	2.3	0/4	33	NA	100	100	25	Ureteral obstruction (25)	3
Smith [29]	2011	33	25	5.75	0/25	16	3.7		97	20	Acute retention (12)	1
											Bladder leak (4)	1
Marchini [18]	2011	66	39	9.2	19/20	15	3	98	92	22	Bladder leak (10)	1
											Ureteral leak (5)	3
											Acute retention (7)	1
Kasturi [17]	2012	300	150	3.6	0/150	24	4	99	99	1	Febrile UTI (1)	2
Chalmers [48]	2012	23	16	6.2	0/17	11.5	2.7	100	91	0	NA	NA
Callewaert [49]	2012	10	5	6.8	0/5	28	4	100	90	40	Acute retention (40)	1
Dangle [50]	2014	40	29	5.38	0/29	At least 4 months	3–5 in 37 ureters. 1–2 in 3 ureters	NA	80	NA	NA	NA

Author	Year										Complications	
Schomburg [51]	2014	35	20	74	0/20	13	2.6	90	100	10	Urine leak (5)	3
											Ureteral stenosis (5)	3
Akhavan [52]	2014	78	50	7.2	0/50	14	3.1	90	92	12	Ureteral obstruction (4)	3
											Ureteral injury (2)	3
											Ileus (4)	1
											Urinary retention (2)	1
Hayashi [32]	2014	15	9	10	0/15	At least 4 months	3.2	100	93	0	n/a	n/a
Grimsby [16]	2015	93	61	6.7	0/61	12	3.3	82	77	10	Ureteral obstruction (5)	3
											Urine leak (3)	3
											Redmission for vomiting (2)	1
Herz [23]	2016	72	54	5.2	0/54	At least 6 months	3.4	94	85	15	Ureteral obstruction (6)	3
											Urinary retention (6)	1
											Ureteral injury (3)	3
Arlen [19]	2016	20	17	9	0/17	16.5 (includes cohort of open reimplants)	3.4	94	100	6	Ileus (6)	1
Gundeti [53]	2016	83	58	5.3	0/58	30 (med)	3.4	NA	82	2	Acute urinary retention (2)	1

(continued)

Table 11.1 (continued)

Study	Year of publication	Number of ureters	Number of patients	Mean age (years)	Intravesical/ extravesical approach	Average follow up (months)	Average preoperative VUR grade from presented data	Clinical success rate	Radiographic VUR resolution	Complication rate (%)	Reported complication (%)	Clavien-Dindo score
Boysen [28]	2017	363	260	6.4	0/260	At least 3 months	3	91.9	87.9	9.6	Acute urinary retention (1.5)	1
											Other grade 1 complication (3.3)	1
											Other grade 2 complication (1.9)	2
											Ureteral obstruction (1.5)	3
											Port site hernia (1)	3
											Urinary leak (1)	3
Srinivasan [55]	2017	127	92		4.00	12.7 (med)	3 (med)	91	67 (VCUG only in select postoperative conditions)	8	Incisional hernia (1)	3
											Urine leak (1)	3
											Grade 1 complication (5.4)	1

Author	Year										Complications
Boysen [26]	2018	199	143	6.6	0/143	7.4	3	NA	93.8	11	Urine leak (2) 3; Ureteral obstruction (1) 3; Port site hernia (1) 3; Foley balloon malfunction (1) 3; Retained portion of drain (1) 3; Acute retention (3) 1; Grade 1 complication (5) 1; Grade 2 complication (1) 2

was no change in voiding function before or after surgery, purportedly from sparing the pelvic plexus [17].

Some later studies had more heterogeneous results [16, 53]. Grimsby et al. reported in a multi-institutional study consisting of three tertiary pediatric hospitals postoperative febrile UTIs in 18% of patients and persistent VUR in 23%. Complications occurred in 10% and a reoperation in 14% [16]. While a large and prospective multi-institutional study reported radiographic success rates of more than 90% overall, postoperative radiographic imaging for persistent VUR was not performed in more than 25%, an issue compounded by their follow-up of 7.4 months [26]. Furthermore, while the paper suggests that having greater experience would improve complication rates, Clavien 1 complications did not improve and Clavien 3 complications increased from 2.7% to 5.6% when compared to their previous study [54]. Other recent reports from high volume RALUR centers report success rates between 82% and 92% [23, 28, 53, 55].

Adoption of RALUR has been slowed due to absence of definitive evidence which demonstrates superiority of this novel technique. Interpretation of existing data is limited by heterogenous or poor reporting of surgical indications for VUR and associated bladder bowel dysfunction and its treatment. While there is no clear evidence that older children are optimal patients for RALUR, average age which children receive surgery appears to be increasing [14]. Furthermore, there may be an ideal body habitus that the RALUR is best suited for, though this has not been well described in the literature [54].

Operative Technique

We perform RALUR in select patients in our institution. Due to the limitations discussed above, we limit this procedure to older children. It is performed only after a complete evaluation and management of bladder bowel dysfunction.

We routinely perform cystoscopy to evaluate for cystitis as well as to identify anomalous anatomy. The patient is then tightly secured, padded, and placed in a 30-degree Trendelenburg position. Pneumoperitoneum is achieved with a Veress needle and pressure set according to the age of the child (8 mmHg for infants, 10 mmHg for preschool, and 12–15 mmHg for school age children to adolescents). A 30 degree downward facing 12 mm camera is placed with a subumbilical incision. Two 8 mm ports are placed laterally, preferably along a line which could be extended to make a Pfannenstiel incision. These trocars are placed cephalad to the umbilical camera port to maximize triangulation, however can be performed in the same horizontal axis according to HIdES principles [42].

The distal ureter is identified and its planned tunnel is measured to be a distance about 5 times the width of the distal ureter. This measurement is performed with the bladder empty. A 3-0 Prolene hitch stitch is placed at the proximal extent of the planned tunnel. The detrusor fibers are then split to expose the underlying mucosa by using blunt dissection and limited spot cautery with the bladder partially distended. It is important to ensure the neoureteral tunnel and ureter within it will have a straight trajectory, without proximal kinking. We find bladder distension and, on occasion, dropping the bladder assist at this point in the case to ensure a straight tunnel. Other groups have described preoperative cystoscopic placement of 4 or 5Fr ureteral catheters in the operative ureter(s) as another method of assisting in ureteral dissection [56]. We attempt to limit dissection of the distal ureter and UVJ to avoid injury to the nerve plexus. Admittedly, this anatomic structure is not clearly seen and instead we maximize conservative tissue handling medial to the UVJ. As the dissection is brought cranially to the holding stitch, we have found that switching the camera to 30 degrees up allows easier dissection superiorly.

The detrusorrhaphy is then completed with 3-0 Vicryl sutures. We regularly perform this starting at the UVJ and moving towards the hitch stitch. The hitch stitch is then removed, and after ensuring a straight course of the ureter, the abdomen is desufflated and all port site fascia and skin is closed. Local anesthetic is then injected. No drain is placed. The foley catheter is then left overnight and the patient is discharged home after documenting acceptable post void residuals.

Conclusion

The role of ureteral reimplantation in the management of VUR has changed remarkably over the past few decades. While RALUR has emerged to expand the laparoscopic approach, the population of children that benefit most from this technique is unclear. Advances in anti-reflux surgery should be assessed by the procedure's ability to decrease morbidity and healthcare costs. RALUR does not convincingly achieve this, and with the limitations with our current literature, should still be considered an investigative surgery.

References

1. DeCotiis KN, Penna FJ, Koyle MA, Caldamone AA. Vesicoureteral reflux: a historical perspective. Afr J Urol. 2017;23:1–4.
2. Edwards D, Normand IC, Prescod N, Smellie JM. Disappearance of vesicoureteric reflux during long-term prophylaxis of urinary tract infection in children. Br Med J. 1977;2(6082):285–8.
3. Garcia-Roig M, Travers C, McCracken CE, Kirsch AJ. National trends in the management of primary vesicoureteral reflux in children. J Urol. 2018;199(1):287–93.
4. Kurtz MP, Leow JJ, Varda BK, Logvinenko T, McQuaid JW, Yu RN, et al. The decline of the open ureteral reimplant in the United States: national data from 2003 to 2013. Urology. 2017;100:193–7.
5. Bowen DK, Faasse MA, Liu DB, Gong EM, Lindgren BW, Johnson EK. Use of pediatric open, laparoscopic and robot-assisted laparoscopic ureteral reimplantation in the United States: 2000 to 2012. J Urol. 2016;196(1):207–12
6. Keren R, Shaikh N, Pohl H, Gravens-Mueller L, Ivanova A, Zaoutis L, et al. Risk factors for recurrent urinary tract infection and renal scarring. Pediatrics. 2015;136(1):e13–21.

7. Abdelhalim A, Khoury AE. Critical appraisal of the top-down approach for vesicoureteral reflux. Investig Clin Urol. 2017;58(Suppl 1):S14–s22.
8. Bandari J, Docimo SG. Vesicoureteral reflux is a phenotype, not a disease: a population-centered approach to pediatric urinary tract infection. J Pediatr Urol. 2017;13(4):378–82.
9. Hoberman A, Greenfield SP, Mattoo TK, Keren R, Mathews R, Pohl HG, et al. Antimicrobial prophylaxis for children with vesicoureteral reflux. N Engl J Med. 2014;370(25):2367–76.
10. Savio LF, Nguyen HT. Robot-assisted laparoscopic urological surgery in children. Nat Rev Urol. 2013;10(11):632–9.
11. Chaudhry R, Stephany HA. Robotic ureteral reimplant-the current role. Curr Urol Rep. 2017;18(4):30.
12. Kutikov A, Guzzo TJ, Canter DJ, Casale P. Initial experience with laparoscopic transvesical ureteral reimplantation at the Children's Hospital of Philadelphia. J Urol. 2006;176(5):2222–5; discussion 5–6.
13. Peters CA, Woo R. Intravesical robotically assisted bilateral ureteral reimplantation. J Endourol. 2005;19(6):618–21; discussion 21–2.
14. Sahadev R, Spencer K, Srinivasan AK, Long CJ, Shukla AR. The robot-assisted extravesical anti-reflux surgery: how we overcame the learning curve. Front Pediatr. 2019;7:93.
15. Bayne AP, Shoss JM, Starke NR, Cisek LJ. Single-center experience with pediatric laparoscopic extravesical reimplantation: safe and effective in simple and complex anatomy. J Laparoendosc Adv Surg Tech A. 2012;22(1):102–6.
16. Grimsby GM, Dwyer ME, Jacobs MA, Ost MC, Schneck FX, Cannon GM, et al. Multi-institutional review of outcomes of robot-assisted laparoscopic extravesical ureteral reimplantation. J Urol. 2015;193(5 Suppl):1791–5.
17. Kasturi S, Sehgal SS, Christman MS, Lambert SM, Casale P. Prospective long-term analysis of nerve-sparing extravesical robotic-assisted laparoscopic ureteral reimplantation. Urology. 2012;79(3):680–3.
18. Marchini GS, Hong YK, Minnillo BJ, Diamond DA, Houck CS, Meier PM, et al. Robotic assisted laparoscopic ureteral reimplantation in children: case matched comparative study with open surgical approach. J Urol. 2011;185(5):1870–5.
19. Arlen AM, Broderick KM, Travers C, Smith EA, Elmore JM, Kirsch AJ. Outcomes of complex robot-assisted extravesical ureteral reimplantation in the pediatric population. J Pediatr Urol. 2016;12(3):169 e1–6.
20. Sillen U. Bladder dysfunction and vesicoureteral reflux. Adv Urol. 2008;2008:815472.
21. Noe HN. The role of dysfunctional voiding in failure or complication of ureteral reimplantation for primary reflux. J Urol. 1985;134(6):1172–5.
22. Higham-Kessler J, Reinert SE, Snodgrass WT, Hensle TW, Koyle MA, Hurwitz RS, et al. A review of failures of endoscopic treatment of vesicoureteral reflux with dextranomer microspheres. J Urol. 2007;177(2):710–4; discussion 4–5.
23. Herz D, Fuchs M, Todd A, McLeod D, Smith J. Robot-assisted laparoscopic extravesical ureteral reimplant: a critical look at surgical outcomes. J Pediatr Urol. 2016;12(6):402 e1–9.
24. Casale P, Patel RP, Kolon TF. Nerve sparing robotic extravesical ureteral reimplantation. J Urol. 2008;179(5):1987–9; discussion 90.
25. Peters CA. Robotically assisted surgery in pediatric urology. Urol Clin North Am. 2004;31(4):743–52.
26. Boysen WR, Akhavan A, Ko J, Ellison JS, Lendvay TS, Huang J, et al. Prospective multicenter study on robot-assisted laparoscopic extravesical ureteral reimplantation (RALUR-EV): outcomes and complications. J Pediatr Urol. 2018;14(3):262 e1–6.
27. Deng T, Liu B, Luo L, Duan X, Cai C, Zhao Z, et al. Robot-assisted laparoscopic versus open ureteral reimplantation for pediatric vesicoureteral reflux: a systematic review and meta-analysis. World J Urol. 2018;36(5):819–28.
28. Boysen WR, Ellison JS, Kim C, Koh CJ, Noh P, Whittam B, et al. Multi-institutional review of outcomes and complications of robot-assisted laparoscopic extravesical ureteral reimplantation for treatment of primary vesicoureteral reflux in children. J Urol. 2017;197(6):1555–61.

29. Smith RP, Oliver JL, Peters CA. Pediatric robotic extravesical ureteral reimplantation: comparison with open surgery. J Urol. 2011;185(5):1876–81.
30. Harel M, Herbst KW, Silvis R, Makari JH, Ferrer FA, Kim C. Objective pain assessment after ureteral reimplantation: comparison of open versus robotic approach. J Pediatr Urol. 2015;11(2):82 e1–8.
31. Dwyer ME, Routh J, Ost MC, Stephany HS, Schneck FX, Gargollo PC, et al., editors. Robot-assisted laparoscopic ureteroneocystostomy carries higher risk of surgical complications than open reimplant: a retrospective analysis of 6,090 cases from 44 children's hospitals. 26th Congress of the European Society for Paediatric Urology, Prague, Czech Republic, 2015.
32. Hayashi Y, Mizuno K, Kurokawa S, Nakane A, Kamisawa H, Nishio H, et al. Extravesical robot-assisted laparoscopic ureteral reimplantation for vesicoureteral reflux: initial experience in Japan with the ureteral advancement technique. Int J Urol. 2014;21(10):1016–21.
33. Neheman A, Strine AC, Concodora CW, Schulte ME, Noh PH. Outpatient robotic unilateral extravesical ureteral reimplantation in the pediatric population: short-term assessment of safety. J Urol. 2019;201(3):615–9.
34. Palmer JS. Extravesical ureteral reimplantation: an outpatient procedure. J Urol. 2008;180(4 Suppl):1828–31; discussion 31.
35. Rodolfo A. Elizondo M, Au JK, Puttmann K, Huang GO, Baek M, et al., editor. Robotic ureteral reimplantation is not associated with increased costs for families and payers: a single institution analysis of hospital charges and outcomes. Pediatric Urology Fall Congress, Montreal, Canada, 2017.
36. Baek M, Koh CJ. Lessons learned over a decade of pediatric robotic ureteral reimplantation. Investig Clin Urol. 2017;58(1):3–11.
37. Mahida JB, Cooper JN, Herz D, Diefenbach KA, Deans KJ, Minneci PC, et al. Utilization and costs associated with robotic surgery in children. J Surg Res. 2015;199(1):169–76.
38. Kurtz MP, Leow JJ, Varda BK, Logvinenko T, Yu RN, Nelson CP, et al. Robotic versus open pediatric ureteral reimplantation: costs and complications from a nationwide sample. J Pediatr Urol. 2016;12(6):408 e1–6.
39. Bennett WE Jr, Whittam BM, Szymanski KM, Rink RC, Cain MP, Carroll AE. Validated cost comparison of open vs. robotic pyeloplasty in American children's hospitals. J Robot Surg. 2017;11(2):201–6.
40. Blinman T. Incisions do not simply sum. Surg Endosc. 2010;24(7):1746–51.
41. Garcia-Roig ML, Travers C, McCracken C, Cerwinka W, Kirsch JM, Kirsch AJ. Surgical scar location preference for pediatric kidney and pelvic surgery: a crowdsourced survey. J Urol. 2017;197(3 Pt 2):911–9.
42. Gargollo PC. Hidden incision endoscopic surgery: description of technique, parental satisfaction and applications. J Urol. 2011;185(4):1425–31.
43. Barbosa JA, Barayan G, Gridley CM, Sanchez DC, Passerotti CC, Houck CS, et al. Parent and patient perceptions of robotic vs open urological surgery scars in children. J Urol. 2013;190(1):244–50.
44. Cost NG, Lee J, Snodgrass WT, Harrison CB, Wilcox DT, Baker LA. Hernia after pediatric urological laparoscopy. J Urol. 2010;183(3):1163–7.
45. Yee DS, Duel BP. Omental herniation through a 3-mm umbilical trocar site. J Endourol. 2006;20(2):133–4.
46. Howell J, Ayanian J. Ernest Codman and the end result system: a pioneer of health outcomes revisited. J Health Serv Res Policy. 2016;21(4):279–81.
47. Lee RS, Sethi AS, Passerotti CC, Peters CA. Robot-assisted laparoscopic nephrectomy and contralateral ureteral reimplantation in children. J Endourol. 2010;24(1):123–8.
48. Chalmers D, Herbst K, Kim C. Robotic-assisted laparoscopic extravesical ureteral reimplantation: an initial experience. J Pediatr Urol. 2012;8(3):268–71.
49. Callewaert PR, Biallosterski BT, Rahnama'i MS, Van Kerrebroeck PE. Robotic extravesical anti-reflux operations in complex cases: technical considerations and preliminary results. Urol Int. 2012;88(1):6–11.

50. Dangle PP, Shah A, Gundeti MS. Robot-assisted laparoscopic ureteric reimplantation: extravesical technique. BJU Int. 2014;114(4):630–2.
51. Schomburg JL, Haberman K, Willihnganz-Lawson KH, Shukla AR. Robot-assisted laparoscopic ureteral reimplantation: a single surgeon comparison to open surgery. J Pediatr Urol. 2014;10(5):875–9.
52. Akhavan A, Avery D, Lendvay TS. Robot-assisted extravesical ureteral reimplantation: outcomes and conclusions from 78 ureters. J Pediatr Urol. 2014;10(5):864–8.
53. Gundeti MS, Boysen WR, Shah A. Robot-assisted laparoscopic Extravesical ureteral reimplantation: technique modifications contribute to optimized outcomes. Eur Urol. 2016;70(5):818–23.
54. Gargollo PC. Editorial comment regarding: prospective multicenter study on robot-assisted laparoscopic extravesical ureteral reimplantation (RALUR-EV): outcomes and complications. J Pediatr Urol. 2018;14(3):263–4.
55. Srinivasan AK, Maass D, Shrivastava D, Long CJ, Shukla AR. Is robot-assisted laparoscopic bilateral extravesical ureteral reimplantation associated with greater morbidity than unilateral surgery? A comparative analysis. J Pediatr Urol. 2017;13(5):494 e1–7.
56. Van Batavia JP, Casale P. Robotic surgery of the kidney and ureter in pediatric patients. Curr Urol Rep. 2013;14(4):373–8.

Chapter 12
Management of Duplication Anomalies

Paul Kokorowski

Partial or complete duplication of the renal collecting system occurs in about one out of 25 individuals [1–3]. The term duplex system is a broad term referring to both partial and complete duplications. A complete duplex system, where separate collecting systems including two ureters inserting independently, is also known as a duplex kidney. A partial duplication can manifest as a bifid system when there are two renal collecting systems that join at the level of the uretero pelvic junction or as bifid ureters with joining of the two ureters prior to insertion distally into the bladder. Duplex kidneys occur at an incidence about 0.8% in the general population [2].

Duplex systems do not necessarily represent a diseased state and individuals may suffer no particular consequences. However, duplex systems are associated with vesicoureteral reflux which is found in 66–72% of complete duplications [1, 4]. Furthermore, some duplex systems are associated obstructive phenomena or renal dysplasia. While the incidence of urinary tract infection (UTI) may not be high among those with duplex systems, the frequency of finding duplications in those who present with UTI is higher than the general population at about 8% [1, 4, 5]. In some individuals, surgical excision or urinary tract reconstruction is warranted. While open surgical management has been well described, minimally invasive surgical techniques have also been developed to manage these cases with similar efficacy and complication rates [6].

P. Kokorowski (✉)
Children's Hospital Los Angeles, Keck School of Medicine, University of Southern California, Division of Pediatric Urology, Los Angeles, CA, USA
e-mail: pkokorowski@chla.usc.edu

© Springer Nature Switzerland AG 2020
P. C. Gargollo (ed.), *Minimally Invasive and Robotic-Assisted Surgery in Pediatric Urology*, https://doi.org/10.1007/978-3-030-57219-8_12

Embryology of Duplication

Both pathogenic and nonpathogenic development of duplex systems originates from early alterations in renal development. It is thought that separate ureteral buds branch off of the Wolffian duct. There is aggregation of the metanephric blastema around each bud resulting in a duplex system. Because each bud inserts separately into the Wolffian duct, there is a differential timing of incorporation of the bud into the genitourinary sinus distally. As the common nephric duct undergoes apoptosis, the more caudally located urinary bud first comes into contact with the urogenital sinus and migrates cranially and laterally, leading to a cranial/lateral displacement of the ureteral orifice. The more cranial ureteral bud incorporates at a later time point, leading to a relatively distal insertion that is sometimes ectopic. As such, it is typical that the upper pole ureter, derived from the more cranially located of the two initial buds, inserts more distally in the genitourinary sinus while the lower pole inserts more proximal. This principle is known as the Wiegert-Meyer rule. As a consequence of ureteral insertion, the lower pole of duplex systems tends to have ureteropelvic junction obstructions and vesicoureteral reflux as the most common pathologic findings. Conversely, the upper pole of duplex kidneys tends to experience more distal obstructive issues with possible ureterocele, dysplasia, or distal ectopic insertion.

An ectopic ureter is "a single or duplex ureter that does not enter the trigone area of the bladder." [7] About 70% of ectopic ureters occur in the setting of ureteral duplication, and about 80% of these cases additionally demonstrate contralateral duplications [5]. In females, a distal ectopic ureter can insert in the bladder neck, urethra, perineum, vagina, uterus, or even the rectum. Since the ureter is a structure derived from the Wolffian duct, insertion into Mullerian structures occurs via a rupture of Gartner's duct or of a Gartner's duct cyst into the vagina. (Fig. 12.1)

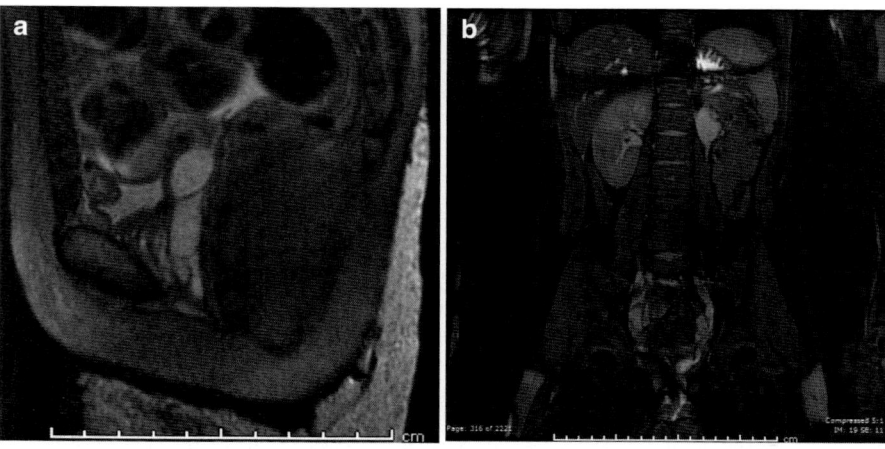

Fig. 12.1 (a, b) MRI of the abdomen and pelvis in a female presenting with lifetime history of continuous incontinence. Coronal and sagittal images demonstrate a left ureter inserting into the vagina with a cystic dilation of the distal portion. This structure represents a Gartner's Duct cyst

In males, sites may include the prostatic urethra, seminal vessels, vas deferens, ejaculatory duct, or an enlarged prostatic utricle.

When ureteral ectopia leads to insertion between the bladder neck and the membranous urethra, there tend to be significant obstructive issues. In the case of severe obstruction, there may be a failure of normal parenchymal development of the upper pole leading to dysplasia of this portion of the kidney.

Ureteroceles

Ureteroceles are cystic dilatations of the distal ureter affecting 0.025–0.2% of individuals based on autopsy studies. Duplex ureters are associated with ectopic ureteroceles in 6–20% of patients [4, 8]. Most patients are Caucasian and are more likely to be female by a factor of 4–7 [5]. About 80% of ureteroceles are associated with the upper pole of a duplicated system and 60–80% have an ectopic location. The classic explanation is a failure to rupture of Chwalle's membrane [3]. Most studies suggest that ureteroceles arise from defective processes occurring at the distal ureter as the ureteric bud detaches from the mesonephric duct [9]. Intravesical ureteroceles are contained within the bladder except perhaps during of voiding, at which time large variants may prolapse into the urethra causing outflow obstruction. Ureteroceles may also be ectopically located at the internal sphincter (sphincteric ureteroceles) or even extend past the bladder neck into the urethra (cecoureteroceles) [10].

As with ectopic ureters, there can be both loss of function and significant dysplasia of the associated upper pole renal parenchyma. When specimens from heminephrectomies are examined histologically, dysplasia is found in up to 70% of cases [11–14]. In addition, there are signs of chronic pyelonephritis in more than half of specimens [14]. Furthermore, hypertension is a theoretical concern in dysplastic kidneys left in situ, though one study with 15 years of follow up found no significant difference in the incidence of high blood pressure (8% vs 9%) between patients undergoing urinary tract reconstruction versus upper pole heminephrectomy [15].

Most ureteroceles are classified as obstructive, though there are some variants including the nonobstructive ureterocele [16]. Furthermore, certain severely obstructed systems can present with ureterocele disproportion which refers to the presence of a ureterocele and a nondilated, dysplastic upper pole that can be easily missed on imaging studies [17].

Clinical Presentation

The clinical presentation of duplication anomalies is wide and varied. Most commonly, duplications are identified during a work-up of a child presenting with a urinary tract infection. In fact, ureteral duplication is ten times more common among children presenting with urinary tract infection when compared to the general population [5]. An incidental finding of hydronephrosis is another typical method of identifying duplication anomalies. With wide spread application of antenatal ultrasonography, many ectopic ureters and ureteroceles are identified before birth [5]. Other presenting symptoms may include incontinence from an ectopically inserting ureter or even from a weakened bladder neck secondary to a large ureterocele. Continuous incontinence in a toilet trained female is suggestive of an ectopic ureter and should be investigated with imaging [18]. There may be pain from obstruction or infection, this being associated with prolapse of the ureterocele in some cases [19, 20].

Imaging

As with many conditions that affect the pediatric urinary system, ultrasound is the first study of choice. In the case of duplex systems, ultrasound can demonstrate the presence of cortical type tissue separating the hyperechoic central portion of the kidney that typifies peripelvic fat and urothelium. Such findings are suggestive of a duplex system (Fig. 12.2).

In the case of obstructive processes, asymmetric dilatation of a portion of the kidney such as the upper pole may be found, often with an associated dilated ureter. In severe cases of distal obstruction there may be a large tortuous ureter that can compress and deform the posterior wall of the bladder as a pseudoureterocele or be confused with small intestine [21]. Large ureters may also cause partial obstructions and varying degrees of hydronephrosis in the 'unaffected' portion of the kidney. In the case of severe obstruction with dysplasia, ultrasound can demonstrate a bundle of cysts where the upper pole of the kidney normally resides.

Voiding cystourethrogram is essential to identify refluxing units and abnormalities of the bladder shape structure. Vesicoureteral reflux into the lower moiety of the

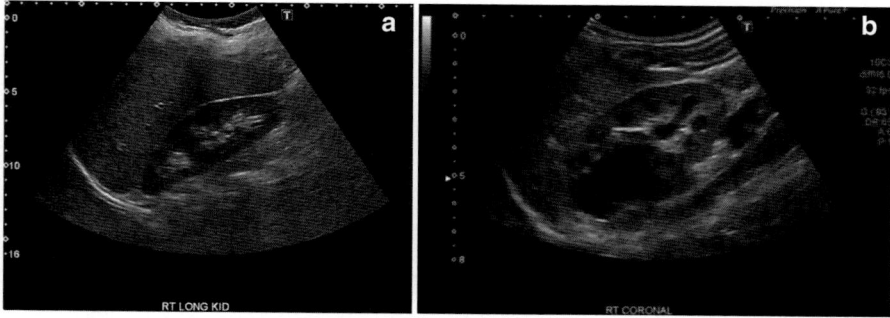

Fig. 12.2 (**a**, **b**) Ultrasound images of duplex kidneys. In image (**a**), duplication is suggested by the hypoechoic parenchyma separating the relatively bright signal from the collecting system and peri-pelvic fat. Image (**b**) demonstrates asymmetric dilatation of the upper portion of the kidney

duplex kidney is present in up to 66% of those presenting with a urinary tract infection [4]. Diverticula can be identified and may need to be managed during surgical reconstruction. Voiding phases are important to identify ectopically inserting ureters that reflux only during the micturition portion of the study.

Nuclear medicine studies are essential for approximating relative function, or in some cases the absence of function certain portions of duplex systems. Parenchymal dysplasia is found in 30–70% of cases at the time of partial nephrectomy [11–13]. Mercaptoacetyltriglycine-3 (MAG-3) Lasix renograms allow for evaluation of upper tract drainage, which plays a role in surgical decision making. Furthermore, MAG-3 scans can be used to identify "yo-yo" or saddle reflux in bifid systems [22, 23]. DMSA scans can be used to specifically evaluate the renal cortex and better estimates the degree of dysplasia and/or renal scaring.

More recently, magnetic resonance imaging is being used to localize specific insertion points of ectopic ureters with predictive values of 75–88% [24]. This modality has the benefit of finer structural details and the ability to create three-dimensional reconstructions of the anatomy of interest.

Principles of Management

General distinctions can be drawn between the management of functional versus non-functional systems. In duplex kidneys with a dysplastic upper pole, observation may be a reasonable strategy. Complete involution is common while in others, only a few cysts remain as remnant features. Should there be concerns about growth of the dysplastic tissue, recurrent infections, uncontrolled hypertension or lower poll partial obstructions related to large dilated ureter, then extirpative surgery is indicated. When specifically considering ureteroceles, endoscopic management is another option for the relief of obstructed or infected systems [10].

Observation is a reasonable strategy when there is a small non-obstructive ureterocele, non-obstructive ectopic ureter without incontinence, low-grade VUR, absence of UTI, and no bladder outlet obstruction [5, 10]. Low grade VUR often resolves with a time course that is delayed when compared to single systems [25]. Typical observational protocols result in surgery for recurrent UTI or obstructive indications in about 30% of cases [26].

Indications for intervention for VUR are similar to those for single systems with a few caveats. First, high grade VUR (gr3–5) has a relatively lower resolution rate in duplex systems as compared to single systems [25]. In addition, sub-ureteric bulking agents seem to have a lower success rate in the setting of duplex systems (50% vs 73%) [27].

When there is an obstructive ureterocele with or without UTI, surgical intervention is indicated. Transurethral incision of the ureterocele (TUI) is a highly effective modality for decompression of the obstructed system with minimal morbidity [10]. This can be a particularly effective therapy in the setting of sepsis involving an obstructed system or in very young patients when other reconstructive options would be challenging. The puncture can be accomplished cystoscopically with a monopolar wire electrode, resectascope, or laser fiber [28]. Typically the incision is made in the dependent portion of the ureterocele and the size of the puncture may relate to the success of decompression and the risk of de novo reflux. One particular laser incision technique involves creating multiple small punctures which reportedly results in similar decompression rates with a reduced risk of secondary vesicoureteral reflux [29]. Overall, the role of TUI is controversial because of high rates of secondary operations. VUR is found immediately after incision of ectopic ureteroceles in about 50% of cases and more commonly with ureteroceles in duplex systems (56% duplex vs 28% single system). In addition, up to 70% require additional procedures including ureteral reimplantations, ureteroureterostomies, or heminephrectomies [10, 28, 30]. Furthermore, the risk of requiring additional procedures is significantly higher with ectopic ureteroceles (64%) as compared to intravesical ureteroceles (18%) and with duplex system ureteroceles in general [10, 31, 32].

In the case of a poorly functioning dilated upper pole in a duplex system, extirpation is an excellent option. This approach minimizes long-term risks of pyelonephritis or hypertension from upper pole renal dysplasia. Laparoscopic, single site laparoscopic, retroperitoneoscopic and robotic/laparoscopic approaches have been described [33–40]. Care must be taken to remove the entire upper system without injuring the collecting system of the lower pole so as to avoid postoperative urinary leaks with possible urinoma formation. With some robotic surgical platforms, selective vascular mapping can be performed with intravenous indocyanine green (ICG) and induced near infrared fluorescence (NIRF) used to assist with identification of the parenchymal portions to be removed [41].

Hemi-nephrectomy can be performed without dissection of the distal ureter (or ureterocele), which reduces the risk of lower pole ureter compromise from direct injury or vascular compromise [42]. On the other hand, leaving ureteral stumps in situ may require reoperation to deal with complications such as reflux or infection [37, 42–47]. Injury to lower pole vascular supply can result in loss of ipsilateral renal function while major intraoperative bleeding can complicate heminephrectomies with a reported risk of 6–10% [37, 38, 48]. Significant bleeding can occur via injury to the robust renal vasculature, however major bleeding can also originate from the ureteral stump [49, 50]. Post-operative urinoma occurs in 5–29% of heminephrectomy cases and can be managed conservatively in most cases [35, 37, 42–44]. One concern with heminephrectomy is the loss of ipsilateral renal function from vascular compromise or injury to lower pole parenchyma. In most cases there is no significant detectable loss of ipsilateral renal function, however a 10% or greater reduction in renal function has been noted in 5–25% of cases [37, 43, 44, 51–53].

For upper tract dilatation associated with relatively preserved function, another option is an upper to lower ureteroureostomy or pyeloureterostomy. In contrast to heminephrectomy, functional loss of the ipsilateral renal unit with a reconstructive procedure is less common with only 11% of patients with greater than 5% or greater functional loss in one study and no patients with greater than 10% loss of ipsilateral renal function in another study [49, 53]. Although traditional teaching has suggested that reconstructive procedures in the presence of poorly functional systems yields inferior outcomes, some have challenged this notion [54].

These procedures have been described using open, laparoscopic and robot assisted techniques. Furthermore, both proximal and distal ureteroureterostomies have been described [55–57]. While the robotic/laparoscopic approach both are feasible, this author prefers the higher anastomosis, especially when there is significant dilatation of the ureter. This allows for removal of a larger portion of the abnormally dilated ureter and less concern for the so called "yo-yo" or saddle reflux from the functioning to non-functioning renal moiety [58].

Removal of the distal ureter can be important to prevent infectious complications, particularly in those who have suffered febrile urinary tract infections in the past. Removing the ureter as distal as possible seems prudent provided that attention is paid to avoiding injury to the good lower pole ureter and other important pelvic structures. The distal remaining segment should be ligated if there's reflux noted on VCUG. Otherwise, the cut end of the ureter can be left open. In the case of an upper pole ectopic ureterocele, complete excision of the intravesical component may not be required in all cases as long as the cut end of the ureter is left open and the ureterocele decompressed.

During reconstructive procedures it is best to use a no touch technique, grasping the adventitia or surrounding tissues while avoiding direct manipulation of the mucosal edges of the anastomosis. Instruments with lower grasping pressures can also reduce the degree of tissue injury, potentially reducing the risk of complications [59].

The typical anastomotic suture size for reconstruction is 5-0 or 6-0. Some prefer the properties of a braided material such as polyglactin while others prefer the sliding ability of monofilaments. Poliglecaprone monofilament suture has faster absorption and doesn't have memory, which can avoid unwanted spiraling. Unfortunately, colored versions on specific needles are subject to availability. Polydioxanone has a color that is easily identifiable during the procedure, but has memory properties and does absorb more slowly, with some surgeons expressing concerns about an increased risk of stone formation.

Positioning and Port Placement

For upper tract procedures the positioning may be anything from completely supine to partially rotated or a complete lateral decubitus position. The advantage of a decubitus position is the ability for gravity to keep intestines out of the field of dissection after releasing from attachments. A straight legged, completely supine position works well for lower tract/pelvic procedures. Lithotomy should be used with caution as there are increased opportunities for pressure injuries including muscular injury or nerve palsies. Lithotomy can be helpful if there will be simultaneous cystoscopic visualization of lesions of interest. All patients should be firmly fixed in position on the bed with circumferential taping and/or multiple well-placed safety straps. Gel rolls and rolled padding may assist in avoiding pressure injuries while maintaining stable patient position. If the table is to be rotated during the procedure this should be tested, prior to draping. Firm fixation of the ports using securing devices and or sutures can reduce the risk dislodging of ports during surgery. Traction on the ports also allows for lower intra-abdominal pressures, minimizing the physiological challenges of pneumoperitoneum.

Traditional port placement for renal/upper tract reconstruction involves in line port orientation. Modifications can be used when performing reconstructive procedures in combination with removal of a distal ureteral segment (Fig. 12.3). The first port should be placed in the umbilical region (supra-, trans-, or infraumbilical are all acceptable based on surgeon preference and experience). Because of the falciform ligament, supraumbilical placement can be slightly more challenging. This port is typically used for the camera while two additional ports (one more cranial in the midline and one more caudal in the midline) can be used for robotic instruments. A 5 mm assistant port can be used in the semilunar line on the contralateral side between the umbilical and cranial robotic ports. If there is an anticipated need to manipulate the upper pole of the kidney, typically for excisional procedures, a fourth robotic arm can be particularly useful. When four robotic ports are used, the

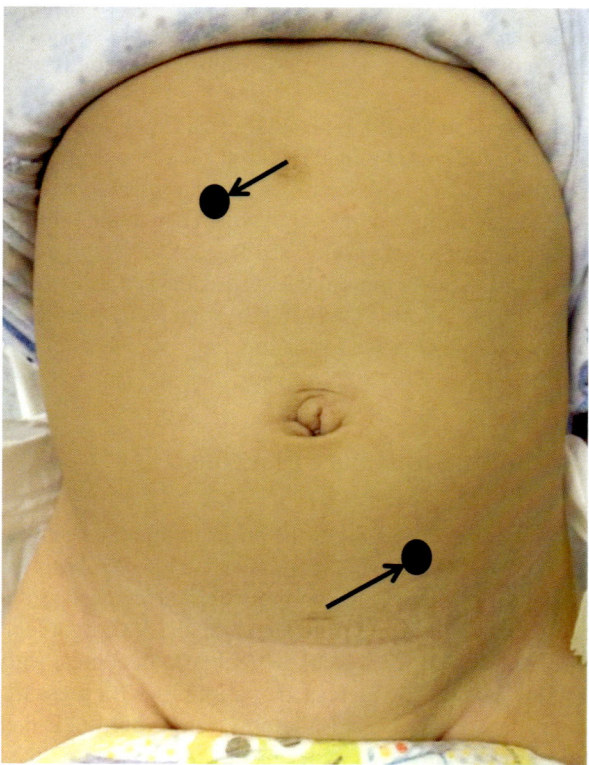

Fig. 12.3 Modification of typical in-line port placement permits improved access to mid and distal ureter, though access to the upper portion of the kidney can be more challenging

camera can be placed in an infraumbilical position and two additional ports placed cranially instead of just one. With larger/older children the caudal port can be placed lateral to midline on the ipsilateral side for a triangulated orientation. Care must be taken to ensure that the port does not end up immediately above the working area. For lower ureteral and reimplantation procedures, a standard setup includes an umbilical port for the camera with right and left abdominal ports lateral and slightly caudal to the umbilical port.

Hidden incision port placement (Figs. 12.4 and 12.5) is especially useful for reconstructive procedures such as high ureteroureterostomies, though access to the upper pole for extirpative procedures can be more challenging [60–63]. The camera angle for hidden incision reconstruction also allows for excellent visualization despite presence of a large liver obscuring portions of the right kidney. A hidden incision upper tract port setup uses the umbilical port as the superior most instrument port while the camera and second instrument port are placed below the belt line (measuring one finger breadth caudal and medial to the anterior superior iliac spine). For these hidden incision ports, initial dissection continues to the anterior fascia. Retractors are then used to identify a point of port passage through the abdominal wall other than directly through the incision. For example, the camera port can be shifted towards the contralateral side and the lateral port can be shifted

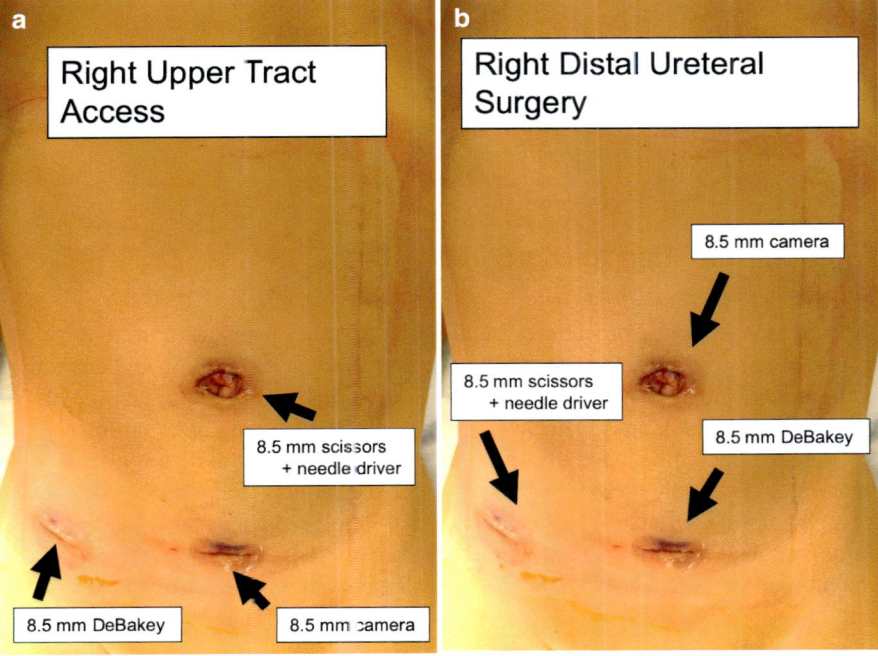

Fig. 12.4 (**a, b**) Hidden incision port placement for upper and lower tract reconstructive procedures. In this case, the same ports were used with different robotic docking positions to perform a multi-quadrant procedure

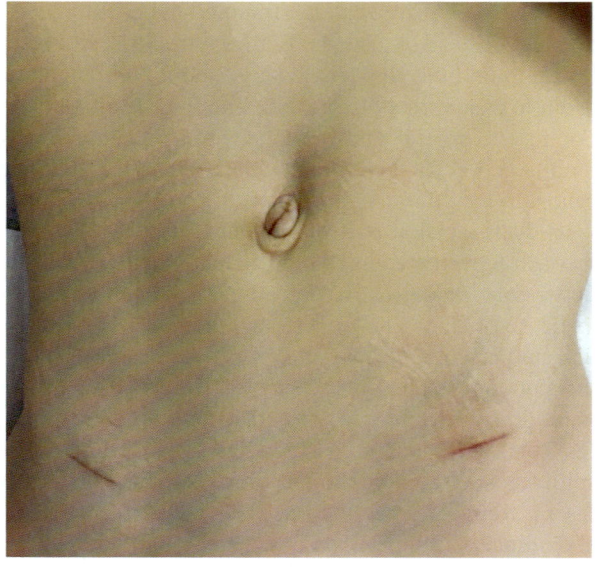

Fig. 12.5 Hidden incisions for pelvic procedures. With traction on the skin incisions, placement of the ports through anterior facia and abdominal layers can be performed superior to the hidden incisions

medially to allow for additional working space. The hidden incision port placement for lower tract/pelvic procedures uses the umbilical incision with two incisions below the belt line as described above. Making fascial penetration cranial to the skin incision typically allows for adequate working space along with preserved cosmetic benefits. Furthermore, multi-quadrant procedures can be accomplished using the same three hidden incisions with re-orientation of the robot docking when transitioning from upper to lower tract portions of the procedure [63].

Technique for High Reconstructions

For high reconstructive procedures such as ureteroureterostomies or ureteropyelostomies, the first step is reflection of the colon medially. Identification and dissection of the ureter(s) begins medial and caudal to the renal parenchyma, just off of the lower border of the kidney. This avoids hilar vessels including aberrant lower pole vasculature. Once the dilated upper pole ureter is identified and distinguished from the normal lower pole ureter, it can be transected obliquely or cut and spatulated on the lateral border. Often times a hitch stitch of 4-0 polypropylene passed through the abdominal wall is helpful to keep the transected and anastomotic portions in view. The normal recipient ureter, which is typically stented, is opened medially. A running or interrupted anastomosis with a wide lumen is performed using 5-0 or 6-0 suture. Polyglactin (Vicryl) poliglecaprone (Monocryl), or Polydioxanone (PDS) sutures may be used (Fig. 12.6).

When excising the distal portion of the disconnected ureter, the goal of dissection is to avoid injury to the 'good' ureter while minimizing residual ureteral tissue

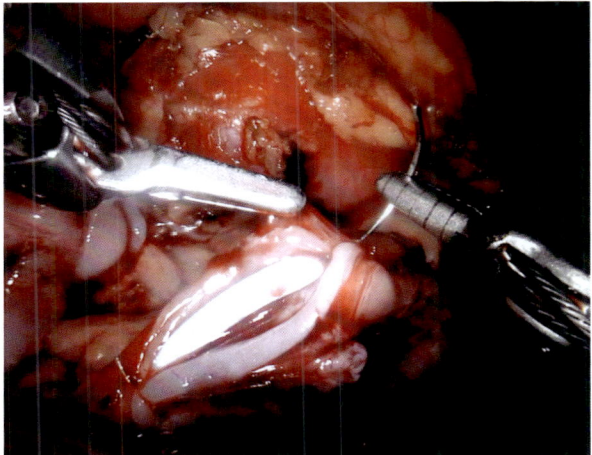

Fig. 12.6 Anastomosis of dilated upper pole ureter to stented lower pole ureter. A large lumen reduces risk of anastomotic stricture

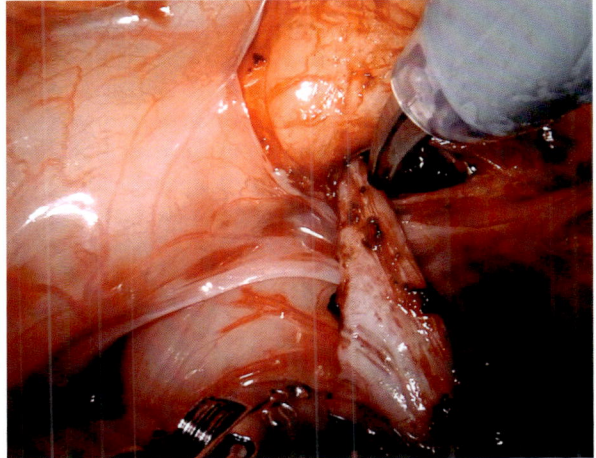

Fig. 12.7 The distal ureter can be traced down into the true pelvis. In this case there was some reflux into the ectopic insertion and the stump was tied off with absorbable suture material

as a nidus for infectious complications. Electrocautery and blunt dissection can be used to separate the two ureters. Most often the adventitial tissue of the dilated ureter to be removed can be gently separated and left in situ alongside the good ureter. This minimizes the risk of disrupting the blood supply to the remaining ureter.

Dissection of the ureter to be excised continues as distally as possible utilizing the initial orientation of the robotic arms and instruments. Adjusting of the direction and degree of abdominal tension can be helpful in reaching further distally. When limitations to further dissection are encountered, re-docking the surgical robot with a modified port placement or by simply switching which ports are used for camera vs arms can afford additional access to the pelvic portion of the dissection (Fig. 12.7).

Care should be taken when dissecting ureters in the pelvis as to avoid important nearby structures. In males the vas deferens can be quite delicate and easily inured.

This structure courses anterior to the ureter as it passes deep in the pelvis and may be situated quite close to the ureterovesical junction. In females the cardinal ligament is particularly vascular, especially in the pubertal/post-pubertal ages. Care should be taken to avoid injury to these vessels as bleeding can be troublesome.

Technique for Low Reconstructions

When performing reconstruction procedures in the pelvis, Trendelenburg position can assist with keeping the intestines out of the way. A redundant sigmoid colon often needs to be gently repositioned out of the true pelvis. This seems to be particularly true among patients with pre-operative bladder bowel dysfunction.

Dissection begins at the level of the ureter as it courses over the iliac vessels in the true pelvis. The peritoneum is incised and the adventitia gently grasped. The ureter is lifted off of the vessels and released circumferentially. Gentle intermittent traction on the ureter cranially and anteriorly can assist in dissection.

For ectopically inserting ureters, the ureter is traced as distally as possible. Closure of the ureteral stump is performed with absorbable suture (4-0 Polyglactin or Polydioxanone PDS) if there is concomitant ureteral reflux on preoperative imaging or if there is a large ureteral orifice in the urethra/bladder neck such that subsequent urethral catheterization is problematic. If the ureter ends in a ureterocele, the contents can be removed with suction and/or filling of the bladder to compress the ureterocele from the inside, as long as the system is non refluxing.

When a reimplantation is to be performed, an appropriate insertion point is identified on the ipsilateral bladder wall. Instillation of irrigation fluid into the bladder can help identify an appropriate location for the detrusor tunnel. A more cranial location to the reimplantation may be required if there are limitations in ureteral length. In addition, the anterior bladder wall can be released to minimize tension on the anastomosis. The detrusor muscle is split leaving mucosa intact. Care should be taken to ensure the presence of a wide portion of visible mucosa such that the submucosal tunnel is not constricting on the reimplanted ureter. Classically, a 5:1 ratio of tunnel is recommended based on normative data [64]; however, a shorter tunnel length (1.5 cm) is theoretically sufficient to prevent urinary reflux [65, 66]. If a hole in the mucosa is inadvertently made, the defect can be closed primarily with 5-0 chromic suture material. The robotic instrument tips can be used to estimate an appropriate tunnel length. When doing so, it is important to rest the reference instrument as close to the tissue as possible to avoid the distorting effects of camera perspective.

When an ectopic ureter needs to be reconnected orthotopically, a small hole in the mucosa at the distal end of the tunnel is made for subsequent anastomosis. The distal ureter is spatulated anteriorly as necessary to allow for a wide lumen. A running or interrupted anastomosis is then performed using 5-0 or 6-0 Polyglactin or poliglecaprone with the first stitch incorporating a portion of detrusor muscle to advance the ureter fully into the tunnel. The tunnel is then closed with interrupted

4-0 Polydioxanone PDS suture. Attention should be paid to the dynamics of the ureter including peristalsis frequency and degree of dilatation with each stitch. Furthermore, the ureteral hiatus should be left wide. The integrity of the closure and the orientation of the ureter is assessed with filling of the bladder with irrigation fluid after the anastomosis is completed.

Post-operative Care

After reconstructive procedures, a single night hospital stay is usually sufficient. An indwelling urinary catheter is typically used for the first night and monitoring for oral liquid/food tolerance along with abdominal exams should alert the surgical team to many early complications. Minimizing narcotic use can enhance recovery of bowel function and there are many options for non-narcotic/enhanced recovery pathways including the use of anti-inflammatory medications, local/regional anesthetic blocks, and early feeding. Typically, patients can go home once tolerating oral hydration and voiding spontaneously [10].

If an indwelling ureteral stent is left in place, it can be removed in 4–6 weeks or after about 1 week if an externalized string is left in place. The first imaging is typically performed about 4 weeks after the procedure or 4 weeks after stent removal (whichever is later).

Complications

Prompt identification and management of complications is important to minimize morbidity. Minor Clavien I/II complications have been shown to occur 28% and 25% of the time respectively with robotic heminephrectomies and ureteroureterostomies [67]. Additionally, urinary tract infections can occur early after reconstructive procedures at a rate of about 33% [68]. This is especially true in those with a history of urinary infection, infected urolithiasis, or obstructed systems. Wound infections are uncommon in pediatric patients. Significant bleeding should also be a rare issue postoperatively, though as noted earlier in this chapter, there are a number of possible bleeding sources. Transfusions are the typical first line treatment unless multiple units of blood are required or if transfusions cannot keep up with ongoing losses.

Urinary leaks are another important complication to look out for, particularly with ureteroureterostomy and other reconstructive procedures. Urinoma formation or anastomotic leaks have been reported in 2.7–13% of UU procedures [49, 69]. Typical signs and symptoms include increasing abdominal distention, nausea, vomiting, and a sudden drop in urine output with increased drain output. Placing an indwelling urinary catheter, leaving externalized drains to gravity and symptomatic medical management will often allow small leaks to resolve within the first 2 weeks

[69]. Overall, the risk of stricture at the anastomotic site is low at 2% [69]. Interventions including ureteral stents, nephrostomy tubes and/or externalized drains may be required in some cases to deal with prolonged urinary leaks or obstruction. Failures do occur with rates of up to 5% [69], however early reoperation is discouraged due to inflammatory changes making tissues challenging to work with and less likely to heal properly. Ureteral stumps can be left in situ, minimizing complications from distal dissection; however, excision for infection is required in 5–7% [14] of minimally invasive cases and up to 12% of open cases [49]. Not surprisingly, larger preoperative ureteral diameter is associated with a higher risk of infectious stump complications postoperatively [49].

Port site herniation should be rare in the pediatric patient, however identification and closure of abdominal wall defects is an important principle [70]. Bowel injury is another rare, potentially catastrophic, event that is best managed with primary closure at the time of injury. Post-operative recognition may be complicated by abscess formation, peritonitis and/or sepsis.

References

1. Nation E. Duplication of the kidney and ureter: a statistical study of 230 new cases. J Urol. 1944;51:456.
2. Whitten SM, Wilcox DT. Duplex systems. Prenat Diagn. 2001;21(11):952–7.
3. Wein AJ, Kavoussi LR, Campbell MF. Campbell-Walsh urology/editor-in-chief, Alan J. Wein; [editors, Louis R. Kavoussi … et al.]. 10th ed. Philadelphia: Elsevier Saunders; 2012.
4. Siomou E, Papadopoulou F, Kollios KD, Photopoulos A, Evagelidou E, Androulakakis P, et al. Duplex collecting system diagnosed during the first 6 years of life after a first urinary tract infection: a study of 63 children. J Urol. 2006;175(2):678–81; discussion 81–2.
5. Michaud JE, Akhavan A. Upper pole heminephrectomy versus lower pole ureteroureterostomy for ectopic upper pole ureters. Curr Urol Rep. 2017;18(3):21.
6. Lee NG, Corbett ST, Cobb K, Bailey GC, Burns AS, Peters CA. Bi-institutional comparison of robot-assisted laparoscopic versus open ureteroureterostomy in the pediatric population. J Endourol. 2015;29(11):1237–41.
7. Glassberg KI, Braren V, Duckett JW, Jacobs EC, King LR, Lebowitz RL, et al. Suggested terminology for duplex systems, ectopic ureters and ureteroceles. J Urol. 1984;132(6): 1153–4.
8. Bisset GS 3rd, Strife JL. The duplex collecting system in girls with urinary tract infection: prevalence and significance. AJR Am J Roentgenol. 1987;148(3):497–500.
9. Mendelsohn C. Using mouse models to understand normal and abnormal urogenital tract development. Organogenesis. 2009;5(1):306–14.
10. Timberlake MD, Corbett ST. Minimally invasive techniques for management of the ureterocele and ectopic ureter: upper tract versus lower tract approach. Urol Clin North Am. 2015;42(1):61–76.
11. Bolduc S, Upadhyay J, Sherman C, Farhat W, Bagli DJ, McLorie GA, et al. Histology of upper pole is unaffected by prenatal diagnosis in duplex system ureteroceles. J Urol. 2002;168(3):1123–6.
12. Perrin EV, Persky L, Tucker A, Chrenka B. Renal duplication and dysplasia. Urology. 1974;4(6):660–4.
13. Abel C, Lendon M, Gough DC. Histology of the upper pole in complete urinary duplication--does it affect surgical management? Br J Urol. 1997;80(4):663–5.

14. Smith FL, Ritchie EL, Maizels M, Zaontz MR, Hsueh W, Kaplan WE, et al. Surgery for duplex kidneys with ectopic ureters: ipsilateral ureteroureterostomy versus polar nephrectomy. J Urol. 1989;142(2 Pt 2):532–4; discussion 42–3.
15. Levy JB, Vandersteer DR, Morgenstern BZ, Husmann DA. Hypertension after surgical management of renal duplication associated with an upper pole ureterocele. J Urol. 1997;158(3 Pt 2):1241–4.
16. Bauer SB, Retik AB. The non-obstructive ectopic ureterocele. J Urol. 1978;119(6):804–7.
17. Share JC, Lebowitz RL. Ectopic ureterocele without ureteral and calyceal dilatation (ureterocele disproportion): findings on urography and sonography. AJR Am J Roentgenol. 1989;152(3):567–71.
18. Wang MH. Persistent urinary incontinence: a case series of missed ectopic ureters. Urol Case Rep. 2015;3(6):223–5.
19. Klauber GT, Crawford DB. Prolapse of ectopic ureterocele and bladder trigone. Urology. 1980;15(2):164–6.
20. Diard F, Eklof O, Lebowitz R, Maurseth K. Urethral obstruction n boys caused by prolapse of simple ureterocele. Pediatr Radiol. 1981;11(3):139–42.
21. Sumfest JM, Burns MW, Mitchell ME. Pseudoureterocele: potential for misdiagnosis of an ectopic ureter as a ureterocele. Br J Urol. 1995;75(3):401–5.
22. Chu WC, Chan KW, Metreweli C. Scintigraphic detection of 'yo-yo' phenomenon in incomplete ureteric duplication. Pediatr Radiol. 2003;33(1):59–61.
23. Ozdogan O, Ates O, Kart Y, Aras F, Olguner M, Akgur F, et al. The diagnosis of yo-yo reflux with dynamic renal scintigraphy in a patient with incomplete ureteral duplication. Mol Imaging Radionucl Ther. 2012;21(3):114–5.
24. Figueroa VH, Chavhan GB, Oudjhane K, Farhat W. Utility of MR urography in children suspected of having ectopic ureter. Pediatr Radiol. 2014;44(8):956–62.
25. Afshar K, Papanikolaou F, Malek R, Bagli D, Pippi-Salle JL, Khoury A. Vesicoureteral reflux and complete ureteral duplication. Conservative or surgical management? J Urol. 2005;173(5):1725–7.
26. Han MY, Gibbons MD, Belman AB, Pohl HG, Majd M, Rushton HG. Indications for nonoperative management of ureteroceles. J Urol. 2005;174(4 Pt 2):1652–5; discussion 5–6.
27. Elder JS, Diaz M, Caldamone AA, Cendron M, Greenfield S, Hurwitz R, et al. Endoscopic therapy for vesicoureteral reflux: a meta-analysis. I. Reflux resolution and urinary tract infection. J Urol. 2006;175(2):716–22.
28. Sander JC, Bilgutay AN, Stanasel I, Koh CJ, Janzen N, Gonzales ET, et al. Outcomes of endoscopic incision for the treatment of ureterocele in children at a single institution. J Urol. 2015;193(2):662–6.
29. Haddad J, Meenakshi-Sundaram B, Rademaker N, Greger H, Aston C, Palmer BW, et al. "Watering Can" Ureterocele puncture technique leads to decreased rates of De Novo Vesicoureteral reflux and subsequent surgery with durable results. Urology. 2017;108:161–5.
30. Jayanthi VR, Koff SA. Long-term outcome of transurethral puncture of ectopic ureteroceles: initial success and late problems. J Urol. 1999;162(3 Pt 2):1077–80.
31. Cooper CS, Passerini-Glazel G, Hutcheson JC, Iafrate M, Camuffo C, Milani C, et al. Long-term followup of endoscopic incision of ureteroceles: intravesical versus extravesical. J Urol. 2000;164(3 Pt 2):1097–9; discussion 9–100.
32. Byun E, Merguerian PA. A meta-analysis of surgical practice patterns in the endoscopic management of ureteroceles. J Urol. 2006;176(4 Pt 2):1871–7; discussion 7.
33. Lee RS, Sethi AS, Passerotti CC, Retik AB, Borer JG, Nguyen HT, et al. Robot assisted laparoscopic partial nephrectomy: a viable and safe option in children. J Urol. 2009;181(2):823–8; discussion 8–9.
34. Tomaszewski JJ, Casel a DP, Turner RM 2nd, Casale P, Ost MC. Pediatric laparoscopic and robot-assisted laparoscopic surgery: technical considerations. J Endourol. 2012;26(6):602–13.
35. Mason MD, Anthony Herndon CD, Smith-Harrison LI, Peters CA, Corbett ST. Robotic-assisted partial nephrectomy in duplicated collecting systems in the pediatric population: techniques and outcomes. J Pediatr Urol. 2014;10(2):374–9.

36. Bansal D, Cost NG, Bean CM, Riachy E, Defoor WR Jr, Reddy PP, et al. Comparison of pediatric robotic-assisted laparoscopic nephroureterectomy and laparoendoscopic single-site nephroureterectomy. Urology. 2014;83(2):438–42.
37. Malik RD, Pariser JJ, Gundeti MS. Outcomes in pediatric robot-assisted laparoscopic heminephrectomy compared with contemporary open and laparoscopic series. J Endourol. 2015;29(12):1346–52.
38. Olsen LH. Robotics in paediatric urology. J Pediatr Urol. 2006;2(1):40–5.
39. Leclair MD, Vidal I, Suply E, Podevin G, Heloury Y. Retroperitoneal laparoscopic heminephrectomy in duplex kidney in infants and children: a 15-year experience. Eur Urol. 2009;56(2):385–9.
40. Zhou H, Ming S, Ma L, Wang C, Liu X, Zhou X, et al. Transumbilical single-incision laparoscopic versus conventional laparoscopic upper pole heminephroureterectomy for children with duplex kidney: a retrospective comparative study. Urology. 2014;84(5):1199–204.
41. Herz D, Smith J, McLeod D, Schober M, Preece J, Merguerian P. Robot-assisted laparoscopic management of duplex renal anomaly: comparison of surgical outcomes to traditional pure laparoscopic and open surgery. J Pediatr Urol. 2016;12(1):44.e1–7.
42. Husmann D, Strand B, Ewalt D, Clement M, Kramer S, Allen T. Management of ectopic ureterocele associated with renal duplication: a comparison of partial nephrectomy and endoscopic decompression. J Urol. 1999;162(4):1406–9.
43. You D, Bang JK, Shim M, Ryu DS, Kim KS. Analysis of the late outcome of laparoscopic heminephrectomy in children with duplex kidneys. BJU Int. 2010;106(2):250–4.
44. Jayram G, Roberts J, Hernandez A, Heloury Y, Manoharan S, Godbole P, et al. Outcomes and fate of the remnant moiety following laparoscopic heminephrectomy for duplex kidney: a multicenter review. J Pediatr Urol. 2011;7(3):272–5.
45. Plaire JC, Pope JC, Kropp BP, Adams MC, Keating MA, Rink RC, et al. Management of ectopic ureters: experience with the upper tract approach. J Urol. 1997;158(3 Pt 2):1245–7.
46. De Caluwe D, Chertin B, Puri P. Fate of the retained ureteral stump after upper pole heminephrectomy in duplex kidneys. J Urol. 2002;168(2):679–80.
47. Cain MP, Pope JC, Casale AJ, Adams MC, Keating MA, Rink RC. Natural history of refluxing distal ureteral stumps after nephrectomy and partial ureterectomy for vesicoureteral reflux. J Urol. 1998;160(3 Pt 2):1026–7.
48. Cabezali D, Maruszewski P, Lopez F, Aransay A, Gomez A. Complications and late outcome in transperitoneal laparoscopic heminephrectomy for duplex kidney in children. J Endourol. 2013;27(2):133–8.
49. Lee YS, Hah YS, Kim MJ, Jung HJ, Lee MJ, Im YJ, et al. Factors associated with complications of the ureteral stump after proximal ureteroureterostomy. J Urol. 2012;188(5):1890–4.
50. Piaggio L, Franc-Guimond J, Figueroa TE, Barthold JS, Gonzalez R. Comparison of laparoscopic and open partial nephrectomy for duplication anomalies in children. J Urol. 2006;175(6):2269–73.
51. Gundeti MS, Ransley PG, Duffy PG, Cuckow PM, Wilcox DT. Renal outcome following heminephrectomy for duplex kidney. J Urol. 2005;173(5):1743–4.
52. Joyeux L, Lacreuse I, Schneider A, Moog R, Borgnon J, Lopez M, et al. Long-term functional renal outcomes after retroperitoneoscopic upper pole heminephrectomy for duplex kidney in children: a multicenter cohort study. Surg Endosc. 2017;31(3):1241–9.
53. Vates TS, Bukowski T, Triest J, Freedman A, Smith C, Perlmutter A, et al. Is there a best alternative to treating the obstructed upper pole? J Urol. 1996;156(2 Pt 2):744–6.
54. McLeod DJ, Alpert SA, Ural Z, Jayanthi VR. Ureteroureterostomy irrespective of ureteral size or upper pole function: a single center experience. J Pediatr Urol. 2014;10(4):616–9.
55. Casale P, Lambert S. Robotic ureteroureterostomy in children with a duplex collecting system. J Robot Surg. 2009;3(3):161.
56. Storm DW, Modi A, Jayanthi VR. Laparoscopic ipsilateral ureteroureterostomy in the management of ureteral ectopia in infants and children. J Pediatr Urol. 2011;7(5):529–33.
57. Grimsby GM, Merchant Z, Jacobs MA, Gargollo PC. Laparoscopic-assisted ureteroureterostomy for duplication anomalies in children. J Endourol. 2014;28(10):1173–7.

58. Smith P, Dunn M. Duplication of the upper urinary tract. Ann R Coll Surg Engl. 1979;61(4):281–6.
59. Mucksavage P, Kerbl DC, Pick DL, Lee JY, McDougall EM, Louie MK. Differences in grip forces among various robotic instruments and da Vinci surgical platforms. J Endourol. 2011;25(3):523–8.
60. Hong YH, DeFoor WR Jr, Reddy PP, Schulte M, Minevich EA, VanderBrink BA, et al. Hidden incision endoscopic surgery (HIdES) trocar placement for pediatric robotic pyeloplasty: comparison to traditional port placement. J Robot Surg. 2018;12(1):43–7.
61. Gargollo PC. Hidden incision endoscopic surgery: description of technique, parental satisfaction and applications. J Urol. 2011;185(4):1425–31.
62. Villanueva CA. Extracorporeal ureteral tailoring during HIDES laparoscopic robotic-assisted ureteral reimplantation for megaureter. J Pediatr Urol. 2015;11(6):362–3.
63. Thaker HKP. Multiquadrant hidden incision endoscopic surgery for pediatric ureteroureterostomy and distal ureterectomy. Videourology. 2019;33:5.
64. Paquin AJ Jr. Ureterovesical anastomosis: the description and evaluation of a technique. J Urol. 1959;82:573–83.
65. Villanueva CA, Nelson CA, Stolle C. Intravesical tunnel length to ureteral diameter ratio insufficiently explains ureterovesical junction competence: a parametric simulation study. J Pediatr Urol. 2015;11(3):144.e1–5.
66. Villanueva CA, Tong J, Nelson C, Gu L. Ureteral tunnel length versus ureteral orifice configuration in the determination of ureterovesical junction competence: a computer simulation model. J Pediatr Urol. 2018;14(3):258.e1–6.
67. Dangle PP, Akhavan A, Odeleye M, Avery D, Lendvay T, Koh CJ, et al. Ninety-day perioperative complications of pediatric robotic urological surgery: a multi-institutional study. J Pediatr Urol. 2016;12(2):102.e1–6.
68. Gonzalez R, Piaggio L. Initial experience with laparoscopic ipsilateral ureteroureterostomy in infants and children for duplication anomalies of the urinary tract. J Urol. 2007;177(6):2315–8.
69. Lashley DB, McAleer IM, Kaplan GW. Ipsilateral ureteroureterostomy for the treatment of vesicoureteral reflux or obstruction associated with complete ureteral duplication. J Urol. 2001;165(2):552–4.
70. Tapscott A, Kim SS, White S, Graves R, Kraft K, Casale P. Port-site complications after pediatric urologic robotic surgery. J Robot Surg. 2009;3(3):187.

Chapter 13
Minimally Invasive Techniques for Management of Urachal Anomalies and Posterior Bladder Pathology

Christopher C. Ballantyne and Sean T. Corbett

Introduction

Advancement of minimally invasive and especially robotic surgery in pediatric urology has resulted in a wider scope of options available for surgical management of various disease conditions. The benefits of robotic surgery are well known; three-dimensional imaging, increased camera magnification, tremor reduction, and an increased range of instrument manipulation not accomplished in standard laparoscopic surgery [1]. As with standard laparoscopy, the ability to observe tissues *in situ* is also advantageous and results in improved anatomical exposure. Enhanced range of motion with robot assistance facilitates more precise suturing [2]. These advantages are readily apparent when dealing with urachal anomalies and the posterior bladder in the pediatric population because it allows for better exposure to anomalies that may be challenging to access in the pediatric pelvis (Figs. 13.1 and 13.2). More common urachal lesions, posterior bladder lesions and deep pelvis structures are listed in Table 13.1. The goals of management of these lesions vary depending on the pathology. In the case of urachal lesions that are symptomatic including pain, infection, or persistent drainage, the goal is to remove the lesion in its entirety. Equally with a bladder diverticulum that may be associated with increased urinary tract infections or altered bladder emptying, the goal in surgical

---

Electronic Supplementary Material The online version of this chapter (https://doi.org/10.1007/978-3-030-57219-8_13) contains supplementary material, which is available to authorized users.

C. C. Ballantyne · S. T. Corbett (✉)
University of Virginia, Department of Urology, Charlottesville, VA, USA
e-mail: ccb6x@virginia.edu; stc2u@virginia.edu

© Springer Nature Switzerland AG 2020
P. C. Gargollo (ed.), *Minimally Invasive and Robotic-Assisted Surgery in Pediatric Urology*, https://doi.org/10.1007/978-3-030-57219-8_13

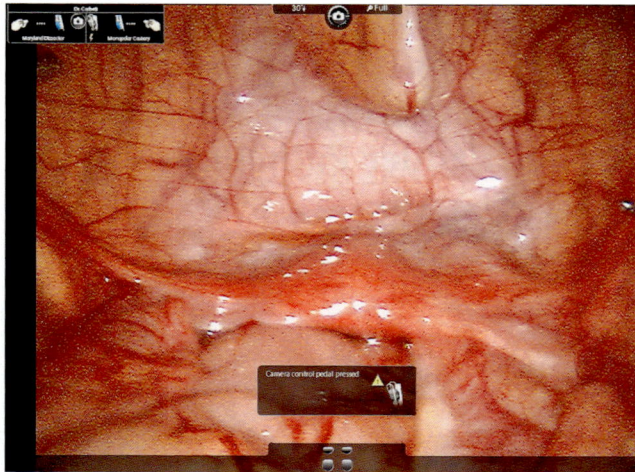

Fig. 13.1 Intraoperative view of urinary bladder and female pelvic structures (uterus, fallopian tubes, and ovaries)

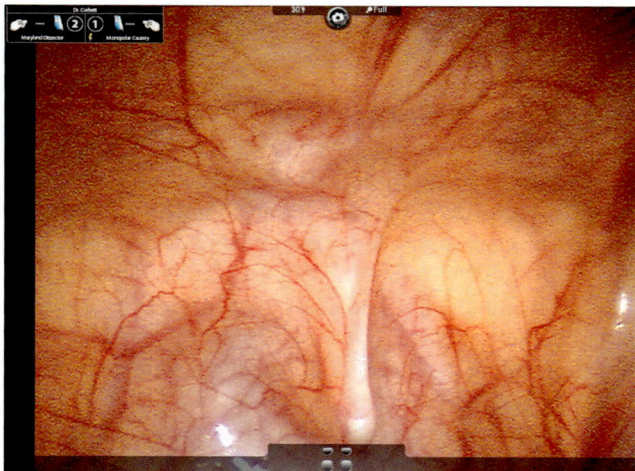

Fig. 13.2 Urachal remnant visualized on anterior abdominal wall. Tip of catheter at bottom of image in decompressed bladder

management is to excise the tic and facilitate more normal emptying. Similarly, in the case of Müllerian duct remnants the goal is for complete excision. This chapter will discuss the minimally invasive surgical approaches for urachal anomalies and other posterior bladder surgeries.

Table 13.1 Urachal and posterior bladder lesions

Urachal anomalies
Patent urachus
Umbilical-urachal sinus
Urachal cyst
Vesicourachal diverticulum
Posterior bladder lesions
Bladder diverticulum
Bladder tumors
Adenocarcinoma
Nephrogenic adenoma
Disorders of sexual differentiation
Persistent Müllerian duct structures

Table 13.2 Urachal anomalies [3, 6, 7, 9]

Patent Urachus (10–48%) – Failure of tract between umbilicus and bladder to obliterate with continued communication between two structures
Umbilical-urachal sinus (18–43%) – Patent portion of urachus in communication with umbilicus but not bladder
Urachal Cyst (31–43%) – Portion of urachal tract is patent that can be located anywhere on tract that is not in communication with either the bladder or umbilicus and is fluid filled
Vesicourachal Diverticulum (3–4%) – Urachus is obliterated everywhere except dome of bladder and can vary in size

Urachus

Urachal Development and Anomalies

The urachus develops from the remnant of the allanotic duct as the bladder descends into the pelvis during the 4th to 5th month of gestation [3]. The allantois continues to narrow over time until only a thick fibrous cord remains, which then becomes the urachus [4]. The urachus, in turn, transitions into the median umbilical ligament and connects the apex of the bladder to the umbilicus [5]. When the communication fails to obliterate there is a urachal remnant and this remnant can present as a patent urachus, umbilical-urachal sinus, vesicourachal diverticulum, or urachal cyst (Table 13.2) [3]. The symptoms can vary depending on the urachal anomaly (Table 13.3). Urachal remnants can have rare malignant degeneration to urachal adenocarcinoma and for this reason can prompt surgical removal. Urachal remnant malignancies are reported as respresenting 0.34% of all bladder cancers and other studies have shown the rate as low as 0.17% [8–10]. Although the likelihood for malignant transformation is rare it does portend a dichotomy in management as some propose an aggressive approach with surgical excision whereas others favor observation. Various imaging modalities are useful to evaluate the urachal remnants (Fig. 13.3).

Table 13.3 Symptoms associated with urachal anomalies

Umbilical drainage
Infection
Pain
Expanding lesion

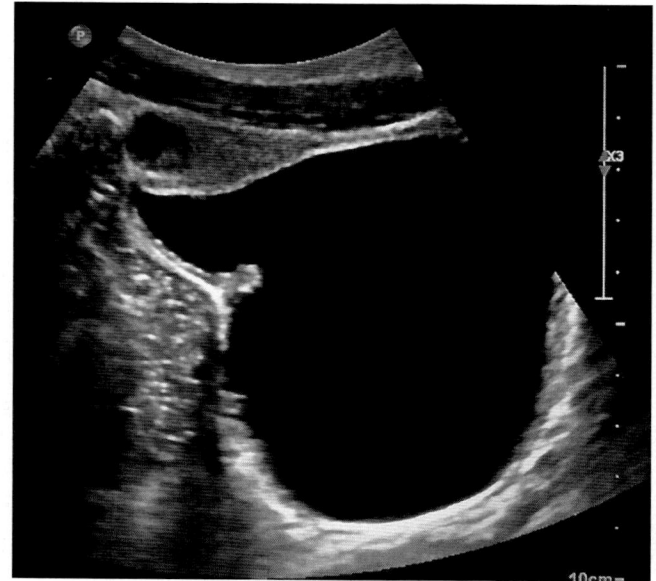

Fig. 13.3 Ultrasound image of a vesicourachal diverticulum

Management

Urachal remnants can be managed conservatively in some cases or by excision in others. Where a conservative approach is applied, the goal is to allow for the remnant to obliterate spontaneously. Progress can be monitored with ultrasound [8]. If infected, antibiotics can be used; however, a delayed surgical approach versus urgent intervention may still be required as infection may be indicative of a failed conservative approach. An operative approach, complete excision, is desirable for patients who have failed conservative management; persistent symptomatic remnants or in some asymptomatic remnants where there is concern for malignancy [11]. Once the decision to proceed with surgery is made there are a variety of approaches available.

Surgical management of urachal remnants requires a wide local excision of the urachus and the extraperitoneal tissues surrounding the urachus [12]. Traditionally this has been through an open approach, which allows for wide local excision of the umbilicus and a cuff of the bladder [13]. The urachus is excised through a lower midline laparotomy incision that carries with it the morbidities of any laparotomy incision such as postoperative pain and slow return to normal function [12]. Laparoscopy has become more commonplace and has been used more frequently by

Table 13.4 Posterior bladder lesions and lesions posterior to the bladder

Bladder diverticula	
Bladder tumors	
	Adenocarcinoma
	Nephrogenic adenoma
Disorders of sexual differentiation	
	Müllerian duct remnants

Table 13.5 Bladder diverticulae [3]

Congenital	Acquired
Solitary, localized herniation	Multiple
In smooth walled bladder	In trabeculated bladders
Dynamic: Intermittent manifestation	Etiologies include:
In children without outlet obstruction	Outlet obstruction
	After bladder surgery, or weakened bladder muscle by infection
	Sequela of neurogenic bladder

surgeons over the laparotomy approach. The laparoscopic approach allows easy identification of the urachal remnant and helps magnify the dissection plane between the extraperitoneal plane and the dome of the bladder in the space of Retzius [12] (Fig. 13.2). Normal laparoscopic excision of the urachal remnants can be difficult if dissection of portions of the bladder or umbilicus is required [13]. With the advancement of robotic-assisted laparoscopic (RAL) surgery more physicians have adopted this approach to excise urachal remnants but there are still surgeons using traditional laparoscopic techniques.

Poster Bladder Lesions and Lesions Posterior to the Bladder

There are various pathologies that can be considered posterior bladder lesions, which, in turn, may lend themselves well to surgical approaches using a minimally invasive technique (Table 13.4).

Bladder Diverticulum

Bladder diverticulae are rare in the pediatric population but can occur in 1.7% of selected children undergoing radiographic evaluation [3]. The etiologies of bladder diverticulae are varied, but they may be congenital or acquired as in the case of bladder outlet obstruction or more commonly as a sequela of a neurogenic bladder (Table 13.5) [3, 14]. Acquired bladder diverticulae occur when there is herniation of bladder mucosa through the detrusor muscle [14]. Congenital bladder diverticulae are most likely caused by congenital defects in the bladder wall and involve both the mucosa and muscular layer of the bladder. Congenital diverticulae are most commonly seen in children with connective tissue diseases such as Ehlers-Danlos, which is commonly diagnosed in childhood [3]. There are times when the bladder diverticulum can involve the ureteral hiatus (Hutch diverticulum).

Various imaging modalities can be utilized to diagnose bladder diverticulae. Ultrasound may be important in the initial detection (Fig. 13.4), but a voiding cystourethrogram (VCUG) remains the gold standard [3]. A VCUG also allow for anatomical and functional imaging of the bladder neck and urethra [15]. Bladder diverticulae are usually discovered during evaluation for infection, hydronephrosis, hematuria, incontinence or obstruction. Diverticulae can be associated with a variety of symptoms (Table 13.6). Congenital diverticulae are dynamic in nature and may not always be present on imaging studies [3].

Management

Bladder diverticulae can be managed with a conservative or surgical approach. Conservative management is desired when the diverticulum is asymptomatic, small, and an incidental finding [3]. Large or symptomatic diverticulae may require surgical intervention. Rarely, a diverticulum can perforate and cause urinary ascites if not managed properly [14].

Similar to urachal lesions, surgical management for bladder diverticulae has traditionally been accomplished through an open approach via a Pfannenstiel incision. Once again, there may be more morbidity associated with this approach, thus alternative options have been developed including, endoscopic resection or fulguration,

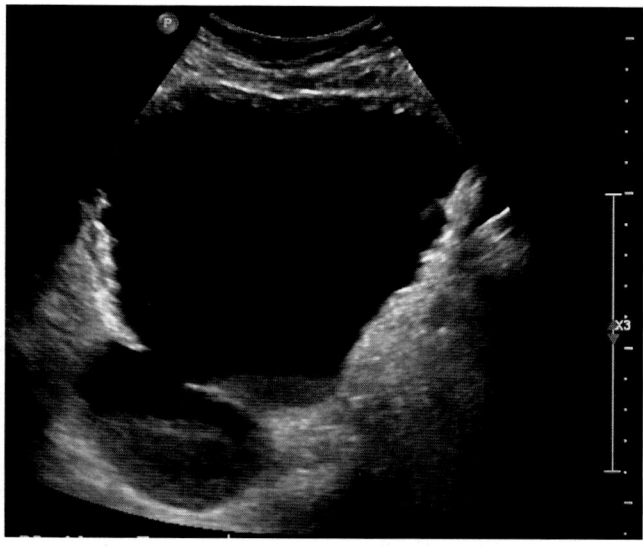

Fig. 13.4 Bladder diverticulum with debris in the diverticulum

standard laparoscopy, or RAL [16]. Laparoscopic diverticulectomy can be performed via a transperitoneal or extraperitoneal approach but may be technically more challenging due to the intracorporeal suturing required to close the bladder after excision of the diverticulum [14, 15]. In this respect the RAL approach has greatly enhanced our ability to repair these in a minimally invasive fashion [15]. If the ureter is associated with the diverticulum and there is the possibility of a ureteral reimplantation in conjunction with excision of the diverticulum then the robot facilitates the complex reconstruction required [17].

Bladder Tumors

Bladder tumors in pediatric patients are exceedingly rare and also rarely amenable to a minimally invasive approach. Rhabdomyosarcoma and urothelial carcinoma are examples of tumors that should not be approached solely with a minimally invasive or RAL approach. For the purpose of this chapter, we will focus primarily on bladder tumors that may be amenable to a minimally invasive approach (Table 13.7). As

Table 13.6 Symptoms associated with bladder diverticulae [16]

Lower urinary tract symptoms refractory to treatment
Bladder or bladder neck obstruction
Presence of tumor or stone in diverticulum
Ureteral obstruction
Voiding dysfunction
Hematuria
Recurrent urinary tract infections

Table 13.7 Bladder tumors [8–10, 18–24]

Bladder adenocarcinoma
Very rare in pediatric populations (approximately 2% of primary bladder neoplasms)
Urachal adenocarcinoma account for 20–39% of bladder adenocarcinomas and 0.17–0.34% of bladder cancers
Can have better outcomes than non-urachal tumors
Can be secondary to metaplasia from chronic infection
Can also be associated with poor outcome because often have metastasized by time of presentation
Treatments include surgery, chemotherapy, and radiation; majority treated with surgical excision
Nephrogenic adenoma
Rare benign metaplastic lesion of urinary tract most commonly bladder without malignant potential
Etiology uncertain but possible causes include: chronic inflammation, irritation, trauma, infection, surgery, and nephrolithiasis
Presents with hematuria, lower urinary tract symptoms, suprapubic pain, flank pain or dysuria
Can mimic variety of malignancies

with tumors in the adult population, these patients may present with a variety of symptoms including hematuria, stones, infections, hydronephrosis, flank pain, dysuria, or outlet obstruction resulting in urinary retention. To minimize radiation exposure, the initial evaluation starts with ultrasound, but additional work-up may require plain film x-ray, CT, and MRI among others. In some cases, transurethral biopsy or resection may be part of the initial evaluation to facilitate diagnosis. Bladder adenocarcinoma, albeit rare, is primarily associated with urachal anomalies. Hence why some surgeons approach any urachal lesion in an aggressive manner; complete excision. These lesions will typically arise at the dome of the bladder and then extend into the urachus. Nephrogenic adenoma is a benign metaplastic lesion without malignant potential. It can develop anywhere within the bladder and unfortunately it can mimic a variety of malignancies and thus requires excision for definitive diagnosis. Fortunately, complete excision is curative for nephrogenic adenoma.

Management

Bladder tumors are not managed conservatively; instead, surgical excision is necessary. Although the gold standard for resection is an open approach, small lesions ideally located may be amenable to a laparoscopic or RAL approach. However, the approach should never compromise the care or tumor management. Wide local excision should be performed. Obviously, repair of the bladder defect will necessitate intracorporeal suturing, which, once again, the robot will facilitate.

Lesions Posterior to the Bladder

We will not focus on ureteral, bladder neck, or urethral lesions, as these will be covered in other chapters. However, gonadal pathology can also be easily addressed using a minimally invasive approach. Aside from undescended testes, there are rare Müllerian or Wolffian pathologies that require surgical management. In general, the need to address disorders of sexual differentiation is beyond the scope of this chapter therefore we will focus primarily on how to perform the procedure as opposed to answering the more complicated questions of when and how.

Müllerian duct remnants are one of the more common pathologies that require intervention. This is a rare genetic disorder where patients have 46 XY karyotype and are phenotypically male but have persistence of Müllerian duct structures. Persistent Müllerian duct syndrome (PMDS) is an autosomal recessive disorder associated with failed regression of Müllerian duct structures secondary to defects in genes for anti-Müllerian hormone (45% of cases) and AMH receptor (39% of cases) [25]. PMDS has three different primary presentations. These presentations are bilateral intra-abdominal testes in positions similar to ovaries (60–70%), single testis in hernia sac or scrotum with contralateral inguinal herni, hernia uteri inguinalis, (20–30%), and both testes in hernia sac with fallopian tubes and uterus (10%)

Table 13.8 Symptoms of MDR [25, 27]

Urinary tract infection
Pain
Post-void incontinence
Palpable abdominal mass
Recurrent epididymitis
Urinary incontinence

Table 13.9 Potential risk associated with MDR [25, 27]

Malignant change of intra-abdominal testis
Endometrial carcinoma
Cyclic hematuria
Urinary stasis
Ejaculatory duct obstruction
Infertility

[26]. Patients typically present with undescended testes, fallopian tubes, uterus, and proximal vagina, which may drain into a prostatic utricle [26]. The enlarged prostatic utricle communicates with the prostatic urethra and stasis of urine here can cause recurrent UTIs, voiding dysfunction, or urinary incontinence [27]. The duct remnants are associated with the base of bladder and prostate, which can make removal difficult [27].

There are various signs and symptoms that can be associated with Müllerian duct remnants (Table 13.8). There are also times when MDRs are asymptomatic and thus detection may be delayed or incidentally diagnosed [25]. MDR can be difficult to visualize with ultrasound and there have been reports where 40% of pelvic ultrasounds have been unable to identify any remnants [25]. Once MDR have been diagnosed there are potential risks associated with leaving Müllerian structures behind, thus (Table 13.9), most surgeons recommend extirpation. There have been 11 malignancies reported in Müllerian remnants, which supports surgical excision [26].

Management

The surgical approach for MDR is generally selected based on surgeon preference, but approaches include transperitoneal, posterior with rectal retraction, posterior and anterior sagittal transrectal, transvesical, laparoscopic and RAL [28]. Once again, the laparoscopic approach allows better visualization and magnification to allow for meticulous dissection and manipulation of tissues. These advantages allow the surgeon to minimize the risk of injury to pelvic nerves and, in turn, hopefully preserve postoperative voiding and bowel function [25]. RAL enhances conventional laparoscopy by improving the visualization and enhancing surgical precision while operating deep in the pelvis [27]. Where there is an undescended intra-abdominal testis or testes, these can be approached concurrently without the need to alter port placement.

Surgical Techniques

For either a laparoscopic or a RAL approach used to address urachal, posterior bladder lesions, or lesions posterior to the bladder the principles are the same. The authors use either approach depending on the pathology due to enhanced visualization, but where more delicate tissue handling and/or suturing is required our preference is a RAL approach. We have divided the approach to the lesions depending on the needs noted above. For simple lesions requiring only excision without delicate tissue handling or suturing, a standard laparoscopic approach is often employed, outlined in Box 13.1.

In the case of more complex lesions where greater tissue handling and/or suturing is required, the authors employ a RAL approach (Box 13.2).

Complications

Rare complications associated with any of these lesions include bladder leak, bladder diverticulum, bladder rupture and the need for reoperation [6]. Conversion to an open approach from a laparoscopic or RAL approach is rare, however, all minimally

---

Box 13.1 Minimally Invasive Approach to Excision of Simple Lesions
1. Supine positioning with the patient's legs slightly frog-legged is preferred. The patient is secured to the operative table after being appropriately padded. Standard laparoscopy is often the norm for straightforward excision of lesions especially those such as urachal lesions not in communication with the bladder.
2. Three ports are placed (the authors prefer 5 mm instruments and camera): A camera port (3, 5, or 10 mm) superior to the umbilicus, can be slightly off midline for better visualization of a lesion extending to the umbilicus. Alternatively, if at the level of the umbilicus can facilitate carrying the dissection out the umbilical incision. Two instrument ports (3, 5, or 10 mm) are placed in the mid-clavicular line bilaterally below the umbilicus or more cephalad depending on where the lesion being addressed is located. (Fig. 13.5)
3. The peritoneum is incised overlying the lesion. Intra-operative ultrasound may facilitate localization of the lesion, especially smaller lesions.
4. The authors prefer utilization of a Maryland grasper and hot scissors for dissection. A stitch can be placed through the lesion to act as a handle unless there is concern for infection. The lesion is completely mobilized proximally and distally. Once again, intra-operative ultrasound can be used to identify that the entire lesion has been excised.

Fig. 13.5 Port placement for laparoscopic and robotic-assisted laparoscopic approach to urachal, posterior bladder, or lesions posterior to the bladder. (*Courtesy of Matthew D. Timberlake, MD, Assistant Professor of Urology and Pediatrics, Texas Tech University Health Science Center, Lubbock, TX*)

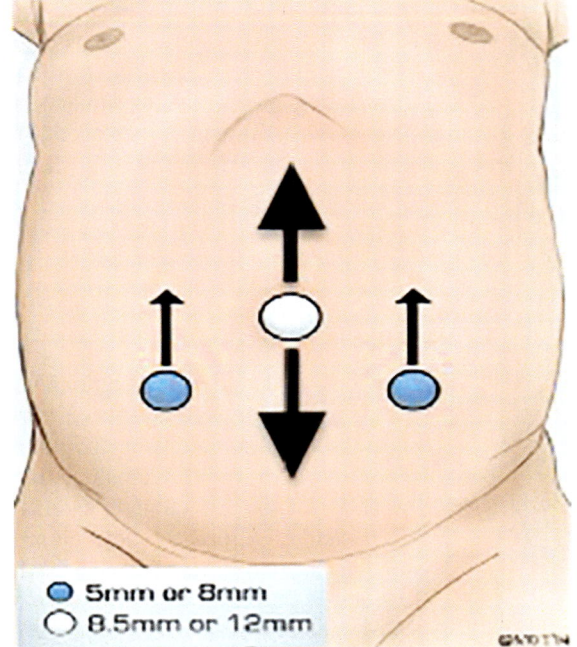

Box 13.2 Minimally Invasive Approach to More Complex Lesions

1. If cystoscopy is required to better define a lesion prior to starting minimally invasive approach the infant/child is positioned appropriately in lithotomy position.
2. The patient can then be repositioned supine and slightly frog-legged, pressure points appropriately padded, and secured to the table. The prep should include the perineum and genitals to allow access intra-operatively. A Foley catheter can be placed onto the sterile field as needed. For an older child or adolescent, the authors would consider using a split leg table and would dock the robot between the legs.
3. The table is placed into Trendelenburg position and can be airplaned either right or left depending on the location of the lesion; however, most are easily accessible with just Trendelenburg.
4. The robot is docked in a modified-side, side-, or end-docked position near the foot of the table.
5. Once again, three ports are placed: A camera port (the authors prefer an 8.5 mm camera port, although a 10 mm can be used as well) superior to the umbilicus, can be slightly off midline for better visualization of a lesion extending to the umbilicus. Alternatively, can place either through the umbilicus to facilitate dissection of the patent urachus or through and

infra-umbilical incision to approach posterior bladder lesions and lesions posterior to the bladder. Two 5 mm (8 mm ports can also be used; the daVinci® Si allows for 5 mm instruments, the Xi only accommodates 8 mm instruments) instrument ports placed in the mid-clavicular line bilaterally below the umbilicus or more cephalad depending on where the lesion being addressed is located. (Fig. 13.1)
6. The peritoneum is incised overlying the lesion. Intra-operative ultrasound can be used to identify smaller lesions.
7. Depending on the lesion dissection will vary:

   (a) Patent urachus (Video 13.1):

      (i) Urachus is identified near umbilicus and dissection using hook cautery and Maryland graspers is performed towards the bladder. Wide excision of the lesion should include a cuff of the bladder. Failure to remove all anomalous tissue can result in recurrence, stone formation, infection, or rarely malignant transformation.
      (ii) The bladder is filled through the pre-placed catheter. Using the urachus the hook cautery can be used to score the bladder cuff for dissection. A combination of sharp dissection with scissors and hook cautery is used to complete excision. The urachus is used as a handle to provide traction on the bladder cuff during excision.
      (iii) The bladder is then repaired in two layers. Depending on the size of the defect created a 3-0 or 4-0 poliglecaprone 25 suture is used in a simple running or in a figure-of-eight fashion to close the mucosa and detrusor muscle using a Maryland grasper and needle driver. The second layer is closed using 3-0 or 4-0 polydioxanone or vicryl. The bladder is then filled to assess for leaks.
      (iv) The remainder of the patent urachus can be dissected to the level of the umbilicus. A suture can be placed through this to aid in identification. A small umbilical incision is made and the suture is grasped and the remaining urachal tissue can be excised.

   (b) Bladder diverticulum or tumor excision:

      (i) As above, except the camera trocar is placed through an infra-umbilical incision. The instrument trocars are infra-umbilical in the mid-clavicular line bilaterally.
      (ii) The bladder is then filled to determine the location of the diverticulum. A hitch stitch or stitches can be placed percutaneously to help provide retraction on the bladder and facilitate resection of lesion involved. Depending on proximity to trigone and ureters ureteral catheters can be placed via cystoscopy prior to docking of the robot. The catheters can facilitate identification of the ureters during dissection to minimize the risk of injury.

(iii) The diverticulum or tumor can be excised again using a combination of sharp dissection with scissors and hook cautery.
(iv) In the case of a tumor, to assure complete excision, a flexible ureteroscope can be used intra-operatively. The scope can be pushed into the lesion or the light shone directly on it to facilitate localization intra-abdominally.
(v) The bladder is then repaired in two layers. Depending on the size of the defect created a 3-0 or 4-0 poliglecaprone 25 suture is used in a simple running or in a figure-of-eight fashion to close the mucosa and detrusor muscle using a Maryland grasper and needle driver. The second layer is closed using 3-0 or 4-0 polydioxanone or vicryl. The bladder is then filled to assess for leaks. A Foley catheter is left in place overnight and removed the following morning.

(c) Lesions posterior to the bladder (Müllerian duct remnants):

(i) As above, the camera trocar is placed through an infra-umbilical incision. The instrument trocars are infra-umbilical in the mid-clavicular line bilaterally.
(ii) Remnants are identified and using Maryland graspers and hook cautery. Dissection is performed with care to avoid injury to the vasa deferentia bilaterally and thus jeopardize potential fertility. There is a rare risk of malignancy in retained Müllerian structures.

8. In all instances above, if additional retraction is required an assistant port can be placed and either a bedside assist can work through this port or another arm on the robot can be deployed.
9. Once resection is completed and depending on the size of the specimens, they can either be retrieved through one of the trocar sites or placed into a laparoscopic specimen bag, which can then be retrieved through the umbilical incision.

invasive surgeons should be prepared and know how to gain exposure in the event that conversion to an open approach is required. Complications that are not typically thought of with an open approach, but should be with a minimally invasive and especially a RAL approach, are those associated with positioning and anesthesia [29]. These include potential pressure areas, the robot itself may push on the patient including on the ET tube, or, in the case of a small child/infant there may be increased robotic arm collisions associated with ports placed in close proximity to one another [30]. Table 13.10 shows common complications that can occur during minimally invasive pediatric urology surgery. A surgeon that plans to approach any of these lesions in a minimally invasive fashion should be well prepared to not only use the tools provided in the minimally invasive toolbox, but also in dealing with any of the complications that may arise.

Table 13.10 Common complications of robotic pediatric urological surgeries [29]

Anesthetic	
	Respiratory
	Cardiovascular
Positioning	
	Orthopedic
	Neurologic
Access	
	Vascular injury
	Viscous injury
	Bladder injury
	Thoracic
	Ex. subcutaneous emphysema
Intraoperative	
	Vascular injury
	Viscous injury
Postoperative	
	Hemorrhage
	Infection
	Incisional hernia

Used with permission of Springer Nature

Postoperative Care and Follow Up

Postoperative care depends on what procedure was performed. In general, for isolated urachal lesions or simple excision of MDR, most of these patients can have their surgery performed in the outpatient setting. However, where reconstructive repair is required including cystotomy closure most of these patients are admitted for overnight observation with an indwelling catheter. In most cases the catheters are removed the following day and a voiding trial is undertaken prior to discharge home. Most patients will present for a postoperative check in 4–6 weeks. Ultrasound can be used to assess the bladder and anterior abdominal wall [11]. A VCUG or additional imaging studies can be included depending on the underlying pathology. Fortunately, complete excision of a nephrogenic adenoma or adenocarcinoma should be curative but follow up with ultrasound can be used for surveillance. Similarly, extirpation of MDR should also be curative and thus not require prolonged follow up. However, surveillance may be required if complete excision was not possible due to proximity to the urethra, prostate, or bladder neck.

Conclusion

Minimally invasive surgical approaches have enhanced our ability to approach and thus manage urachal lesions, posterior bladder lesions, and lesions posterior to the bladder. The robot has vastly improved on standard laparoscopy and broadened the applicability of the minimally invasive approach to those less skilled with standard laparoscopy. The surgeon should never compromise patient care/outcomes purely because of technology. However, for surgeons well versed in minimally invasive techniques these tools complement our current armamentarium well. Continued technological advances should enhance our ability to manage more complex lesions.

Key Points
- Robotic assisted surgery facilitates better access, enhanced range of motion, and precise suturing in the pediatric pelvis
- Urachal remnants operated on where patients failed conservative management, persistent symptomatic remnants or concern for malignancy
- Bladder diverticulae are rare but can be managed surgically when large or symptomatic
- Bladder tumors are rarely amenable to a minimally invasive surgical approach
- Common complications can be seen with anesthesia, positioning, access, and can be further subdivided into intraoperative and postoperative

References

1. Kim C. Robotic urologic surgery in infants: results and complications. Front Pediatr. 2019;7:187. Published online 2019 May 13.
2. Mizuno K, Kojima Y, et al. Robotic surgery in pediatric urology: current status. Asian J Endosc Surg. 2018;11(4):308–17.
3. Frimberger D, Kropp BP. Bladder anomalies in children. In: Wein AJ, editor. Campbell-Walsh urology. Philadelphia: Elsevier; 2015. p. 3173–3181.E2.
4. More KL. Urogenital system. In: Moore KL, editor. The Developing Human: Clinically Oriented Embryology. 11th ed. Philadelphia: Saunders; 2019. p. 223–62.e1.
5. Nix JT, Menville JG, Alber M, et al. Congenital patent urachus. J Urol. 1958;79:264–73.
6. Destri L, Schillaci D, Latin R, et al. The urachal pathology with umbilical manifestation: overview of laparoscopic technique. J Laparoendosc Adv Surg Tech A. 2011;21(9):809–14.
7. Naiditch JA, Radhakrishnan J, Chin AC. Current diagnosis and management of urachal remnants. J Pediatr Surg. 2013;48(10):2148–52.
8. Stopak JK, Azarow KS, et al. Trends in surgical management of urachal anomalies. J Pediatr Surg. 2015;50(8):1334–7.
9. Widni E, Hollwarth M, Haxhija E. The impact of preoperative ultrasound on correct diagnosis of urachal remnants in children. J Pediatr Surg. 2010;45(7):1433–7.
10. Sheldon CA, Clayman RV, Gonzalez R, et al. Malignant urachal lesions. J Urol. 1984;131:1–8.
11. Chiarenza SF, Scarpa MG, et al. Laparoscopic excision of urachal cyst in pediatric age: report of three cases and review of the literature. J Laparoendosc Adv Surg Tech A. 2009;19(Suppl 1):S133–6.
12. Sukhotnik I, Aranovich I, Mansur B, et al. Laparoscopic surgery of urachal anomomalies: a single-center experience. Isr Med Assoc J. 2016;18(11):673–6.
13. Rivera M, Granberg CF, et al. Robotic-assisted laparoscopic surgery of urachal anomalies: a single-center experience. J Laparoendosc Adv Surg Tech A. 2015;25(4):291–4.
14. Meeks J, Hagerty J, et al. Pediatric robotic-assisted laparoscopic diverticulectomy. Urology. 2009;73(2):299–301.
15. Christman M, Casale P. Robot-assisted bladder diverticulectomy in the pediatric population. J Endourol. 2012;26(10):1296–300.

16. Eyraud R, Laydner H, et al. Robot-assisted laparoscopic bladder diverticulectomy. Curr Urol Rep. 2013;14(1):46–51.
17. Noh P, Bansal D. Pediatric robotic assisted laparoscopy for paraureteral bladder diverticulum excision with ureteral reimplantation. J Pediatr Urol. 2012;9(1):28–30.
18. Maemoto R, Matsuo S, et al. Umbilical resection during laparoscopic surgery for urachal remnants. Asian J Endosc Surg. 2019;12(1):101–6.
19. Sakata S, Gruny J, et al. Urachal-sigmoid fistula managed by laparoscopic assisted high anterior resection, primary anastomosis and en bloc resection of the urachal cyst and involved bladder. Asian J Endosc Surg. 2016;9(2):201–3.
20. Hong S, Kim J, et al. Laparoscopic partial cystectomy with en bloc resection of the urachus for urachal adenocarcinoma. Int J Urol. 2007;14(10):963–5.
21. Gleason J, Bowlin P, et al. A comprehensive review of pediatric urachal anomalies and predictive analysis for adult urachal adenocarcinoma. J Urol. 2015;193(2):632–6.
22. Turcan D, Acikalin M. Nephrogenic adenoma of the urinary tract: a 6-year single center experience. Pathology. 2017;213(7):832–5.
23. Ozcift B, Kacar A, et al. Recurrence of childhood nephrogenic adenoma in urinary bladder developed four years after previous surgery despite intravesical sodium hyaluronte therapy. Turk J Urol. 2016;42(4):303–6.
24. Natale C, Leinwand G, et al. Reviewing the demographic, prognostic, and treatment factors of primary adenocarcinoma of the bladder: a SEER population-based study. Clin Genitourin Cancer. 2019;17:380–8.
25. Raicevic M, Saxena A. Laparoscopic management of mullerian duct remnant in paediatric age: evidence and outcome analysis. J Minim Access Surg. 2018;14(2):95–8.
26. Diamond D, Yu R. Disorders of sexual development: etiology, evaluation, and medical management. In: Wein AJ, editor. Campbell-Walsh urology. Philadelphia: Elsevier; 2015. p. 3469–3497.E6.
27. Lima M, Maffi M, et al. Robotic removal of mullerian duct remnants in pediatric patients; our experience and review of literature. Pediatr Med Chir. 2018;40(1) https://doi.org/10.4081/pmc.2018.182.
28. Okur H, Gough D. Management of mullerian duct remnants. Urology. 2003;61(3):634–7.
29. Corbett ST. Complications of laparoscopic and robotic pediatric urologic surgery. In: Ghavamian R, editor. Complications of laparoscopic and robotic urologic surgery. New York: Springer; 2014. p. 277–91.
30. Dangle PP, et al. Ninety-day perioperative complication of pediatric robotic urological surgery: a multi-institutional study. J Pediatr Urol. 2016;12(2):102.e1–6.

Chapter 14
Robotic Appendicovesicostomy

Carlos A. Villanueva Del Rio

Preoperative Considerations

Indications

An appendicovesicostomy (APV), also known as the Mitrofanoff procedure, is indicated in cases where clean intermittent catheterization (CIC) through the urethra is not possible or practical –due to pain, strictures, false passages, or body habitus.

For patients not ready to start CIC through an APV who are in need of a diverting procedure, a permanent catheter that is exchanged periodically could be left in the APV long term until the child is ready for CIC with no harm to the APV (https://doi.org/10.1016/j.jpurol.2019.02.011).

Postoperative Urodynamic Changes Induced by the APV Procedure

In patients with neurogenic bladder with adequate continence who are candidates for an isolated APV, thought should be given to the possible effects of the APV on bladder dynamics. For example, a patient able to stay dry with intermittent catheterization every 4 hours who has low detrusor leak point pressure (DLPP), might start leaking after the APV. Consideration for concomitant bladder augmentation/bladder neck sling or reconstruction should be given for these patients. In Nguyen et al. robotic APV series [1], one out of the 10 patients developed marked changes in bladder compliance causing bilateral VUR and incontinence from the APV stoma, eventually requiring bladder augmentation.

C. A. Villanueva Del Rio (✉)
Phoenix Children's Hospital, Phoenix, AZ, USA

An isolated APV is best suited for bladders with normal capacity, compliance, and bladder outlet.

No Appendix

This chapter assumes a healthy usable appendix is available. How to perform a robotic Monti will not be covered in the chapter.

Operative Considerations

Bowel and Antibiotic Prep

Guidelines from the American Urologic Association (https://www.auanet.org/guidelines/optimizing-outcomes-in-urological-surgery-pre-operative-care-for-the-patient-undergoing-urologic-surgery-or-procedure) recommend against a mechanical bowel prep before urologic surgery for the purpose of preventing surgical site infections. An antibiotic oral prep was recommended for colon surgery but not specifically for isolated use of the appendix. Preoperative treatment of constipation might facilitate surgical exposure and manipulation of the bowel and should be considered.

Preoperative Systemic Antibiotics

The American Urologic Association (AUA) antibiotic guidelines (https://www.auanet.org/guidelines/antimicrobial-prophylaxis-2008-reviewed-and-validity-confirmed-2011-amended-2012) do recommend preoperative systemic antibiotics for urologic surgery entering the urinary tract and bowel:

- 1st line: 2nd/3rd gen. Cephalosporin – Aminoglycoside (Aztreonam) + Metronidazole or Clindamycin
- 2nd line: – Ampicillin/Sulbactam – Ticarcillin/Clavulanate – Piperacillin/Tazobactam – Fluoroquinolone

The AUA guidelines endorse continuing antibiotics for 24 h. However, the American College of Surgeons recommends stopping all prophylaxis after incision closure [2].

14 Robotic Appendicovesicostomy

Positioning

Patient is positioned supine in frog leg, with rolled towels under the knees and secured to the bed with tape at the chest and legs. A bean bag can be used under the patient to facilitate rotation to the left side if the appendix is found high in the right upper quadrant.

Some Trendelenburg might help moving the bowel superiorly during the bladder anastomosis. However too much Trendelenburg could also move the cecum and appendiceal mesentery superiorly making the anastomosis more difficult.

Foley catheter is placed on the field to allow for regulation of bladder filling. Orogastric tube is placed by anesthesia to decompress the stomach before accessing the abdomen.

Port Configuration

Robotic 8 mm trocars at umbilicus, both ends of the bikini line (ports higher in the fascia), and right upper quadrant/subxiphoid area (positioning this last trocar on the right side might decrease interference with the umbilical trocar). A V flap with the base inferior is marked, incised, and developed in the umbilicus before placing the 8 mm robotic trocar in this location (Fig. 14.1).

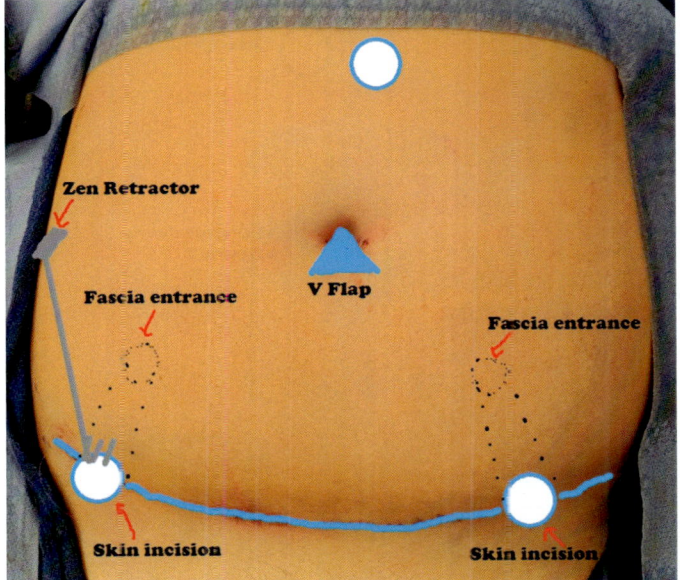

Fig. 14.1 Port placement for robotic APV

Appendix Harvesting

Instruments are positioned as follows: Camera at the umbilicus, left arm DeBakey forceps at the left bikini line, right arm monopolar scissors at right upper quadrant/subxiphoid location. The right lower quadrant trocar can be used to assist holding the appendix. Patient is rotated to the left side and then the robot is docked along a line going from the umbilicus to the right lower quadrant trocar (Fig. 14.2).

The right colon and appendix are mobilized as needed. The appendix is assessed for usability: a minimum of 6–7 cm seems to be adequate to perform the procedure. This step is very important as the 10-× magnification provided by the robotic camera can be misleading: significant time can be wasted trying to reimplant an unusable appendix just to convert to an open Monti procedure at the end.

Vascular arcade is identified and preserved. The appendix can be divided with staples with or without taking a cuff of cecum (to be used to extend the length of the appendix for obese patients or short appendix). The appendix can also be divided with scissors and then closed in two layers with absorbable suture.

The tip of the appendix is cut distally at the center, creating anterior and posterior flaps (fish mouth, Fig. 14.3). This incision is extended proximally until the appendix caliber is adequate.

A 10 Fr feeding tube is cut to 10–12 cm. The tapered end of the feeding tube is advanced from the appendix cuff towards the appendix tip, letting 2 cm of the tube

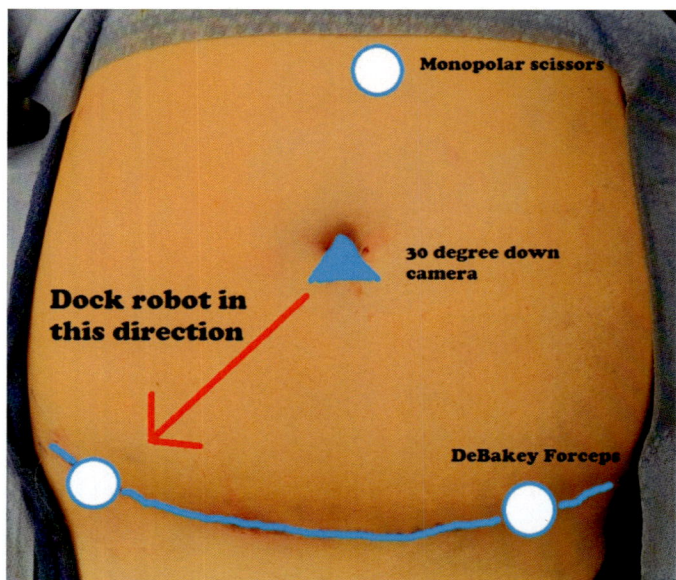

Fig. 14.2 Port placement and docking for appendix harvesting

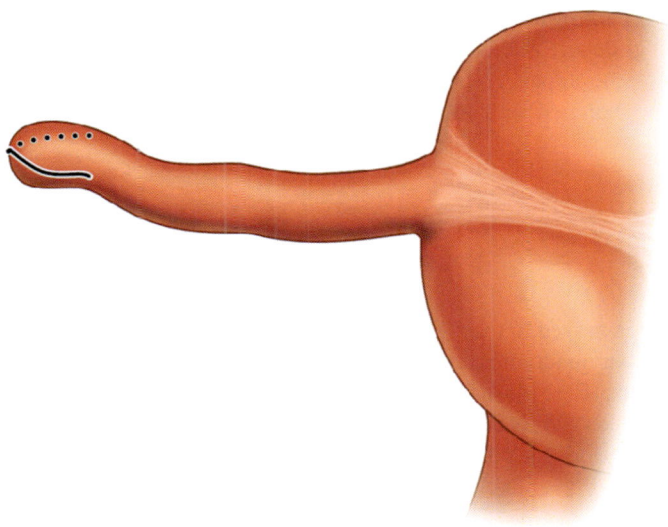

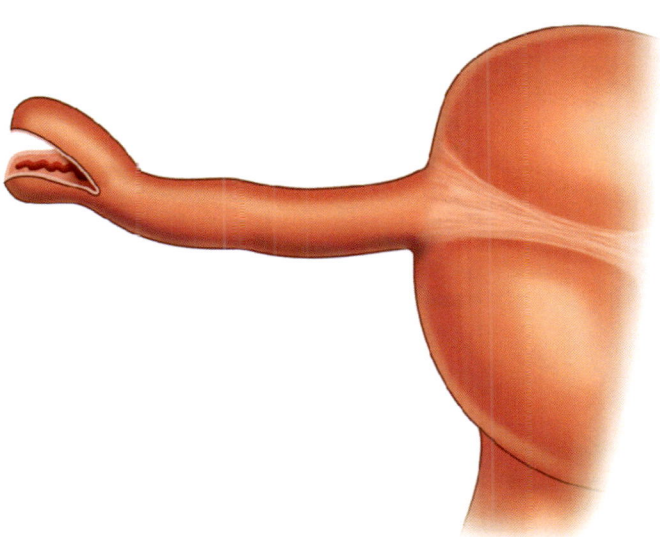

Fig. 14.3 Distal configuration of the cut appendix

stick out of the tip of the appendix. At this point the tip of the tube is cut to allow passage of a glidewire at the end of the case. Using a 2-0 suture, the tube is secured proximally to the appendix by passing the suture through the tube, through the appendix, and then tied with an air not. Now the appendix can be manipulated using the tube.

APV

The right arm is moved to the right lower quadrant port and the assistant arm moves to the right upper quadrant/subxiphoid area. The robot is re-docked now pointing in between the legs (Fig. 14.4).

For an isolated APV, is best to stay extravesical. The bladder implantation can be approached anteriorly or posteriorly.

Anterior Implantation

With the anterior reimplantation the bladder is mobilized anteriorly (drop the bladder like the start of a robotic prostatectomy). The dome of the bladder is held by the assistant port to stretch the anterior bladder dome and a 3–4 cm extravesical tunnel is marked. The bladder is filled as needed to be able to make the detrusorotomy.

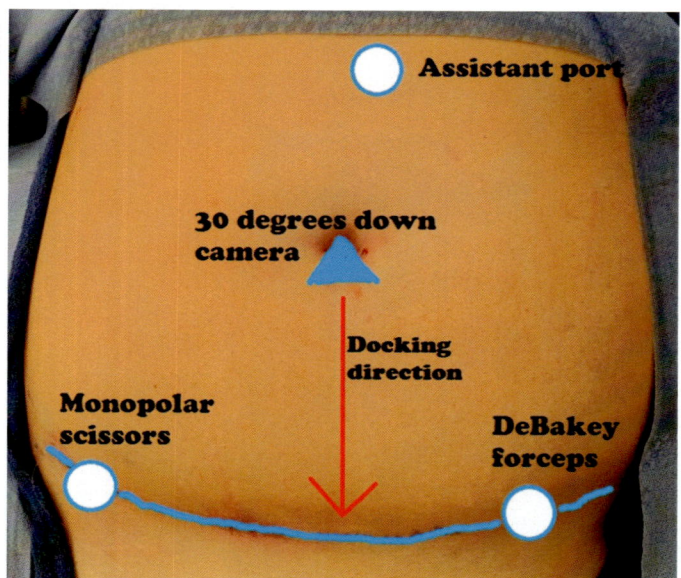

Fig. 14.4 Port placement and docking for APV

Monopolar scissors are used doing small cuts, in a similar fashion as when doing an extravesical reimplant. Once a 3–4 cm tunnel is made the distal mucosa is opened bluntly using 2 robotic Black Diamond forceps followed by an anchoring suture using 4-0 polyglactin of the anterior flap of the fish mouth to the apex of the detrusorotomy, mucosa and muscle. The posterior flap of the fish mouth is sutured to the mucosa only. With these two anchoring sutures, each side of the opened mucosa is sutured to the appendix with a running 5-0 polyglactin suture. To avoid all this suturing, the modified Shanfield technique can be used (see below). The tunnel is then closed with 3–0 polyglactin interrupted sutures from distal to proximal.

Posterior Implantation

With the posterior approach the bladder is not "dropped" or mobilized. The tunnel is made in the posterior bladder wall with the appendix insertion at the inferior end of the detrusorotomy. The anastomosis is similar only that the posterior flap of the fish mouth is the one that is anchored to the muscle instead of the anterior flap. When closing the tunnel with 3-0 polyglactin, the first suture is distal then moving proximally with each new suture −3 to 4 of them.

Anterior Versus Posterior Implantation

The anterior wall anastomosis is technically easier to perform and reduces the amount of appendix needed to reach the surface [3]. The posterior anastomosis might allow better emptying of the bladder with less chance of UTI and possible stones [4].

Direction of Detrusorotomy

For umbilical stomas the detrusorotomy is kept in the midline, whereas with right lower quadrant stomas the detrusorotomy is angled to align the appendix with the stoma location.

Anastomosis of Appendix to Bladder

The anti-reflux mechanism of the APV is predicated to depend on Paquin's 5/1 ratio of ureteral diameter to intravesical tunnel length. The intravesical configuration of the ureteral orifice was also thought to be important by Paquin and then by Lyons, but their ideas about the ureteral orifice were never incorporated into modern reimplantation techniques. Recently on computer models, we demonstrated that the intravesical configuration of the ureteral orifice was important at preventing reflux

[5]. Decades ago, Shanfield showed that in dog ureteral reimplants, just protruding the ureter into the bladder -no tunnel – prevented reflux [6].

Weller et al. [7] initially described in 2013 a series of six laparoscopic APV procedures using the Shanfield technique to reimplant the appendix into the bladder. More recently, the group from Great Ormond Street published a video demonstrating Shanfield's technique for the laparoscopic APV [8]. The Shanfield's anastomosis greatly simplifies the most technical difficult part of a laparoscopic APV.

However, Weller et al. [7] experienced postoperative bleeding when using the Shanfield's technique, likely from the lack of mucosa to mucosa sutures.

With robotic assistance, the difficulty of the mucosa to mucosa anastomosis is greatly reduced and it does not seem worth it to omit it due to the risk of bleeding. That been said, a Shanfield anchoring suture can be placed and not sutured, followed by the mucosa to mucosa anastomosis, subsequently tying the Shanfield suture to provide intravesical protrusion of the appendix which could decrease the chance of difficulties with catheterization and incontinence.

Hitch Sutures

To prevent problems with catheterization it is imperative to keep the extravesical segment of the appendix the shortest possible. Hitch sutures that secure the appendix hiatus area of the bladder to the peritoneum can prevent kinking that occurs with bladder filling.

That been said, some surgeons do not fix the bladder to the anterior abdominal wall [3].

Stoma Location

Stoma should be placed where it would be easily catheterized by the dominant hand of the patient (if placed in the lower abdomen) or the umbilicus. Ideally, exposed mucosa is to be avoided due to its mucus production and its tendency to bleed.

At the umbilicus, a V flap is marked with a caudal base (apex directed at the head of the patient) and dissected down to rectus fascia. The appendix is then secured to the fascia with polyglactin sutures. The appendix is spatulated ventrally. The apex of the spatulation is anastomosed with interrupted absorbable sutures to the apex of the flap. Then each side of the spatulation is sutured to each side of the flap. Finally, the non-spatulated appendix is sutured to the superior umbilical edge.

For implantation in the lower abdomen, the VQ technique is associated with low rates of stenosis and good concealment of the mucosa, with less scarring compared to the VQZ flap [9].

Once the appendix has been matured to the skin, a glidewire is passed through the 10 Fr feeding tube and then the feeding tube is removed. Alongside the glidewire, a 12 Fr feeding tube is placed. If the cathing is easy, the tube is secured at the skin level and the glidewire removed. If the cathing was difficult, the glidewire can be used to pass the 12 Fr feeding tube.

Testing for Easy catheterization at Every Step?

Some surgeons recommend testing the conduit to make sure it catheterizes easily at every step during the surgery and with different bladder volumes. Because laparoscopic insufflation distorts things, testing cannot be done in the same fashion as when doing open surgery.

We do not routinely test for catheterization ease during surgery.

Port Closure

All ports are closed at the fascia with 2-0 polyglactin

Catheters

When a urethral catheter can be left in place, no suprapubic tube is necessary. Both the urethral and APV catheters are left open after surgery and the urethral catheter is left open at discharge (capping the APV catheter).

If a suprapubic catheter is needed, an 8–10 Fr percutaneous nephrostomy tube can be placed into a full bladder with robotic assistance into the anterior wall (avoid posterior placement of a suprapubic catheter to prevent an internal hernia).

Postoperative Care

Length of Catheter Duration

For an isolated APV procedure, most series report leaving a catheter in the conduit for 3–4 weeks and then starting CIC. A safety catheter is left in the urethra or through the skin as a suprapubic tube until CIC is established. Leaving a catheter overnight or an L stent at least initially could help prevent stomal stenosis.

Diet

A regular diet can be started in the immediate postoperative period.

Antibiotic Prophylaxis

Many times, patients having an APV have indwelling urethral or suprapubic catheters before surgery. These catheters are usually infected with bacteria which cannot be eradicated before surgery, but which can be suppressed. The AUA guidelines recommend a treatment course (not prophylactic) of antibiotics targeted at the preoperative urine cultures.

Otherwise in patients with clean preoperative urine cultures, despite minimal evidence, a common practice is to prescribe antibiotic prophylaxis until CIC through the APV is established.

Postoperative Complications

Early postoperative complications include bowel obstruction, infections and urinary leak. Long term and more specific to APV, stomal stenosis, incontinence and difficulties with catheterization are the main complications.

Stomal Stenosis

Stomal stenosis can be easily prevented using an ACE stopper in between catheterizations and/or overnight, when catheterizations start to become difficult or as a preventative measure in the first few months after surgery [10].

Alternatively, an L stent plus minus steroids can be used to treat or prevent stenosis [11].

Incontinence

Incontinence should be initially be addressed with urodynamics, as bladder compliance and dynamics could have changed because of the surgery. If the incontinence is found to be due to APV incompetence, hyaluronic acid/dextranomer can be tried before attempting an open revision.

Difficulties with Catheterization

If the problem is due to kinking of an intraabdominal segment of appendix, an open revision with bladder hitching could be required.

Outcomes

Gundeti's group reported on 8 Mitrofanoff with anterior implantation with 100% continence rate and 1/8 stomal stenosis [3]. Nguyen reported on 10 robotic APV with 1/10 developing incontinence requiring a revision and another one requiring hyaluronic acid/dextranomer injection [1].

A multi-institutional study with 33 isolated robotic APV, reported at 90-days 2 small bowel obstructions, 3 UTI's, 2 surgical site infections, 3 ileus for a total of 8 complications (24%). Their mean operative time was 5.2 h [12].

References

1. Nguyen HT, Passerotti CC, Penna FJ, Retik AB, Peters CA. Robotic assisted laparoscopic Mitrofanoff appendicovesicostomy: preliminary experience in a pediatric population. J Urol. 2009;182(4):1528–34.
2. Ban KA, Minei JP, Laronga C, Harbrecht BG, Jensen EH, Fry DE, et al. American College of Surgeons and Surgical Infection Society: surgical site infection guidelines, 2016 update. J Am Coll Surg. 2017;224(1):59–74.
3. Famakinwa OJ, Rosen AM, Gundeti MS. Robot-assisted laparoscopic Mitrofanoff appendicovesicostomy technique and outcomes of extravesical and intravesical approaches. Eur Urol. 2013;64(5):831–6.
4. Berkowitz J, North AC, Tripp R, Gearhart JP, Lakshmanan Y. Mitrofanoff continent catheterizable conduits: top down or bottom up? J Pediatr Urol. 2009;5(2):122–5.
5. Villanueva CA, Tong J, Nelson C, Gu L. Ureteral tunnel length versus ureteral orifice configuration in the determination of ureterovesical junction competence: a computer simulation model. J Pediatr Urol. 2018;14(3):258.e1–6.
6. Shanfield I. New experimental methods for implantation of the ureter in bladder and conduit. Transplant Proc. 1972;4(4):637–8.
7. Weller S, Bortagaray JI, Corbetta JP, Corro RJ, Duran V, Sager C, et al. Laparoscopic Mitrofanoff procedure using single 'U-Stitch' anastomosis: a way to make it simple. J Pediatr Urol. 2013;9(4):432–6.
8. Papageorgiou E, Cherian A. Laparoscopic posterior appendix Mitrofanoff using the modified Shanfield anastomosis. J Pediatr Urol. 2019;15:419–20.
9. England RJ, Subramaniam R. Functional and cosmetic outcome of the VQ plasty for Mitrofanoff stomas. J Urol. 2007;178(6):2607–10; discussion 2610.
10. Lopez PJ, Ashrafian H, Clarke SA, Johnson H, Kiely EM. Early experience with the antegrade colonic enema stopper to reduce stomal stenosis. J Pediatr Surg. 2007;42(3):522–4.
11. Mickelson JJ, Yerkes EB, Meyer T, Kropp BP, Cheng EY. L stent for stomal stenosis in catheterizable channels. J Urol. 2009;182(4 Suppl):1786–91.
12. Gundeti MS, Petravick ME, Pariser JJ, Pearce SM, Anderson BB, Grimsby GM, et al. A multi-institutional study of perioperative and functional outcomes for pediatric robotic-assisted laparoscopic Mitrofanoff appendicovesicostomy. J Pediatr Urol. 2016;12(6):386.e1–5.

Chapter 15
Complex Bladder Reconstruction

Daniel G. DaJusta and Molly E. Fuchs

Introduction

Robotic surgery has allowed for expanded indications of laparoscopic surgery especially in the area of complex reconstructive surgery. While standard laparoscopy has become the gold standard for a variety of straight forward procedures such as cholecystectomy and nephrectomy, its use for complex reconstructive surgery was limited to a select few of extremely skilled surgeons and was associated with prolonged operative times and steep learning curves. With the adoption of robotic assisted laparoscopy, a number of advantages have been noted including ease of suturing and improved mobility in limited working space. As a result, complex surgical procedures are now being performed more commonly with comparable success as open techniques. Robotic surgery has also helped reduce operative time and learning curves for these complex reconstructions. Other known benefits are decrease blood loss, faster recovery and improve cosmesis. An important example of the adoption of robotic assisted laparoscopy is radical cystectomy with intra-corporeal neobladder creation. This procedure has gained popularity in recent years and initial reports showing feasibility failed to demonstrate a clear benefit. However, over time, the robotic technique has been able to match the open cystectomy technique in oncological outcomes and complication profile but showed advantages of decreased blood loss and shorter hospital stay [1].

Robotic complex bladder reconstruction in pediatric urology has followed suit in this trend. Procedures such as Mitrofanoff, bladder neck reconstruction, and augmentation, are now able to be completed laparoscopically with the aid of the robot and their feasibility has been clearly established. Outcomes for these surgeries performed with the robot have been comparable to their open technique counterparts. However, the number of published series in the literature is still small, which has hindered the ability to demonstrate the well know benefits of robotic surgery. While only a small number of institutions world wide are performing such procedures, the adoption of robotic technique continues to grow as more pediatric urologists gain experience with complex reconstruction.

The purpose of this chapter is to discuss complex robotic reconstruction techniques such as bladder neck reconstruction, Mitrofanoff creation (Appendicovesicostomy or MONTI) and bladder augmentation. It is important to point out that the robotic procedure tends to mimic the technique of the open procedure, thus the robotic techniques described herein will have similar steps to each procedure's open counterpart.

Indications

Indications for complex reconstructive surgery vary widely. In the pediatric urology population, however, the indication is typically related to achieving continence in patients with neurogenic bladder. This is typically seen in children with a number of common urologic conditions: myelomeningocele, bladder exstrophy complex, cloacal anomalies, spinal cord injury, posterior urethral valves, and prune belly syndrome among others. Regardless of the underlying cause of neurogenic bladder, these children may have incontinence secondary to bladder outlet incompetence, bladder overactivity, or a combination of the two problems. Bladder outlet incompetence is characterized by urine leakage at low leak point pressures in the absence of detrusor contraction. Children with neurogenic bladder and poor outlet resistance, will not be dry despite appropriate therapy with clean intermittent catheterization and anticholinergic pharmacotherapy. Common urodynamic findings will be consistent with detrusor areflexia and detrusor leak point pressures lower than 50 cm H_2O. Usually, a smooth-walled bladder with an open bladder neck is observed during voiding cystography. In this population, bladder neck procedures are usually indicated along with the creation of a catheterizable channel as performing intermittent catheterization (CIC) through the reconstructed bladder neck should be avoided. In addition to the bladder outlet procedure and the catheterizable channel creation, it may also be necessary to perform a bladder augmentation simultaneously. The dilemma of whether to perform an augmentation cystoplasty at the time of reconstruction continues to be a highly debated topic. In a recent series of open bladder neck reconstruction without simultaneous augmentation cystoplasty, up to 40% of the patients developed bladder decompensation and ultimately required augmentation [2]. Unfortunately, no pre-operative parameter was identified to predict the future need for augmentation. Thus, appropriate pre-operative counseling should be undertaken with the child and family about the future need for augmentation after a bladder neck procedure alone. Additionally, close post-operative follow up should be undertaken to evaluate renal and bladder function. The authors recommend obtaining urodynamic testing in these patients within 6 months after surgery as prompt recognition of bladder deterioration is critical in order to intervene early and prevent renal damage.

Bladder overactivity is characterized during urodynamic studies by multiple bladder uninhibited contractions loss of bladder compliance is evidenced by quickly-rising baseline bladder pressures during the filling phase. Uninhibited bladder contraction can be treated medically with anticholinergic pharmacotherapy. This class of medication is associated with significant side effects such as dry mouth, flushing, and constipation. More recently, intra-detrusor injection of Onobotulinumtoxin-A (Botox™) has been utilized and is accepted as an alternative to anticholinergics with a more acceptable side-effects profile. It is important to note that bladders with loss of compliance tend to be less responsive to medical therapy. Nevertheless, once medical therapy is no longer effective in managing incontinence, surgical intervention becomes necessary, typically in the form of augmentation cystoplasty. This can be performed in isolation, in patients whose bladder outlet is normal and there is no difficulty with CIC per urethra. An incontinent diversion, such as an ileo-vesicostomy, can also be an option for select cases in which the patient does not wish to or cannot perform CIC. Finally, in patients with incompetent bladder outlet and with reduced compliance, a combination of bladder neck reconstruction with Mitrofanoff and augmentation becomes necessary.

The overall goal of the bladder reconstruction for the neurogenic bladder is to achieve continence. While the definition of continence varies across published literature of open and robotic surgery, in general, these procedures can achieve good rates of continence. However, one cannot lose sight of the long-term risks that come with these procedures, which will be discussed in details later in the chapter. Needless to say, families and patient need to be aware of the risks and must be prepared to adhere to the demanding post-operative routine in order to prevent complications.

Surgical Techniques

Whether performing a bladder neck reconstruction and Mitrofanoff with or without augmentation or performing an ileo-vesicostomy, most complex robotic bladder reconstruction procedures share a few similarities. An initial cystoscopy is usually performed in order to inject Botox™, which has been shown to be helpful in the post-operative pain control. Additionally, externalized ureteral stents can be placed cystoscopically in order to identify the ureters during bladder neck reconstruction. Patient position and port placement are also quite similar amongst these procedures. Thus, these initial steps will be described separately followed by specifics of each procedure including reported outcomes and comparison to open techniques when available.

While bowel preparation for open reconstructive surgeries using ileum is no longer a necessity, in robotic surgery, the authors continue to recommend pre-operative mechanical bowel preparation prior to the surgery. The primary reason for this recommendation is not to decrease the intestinal bacterial burden, but rather, to provide extra intra-abdominal space during the surgery. Patients undergoing these operations often have neurogenic bowel and can have a significant degree of fecal impaction with a dilated colon. This issue, if not addressed preoperatively will make any laparoscopic surgery difficult if not impossible to complete. This Bowel preparation can be accomplished at home, eliminating the need for pre-admission, particularly in patients on an enema regimen, either retrograde or antegrade. If the patient is not on an enema bowel regimen, pre-admission with mechanical bowel prep may be required for adequate colonic decompression.

Initial Cystoscopy

While not always necessary, most of the cases done in our institution begin with a cystoscopy, as we do perform Botox™ bladder injection in all patients with neurogenic bladder prior to bladder reconstruction. We have shown that this does decrease the need for anticholinergic and narcotic pain medication post-operatively. It also seems to shorten hospital stay. For bladder neck reconstruction cases, especially for a surgeon at the beginning of the learning curve, placement of the temporary external ureteral catheter is recommended to aid in ureteral orifice identification. The authors recommend 5 Fr open ended catheters for these temporary ureteral stents.

Patient Position

Once the cystoscopy is completed the patient can then be placed supine in the table. A bean bag can be used but is not a necessity. If a bean bag is used, extra padding between the bean bag and the patient is a must. Additional padding should be provided to any pressure point including IV tubing and the patient should be secured to the table using a wide silk tape (Fig. 15.1). While not so important with the new generation of the robot, placing the shorter end of the operative table in relation to its base towards the patient feet allow for easier docking from the feet. A movement test of the table should be conducted prior to prepping and draping to confirm the patient is well secured. After this, the patient can be prepped and draped. The table should be tilted to the left during dissection of the colon to mobilize the appendix and colon for the MItrofanoff. Trendelenburg position is recommended during the robotic portion of the procedure.

Abdominal Access, Port Position, and Docking

Whether Hassan or Veress needle technique, the choice of abdominal access is determined based on the surgeon's preference, and further discussion is beyond the scope of the chapter. The initial port is usually placed in the umbilicus. If a Mitrofanoff is being performed an inverted V-shaped incision is created for later

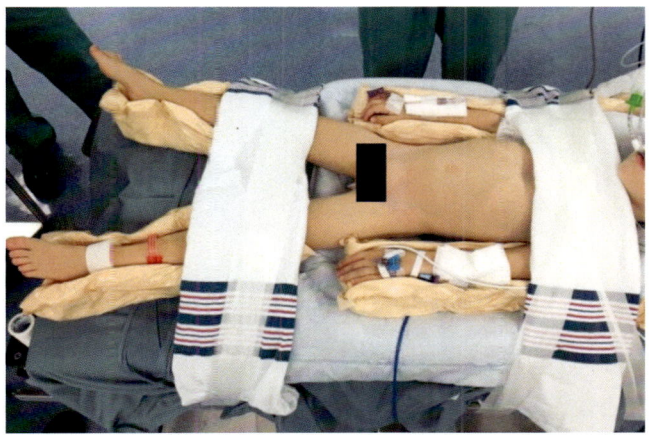

Fig. 15.1 Patient position

anastomosis with the channel in order to prevent stenosis. If the patient has a prior history of abdominal surgery with a scar involving the umbilicus, an alternative initial port should be selected such as the left upper quadrant where an assist port will usually be placed. Following the initial 5 mm port placement, the robot arms port can be placed under direct vision. The authors recommend using 8 mm ports. One port should be placed on each side of the camera slightly below or at the same level of the umbilicus. If using a 4th robotic arm, the port should be placed in the right lower quadrant. Finally, a 12 mm assist port can be placed in the left upper quadrant in between the umbilicus and robotic arm port (Fig. 15.2).

The robot can be docked from the foot of the bed either in the middle or coming from the right side of the patient and straddling the corner of the bed base. Having the shorter end of the operative table in relation to its base towards the patient feet will make docking easier. The new XI robot model can be docked coming from either side of the bed.

Mitrofanoff (Appendicovesicostomy/MONTI)

This procedure should begin with mobilization of the right colon up to the hepatic flexure in order to allow enough mobility for the cecum to reach the pelvis. The appendix is then evaluated for length to make sure it is suitable for the MItrofanoff. Again, if using the XI model, this can be done with the robot as it has greater mobility. If using the SI this will require re-docking from a different position, thus the authors recommend performing this mobilization with standard laparoscopic instruments in order to avoid the need for re-docking. A suitable appendix needs to be long enough to allow for a 3 cm tunnel in addition to length to traverse the abdominal wall on the desired location. If the distance between the bladder and umbilicus is too great, a right lower quadrant stoma position can be selected.

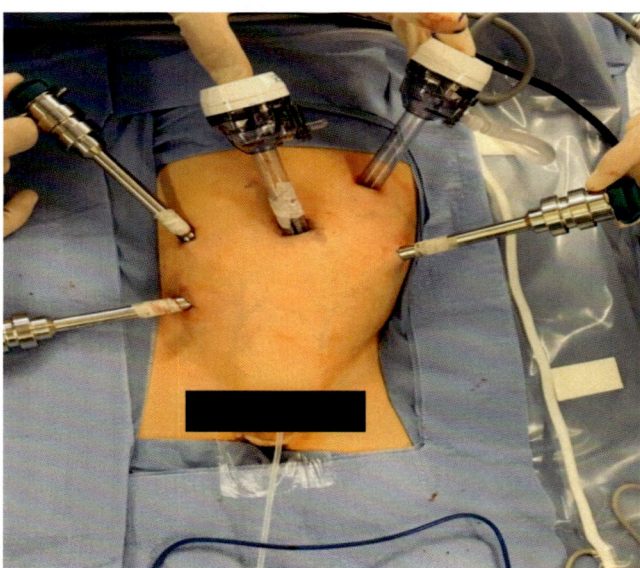

Fig. 15.2 Port position

Once the appendix is appropriately dissected it can be transected at its junction with the cecum. The stump can be ligated with an absorbable suture and imbricated using a silk purse string in a similar fashion of an open appendectomy. The appendix is then cannulated with a 12 French catheter cut to 10–12 cm after opening the distal end of it. It should be secured in place with a stitch at the proximal end.

The bladder should be dissected from the anterior abdominal wall up to the pubic bone and hitched back up to the anterior abdominal wall close to the umbilicus. This is done in order to decrease the distance between the bladder and the umbilicus. The bladder can now be partially filled and a trough in the detrusor muscle down to the mucosa can be created for about 3.5–4 cm. The mucosa should be easy to identify as it should bulge out as the detrusor muscle is incised. Detrusor flaps should be elevated on each side of the trough (Fig. 15.3a). A small opening in the bladder mucosa is then created at the most caudal portion of the tunnel in order to create the anastomosis with the appendix. A mucosa to mucosa anastomosis between the distal end of the appendix and the bladder mucosa can then be created using absorbable sutures over the previously placed catheter. Next, the detrusor flaps can be brought together behind the appendix using absorbable sutures in a similar fashion of the technique for extra-vesical ureteral reimplantation (Fig. 15.3b). At this point, the robot is undocked and using laparoscopic instruments the proximal end of the appendix can be brought up to the umbilical port and the stoma matured.

The technique to create a MONTI small bowel channel is similar except for the need to harvest the 2–3 cm segment of small bowel which can be done using endoscopic staplers. A standard stapler or sewn bowel anastomosis is done to recreate

Fig. 15.3 (**a**) Detrusor tunnel with bulging mucosa; (**b**) Implanted Mitrofanoff with detrusor tunnel closed

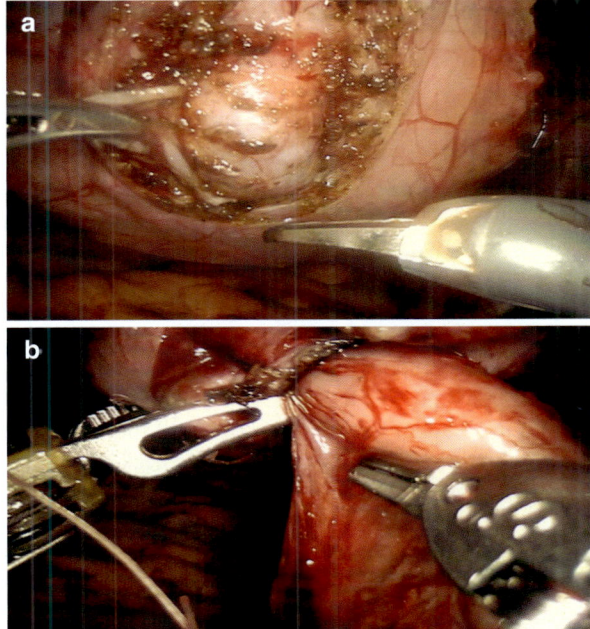

bowel continuity. Following that, the bowel segment is detubularized along the antimesenteric border. This should be performed slightly off the midline to create a longer channel limb to be implanted in the bladder. The segment should then be retubulirized longitudinally in order to create a longer, narrower channel, over a 12 or 14 French catheter. Then, the implantation into the bladder can be performed in a similar manner as described before.

At this time there is good evidence to support the robotic-assisted technique as not just a feasible option, but with a reasonable amount of benefit. Of all the bladder reconstruction techniques, the robotic mitrofanoff is the one with the larger number of cases in the literature. Gundeti et al. performed a multicenter study that included 88 patients undergoing robotic Mitrofanoff with a follow up of 29.5 months [3]. Their results showed that the technique is reproducible and has comparable complication rates as well as functional outcomes. Grimsby et al. compared 28 patients who underwent open versus 39 robotic appendicovesicostomy procedures with a mean follow up of 2.7 years [4]. There was no difference in the number of postoperative complications or reoperation in both groups during the follow-up period. Due to the fact that many patients underwent concomitant procedures, such as bladder neck reconstruction and augmentation, a comparison to evaluate the benefits of the robotic technique such as shorter hospital stay could not be done. Ultimately, as a stand-alone procedure, robotic Mitrofanoff should be the surgery of choice for the less experienced surgeon to begin building his experience with complex robotic bladder reconstruction.

Bladder Neck Repair (BNR) with Sling

The patients undergoing this procedure will always need a concomitant MItrofanoff as they will no longer be able to perform CIC per urethra. This is done in a similar fashion as discussed above, thus there is no need to describe this portion once again. Once the robot is docked after already doing cystoscopy and placing stents for ureteral orifice identification and mobilizing the cecum, the bladder should be freed from the anterior abdominal wall. This should be done down to the endopelvic fascia. The endopelvic fascia should then be opened on each side of the urethra. Some surgeons may find dissecting behind the bladder first in order to reach the bladder neck from behind and create the space in between the bladder neck and posterior structure easier. Identification of the bladder neck is accomplished by the movement of the Foley catheter balloon. Irrespective of the approach, the goal is to dissect around the bladder neck completely until there is enough space to place the instrument behind the bladder neck. Another trick to help with this dissection is to open the urethra and raise the anterior urethral flap first. This will allow for dissection behind the urethra under direct vision, thus, preventing potential back walling of the urethra. Once the instrument can be passed around the bladder neck the sling can be passed behind the bladder neck and pulled up to aid with the bladder neck repair. If not done already, an anterior flap of the urethra should be raised from 10 to 2 o'clock position and dissected cranially into the bladder neck up to the ureteral orifice (Fig. 15.4a). The resultant defect left by raising the flap should be closed with two layers using an absorbable suture. This is done after removing the Foley catheter and the stents and replacing them with a 5 Fr feeding tube which the urethra is closed over (Fig. 15.4b). The sling is them wrapped around the bladder neck in a 360-degree fashion and tightened. The sling should be secured to itself on each side of the bladder with a non-absorbable stitch. Each end of the sling is then secured to the pubic bone using two 2-0 prolene stitches on each side (Fig. 15.4c). The sling should be under enough tension to kink the urethra slightly. At this point, the steps for implanting the Mitrofanoff on the back of the bladder should be undertaken as previously described.

The technique described here for the bladder neck reconstruction mimics the open Mitchel bladder neck repair with sling described by Snodgrass et al. [5] The main reason the authors adopted this technique was due to the superior continence success described of the open combine technique when compared to bladder neck reconstruction or sling alone. Ultimately, while the robotic-assisted procedure described has been shown to be safe and feasible [6], future evaluation must be performed to show that the functional outcomes for a new robotic or laparoscopic technique are similar to open surgery.

Grimsby et al. compared 19 patient undergoing the robotic bladder neck reconstruction with sling and Mitrofanoff procedure to 26 patients who had the very same procedure done open [7]. The operative time was significantly longer in the robotic group. Complication rate within 30 days from surgery was similar in both groups. The overall need for a revision procedure due to incontinence was similar in both groups showing a similar functional outcome for both procedures. Hospital length

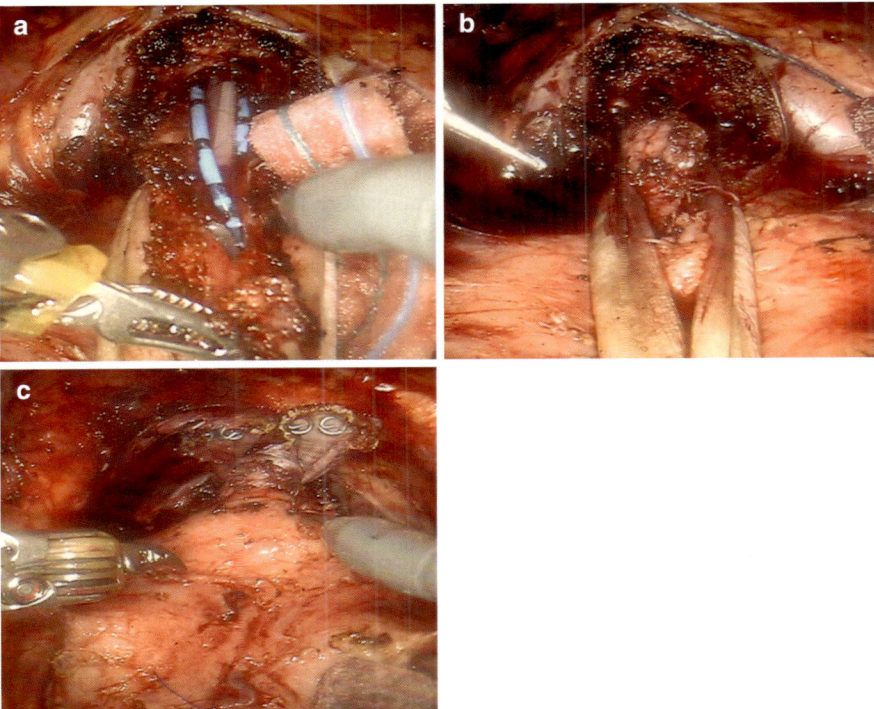

Fig. 15.4 (**a**) Dissected bladder neck with raised anterior urethral flap, urethral catheter and ureteral open ended visible; (**b**) Reconstructed bladder neck; (**c**) Sling wrapped around bladder neck reconstruction and secured to the pubic bone

of stay was similar, thus there was no specific benefit to the robotic technique. However, it is important to consider that this is a comparison of the initial experience with complex robotic reconstruction versus a well established open technique. With additional experience and larger numbers, one could expect to show potential benefits demonstrated by other types of robotic-assisted procedures.

Bladder Augmentation

Bladder augmentation can be done as a standalone procedure in a patient who can perform CIC per urethra but have lost of compliance or significant overactivity as the reason for urinary incontinence. It can also be performed in combination with the above mention procedures. As described before, the initial steps are similar and there is no need to discuss it once again.

One of the most important steps of the augmentation is the selection of a mobile bowel segment of about 20 cm in length about 15 cm away from the ileal cecum valve. The segment is isolated using a laparoscopic endo-GIA. A standard stapled bowel anastomosis can be performed using the laparoscopic endo GIA or a sewn anastomosis can be done. The mesentery is also reapproximated to prevent space for a potential internal hernia. The bowel can then be open on its antimesenteric border. It can be reconfigured in a U but augmentation without reconfiguration can also be performed.

The bladder is then dissected from the anterior abdominal wall and a cystotomy created in a similar fashion of an open augmentation. The detubularized bowel segment edges can them be sewn to the edges of the cystostomy using absorbable stitches. In this case, using a barb type suture may be beneficial in order to decrease operative time. A suprapubic tube should be brought into the bladder through a puncture site in the abdominal wall and place into the bladder for additional drainage.

Feasibility for robotic bladder augmentation is now well established in the literature [8]. Additionally, functional outcomes on the series reported so far are similar to the open technique. Cohen et al. reported in a comparison between 15 robotic augmentations versus 17 open procedures [9]. The analysis showed a similar increase in bladder capacity, narcotic use and complication rates between groups. Length on surgery was longer for robotic (627 min versus 265) while the length of stay was one day shorter for the robotic cohort, though this was not significant. Thus, the usual benefits of using a robotic technique such as shorter hospital stay and decrease post-operative pain have no pan out as expected. This, again, could be related to the limited number of cases done so far as well as early surgeon experience.

Ileo-Vesicostomy

In a select group of patients who do not have the ability to perform CIC or do not wish to do so, an incontinent diversion may be selected as the reconstruction option. Techniques such as ileo-vesicostomy and ileal conduit have all been performed successfully robotic. These procedures offer safe low-pressure bladder drainage into a urostomy bag. Having to wear a bag can be considered an inconvenience, and may be viewed as an inferior option compared to the previously discussed forms of reconstruction. However, patients who undergo these procedures will be dry from below and able to wear underwear. They will also have a less demanding post-operative routine as they will not need to cath at regular schedules. This form of reconstruction is extremely safe for the kidneys as if offers continue low-pressure drainage. This urinary diversion is particularly prone to require revision if a patient's body habitus changes either from somatic growth or weight gain.

The procedure begins in a similar fashion as described above. We do recommend doing cystoscopy with Botox™ at the beginning and placing a Foley catheter. The port position is similar as previously described but one of the robotic arm ports should be position close to the site pre-operative marked for the stoma, in order to incorporate the port site in the stoma incision. Patient position and docking are also similar.

After the robot is docked the initial step consists of accessing the terminal ileum. A 10–15 cm segment of mobile distal ileum, depending on patient body habitus, should be select at least 15 cm away from the ileocecum valve. A laparoscopic endo GIA can be used to isolate the segment and the robotic vessel sealer can be used to incise the mesentery on each side in order to obtain additional mobility. A standard stapled bowel anastomosis can be performed using the laparoscopic endo GIA, but a sewn anastomosis can also be done.

At this point, the bladder can be dissected from its anterior abdominal wall until the pubic bone is reached. With the bladder partially full an inverted U flap incision should be created in the anterior wall of the bladder. This should create a large opening in the bladder with a base of at least 3 cm wide. The stapled proximal end of the isolated bowel segment is removed and the bowel irrigated clean. The end should them be spatulated on the antimesenteric border. This is then sewn to the bladder opening with the U shape flap sewn to the spatulated portion. Suturing should begin in the inferior portion (mesenteric side). The type of suture should be the surgeon's choice but the authors use a barbed type suture starting on the inferior portion and running one suture to each side of the anastomosis. Once the ileo-vesical anastomosis is completed it can be tested by filling the bladder through the previously placed Foley catheter.

The robot can then be undocked and the stoma incision is then created. A laparoscopic grasper can be used to bring the proximal end of the bowel segment to the skin, under direct vision to prevent any twisting of the mesentery. The stoma can them be matured to the skin in a rosebud configuration. A large size Foley catheter can be passed down the ileo-vesicostomy into the bladder and left in place for drainage. The catheter is usually left in place for 3 weeks.

To this date, most of the literature on this procedure is based on case reports and one video presentation. The technique is feasible, yet the biggest risk of the procedure involves the creation of an intracorporeal bowel anastomosis. The authors have performed this procedure in three patient, two of each had a very short hospital stay of 4 days and excellent functional results. One patient did experience an anastomosis leak and had a prolonged hospital stay, but ultimately did well.

Bladder Reconstruction in Patients with Prior Abdominal Surgery

In the past, prior intraabdominal surgery was considered a relative contraindication for laparoscopic procedures. There was an increase in the complication and conversion to open rates associated with prior intraabdominal surgery. Over time, as surgeons became more comfortable with the laparoscopic and robotic-assisted technique, this concern has lessened. This is similar in complex robotic-assisted bladder reconstruction techniques. Often patient undergoing this procedure have had surgery in the past, this is usually the case in the myelomeningocele population which often have had multiple ventriculoperitoneal shunt revisions. As the experience with these cases increased, so did the number of patients operated, on who prior intraabdominal surgery had been performed. Again, recent data has come forward to suggest that even in this population, the technique is safe and feasible. Gargollo et al. described a cohort of 36 patients with prior intraabdominal open surgery who underwent robotic complex bladder reconstruction [10]. There was an increase in the operative time which eventually improved with surgeons experienced. There was also a slight increase chance of conversion to open, especially in patients with multiple shunt revision.

Bowel Management Consideration

Many patients undergoing the above mention procedures have a concomitant neurogenic bowel that may benefit from an antegrade enema option. This is often offered to patients undergoing an open procedure as part of the surgical plan. Either placement of a cecostomy tube, creation of a Malone or neo-Malone channel may be options that can be offered to the patient in order to better manage their neurogenic bowel via antegrade enema. All of these options have been performed successfully and safely utilizing the robotic technique in combination with the above-described surgeries [11]. Thus, whenever indicated these surgeries should be combined with the above mention techniques in order to avoid separate interventions.

Post-Operative Considerations

Continue bladder drainage is paramount in almost all of the above mentioned procedure in the immediate post-operative period. Maintaining bladder drainage is done by leaving catheters in place through channels for at least 3 weeks postoperatively prior to the start of any catheterization regimen. During this period family should be taught to irrigate catheter in order to keep the patent. This is especially important in the robotic BNR, sling and Mitrofanoff procedure as there is often only one catheter draining the bladder through the created Mitrofanoff since suprapubic catheters are typically not placed during robotic bladder reconstruction unless a bladder augmentation is performed.

After patients are taught to perform CIC, follow up should be similar to open cases. The authors will often have a renal and bladder ultrasound and serum renal function panel performed about 6 weeks after the beginning of CIC. Consideration for early urodynamic evaluation should be given for patient undergoing a bladder neck procedure without augmentation. The authors recommend urodynamic testing within 6 months of surgery in order to evaluate for loss of bladder compliance that is known to be seen in up to 40% of patients undergoing this operation. This loss of compliance can lead to loss of renal function in a silent manner. While most of the time the loss of compliance and increase in bladder pressure will lead to renal US changes. Relying upon only renal ultrasound changes may lead to irreversible renal function loss.

Summary

Robotic-assisted bladder reconstruction procedures continue to gain popularity among pediatric urologist. Feasibility and safety for most of these surgeries are now well established. Unfortunately, in contrast to our adult colleagues, pediatric urologists suffer from a low volume of cases which hinders our ability to advance the technique in an expedited manner. This lack of volume is the primary reason that the benefits of robotic surgery that have been proven in adult robotic procedures have not yet been realized in pediatric bladder reconstruction procedures. This is also due to the fact these are complex cases with a significant learning curve resulting in a limited number of pediatric urologist performing these procedures. Once the learning curve has been surpassed it is likely that the usual benefits that are demonstrated in other complex robotic cases when compared to open techniques should be attained.

References

1. Sathianathen NJ, Kalapara A, Frydenberg M, Lawrentschuk N, Weight CJ, Parekh D, Konety BR. Robotic assisted radical cystectomy vs open radical cystectomy: systematic review and meta-analysis. J Urol. 2019;201(4):715–20.
2. Grimsby GM, Menon V, Schlomer BJ, Baker LA, Adams R, Gargollo PC, Jacobs MA. Long-term outcomes of bladder neck reconstruction without augmentation cystoplasty in children. J Urol. 2016;195(1):55–61.
3. Gundeti MS, Petravick ME, Pariser JJ, Pearce SM, Anderson BB, Grimsby GM, Akhavan A, Dangle PP, Shukla AR, Lendvay TS, Cannon GM Jr, Gargollo PC. A multi-institutional study of perioperative and functional outcomes for pediatric robotic-assisted laparoscopic Mitrofanoff appendicovesicostomy. J Pediatr Urol. 2016;12(6):386.e1.
4. Grimsby GMJM, Gargollo PC. Comparison of complications of robot-assisted laparoscopic and open appendicovesicostomy in children. J Urol. 2015;194(3):772–6.
5. Snodgrass W, Barber T. Comparison of bladder outlet procedures without augmentation in children with neurogenic incontinence. J Urol. 2010;184(4 Suppl):1775–80.
6. Bagrodia A, Gargollo P. Robot-assisted bladder neck reconstruction, bladder neck sling, and appendicovesicostomy in children: description of technique and initial results. J Endourol. 2011;25(8):1299–305.
7. Grimsby GM, Jacobs MA, Menon V, Schlomer BJ, Gargollo PC. Perioperative and short-term outcomes of robotic vs open bladder neck procedures for neurogenic incontinence. J Urol. 2016;195(4 Pt 1):1088–92.
8. Murthy P, Cohn JA, Selig RB, Gundeti MS. Robot-assisted laparoscopic augmentation ileocystoplasty and Mitrofanoff appendicovesicostomy in children: updated interim results. Eur Urol. 2015;68(6):1069–75.

9. Cohen AJ, Brodie K, Murthy P, Wilcox DT, Gundeti MS. Comparative outcomes and perioperative complications of robotic vs open cystoplasty and complex reconstructions. Urology. 2016;97:172–8.
10. Gargollo PC, Granberg C, Gong E, Tu D, Whittam B, Dajusta D. Complex robotic lower urinary tract surgery in patients with history of open surgery. J Urol. 2019;201(1):162–8.
11. Halleran DR, Wood RJ, Vilanova-Sanchez A, Rentea RM, Brown C, Fuchs M, Jayanthi VR, Ching C, Ahmad H, Gasior AC, Michalsky MP, Levitt MA, DaJusta D. Simultaneous robotic-assisted laparoscopy for bladder and bowel reconstruction. J Laparoendosc Adv Surg Tech A. 2018;28(12):1513–6.

Chapter 16
Bladder Augmentation Procedures

Brittany L. Adamic, Lakshmi Kirkire, Ciro Andolfi, and Mohan S. Gundeti

Introduction

Augmentation ileocystoplasty is necessary to protect the upper tract and provide social continence in neurogenic bladder patients who fail conservative management. Augmentation allows for decreased voiding pressures, increased bladder capacity and continence. The majority of patients requiring this procedure have neurogenic bladder often due to spinal dysraphism, valve bladder due to posterior urethral valves or Arnold-Chiari malformation [1, 2]. Often, concomitant procedures such as a catheterizable channel, antegrade continent enema channels and bladder neck procedures are required in this patient population for achieving social urinary and fecal continence.

Augmentation ileocystoplasty was traditionally performed as an open procedure. The morbidity and pain associated with open laparotomy incision have led to interest in performing this surgery in a minimally invasive fashion. Decreased

---

B. L. Adamic
University of Chicago, Department of Surgery, Section of Urology, Chicago, IL, USA
e-mail: brittany.adamic@uchospitals.edu

L. Kirkire
University of Chicago, Pritzker School of Medicine, Chicago, IL, USA
e-mail: lakshmi.kirkire@uchospitals.edu

C. Andolfi
University of Chicago Medical Center, Department of Surgery, Sections of Adult and Pediatric Urology, Chicago, IL, USA

Comer Children's Hospital, Department of Surgery, Section of Urology, Chicago, IL, USA
e-mail: candolfi@surgery.bsd.chicago.edu

M. S. Gundeti (✉)
The University of Chicago Medicine, Department of Urology, Chicago, IL, USA
e-mail: mgundeti@surgery.bsd.uchicago.edu

© Springer Nature Switzerland AG 2020
P. C. Gargollo (ed.), *Minimally Invasive and Robotic-Assisted Surgery in Pediatric Urology*, https://doi.org/10.1007/978-3-030-57219-8_16

ost-operative pain, improved cosmesis, decreased convalescence and improved tissue handling without compromising outcomes has led to surgeons favoring a minimally invasive approach across many pediatric operations [3–5]. In regards to augmentation ileocystoplasty, this complex, time consuming and challenging operation has been described laparoscopically, however the steep learning curve has prevented its incorporation into widespread practice [6, 7]. The robotic platform allows urologists to perform complex reconstructive procedures with a shorter learning curve [8]. Advantages of the robotic approach include seven degrees of freedom, high resolution 3D picture, direct view movement and limiting tremor. The robotic-assisted laparoscopic ileocystoplasty (RALI) has proven to be a desirable alternative to straight laparoscopy. The RALI has shown to be safe and just as effective as open approach since its inception in 2008 [1, 9].

Patient Selection and Pre-operative Work Up

Patients who fail medical management, have persistent severe hydronephrosis or who have concerning urodynamic findings (reduced bladder compliance, ALPP >40 cm H_2O) are often considered for this procedure. The EAU guidelines state this procedure is indicated to decrease bladder pressure and increase bladder capacity when more conservative measures have failed [10]. Patients require videourodynamics to determine detrusor leak point pressure, compliance, and capacity prior to surgical management. Videourodynamics may also be helpful to evaluate the bladder neck competency and identify patients who may benefit from bladder neck reconstruction. A urinalysis should be obtained prior to surgery. If suspicious, a culture should be obtained and a urinary tract infection should be treated prior to surgery. DMSA [technetium-99m dimercaptosuccinic acid] can be obtained to identify renal scarring in those at risk. In patients with known vesicoureteral reflux (VUR), we prefer not to perform concomitant ureteral reimplant as the VUR often resolves with improvement in bladder pressures.

Patients and family members must understand the commitment to lifelong catheterization, via either urethra or a continent cutaneous channel. This can be taught to patients, parents and care givers pre-operatively. Expectations regarding post-operative pain, recovery and complications should be managed. Stoma site preference can be discussed with family, we often choose the umbilicus or right iliac fossa.

Pre-operative Considerations

The robotic approach is reserved for patients 6 years of age or older due to the small intra-abdominal space in younger children, precluding the movement of robotic arms. We recommend pre-operative consultation with neurosurgery for patients with ventriculoperitoneal (VP) shunts and those with spinal dysraphism to rule out possibility of secondary tethered cord and ensure spinal anatomy is appropriate for prolonged lithotomy.

Contraindications

Generalized contraindications to ileocystoplasty include patients with compromised renal function (who may be unable to compensate for metabolic derangements postoperatively, with the exception of patients awaiting renal transplant), renal tubular acidosis, hepatic failure, inflammatory bowel disease, short bowel syndrome and poor compliance with intermittent catheterization. The ileum is the preferred bowel segment when performing a laparoscopic or robotic assisted laparoscopic bladder augmentation due to the length of the mesentery, ease of handling and fewer metabolic derangements.

Relative contraindications include severe kyphosis limiting intra-abdominal space and multiple prior surgeries, as this may require open conversion due to dense adhesions [11]. Specifically, spina bifida patients may have unsuitable anatomy for abdominal insufflation and allow enough room for adequate exposure. VP shunts are not a contraindication to laparoscopic surgery, however the surgical team must be aware of possible complications regarding the VP shunt including VP shunt failure due to obstruction caused by peritoneal insufflation [12]. If present, a VP shunt can be placed into an endoscopic pouch for the duration of the operation.

Peptic ulcer disease would be a contraindication to a gastric augmentation, however this cystoplasty patch is rarely used today. A history of pelvic radiation, diverticulitis and ulcerative colitis may lead to a more difficult operation, and would be considered relative contraindications to a robotic approach. Early in the learning curve, patients who have had prior appendectomy may be best suited with an open catheterizable channel creation. An experienced robotic surgeon may be required to perform a Monti Catherizable channel robotically.

Preoperative Preparation

Mechanical bowel prep is not recommended for small bowel procedures [13–15]. A mechanical bowel prep can be safely omitted without increase in intra-abdominal infections [16].

Pre-operative weight-based cefazolin, metronidazole and gentamicin are administered within 30 min before skin incision and are continued for 24–48 h. Patients with ventriculoperitoneal shunts receive one dose of prophylactic vancomycin preoperatively and cefazolin is omitted.

Surgical Technique

With the declining favorability of the purely laparoscopic approach, we will discuss the robotic approach.

Patient Positioning, Port placement and Robot Docking

The patient is positioned in a supine semilithotomy with a slight 10° Trendelenburg. The patient's arms are tucked to the sides. Pneumatic deep venous compression devices are used throughout the operation to prevent deep venous thrombosis. An orogastric tube is inserted for the duration of the surgical procedure. We pad the patient's head and face with foam padding. A urethral foley catheter is placed sterilely on the field. We do not place ureteral catheters routinely for ureteric orifice identification, however a novice surgeon may wish to do so to avoid ureteral injury. A 12 mm camera port is placed in a supraumbilical position with Hasson's technique. We have previously described umbilical camera port placement; however, this does not allow for the identification and dissection of the appendix and bowel. If utilizing the DaVinci X® robot, an 8 mm camera port is placed similar position. Additionally, the 8 mm robotic port can be placed within a 12 mm Hasson port if desired. After establishing pneumoperitoneum, the 8 mm robotic working arm ports are placed laterally at the level of the umbilicus in the mid clavicular line. A 5 mm assistant port is placed in the left upper quadrant, inferior to the costal margin and in the midclavicular line. A larger assistant port can be utilized if performing a stapled bowel anastomosis to accommodate the stapler. A fourth arm robotic working arm port can be placed at the site of stoma creation in the right iliac fossa for patients who are greater than 12 years of age or 5 feet tall due to restriction of the space. If an umbilical stoma creation is planned the right robotic arm port can be placed below the costal margin in the mid clavicular line to mirror the left robotic arm port.

Diagnostic Peritonoscopy

We recommend beginning the case with diagnostic peritonoscopy and lysis of adhesions if necessary. The appendix is identified, ensuring adequate length and vascularity to allow for successful appendicovesicostomy. This step facilitates the ease of appendix isolation, especially in patients with VP shunts when the appendix may be in a suprahepatic location. The evaluation of the appendix and intra-abdominal anatomy allows for conversion to open if required prior to docking the robot or creation of the Monti channel if appropriate expertise is available.

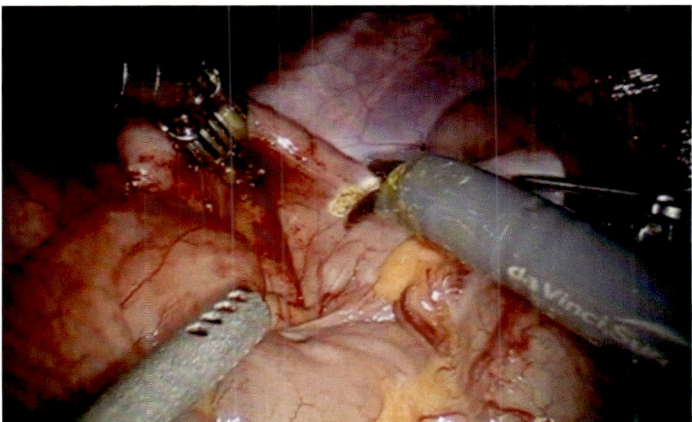

Fig. 16.1 Division of the appendix

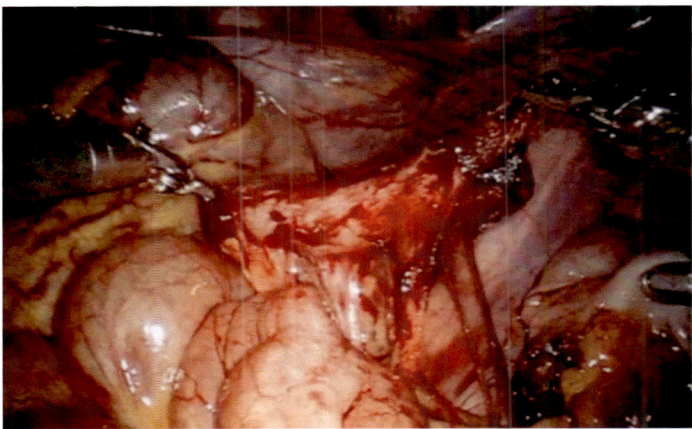

Fig. 16.2 Evaluation of the appendiceal mesentery and mobility

Appendiceal Isolation and Harvest

A traction suture can be placed at the tip of the appendix to aid in dissection and manipulation while minimizing tissue handling. A 4-0 Vicryl suture (polyglactin) is placed as a stay suture and a mesenteric window with adequate blood supply is developed. The appendix is then excised from the cecum (Fig. 16.1). If a short appendix is noted, a cecal flap can be taken to ensure adequate length and avoid stomal stenosis (Fig. 16.2). In those who require antegrade continence enema channel creation, the length of the appendix will determine the need for split technique versus a cecal flap. A large defect in the bowel is closed in two layers, while a small defect may be secured with a purse string suture (Fig. 16.3). We do not fenestrate the mesentery as described by other authors [8].

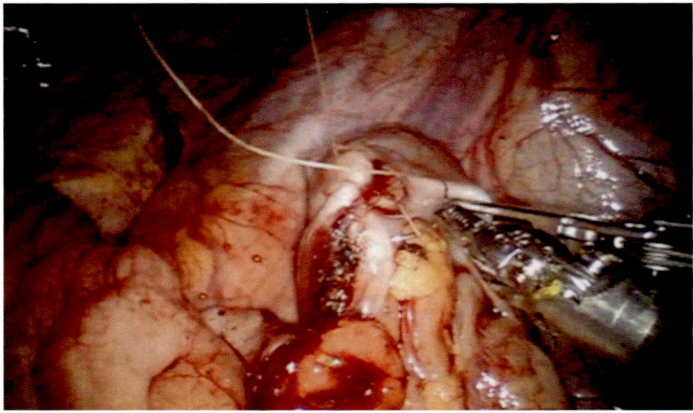

Fig. 16.3 Hand sewn closure of large bowel defect

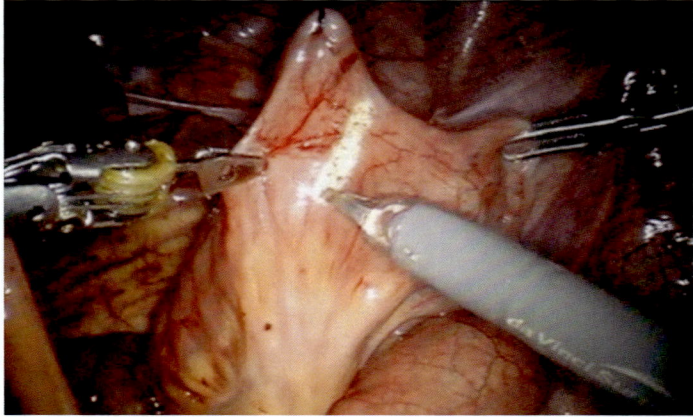

Fig. 16.4 Electrocautery division of the ileum

Ileal Loop Isolation and Anastomosis

A 20 cm ileal segment is isolated 20 cm proximal to the ileocecal junction for the cystoplasty patch. Percutaneous stay sutures on a keith needle (3-0 silk) are placed in the proximal and distal ends of the bowel. This maneuver provides traction of the bowel and allows for easier isolation and anastomosis. A pre-measured umbilical tape is used to ensure accurate measurement of the bowel segments. After ensuring mesenteric length and that the ileal segment will reach the bladder, the ileal loop is transected (Fig. 16.4). Division of the mesentery is performed with the Harmonic scalpel® and bipolar forceps to reduce bleeding and facilitate the dissection (Fig. 16.5).

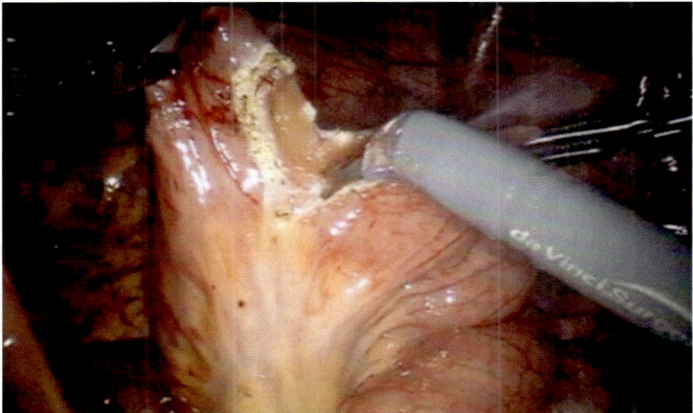

Fig. 16.5 Monopolar division of the ileum

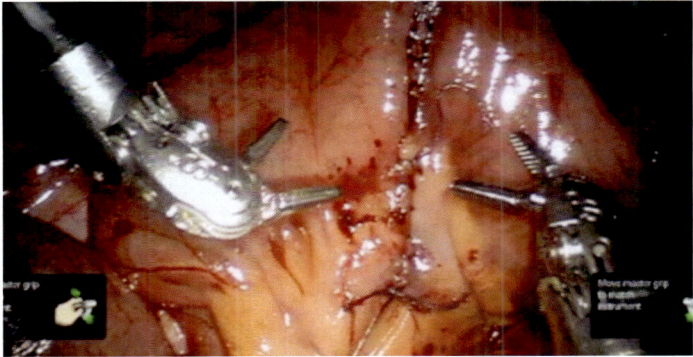

Fig. 16.6 Completed hand sewn bowel anastomosis

Bowel continuity is re-established by hand sewn single layer seromuscular anastomosis using 5-0 PDS in children, or 4-0 PDS in the adult (Fig. 16.6). We start the anastomosis on the antimesenteric border using a running stitch toward the mesentery on the posterior wall. On the anterior wall of the bowel, a separate stitch is run from the mesenteric border toward the antimesenteric border. The mesenteric defect is closed to prevent the possibility of closed loop bowel obstruction. Alternatively, a stapled bowel anastomosis can be performed. Appropriate precautions should be taken to account for the small diameter of the pediatric bowel pediatric and feasibility of the generic staplers to prevent any leaks.

Detrusorotomy and Extravesical Appendicovesicostomy

We suggest using the intravesical approach to performing the appendicovesicostomy to reduce operative time. In cases of a short appendiceal length, the extravesical approach may be required. The bladder is distended with normal saline. A submucosal tunnel is created with monopolar scissors. The detrusorotomy can be made in the coronal plane to reduce bleeding. A midline detrusorotomy is made for umbilical stoma location, otherwise a right sided oblique detrusorotomy is made for right iliac fossa stoma creation. When performing the intravesical approach, the appendix is brought to the posterior wall, and orientation of the appendix is

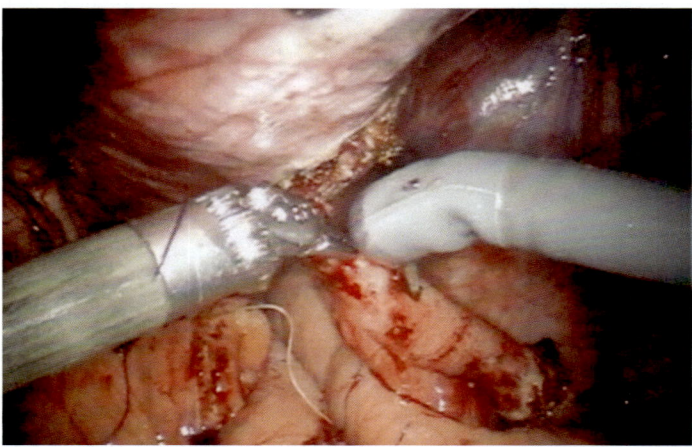

Fig. 16.7 Spatulation of the appendix

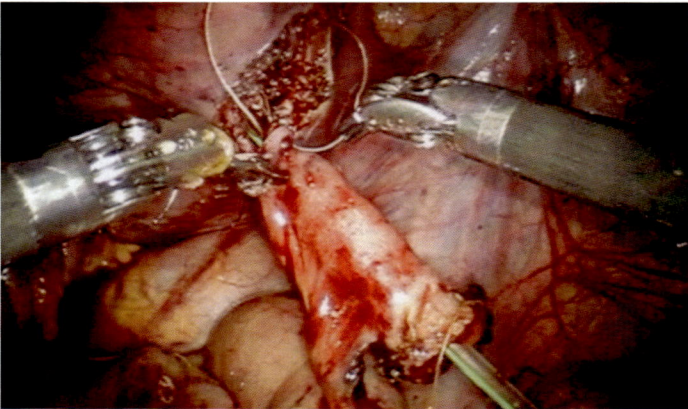

Fig. 16.8 Appendicovesicostomy anastomosis

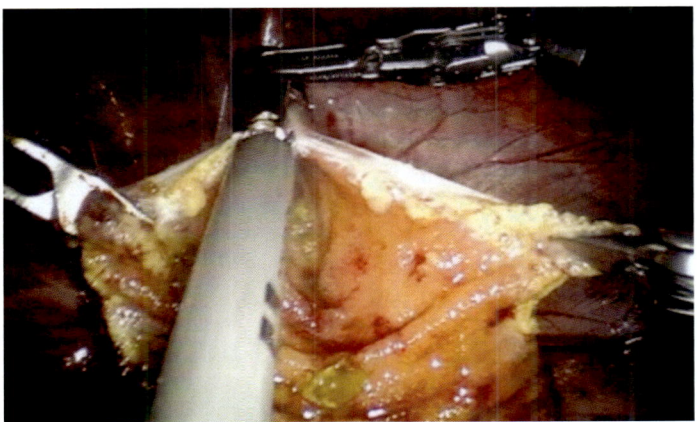

Fig. 16.9 Detubularization of the ileum with harmonic scalpel

organized according to planned stoma site creation to avoid angulations which may lead to difficult catheterization. For umbilical stomas this should be in the craniocaudal direction, while iliac fossa stomas can be oriented in a lateral direction. The previously placed stay suture at the tip of the appendix allows for easy manipulation while minimizing direct handling of the appendix. The appendix is spatulated and anastomosed to the bladder mucosa (Fig. 16.7). An 8 French feeding tube is placed within the appendix. A few crotch sutures can be placed in an interrupted fashion with 4′0 PDS II® Medline Industries (polydioxanone) suture, and the remainder of the anastomosis can be run in a circular fashion (Fig. 16.8). The catheter can be moved back and forth to ensure smoothness of passage and ensure no erroneous suture placement. We suture the feeding tube to the bladder mucosa with an absorbable monofilament suture to prevent dislodgement.

Ileal Detubulrization

The previously isolated ileal segment is now detubularized along the antimesenteric border with a harmonic scalpel (Fig. 16.9). The use of harmonic scalpel allows for a reduction in operative time. We do not utilize a bowel prep. Stay sutures are placed at the proximal and distal ends of the ileal patch.

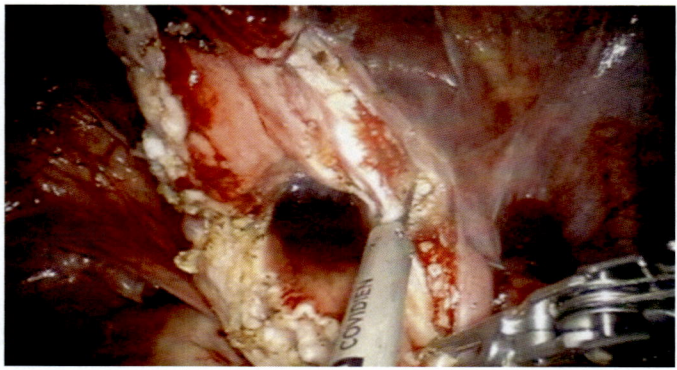

Fig. 16.10 Cystotomy with harmonic scalpel

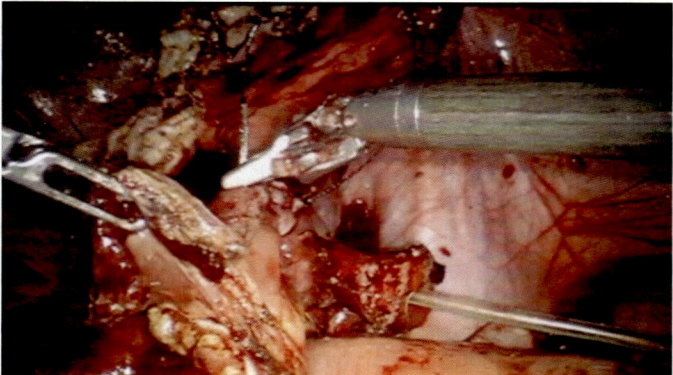

Fig. 16.11 Patch ileocystoplasty

Cystotomy and Patch Ileoystoplasty

The cystotomy is performed in the coronal plane. A thick-walled bladder is often encountered, and we find the harmonic scalpel aids in hemostasis and decreases operative time compared to our previous use of monopolar scissors (Fig. 16.10). Attention is turned to the bladder augmentation with ileal patch. The detubularized bowel is sutured to the apices of the cystotomy. Utilization of the 4th arm can aid in retraction and exposure. The posterior edge of the cystotomy is anastomosed first to the ileal segment using a single layer running suture. A modification to our previously described technique is the use of a barbed quill suture to perform the posterior bowel bladder anastomosis in a continuous fashion (Fig. 16.11). We utilize either a 2-0 Quill™ suture (Surgical specialties corporation), Vicryl or polydioxanone (PDS). Our experience is that placement of only one suprapubic catheter often leads to dislodgement and clogging, therefore two suprapubic catheters can be placed

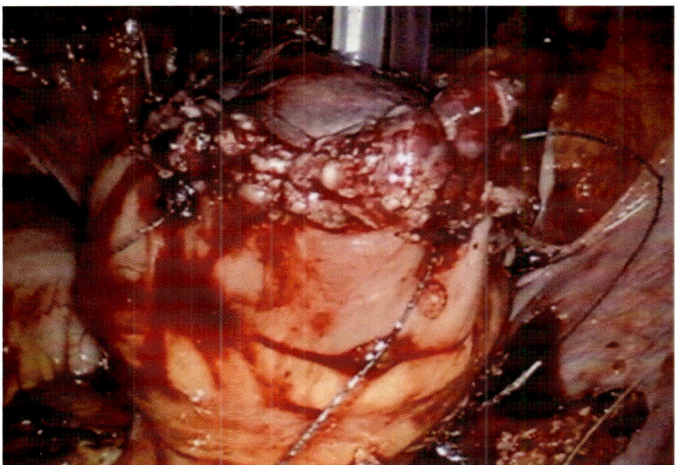

Fig. 16.12 Leak test

percutaneously to provide maximal drainage. Ureteral catheters are removed at this time if they were placed. The anterior bladder bowel anastomosis is performed working from the apices toward the midline. Lapra-Ty clips are applied during the ileovesical anastomosis to decrease tension on the suture line. The augmented bladder is filled with sterile water to identify leakage (Fig. 16.12). We do not reconfigure the bowel segment into U cup prior to anastomosis to the bladder. We have found that during the anastomosis, the differences in length can be remedied by utilizing an imbricated suture on the intestine.

We do not leave a drain for this procedure. The VP shunt can be removed from the endoscopic pouch, and presence of cerebrospinal fluid indicates functionality of the shunt.

Maturation of APV Stoma

The appendix can be brought to the right iliac fossa through the 4th arm robotic port with the assistance of a stay suture. If an umbilical location is desired, this incision can be made and the appendix and tubing brought through the skin. A skin flap (V, VQ, VQZ technique) is created and anastomosed to the microfanoff appendicovesicostomy (MAPV) using 5-0 PDS II® Medline Industries (polydioxanone) suture. The fascia of the remaining port sites is closed with 2-0 Vicryl suture under direct vision and the skin is closed with 5-0 Monocryl® Ethicon (poliglecaprone) or equivalent suture.

Post-operative Management

Orogastric tube is removed prior to extubation. We immediately begin a clear liquid diet which can be advanced as tolerated. The suprapubic catheters and urethral catheter are left freely draining for 4 weeks. The MAPV catheter is capped and taped to the abdomen. At 4 weeks post-operatively, the MAPV and urethral catheters are removed and the SPTs are capped. The patient/family is taught clean intermittent catheterization (CIC). We do not perform routine cystograms unless there is a specific concern. The suprapubic catheters are removed after the patient/family has shown competence in performing CIC. We continue antibiotic prophylaxis for 4 weeks while the catheters are indwelling.

Reducing Operative Time

The longer operative time in minimally invasive lower urinary tract reconstruction remains the leading limitation. The bowel anastomosis is often time consuming [11] and stapled bowel anastomoses would likely reduce operative time. Retrospective pediatric surgery literature has shown similar outcomes when performing stapled bowel anastomoses when compared to the hand-sewen technique, without increased obstruction, stricture or leak [17–19]. There is little urologic research on this subject, however, in performing RALIMA in a porcine model, the hand-sewn technique may be associated with lower incidence of bowel leak [8]. We prefer a hand-sewn bowel anastomosis as we have not had bowel anastomotic complications with the single layer seromuscular closure technique [16].

Published laparoscopic ileocystoplasty operative time ranges from 202–480 min when the bowel anastomosis is performed in an extracorporeal fashion [20–23]. Lorenzo et al. described a completely intracorporal laparoscopic ileocystoplasty in 2007, however operative time was not reported [6]. In the adult literature, robotic augmentation enterocystoplasty with continent catheterizable channel has been described on average operative time 365 minutes (ranging from 220–788) [24]. In the pediatric population, robotic approach operative time ranges from 320–659 min [1, 25, 26]. Contemporary open augmentation ileocystoplasty operative times are not readily available in the literature. One group noted an average of 234 min for extraperitoneal approach and 336 min for intra-peritoneal approach [27]. Analysis of the NSQIP data by McNamara et al. revealed a median operative time of 426 min for augmentation ileocystopasty with appendicovesicostomy, 318 min for an augmentation alone and 234 min for only the appendicovesicostomy [28]. Although operative time remains the criticism of the robotic approach, with increasing experience the robotic assisted approach likely will have a similar operative time as an open approach.

Complications

Surgical Complications

Complications with any intra-abdominal surgery such as vessel injury, bowel injury, VTE can occur after a minimally invasive augmentation cystoplasty. Inadvertent damage to the ureteral orifices is possible and ureteral stenting may be advised for the novice surgeon. Bowel related complications such as ileus, bowel leak, sepsis, metabolic abnormalities may occur, as well as surgical site infections. Integrity of a VP shunt can be compromised in patients with these devices. We often observe that patients have difficulty with clogged catheters or catheter dislodgment after this procedure, therefore it is reasonable to place two suprapubic catheters.

Short Term Complications

In general, the 30-day readmission rate in a large national database after cystoplasty was noted to be 19.6%, with readmissions most commonly for c. diff, ileus, bowel obstruction, constipation, UTI, pyelonephritis, surgical site infection and wound dehiscence [29]. Readmissions were noted for gastrointestinal complications (19.6%), UTI (14.1%) and wound complications (11.2%) [29].

Long Term Complications

Long-term sequalae include bladder stones, UTIs, bladder perforation, stomal stenosis, managing mucous production and metabolic abnormalities. Literature for RALI long term outcomes is lacking. Open augmentation ileocystoplasty 10-year complications include bladder rupture (2.9–6.4%), small bowel obstruction (5.2–10.3%), bladder stones (13.3–36.0%), pyelonephritis (16.1–37.1%), and reaugmentation (5.2–13.4%). Bladder neck surgery and stoma creation at time of AC were associated with an increased hazard of bladder rupture (HR 1.9) and bladder stones (HR 1.4) respectively [30].

Stone Formation

These patients are at high risk for developing bladder stones, thought to be due to mucous production, chronic bacterial colonization and metabolic abnormalities. Mucous is thought to bind calcium from urine and become a nidus for stone formation. These stones are often infectious stones, with reports of 69.2% of bladder stones being infectious in nature (struvite, carbonate apatite, ammonium acid ureate, mixed calcium phosphate) [31]. Additional proposed mechanisms include contraction alkalosis due to dehydration leading to stone formation [32].

Mucous Production

Mucous can be managed with daily irrigations and mycolytics. Proposed agents include N-acetylcysteine, octreotide, aspirin and ranitidine. The efficacy of these agents is questionable and further, high quality studies are required [33, 34].

Neoplasia

The risk of secondary malignancy in patients undergoing augmentation cystoplasty ranges between 1.2% and 4.5% with a median latency interval between 19–32 years [35, 36]. Patients who are immunosuppressed, such as valve bladder patients who require renal transplant may have an even higher risk, with 13% developing a secondary malignancy with a latency of 22–25 years in a small series [35]. This risk should be discussed with patients prior to surgery.

Metabolic Deranagments

When small bowel is incorporated into the urinary tract, reabsorption of water, sodium, hydrogen, ammonium and chlorite while increased loss of potassium and bicarbonate can occur. The overall constellation may lead to a hyperchloremic metabolic acidosis [37]. Although rarely symptomatic, patients may require oral bicarbonate supplementation. A study looked at cystoplasty including gastrocystoplasty and colocystoplasty, 22.5% of patients were noted to have a metabolic acidosis and 15–16% of patients required oral bicarbonate [38, 39].

B12 Deficiency

Five years after the use of ileum for cystoplasty, we recommend obtaining a B12 level annually and repleting orally if necessary [40].

Outcomes

Comparing outcomes to an open approach, RALI may offer a decreased length of stay by 2 days in one study [11]. There are concerns that patients with spinal dysraphism may not be suitable candidates for epidural and have increased post-operative narcotic requirements. However, narcotic use and post-operative complications did not differ between the RALI and OAI groups in this small study. Further research directly comparing the two approaches is needed.

One study comparing the open to robotic augmentation ileocystoplasty showed similar rates of 30 day (52.9% vs 46.7%) and 90 day (23.5% vs 27%) complications [2].

Conclusion

With appropriate patient selection, robotic assisted laparoscopic ileocystoplasty is feasible and may decrease post-operative pain and length of stay. And the outcomes when compared to the open alternative are at par.

Conflicts of Interest Dr. Mohan S. Gundeti is co-director for the NARUS course. The other authors have no conflicts of interest to declare.

References

1. Gundeti MS, Petravick ME, Pariser JJ, et al. A multi-institutional study of perioperative and functional outcomes for pediatric robotic-assisted laparoscopic Mitrofanoff appendicovesicostomy. J Pediatr Urol. 2016;12(6):386–e1.
2. Cohen AJ, Brodie K, Murthy P, Wilcox DT, Gundeti MS. Comparative outcomes and perioperative complications of robotic vs open cystoplasty and complex reconstructions. Urology. 2016;97:172–8.
3. Sorensen MD, Delostrinos C, Johnson MH, Grady RW, Lendvay TS. Comparison of the learning curve and outcomes of robotic assisted pediatric pyeloplasty. J Urol. 2011;185:2517–22.
4. Barbosa JABA, Barayan G, Gridley CM, et al. Parent and patient perceptions of robotic vs open urological surgery scars in children. J Urol. 2013;190:244–50.
5. Baek M, Koh CJ. Lessons learned over a decade of pediatric robotic ureteral reimplantation. Investig Clin Urol. 2017;58(1):3–11.
6. Lorenzo AJ, Cerveira J, Farhat WA. Pediatric laparoscopic ileal cystoplasty: complete intracorporeal surgical technique. Urology. 2007;69:977–81.
7. Docimo SG, Moore RG, Adams J, et al. Laparoscopic bladder augmentation using stomach. Urology. 1995;46:565–9.
8. Passerotti CC, Nguyen HT, Lais A, et al. Robot-assisted laparoscopic ileal bladder augmentation: defining techniques and potential pitfalls. J Endourol. 2008;22:355–60.
9. Gundeti MS, Eng MK, Reynolds WS, Zagaja GP. Pediatric robotic-assisted laparoscopic augmentation ileocystoplasty and Mitrofanoff appendicovesicostomy: complete intracorporeal–initial case report. Urology. 2008;72:1144–7.

10. Blok B, Pannek J, Castro-Diaz D, et al. EAU guidelines on neuro-urology, 2017. Available at: http://uroweb.org/guideline/neuro-urology. Accessed Aug 2019.
11. Murthy P, Cohen JA, Selig RB, Gundeti MS. Roboti-assisted laparoscopic augmentation ileocystoplasty and mitrofanoff appendicovesicostomy in children: updated interim results. Eur Urol. 2015;68(6):1069–75.
12. Baskin JJ, Vishteh AG, Wesche DE. Ventriculoperitoneal shunt failure as a complication of laparoscopic surgery. JSLS. 1998;2:177–80.
13. Gundeti MS, Godbole PP, Wilcox DT. Is bowel preparation required before cystoplasty in children? J Urol. 2006;176(4):1574–7.
14. Shah M, Ellis CT, Phillips MR, Marzinsky A, Adamson W, Weiner T, Erickson K, Lee S, Lange PA, SE ML. Preoperative bowel preparation prior to elective bowel resection or ostomy closure in the pediatric patient population has no impact on outcomes. A prospective randomized study. Am Surg. 2016;82(9):801–6.
15. Leys CM, Austin MT, Pietsch JB, Lovvom HN. Elective intestinal operations in infants and children without mechanical bowel preparation: a pilot study. J Pediatr Surg. 2005;40(6):978–81.
16. Gundeti MS, Wiltz AL, Zagaja GP, Shalhav AL. Robot-assisted laparoscopic intracorporeal hand-sewn bowel anastomosis during pediatric bladder reconstructive surgery. J Endourol. 2010;24(8):1325–8.
17. Hintz GC, Alshehri A, Bell CM, Butterworth SA. Stapled versus hand-sewn pediatric intestinal anastomoses: a retrospective cohort study. J Pediatr Surg. 2018;53(5):959–63.
18. Kozlov Y, Novogliov V, Podkamenev A, Wber I. Stapled bowel anastomoses in newborn surgery. Eur J Pediatr Surg. 2013;23(1):63–6.
19. Wrighton L, Curtis JL, Gollin G. Stapled intestinal anastomoses in infants. J Pediatr Surg. 2008;43(12):2231–4.
20. Gill IS, Rackley RR, Meraney AM, et al. Laparoscopic enterocystoplasty. Urology. 2000;55:178–81.
21. Noguera RJS, Astigueta JC, Carmona O, et al. Laparoscopic augmentation enterocystoplasty through a single trocar. Urology. 2009;73:1371–4.
22. Rackley RR, Abdelmalak JB. Laparoscopic augmentation cystoplasty. Surgical technique. Urol Clin North Am. 2001;28:663–70.
23. El-Feel A, Abedl-Hakim MA, Abouel-Fettouh H, Abdel-Hakim AM. Laparoscopic augmentation ileocystoplasty: results and outcome. Eur Urol. 2009;55(3):721–7.
24. Flum AS, Zhao LC, Kielb SJ, Wilson EB, Shu T, Hariston JC. Completely intracorporeal robotic-assisted laparoscopic augmentation enterocystoplasty with continent catheterizable channel. Urology. 2014;84(6):1314–8.
25. Wiestma AC, Estrada CR, Cho PS, Hollis MV, Yu RN. Robotic-assisted laparoscopic bladder augmentation in the pediatric patient. J Pediatr Urol. 2016;12(5):313.e1–2.
26. Kibar Y, Yalcin S, Kaya E, Kopru B, Ebiloqlu T, Tomruk H. Our experiences with robot-assisted laparoscopic surgery in pediatric patients: the first case series from Turkey. Turk J Urol. 2017;43(3):355–60.
27. Reyblat P, Chan KG, Josephson DY, Stein JP, Freeman JA, Grossfeled GD, Esrig D, Ginsperg DA. Comparison of extraperitoneal and intraperitoneal augmentation enterocystoplasty for neurogenic spinal cord injury patients. World J Urol. 2009;27:63.
28. McNamara ER, Kurtz MP, Schaeffer AJ, Logvinenko T, Nelson CP. 30-day morbidity after augmentation enterocystoplasty and appendicovesicstomy: a NSQIP pediatric analysis. J Pediatr Urol. 2015;11:209.e1–6.
29. Maldonado N, Michel J, Barnes K. Thirty-day hospital readmissions after augmentation cystoplasty: a nationwide readmissions database analysis. J Pediatr Urol. 2018;14(6):533e1–9.
30. Schlomer BJ, Copp HL. Cumulative incidence of outcomes and urologic procedures after augmentation cystoplasty. J Pediatr Urol. 2014;10:1043–50.

31. Szymanski KM, Misseri R, Whittam B, Lingeman JE, Amstutz S, Ring JD, Kaefer M, Rink RC, Cain MP. Bladder stones after bladder augmentation are not what they seem. J Pediatr Urol. 2016;12(2):98.e1–6.
32. Shepard CL, Wang C, Hopson BD, Bunt EB, Assimos DG. Urinary tract stone development in patients with myelodysplasia subjected to augmentation cystoplasty. Rev Urol. 2017;19:11–5.
33. Covert WM, Westin SN, Soliman PT, Langley GD. The role of mucoregulatory agents after continence-preserving urinary diversion surgery. Am J Health Syst Pharm. 2012;15:483–6.
34. Khorrami MH, Javid A, Izadpanahi MH, Alizadeh F, Zargham M, Khorrami F. Efficacy of long-acting octreotide on reducing mucus production in patients with ileal neobladder. Clin Genitourin Cancer. 2017;15(1):e9–e13.
35. Husmann DA, Rathbun SR. Long-term follow up of enteric bladder augmentations: the risk for malignancy. J Pediatr Urol. 2008;4(5):381–5.
36. Soergel TM, Cain MP, Misseri R, Gardner TA, Koch MO, Rink RC. Transitional cell carcinoma of the bladder following augmentation cystoplasty for neuropathic bladder. J Urol. 2004;172:1649–52.
37. Nurse DE, Mundy AR. Metabolic complications after cystoplasty. Br J Urol. 1985;63:165–70.
38. Cheng K, Kan C, Chu PS, Man C, Wong BT, Ho L, Au W. Augmentation cystoplasty: urodynamic and metabolic outcomes at 10-year follow-up. Int J Urol. 2015;22:1149–54.
39. Greenwell TJ, Venn SN, Mundy AR. Augmentation cystoplasty. BJU Int. 2001;88:511–25.
40. Steiner MS, Morton RA, Marshall FF. Vitamin B12 deficiency in patients with ileocolic neobladders. J Urol. 1993;149:255–7.

Part IV
Endoscopy and Percutaneous Surgery

Chapter 17
Endoscopic Treatment of Vesicoureteral Reflux

Angela M. Arlen and Andrew J. Kirsch

Introduction

Vesicoureteral reflux (VUR) is one of the most common urologic diagnoses in the pediatric population, yet optimal management remains a source of controversy and ongoing debate. Treatment options include observation with or without continuous antibiotic prophylaxis and surgical correction. The key to selecting children for surgical correction is identifying those patients at greatest risk for recurrent pyelonephritis and reflux unlikely to spontaneously resolve over time. Once it is determined a given child may benefit surgical intervention, options include endoscopic, laparoscopic/robotic, and open repairs.

Given the minimally invasive nature of Dx/HA, the initial frequency of endoscopic VUR management increased rapidly following FDA approval in 2001 [1, 2]. More recently, a steady decline in all anti-reflux surgeries has been observed, including Dx/HA injection, [3] likely as a result of the shifting emphasis to prevent recurrent urinary tract infection (UTI) and progressive renal scarring, while minimizing resource utilization and overtreatment. Published success rates vary widely between surgeons and techniques [4, 5]. Aggregate literature suggests that endoscopic therapy is relatively effective for the treatment of most primary VUR, while stressing the importance of reflux grade and structural/functional bladder anomalies on ultimate success rates. In a systematic meta-analysis evaluating Dx/HA for pediatric VUR, the estimated aggregate success rate for endoscopic therapy was 72% with 89% success for grade I, 83% for grade II, 71% for grade III, 59% for IV and

---

A. M. Arlen
Yale University School of Medicine, Department of Urology, New Haven, CT, USA
e-mail: angela.arlen@yale.edu

A. J. Kirsch (✉)
Emory University, Children's Healthcare of Atlanta, Atlanta, GA, USA

62% for grade V reflux [4]. Modifications to injection technique, described below, have led to much higher success rates with limited associated morbidity.

Indications

Primary VUR in infants and young children tends to spontaneously improve and often completely resolve over time, however a cohort remains who are at risk for recurrent pyelonephritis and the potential harmful sequela of renal scarring. Surgical intervention may be necessary in children with persistent reflux, renal scarring and/or recurrent febrile UTI. Families/caregivers should be thoroughly counseled regarding the potential pros and cons of various VUR management options, and all children should undergo screening for and treatment of any co-existing bowel-bladder dysfunction. The 2010 AUA Reflux Guidelines recommend management of any suspected voiding dysfunction, preferably prior to surgical intervention, as these children are known to have increased surgical complications as well as higher failure rates [6]. While endoscopic injection initially focused on the treatment of primary VUR, over time Dx/HA has emerged as a potential treatment option for VUR associated with anatomic abnormalities such as paraureteral diverticula, ectopic ureters, and megaureters, depending on both surgeon experience and parental preference [7–9].

General Surgical Principles

- Child is placed in dorsal lithotomy position; the ability to rotate cystoscope over the thighs is crucial in order to visualize and inject laterally displaced orifices.
- Pediatric rigid cystoscope with at least a 4 French working channel is required; an off-set lens should be utilized to allow passage of the needle in line with ureter.
- Tower/monitor should be positioned so that the surgeon can easily visualize the screen and assess injection progress.
- Bladder should be decompressed during injection and the needle primed with Dx/HA prior to insertion.
- Hydrodistention is performed bilaterally prior to injection with the tip of the cystoscope placed at the ureteral orifice; a pressured stream is achieved by placing the irrigation bag approximately 1 m above the pubic symphysis on full flow. Ureteral hydrodistention is graded according to distensibility of the orifice (Table 17.1), and allows for ongoing visualization of tandem intraluminal and orifice injection sites as well as ensuring adequate coaptation.
- Surgeon should inject the implant, this allows control of the volume and pressure during injection, whilst viewing the appearance of the implant mound. Dx/HA should be injected slowly; if the orifice is difficult to inject, ensure that the bladder is not over-distended and the needle is not occluded.

Table 17.1 Hydrodistention grading

Ureteral hydrodistention grade	Endoscopic findings
H0	No orifice distension
H1	Orifice opens, intramural tunnel not evident
H2	Intramural tunnel evident, extramural tunnel not visualized
H3	Extramural tunnel visualized/ureter can accept the cystoscope

- Dx/HA is typically an ambulatory procedure and all patients receive preoperative antibiotic prophylaxis, which is continued until clinical follow-up.
- Renal-bladder ultrasound is obtained 4–6 weeks postoperatively to assess for asymptomatic hydronephrosis and implant integrity.
- AUA Reflux Guidelines also recommend a postoperative voiding cystourethrogram (VCUG) following Dx/HA injection though surgeon's clinical experience and success rate can be taken into consideration [6].

Endoscopic Injection Techniques

STING Technique

With the traditional STING method, the needle is introduced under the bladder mucosa at the 6 o'clock position 2–3 mm *below* the refluxing orifice. Dx/HA is injected until there is a sufficient bulge present, with the orifice assuming a crescent-like shape [10]. The bulking agent augments tissue below the ureteral orifice, providing support to the refluxing orifice. Submucosal ureteral length is thereby potentially increased, the valve mechanism enhanced, thus preventing retrograde flow of urine into the upper tract [11]. The relatively low success of the STING method compared to ureteral reimplantation ultimately led to development of the HIT and Double HIT methods.

HIT and Double HIT Methods

Double hydrodistention implantation technique (HIT) differs from the STING method in that it utilizes tandem intramural injections with goal of achieving both ureteral and orifice coaptation. Hydrodistention is performed with the cystoscope directed at the ureteral orifice. Hydrodistention allows for visualization of the intraluminal injection site as well as ongoing assessment of injection progress. Classification is as follows: H0 – no hydrodistention, H1 – ureteral orifice open but tunnel is not evident, H2 – intramural tunnel visualized, and H3 – extramural ureter is visualized [12] (Table 17.1). Ureteral hydrodistention causes the refluxing orifice and ureter to initially open but following successful injection, the ureter and orifice should achieve coaptation (i.e., H0 grade).

In the Double HIT method, the needle is placed into the distended ureteral orifice and inserted in the mid-ureteral tunnel at the 6 o'clock position (rather than *below* the orifice as in the STING method). Dx/HA is injected until a sufficient bulge is produced, which coapts the detrusor tunnel. A second injection at the distal most aspect of the intraureteral tunnel results in coaptation of the ureteral orifice. HD is performed following each injection to monitor progress and ensure adequate ureteral coaptation (Fig. 17.1). Patients with high grade VUR occurring early in the bladder cycle are more likely to have abnormal ureteral hydrodistention, and are more likely to require an increased volume of Dx/HA to achieve satisfactory coaptation of the ureteral tunnel and orifice [13].

Advantages of HIT over STING include improved visualization of the distal ureteral lumen with the aid of hydrodistention, allowing accurate placement of the needle at the desired position within the distal ureter as well as better visualization of ureteral lumen throughout injection – Dx/HA can be visualized tracking proximally in Waldeyer's sheath. Unlike the STING technique were coaptation is directed

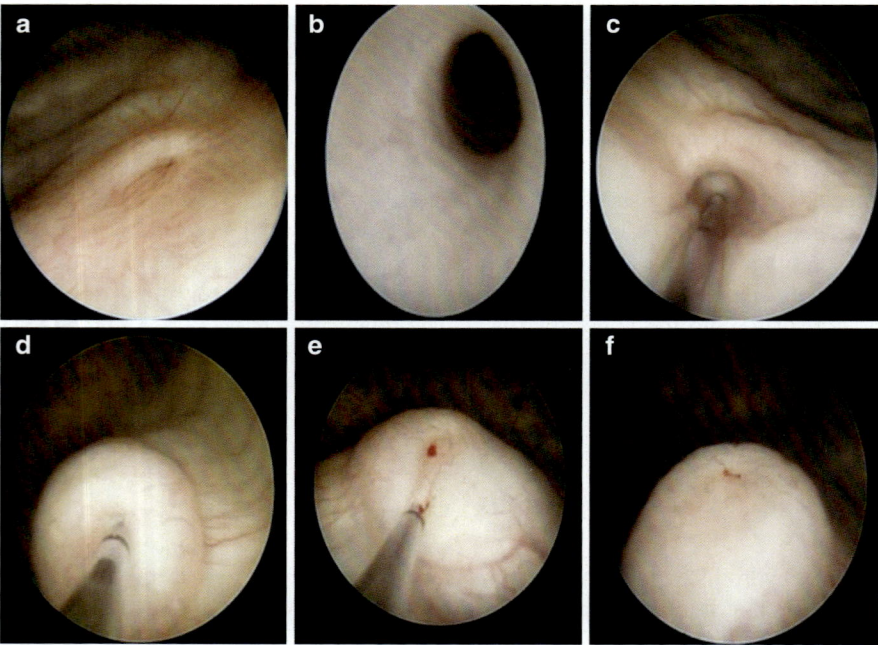

Fig. 17.1 Double HIT Method. Bladder is emptied and ureteral orifice visualized (**a**), followed by hydrodistention, and in this case the extramural ureter is visualized (**b**). Proximal HIT is then performed with the needle inserted into mid-ureteral tunnel at the 6 o'clock position (**c**) and sufficient bulking agent is injected to produce a bulge which coapts the tunnel (**d**). Distal HIT is then performed (**e**) and leads to coaptation of the ureteral orifice (**f**)

only at the orifice, with Double HIT the coaptation involves the intramural ureter as well as the orifice [11]

Outcomes/Complications

Endoscopic repair confers several advantages, in that is a brief ambulatory procedure with minimal postoperative pain and limited restrictions. Significant complications are rare but warrant prompt attention (Table 17.2). Early complications occur within the initial 2–3 perioperative days. Less than 4% of children undergoing Dx/HA injection report transient renal colic symptoms, and the majority resolve with time and analgesics. Approximately 0.6% of children experience ureteral obstruction following endoscopic injection. Obstruction is frequently associated with untreated voiding dysfunction or megaureters requiring a large volume of bulking agent [6, 11]. Persistent, high-grade obstruction requiring an indwelling ureteral stent or percutaneous nephrostomy tube placement is rare.

The most common complication following endoscopic therapy is febrile UTI. Preoperative urinalysis, with culture/treatment when appropriate, significantly reduces risk of perioperative infection. In patients with a symptomatic UTI, surgery should be delayed until a course of appropriately antibiotics has been completed. The incidence of febrile and non-febrile UTI following endoscopic injection in long-term studies ranges from 0–21% to 5.6–25%, respectively, with most infections occurring in the 3–4 years following injection [5, 14–18].

Success rates, while up to 94% with the Double HIT method, [18–20] are known to vary widely with reported treatment failure rates of 6–50%; outcomes are dependent upon the technique utilized, injected material, VUR grade and surgeon experience [7]. Acknowledging endpoints of injection are also key to a successful implantation. After Dx/HA injection, the bladder should be drained and hydrodistention again performed to confirm absence of ureteral distensibility (i.e., H0 ureter). Failures may result from Dx/HA displacement (implant migration), disruption (mucosal breach) or dissolution (decrease in implant volume). Patients with a previous history of voiding dysfunction are particularly susceptible to failure, and thus must be encouraged to continue a voiding and bowel regimen postoperatively.

Length of follow-up also has an impact on success rates, studies (not utilizing the Double HIT method) with longer clinical follow-up suggests that results may not be

Table 17.2 Complications of endoscopic Dx/HA injection

Complications of endoscopic injection	
Persistent VUR	Ranges from 6% to 50% depending on technique, grade, surgeon
Ureteral obstruction	Occurs in <1%
UTI	5–25%; most immediate UTIs can be avoided with preop UA/culture
Renal colic	2% nausea/flank pain; majority resolve spontaneously

durable. Radiographic recurrence of reflux after initial successful endoscopic injection appears to be around 15–20% within several years and is stable thereafter [14–16]. In our long-term data, success has remained greater than 90% with greater than 96% parental satisfaction. 250) [21]. Late failures are hypothesized to be secondary to the biodegradable nature of Dx/HA; the clinical significance of late recurrent VUR in the absence of symptomatic infections is unclear.

Conclusions

Dx/HA injection is a safe and effective minimally invasive alternative to ureteroneocystostomy, with Double HIT achieving the highest success rates. Treating bladder-bowel dysfunction preoperatively and achieving ureteric tunnel and orifice coaptation with loss of hydrodistention are keys to success injection. Postoperative febrile UTI is the most common complication with rates comparable to other antireflux surgery.

References

1. Lendvay TS, Sorensen M, Cowan CA, Joyner BD, Mitchell MM, Grady RW. The evolution of vesicoureteral reflux management in the era of dextranomer/hyaluronic acid copolymer: a pediatric health information system database review. J Urol. 2006;176:1864–7.
2. Nelson CP, Copp HL, Lai J, Saigal CS. Is availability of endoscopy changing initial management of vesicoureteral reflux? J Urol. 2009;182:1152–7.
3. Garcia-Roig M, Travers C, McCracken CE, Kirsch AJ. National trends in the management of primary vesicoureteral reflux in children. J Urol. 2018;199(1):287–93.
4. Routh JC, Inman BA, Reinberg Y. Dextranomer/hyaluronic acid for pediatric vesicoureteral reflux: systemic review. Pediatrics. 2010;125:1010–9.
5. Yap TL, Chen Y, Nah SA, Ong CCP, Jacobsen A, Low Y. STING versus HIT technique of endoscopic treatment for vesicoureteral reflux: a systemic review and meta-analysis. J Pediatr Surg. 2016;51(12):2015–2.
6. Peters CA, Skoog SJ, Arant BS Jr, Copp HL, Elder JS, Hudson RG, et al. Summary of the AUA guideline on management of primary vesicoureteral reflux in children. J Urol. 2010;184:1134–44.
7. Routh JC, Bogaert GA, Kaefer M, Manzoni G, Park JM, Retik AB, et al. Vesicoureteral reflux: current trends in diagnosis, screening, and treatment. Eur Urol. 2012;61:773–82.
8. Kurtz MP, Leow JJ, Varda BK, Logvinenko T, McQuaid JW, Yu RN, et al. The decline of the open ureteral reimplant in the United States: national data from 2003 to 2013. Urology. 2017;100:193–7.
9. Häcker FM, Frech-Dörfler M, von Rotz M, Rudin C. Endoscopic hyaluronic acid/dextranomer gel implantation is effective as first-line treatment of vesicoureteral reflux (VUR) in children: a single centre experience. Eur J Pediatr Surg. 2011;21:299–303.
10. O'Donnell B, Puri P. Treatment of vesicoureteral reflux by endoscopic injection of Teflon. Br Med J. 1984;289:7–9.
11. Lackgren G, Kirsch AJ. Endoscopic treatment of vesicoureteral reflux. BJU Int. 2010;105:1332–47.

12. Kirsch AJ, Kaye JD, Cerwinka WH, Watson JM, Elmore JM, Lyles RH, et al. Dynamic hydrodistention of the ureteral orifice: a novel grading system with high interobserver concordance and correction with vesicoureteral reflux grade. J Urol. 2009;182:1688–92.
13. Arlen AM, Broderick KM, Huen KH, Leong T, Scherz HC, Kirsch AJ. Temporal pattern of vesicoureteral reflux on voiding cystourethrogram correlates with dynamic endoscopic hydrodistention grade of ureteral orifice. J Urol. 2014;192:1503–7.
14. Brandstrom P, Esbjorner E, Herthelius M, Swerkersson S, Jodal U, Hansson S. The Swedish reflux trial in children: III. Urinary tract infection pattern. J Urol. 2010;184:286–91.
15. Läckgren G, Wåhlin N, Sköldenberg E, Stenberg A. Long-term followup of children treated with dextranomer/hyaluronic acid copolymer for vesicoureteral reflux. J Urol. 2001;166(5):1887–92.
16. Friedmacher F, Colhoun E, Puri P. Endoscopic injection of dextranomer/hyaluronic acid as first line treatment in 851 consecutive children with high grade vesicoureteral reflux: efficacy and long-term results. J Urol. 2018;200(3):650–5.
17. Kamdem F, Galli G, Aubert D. Long-term incidence of febrile UTI after DxHA treatment of VUR. J Pediatr Urol. 2014;10(1):56–61.
18. Arlen AM, Scherz HC, Filimon E, Leong T, Kirsch AJ. Is routine voiding cystourethrogram necessary following double hit for primary vesicoureteral reflux. J Pediatr Urol. 2015;11(1):40–5.
19. Kaye JD, Srinivasan AK, Delaney C, Cerwinka WH, Elmore JM, Scherz HC, et al. Clinical and radiographic results of endoscopic injection for vesicoureteral reflux: defining measures of success. J Pediatr Urol. 2012;8:297–303.
20. Kalisvaart JF, Scherz HC, Cuda S, Kaye JD, Kirsch AJ. Intermediate to long-term follow-up indicates low risk of recurrence after Double HIT endoscopic treatment for primary vesicoureteral reflux. J Pediatr Urol. 2012;8:359–65.
21. Lightfoot M, Bilgutay AN, Tolin N, Eisenberg S, Weiser J, Bryan L, Smith E, Elmore J, Scherz H, Kirsch AJ. Long-Term clinical outcomes and parental satisfaction after Dextranomer/Hyaluronic Acid (Dx/HA) injection for primary vesicoureteral reflux. Front Pediatr. 2019;7:392. PMID 31612121.

Chapter 18
PCNL

Matthew T. Migliozzi, Mark G. Biebel, and Michael P. Kurtz

Introduction

Percutaneous nephrolithotomy (PCNL) is the gold-standard treatment of large renal stone burden in children, and has several unique technical considerations related to age. The first is the enriched population of patients with spinal dysraphism compared with an adult practice. Patients with spina bifida are both more likely to require PCNL and have a 50–210% higher risk of every measurable complication based on national data [1]. Such complexity is reflected in stone scores, addressed below, and surgeons should expect poorer stone clearance [2].

Secondly, while lower skin-to-stone distance in children facilitates initial puncture, the kidney is more mobile. This is true in our experience and is present in numerous reports, even for less technical procedures such as pediatric nephrostomy tube placement [3]. This makes tract dilation more precarious as the kidney tends to slide with the instrument [3, 4].

Lastly, blood loss is a concern. While children have proportionally higher in red cell volume than adults, total circulating volume is lower. For bedside approximation, blood volume 7–8% of total body weight is reasonably accurate for term newborns through adolescents [5]. For the most precise calculations, lean body mass is

M. T. Migliozzi
Boston Children's Hospital, Department of Urology, Boston, MA, USA
e-mail: mmiglioz2@student.touro.edu

M. G. Biebel
Boston Medical Center/Boston University School of Medicine, Department of Urology, Boston, MA, USA
e-mail: Mark.Biebel@bmc.org

M. P. Kurtz (✉)
Harvard Medical School, Boston Children's Hospital, Department of Urology, Boston, MA, USA
e-mail: michael.kurtz@childrens.harvard.edu

© Springer Nature Switzerland AG 2020
P. C. Gargollo (ed.), *Minimally Invasive and Robotic-Assisted Surgery in Pediatric Urology*, https://doi.org/10.1007/978-3-030-57219-8_18

most closely associated with total circulating volume [6]. As children are smaller, hemodynamically significant blood volumes may be lost quickly, and 30% blood loss may present with only mild tachycardia and no hypotension [5]. Pediatric anesthesiologists will be able to rescue the patient with a transfusion, and it is for this reason that pediatric PCNL should take place in a setting with intensive care units available and prompt angiography capability.

This chapter is organized as a procedure would be performed sequentially, describing preoperative stone scoring systems, patient positioning, imaging and renal access, size of the tract and instrumentation, and complications. At the end we share our approach.

Stone Scoring Systems

Several stone scoring systems exist to help predict outcomes of PCNL preoperatively. These can be useful in counseling patients and in pre-operative planning for the surgeon. The three most commonly used systems are (1) Guy's stone score, (2) STONE score, and (3) CROES nomogram. These scoring systems primarily depend on evaluation of a non-contrast CT scan.

Guy's stone score grades the complexity of planned PCNL as shown below. The initial study in 2010 by Thomas, et al. showed that this score was reproducible and could independently predict stone-free rate after PCNL [7].

- Grade I: Solitary stone in mid/lower pole or solitary stone in the pelvis with simple anatomy.
- Grade II: Solitary stone in upper pole or multiple stones in a patient with simple anatomy or a solitary stone in a patient with abnormal anatomy.
- Grade III: Multiple stones in a patient with abnormal anatomy or stones in a caliceal diverticulum or partial staghorn calculus.
- Grade IV: Staghorn calculus or any stone in a patient with spina bifida or spinal injury.

The *STONE nephrolithometry score* is an acronym for **S**tone size (in mm^2), **T**ract length (skin-to-stone distance), degree of **O**bstruction (presence of hydronephrosis), **N**umber of involved calices, and stone **E**ssence (stone density). Each of these variables is assigned a score and the overall summed score is used to predict outcomes. The initial study of this scoring system in 2013 by Okhunov, et al. showed it to be significantly predictive for stone-free rate, operative time, hospital length of stay, and blood loss [8].

The ***CROES (Clinical Research Office of the Endourological Society) nomogram*** is a predictive model based on a large multi-center study that considers surgeon case volume, prior treatment, stone burden, stone location, and number of stones. The summative score can be correlated with a percentage score signaling the likelihood of treatment success (stone free) after PCNL [9].

When comparing these scoring systems, several studies have shown them to be equivalent in predicting PCNL stone-free rate. Guy's score was the only system that could significantly predict complications in a meta-analysis by Jiang et al. [10, 11]

Aldaqadossi et al. evaluated if these scoring systems, initially formulated with adult patients, could be applicable to the pediatric world. In a retrospective study of 125 children who underwent PCNL, Guy's, STONE, and CROES scores were calculated. STONE score was the most accurate in predicting stone-free rate. Guy's score was the only score significantly associated with complication rate. Despite these findings, further research is needed to more accurately modify scoring system measurement values based on patient size and age [12].

Patient Positioning

Traditionally, PCNL has been performed in the prone position to allow for easy access to the posterior calyces of the kidney. However, prone surgery may add operative time for positioning and has a higher risk of injury of the cervical spine, eyes, and arms if not positioned properly [13, 14]. Additionally, it can be more difficult for the anesthesia team to troubleshoot airway concerns intra-operatively, which can be particularly problematic in morbidly obese patients. Despite these factors, prone positioning can be safely executed with no increase in complications as compared to other positions with careful positioning and planning [15, 16]. It remains the most common PCNL position amongst urologists. A slight modification to this position is the prone split-leg position using a split leg table, which allows easier access for cystoscopy and retrograde ureteroscopy.

In 1987, Valdivia et al. described the first supine PCNL. Later they presented a series of 557 patients who underwent supine PCNL and showed it to be safe and effective [17]. Since that time, studies have compared prone and supine positioning for PCNL. In general, operative time is less for the supine position, but all other parameters including blood loss, hospital length of stay, and complications were not significantly different. Stone-free rate has been reported as either equivalent or better in the supine group, depending on the study [15, 16, 18]. Gamal et al. analyzed supine PCNL in a series of children (mean age 6.8 years old) and found it to be safe and effective as well. For positioning, the posterior axillary line was marked preoperatively with the child standing. In this study, a ureteric catheter was placed in the lithotomy position initially, and then the legs were returned to the straight position, although some surgeons maintain the lithotomy position throughout the case. Then, two saline bags were placed under the ipsilateral hip and shoulder to expose the working area [19].

The flank-free modified supine position has also been used successfully in children. For this position, a bag is placed under the ipsilateral shoulder and the ipsilateral arm is crossed over the chest. The ipsilateral leg is extended and crossed over the flexed contralateral leg. This position increases the distance between the costal margin and iliac crest, allowing for a slightly wider working space [20].

Another slight modification is the Galdakao-modified supine Valdivia position, proposed in 2007 by Ibarluzea, et al. This positioning involves similar crossing of the arm and bumping of the ipsilateral shoulder. The difference is the legs are kept in lithotomy position with slight rotation towards the contralateral side. This allows for easy simultaneous antegrade and retrograde access [21]. This position has been used in small series of pediatric patients with success [22]. A slight modification of this position is termed "Giusti's position" and involves a straight, flat ipsilateral leg and the contralateral leg in a single stirrup [23].

Lateral decubitus position on a flexed table has also been used for PCNL. Jian Wei Gan et al. described this in 347 adult patients and found it to be safe and effective [24]. No direct comparative studies have been done, but the advantages of this position include decreased anesthetic and eye risks (as compared to prone) and a larger space to work in for renal access with the table flexion opening the space between the costal margin and iliac crest. This position has not been studied in the pediatric population.

Overall, there are many options for PCNL position in both adults and children. The traditional prone position is still the most commonly used, but other positions described may offer similar efficacy, shorter operative times, and decreased risks. Further comparative studies are needed to determine the optimal position. At this point, surgeon preference and experience dictate the position chosen.

Importantly, if there are any concerns for extremity contractures or limited range, we recommend ranging the patient's limbs in the office or the preoperative area. Hips and shoulders are the most critical extremities to examine. This way, the patient can report discomfort or tightness and reduce the risk of injury during anesthetized positioning.

Imaging During PCNL Procedure

Selection of a particular renal calyx for access helps with treatment of the stone depending on its size and location within the kidney. In general, a lower pole posterior calyx is preferred. Skin puncture sites posterior to the posterior axillary line are safest. Entry of the anterior calyces can be associated with increased complications, including bleeding and even bowel injury [25]. Some studies have shown benefit to upper pole access as well. However, upper pole access can have a higher risk of pleural injury if it is performed above the costal margin [26]. There are several techniques described for percutaneous renal access, which will be described below. No technique has been shown to be superior to another, therefore surgeon comfort and experience should direct which technique is used [27].

To assist with percutaneous access of a particular calyx, it is helpful to place a retrograde ureteral catheter via cystoscopy so that the calyces can be outlined with contrast, or distended with saline for ultrasound, before proceeding with the techniques below.

Eye of the Needle/Bull's Eye Technique

With the patient in prone position, this technique begins with placing the C-arm 20–30 degrees towards the side of the kidney being accessed. This mimics the angle of the posterior calyces. The needle is also placed at 20–30 degrees and the tip of the needle is directed over the appropriate posterior calyx. The needle appears as a dot on fluoroscopy since the X-ray beam is parallel to it. The calyx appears as a circle surrounding this dot since it is being viewed end-on. At this angle, the X-ray beam, needle, and calyx are all parallel. The C-arm is then rotated back to a vertical position (zero degrees) to view needle depth. It is advanced using a needle driver until the needle tip is overlying the end of the calyx. At this point the needle tip should be in the calyx and this can be confirmed by aspiration of urine. If it is not in position, the C-arm can be rotated between these two angles to make the necessary adjustments [25, 28].

Triangulation Technique

This technique uses biplanar fluoroscopy with the planes parallel to and oblique to the line of puncture. When in the parallel plane, only medial and lateral adjustments are made. When in the oblique plane, only superior and inferior adjustments are made. Once the needle tip is aligned with the proper calyx, ventilation is suspended by anesthesia and the needle is advanced under fluoroscopy into the calyx until urine can be aspirated [25, 29].

Hybrid Technique

This technique uses a combination of the prior two techniques and some mathematical calculation. To begin this technique, the patient is prone and the C-arm is kept in the vertical position and the skin over the target calyx is marked (triangle point 1). The C-arm is then rotated 30 degrees towards the surgeon and the skin is marked at the point where the desired calyx appears end-on (triangle point 2). The distance between points 1 and 2 is measured (x). The distance from the skin to the target calyx (R) can be calculated using the eq. $R = 12x / 6.28$. The third point of the triangle is marked inferiorly to the line between points 1 and 2 at a distance that forms an equilateral triangle. The needle is inserted into the skin at point 3, aiming superiorly towards the plane created by points 1 and 2. The needle should be advanced a distance calculated by R earlier to achieve access into the target calyx. Again, aspiration of urine can be used to confirm proper position [29].

Cross-Table Lateral Bull's Eye Technique

This technique has been described for access in supine or modified supine positions. To begin a zero-degree retrograde pyelogram is taken. Then the C-arm is rotated so that a cross-table lateral image is taken from the contralateral side of the table. In this view the location of the desired calyx is marked on the skin. The C-arm is rotated back to zero-degrees and the needle is advanced parallel to the floor and in line with the calyx. Movement should only occur in the superior or inferior directions. If there is no urine return, the C-arm is rotated cephalad to adjust the depth of puncture [23].

Ultrasound-Guided Access

The obvious advantage of this technique is the elimination of radiation exposure during access and real-time visualization during the full procedure. Additionally, Doppler flow imaging can be used to avoid major vascular injury and surrounding viscera (spleen, liver, bowel) can be seen. Retrograde ureteral catheter placement is not typically needed prior to this technique. This technique works best in non-obese patients. A curvilinear or curved array probe should be used in most cases; linear probes are often best for infants or toddlers. Once the target calyx is identified on ultrasound, the needle is advanced alongside the probe such that it can be seen puncturing the calyx in real time; a needle guide may be helpful to fix the needle in the plain of the transducer array. Once the needle is in the desired calyx, wire advancement and tract dilation have also been performed under ultrasound guidance, but a combination of both ultrasound and fluoroscopy have also been used [30, 31]. Ultrasound guidance is often used in combination with some of the above fluoroscopic access techniques.

Cone-Beam CT

Interventional radiologists have long used the combination of CT and fluoroscopy, in a single machine, to access difficult anatomic structures. Recently, urologists have started to do the same. In brief, a motorized c-arm rotates and acquires a CT of the relevant anatomy [32, 33]. The C-arm then can be positioned in eye-of-the-needle or orthogonally to judge depth. We use this for our most complex cases. Such radiologic tools are complex, mostly mounted within a single room, and fluid must be kept separate from electronic elements in the unit base. In our cases, radiation from a cone-beam CT is higher than that of non-contrast stone CTs obtained on standard multidetector machines.

Risk from Fluoroscopy

Radiation doses in PCNL for both patient and staff are some of the highest in of all endourologic cases [34, 35]. Strategies to reduce radiation to a dose as low as reasonably achievable (ALARA) are important considerations for pre- and post-procedure diagnostic imaging as well as for intraoperative guidance.

Radiation exposure to staff from PCNL is within safe range – 4 min of fluoroscopy leads to approximately 0.04 mSv for staff per case which is far below the 50 mSv annual occupational dose limit [36]. This matches with prior studies, although finger dose is about tenfold higher than for the rest of the body [35]. We do not wear radiation reducing gloves (RRGs). Even if the operator wears RRGs, placing a hand in the field causes the dose to the patient to increase 2.8-fold or more [37] and while scatter radiation is reduced, protection of the hands is so limited that national and international guidelines recommend against use of RRGs when the hands are in the primary beam [38]. It's also easy to be fooled – a hand in an RRG appears more protected than it truly is, as both sides of the glove attenuate the beam on the image, but only one side of the glove actually protects the hand. The simple message is that it is critical to keep the hands out of the field of view when using the c-arm. Distance has an enormous effect; dose to the fingers in the primary beam is over 100 times greater than if the fingers are just 15 cm away from the beam [39].

We also note that flat panel detectors seem to be associated with dramatically lower dose than traditional image intensifiers with pediatric ureteroscopy [40]. Dose is reduced when the image detector as close to the patient as possible. There are practical limits on this with prone PCNL, as the detector will often be limited by the back of the needle, the sheath, or the rigid endoscope, but lowering it as much as possible is advised.

Reducing patient radiation exposure is a critical principle, and should be integrated as a part of, but not superseding, safe and effective surgery for stone. We should also be realistic about what the known harms of low-dose radiation exposure are, as professional organizations do not support extrapolation of cancer risk for doses below 100 mSv [41]. Nearly all PCNLs will be in this range. For this reason, we advocate focusing on overall safety, from a procedural and dosimetry standpoint. We perform fluoroscopic time-outs for every urologic procedure using a c-arm, standardizing commands, positioning of the unit, and machine settings.

Instrumentation and Tract Size

Standard PCNL

Over the past several decades the practice of removing large renal stones has evolved to include advances in technology and a variety of approaches. These approaches fall within four major categories: Standard PCNL, Mini PCNL, Ultra-mini PCNL, and Micro PCNL [42–46]. Generally, each approach is defined by the access sheath caliber. In turn, individual approaches vary regarding nephroscope caliber, dilation method, fragmentation source, and options for debris removal.

Standard PCNL dilatation is used to create access tracts ranging from 24-30F. There are several options for dilatation of the access tracts including serial Alken metal telescope dilators, semi-rigid Amplatz fascial dilators, and balloon dilators. Although Amplatz dilators are still widely used, balloon dilation is associated with a decreased incidence of hemorrhage, fewer blood transfusions, and a shorter operative duration and recovery period [47, 48]. The one drawback to balloon dilation is the relatively high cost. Several recent prospective studies have yielded promising data where access tract dilation was achieved using a single step Amplatz technique with similar outcome and safety profiles to the more expensive balloon approach [45, 49].

Due to these large caliber tracts, options for visualization include a variety of flexible and rigid nephroscopes. Popular options include digital and fiberoptic nephroscopes with numerous ergonomic features, internal vs. external light sources, and weight profiles. As the image quality of endoscopes continues to improve, their size continues to decrease in order to improve maneuverability and increase working channel calibers [50].

Mini and Ultramini PCNL

The relative difference in anatomy between adults and the pediatric population drove the development of mini PCNL (miniperc) in order to reduce morbidities associated with standard PCNL in children. In 1997 Helal et al. developed the mini PCNL technique, using a 15F Hickman catheter introduction set and a 10F pediatric cystoscope [51]. The smaller diameter, peel-away sheath was easier to maneuver with pediatric instruments and avoided excessive dilation of parenchymal tracts. The following year Jackman et al. developed the first ultramini PCNL using an 11F peel-away vascular access sheath with either a 7F rigid pediatric cystoscope or 9.5F flexible ureteroscope [46].

There are several major differences between mini and ultramini PCNL. Although mini PCNL may use the same fragmentation modalities as standard PCNL (holmium laser, pneumatic, and ultrasonic), ultramini PCNL is limited to holmium laser fragmentation [43]. Methods of fragment removal also differ. Here again, mini PCNL is similar to standard PCNL where options include irrigation, suction, and/or removal by grasping devices. Ultramini PCNL removes fragments upon rapid removal of the endoscope, creating a "vortex" that effectively flushes out any residual debris.

Stone free rates (SFR) are generally comparable between standard and mini/ultramini PCNL approaches. An improved SFR was observed when mini PCNL was performed to clear staghorn calculi [52] and in instances of multiple caliceal stones [53]. However, there remains much debate as to whether or not mini and ultramini approaches significantly decrease morbidity when compared to standard PCNL. Initial small series using mini PCNL in pediatric populations claimed the use of smaller tracts led to less parenchymal trauma [54–56]. Although, further series observed no difference in acute phase reactants [57], renal injury [58], or renal scar volumes [58] between mini/ultramini and standard PCNL techniques. The true advantage of mini and ultramini PCNL is decreased perioperative bleeding [53, 59–61], decreased pain postoperatively, [62] and overall shorter hospital durations [60, 62].

The most common disadvantage associated with Mini and Ultramini PCNL was the relatively longer intraoperative time when compared with that of standard PCNL. These longer intraoperative periods are associated with a prolonged intracorporal lithotripsy periods required to create fragments small enough to pass through smaller diameter sheaths [60] along with decreased visibility [63]. However, issues with visibility may correlate with surgeon experience and prolonged lithotripsy periods may decrease with improvements/miniaturization of current suction devices.

When considering the outcomes of the aforementioned studies, mini and ultramini PCNL are reasonable options for adult patients with stones ranging from 1.5–2.0 cm and for children with relatively large stones [42, 59, 64]. When compared with standard PCNL, both mini and ultramini PCNL have similar SFR rates as standard PCNL and have lower complications in some reports [65].

Micro PCNL

As the mini and ultramini PCNL approaches improved and the benefits of smaller access tracts were observed, one question lingered: what is the smallest feasible caliber access tract for PCNL? In 2011 Desai et al. were the first to describe the micro PCNL (microperc) approach [66]. Micro PCNL utilizes a single step approach where access is created under direct visualization using a 4.85F (16-gauge) all-seeing needle. The needle sheath provides access for the flexible telescope and 200 μm holmium laser fiber. A three-way connector attached to the end of the needle sheath allows for the passage of irrigation, telescope, and laser fiber [66]. This approach does have a drawback. Due the small caliber access tracts, stones must be sufficiently vaporized as the approach does not allow fragment removal. Another difference between micro PCNL and other PCNL techniques is the use of a pressurized irrigation system to remove vaporized debris from the tracts.

The primary advantage of micro PCNL is decreased perioperative bleeding. Bleeding is typically correlated with access tract caliber and trauma introduced during tract dilation. In a study of 140 renal units, Hatipoglu et al. reported an SFR of 82%, no postoperative complications, and 0.71% of patients requiring transfusion due to significant blood loss [67]. Single step access provides additional benefit as the all-seeing needle allows the operator direct visualization of the anatomy and the ability to avoid critical structures during tract creation. This is particularly useful when entering ectopic renal systems where the possibility of damaging nearby bowel is increased [59]. The small caliber tracts have also been shown to decrease the need for post-operative percutaneous nephrostomy drainage in favor of a tubeless procedure which may lead to decreased hospital recovery periods and improved healing [59, 68].

Micro PCNL is favored when the stone burden consists of a single stone or multiple stones with a cumulative diameter less than 1.5 cm [59]. It may also prove beneficial when precision is required as in cases of ectopic renal systems, horseshoe kidneys, and stones located within calyceal diverticula [66].

Energy Sources for Stone Fragmentation

Fragmentation devices fall into one of several categories including electrohydraulic (EHL), ultrasonic, laser, and pneumatic. The energy source and manner of fragmentation are the distinguishing factors, each associated with its own advantages and disadvantages. Ultrasonic and pneumatic lithotripters were the favored options prior to the development of the holmium laser. EHL has largely fallen out of favor.

Electrohydraulic

First developed by Yutkin in 1955, EHL was the first lithotripsy device used for PCNL. It is generally cheaper than other lithotripsy devices but considered to be the least safe [69]. The device works via spark-gap technology: a spark created at the probe-stone interface vaporizes fluid, creating a shockwave. The force of repeated shockwaves causes stone fragmentation. Since its initial development, EHL technology has improved and miniaturized to provide more precision during the process but it still maintains the worst complication profile when compared to other lithotripsy devices. In a study accessing the safety of EHL and pneumatic devices, Hofbauer et al. describes 34 patients who underwent EHL and 38 who underwent pneumatic lithotripsy. Although the efficacy was similar, perforations occurred at a much higher rate with EHL (17.6%) than with pneumatic lithotripsy (2.6%) [70]. Even newer EHL models have been known to damage ureteroscope lenses and collecting systems and cause major intrarenal bleeding if the spark is discharged while not in contact with the stone [71].

Ultrasonic

Ultrasonic lithotripsy relies on mechanical vibration created by piezo-ceramic elements that is transmitted to rigid probes resulting in a drilling motion [72, 73]. The device allows for simultaneous aspiration of smaller stone fragments through a hollow inner lumen during lithotripsy, requiring less retrieval for these smaller fragments than other lithotripters. Ultrasonic lithotripters are considered safe, as contact with surrounding tissue only results in superficial abrasions rather than perforations [69]. Disadvantages of ultrasonic lithotripsy include the need for continuous irrigation to prevent the probe from overheating and unfavorable efficacy with hard and smooth surfaced stones. For this reason, ultrasonic lithotripsy is ideal for stones with a soft matrix such as phosphate stones. Recent improvements in ultrasonic lithotripsy include a dual ultrasonic lithotripter with separate probes vibrating at different frequencies. *In vitro* trials have shown this device to be as efficacious as older versions of ultrasonic lithotripters with potentially faster fragmentation rates and fewer instances of overheating [50, 74]. Clinical trials are needed to assess outcomes and complications *in vivo*.

Pneumatic Lithotripsy

In pneumatic lithotripsy, compressed carbon dioxide propels a projectile into a solid, rigid, probe which chisels renal calculi similarly to the mechanical action of a jackhammer. Unlike most other lithotripsy modalities, this process does not create heat [75]. Damage to nearby tissue consists of superficial abrasions, similar to that of ultrasonic lithotripters [76], but with the potential to cause significant hemorrhage when fragmenting granulation tissue, encased stones, or stones impacted in the calyceal neck [69]. Retrograde displacement of stones is also a consideration, necessitating the need for precise positioning using either a rigid or semirigid endoscope in order to avoid tissue damage. Although the potential for these complications exist, they are rare with careful use and experience. Pneumatic lithotripsy can fragment stones of any composition and size with great efficacy and is the least expensive of the lithotripsy options. Stone fragments tend to be large and must be removed manually with grasping devices, a process that may increase operative time.

Combined Pneumatic and Ultrasonic Lithotripsy

A device containing both pneumatic and ultrasonic capabilities combines the benefits of these two modalities while minimizing their disadvantages. The pneumatic probe is able to fragment most stones regardless of size and composition while the ultrasonic probe provides further fragmentation of smaller pieces [77]. The ultrasonic probe's negative pressure suction is able to clear debris without requiring tedious periodic washings (withdrawal and insertion) of the nephroscope. This in turn reduces intra- and post-operative complication rates, increases SFR, reduces operative time, and reduces the risk of bacterial infections [69]. Studies have shown this combination results in significantly faster stone fragmentation and clearance rates when compared to either pneumatic or ultrasonic devices alone [78].

Holmium YAG Laser Lithotripsy

The holmium:yttrium-aluminum-garnet laser (Ho:YAG) is a high-energy pulse solid-state laser and has been the gold standard for lithotripsy for the past 20 years. Laser lithotripsy is especially effective for fragmenting most types of large stones with few complications and all stones can be treated [79, 80]. Teichman et al. observed that laser lithotripsy yielded smaller stone fragments (average < 1 mm in diameter) that could be easily passed [81]. Additionally, laser fibers are small enough to be used in most flexible endoscopes and the small caliber access tracts used in ultramini and micro PCNL. Several disadvantages associated with laser lithotripsy include potential perforation and bleeding with inadvertent tissue exposure, the need for grasping device removal of large fragments, and the relatively high cost of the higher-powered laser system.

Thulium Fiber Laser Lithotropsy

Thulium fiber laser (TFL) is a promising new form of laser lithotripsy which will reach the US market in early 2020; we have yet to have hands-on experience. Proponents suggest it may revolutionize laser lithotripsy, with improved dusting, less retropulsion, and higher efficiency [82].

Compared to the best Ho:YAG systems, a TFL produces more dust, and does so more quickly [83, 84]. Whereas the Ho:YAG emits at 2100 nm, this TFL emits at 1940 nm, which allows for energy to be absorbed with 4 times greater efficiency in water. As it is not dependent on a flash lamp and instead uses diodes, it is possible to run this laser at a 2200 Hz, a staggering number for those accustomed to the Ho:YAG [85]. It is not clear if it will be applied clinically as such. TFL is also available in a 50 µm fiber which allows for greater instrument deflection, better irrigation, and improved visibility [86]. Clinical trials are needed to determine efficacy *in vivo*, and optimal settings and fiber combinations are not known.

Post-operative Drainage and Hemostasis

After the surgery is complete, the surgeon must decide which tubes to leave in place temporarily. Leaving a nephrostomy tube in place serves to both tamponade the tract (theoretically, although tract diameter often greatly exceeds tube diameter) and drain the collecting system in the immediate post-operative period, which helps prevent urinary extravasation and bleeding. A nephrostomy tube also allows for easier access back into the renal pelvis if repeat surgery or a second look is required. For pediatric patients, the size of the nephrostomy tube will depend on how large the tract was dilated to during the initial steps of the surgery [87]. Occasionally, a double J ureteral stent will be placed over a wire as well. This is typically preferred if there are many stone fragments remaining, or in cases of solitary kidneys or bilateral procedures [87]. Lastly, a urethral catheter is usually left in place after surgery.

In a standard PCNL, a nephrostomy tube and urethral catheter (sometimes an additional JJ ureteral stent as well) will remain in place for 1–2 days after surgery. More recently, "tubeless" and "totally tubeless" PCNLs have been performed. The goal of tubeless PCNL (no nephrostomy tube left in place) is to decrease patient discomfort post-operatively and shorten hospital length of stay, while ensuring no increased risk of bleeding or urinary extravasation. In tubeless PCNL, typically a ureteral JJ stent will be left in place for renal drainage. Tubeless PCNL was compared in a randomized controlled trial (RCT) to standard PCNL in children under 3 years old by Song. et al. in 2015. With 35 patients in each group, there were no differences in post-operative complications including hemorrhage, fever, or urinary extravasation. Tubeless PCNL resulted in shorter hospital stay [88].

Totally tubeless PCNL (no ureteral JJ stent or nephrostomy tube post-operatively) was first described in 1984 by Wickham et al. in patients who, at the end of the procedure, had intact collecting systems, were deemed stone-free, and had minimal visible bleeding. Post-operative hemorrhage and urinary extravasation were two of the more common complications [89]. These complications have decreased as available instruments become smaller and smaller.

In 2012, Aghamir et al. performed a prospective RCT comparing totally tubeless PCNL to standard PCNL in children under 14 years old. Operative time, hemoglobin drop, and complications were not significantly different in the groups. The totally tubeless group had significantly shorter hospital stays and lower narcotic use [90]. Ozturk et al. in 2010 showed similar results in younger, preschool children (mean age 56 months) [91].

Some have investigated the utility of applying hemostatic agents into the PCNL tract instead of using tubes for tamponade and drainage effect. These studies are primarily in the adult population. Nagele et al. studied using gelatin matrix hemostatic sealant, Floseal Hemostatic Matrix (Baxter International Inc., Deerfield, Illinois, USA) in the tract after mini-PCNL (in addition to a JJ ureteral stent) in adult patients. The benefit of Floseal is that it can expand in volume up to 20%. In comparison to the control group, there was no increased risk of bleeding or evidence of urinary extravasation on ultrasound in the tubeless group. The length of hospital stay was slightly shorter in the tubeless group [92]. Other adult studies have investigated the use of electrocautery and fibrin glue, Tisseel Fibrin Sealant (Baxter International Inc., Deerfield, Illinois, USA) in the PCNL tract instead of a nephrostomy tube. Fibrin glue use decreased hospital stay when compared to use of nephrostomy tube, and had no difference in post-operative bleeding [93]. Use of electrocautery of visible bleeding points controlled post-operative bleeding well, but the risk of transient urinary leakage was slightly higher [94]. Use in the pediatric population and the risk of urinary obstruction caused by application of these agents is not yet well studied.

Overall, tubeless and totally tubeless PCNL have been shown to be safe and effective in well selected pediatric patients. Not having a nephrostomy tube post-operatively can decrease patient discomfort, narcotic use, and hospital length of stay. Leaving a ureteral JJ stent (tubeless PCNL) will ensure renal drainage and prevent obstruction by residual fragments, but will not prevent bleeding. At the end of any PCNL, the risk of post-operative bleeding and/or urinary extravasation must be assessed by the surgeon. If the risk is deemed higher based on the proceedings of a particular case or patient characteristics, a nephrostomy tube should be considered.

Outcomes

The main goal of PCNL in children is to clear a large stone burden with a single operation. Studies have shown that in general the stone-free rate (varying definitions amongst studies) after PCNL in the pediatric population ranges from 87–100% [64, 95]. No differences were seen in stone-free rate between mini-PCNL and standard PCNL, however operative times were longer for mini-PCNL [55, 96]. Stone-free rates were higher for PCNL when compared to both SWL for stones larger than 10 mm and retrograde ureteroscopy/lithotripsy for stones larger than 20 mm [64].

A fluoroscopic X-ray at the end of the procedure can confirm that there are no large radiopaque stones remaining. Performing flexible nephroscopy at the end of the procedure is commonplace to ensure all large stone fragments have been removed.

Risks, Probabilities, and Management of Complications

PCNL is a safe procedure with uncommon minor complications and rare major complications. The CROES PCNL Global Study reviewed cases for 5803 patients at 96 centers and found complications occurred in 20.5% [97]. These complications were categorized using the Clavien-Dindo Classification: low-grade (I-II) 16.4%, medium-grade (IIIa-IIIb) 3.6%, and severe-grade (IV-V) 0.5% [97]. The most important complications include bleeding, infection, injury to adjacent organs, and renal pelvis perforation. Mortality in PCNL has been reported between 0.04–0.8% [98].

Bleeding

Bleeding requiring transfusion is reported in 0–20% of patients and is primarily related to BMI, multiple punctures, the use of large dilators, stone size, extended operative periods, and the degree of preoperative hydronephrosis [99]. For hemorrhages occurring during dilation, a larger sized Amplatz sheath or balloon dilator may be inserted to tamponade or a nephrostomy tube may be inserted and clamped [100]. If bleeding becomes too severe, renal angiography and arterial embolization may be necessary to reduce renal loss [101]. In a review of 370 patients who underwent PCNL, Kuk Lee et al. found 43 (11.6%) required transfusion and only 9 (2.4%) required angioembolization following surgery [99].

Infection

Infection is a relatively common complication of PCNL, with fever affecting anywhere from 2.8–32.1% of patients [102]. In a study of 698 patients receiving PCNL, postoperative sepsis occurred in 4 (0.4%) patients [103]. Several factors predisposing patients to infection include preoperative bacteriuria, degree of urinary tract obstruction, high operative intrarenal pressure due to high flow isotonic solutions, stone size, renal anomalies, neurogenic bladder dysfunction, and extended operative periods [104]. When compared to retrograde intrarenal surgery (RIRS), PCNL tends to have higher rates of fever [105], but in our experience the lower pressure seems to reduce the risk of sepsis. That said, massive fluid absorption can occur in standard PCNL, with over 1 L of irrigant absorbed in 28% of patients [106].

Adjacent Organ Injury

Injury to adjacent organs is incredibly rare in PCNL. The rate of injury to the colon may occur in 0.2–1% patients [105, 107] and is associated with left percutaneous renal access, female sex, thin body habitus, in the setting of a horseshoe kidney or prior bowel or renal surgery with heterotopic positioning of the bowel [102, 108]. Preoperative CT scans to assess for retrorenal colon in patients with either a horseshoe kidney or jejunalileal bypass and avoiding access lateral to the posterior axial line can prevent colon injury [100]. If colon injury occurs and is extraperitoneal without peritonitis, insert an indwelling ureteral stent, pull the nephrostomy tube into the colon, give broad spectrum antibiotics, and perform a CT with contrast in 2 weeks to confirm tract closure. If the injury is intraperitoneal or peritonitis is present, proceed to exploration, diverting colostomy and urinary drainage with antibiotics [100].

Injury to nearby solid organs (spleen, liver) occurs <1% of patients, and the reported rate of pleural injury during percutaneous access is 0.3–1% [107]. Due to the proximity of the diaphragm and the upper poles of the kidneys, injury is more common with upper pole supracostal access. Injuries can result in either hydrothorax, pneumothorax, or hydropneumothorax and may require chest tube placement in 64% of these patients [109].

Perforation of the Renal Pelvis and Collecting System

Injury to the renal collecting system may occur in up to 8% of patients. This may lead to electrolyte abnormalities, mental status changes, or intravascular volume overload due to extravasation and absorption of irrigation fluid [107]. Of particular concern is perforation of the renal pelvis. In one study of 582 patients who underwent PCNL, 4 (0.7%) required immediate surgery for laceration of the renal pelvis [110]. Perforation of the renal pelvis can be prevented by avoiding aggressive tract dilation, and medial displacement of the sheath [100]. If perforation is suspected, assess drainage of the renal pelvis, place a reentry nephrostomy or double-J stent, perform a nephrostogram prior to removal of the stent and nephrostomy, and give antibiotics.

Our Preferred Technique

For the most complex cases, with a thoracic or abdominal kidney, renal access becomes hazardous under fluoroscopic or ultrasound guidance alone. In these cases we prefer DynaCT, as described above, both for access and confirmation of stone-free status with intraoperative 3D imaging. For all other cases we prefer an ultrasound guided puncture in the prone position as it allows for the shortest access tract, fluoroscopic dilation, and we pre-place a ureteral catheter to allow for gentle renal dilation with saline prior to puncture.

For equipment size, in general we adhere to the chart shown in Table 18.1; note that this indicates the largest equipment used, and smaller stones and lower stone scores may allow for smaller equipment.

We prefer to puncture with a 21 g needle as part of a MAK-NV system (Fig. 18.1). Note that the largest wire possible through a 21 g system is 0.018. We prefer the smaller needle because, it retains the benefits of a larger needle in that it is easy to see on ultrasound and has "feel" for the parenchyma, while less force is required for introduction. In our experience if the initial puncture is imperfect and the 21 g needle repositioned, we have never seen a hematoma within or around the kidney on ultrasound. The downside is that 21 g renal access requires an additional step. It is not recommended, and likely impossible, to pass an open-ended catheter over the 0.018 wire; dilation with included tapered cannula and introducer is necessary and easy. Antegrade pyelography through the introducer with the 0.018 wire in place is possible, and commonly used by interventional radiologists. Once positioned, the introducer allows a stiff 0.038 wire to be passed alongside, keeping the 0.018 wire in place at the same time.

We then dilate in the standard fluoroscopic manner, and use the equipment above. 11–13 and 16Fr sheaths are placed with one-step dilation. The 24Fr size is a balloon/sheath system. We note also that in our experience, use of the 19.5Fr rigid nephroscope has excellent optics, and has a 12.4Fr working channel. While this is

Table 18.1 Equipment default selections based on age

Age range	Largest sheath	Endoscope Rigid	Endoscope Flexible	Lithotripter
Infants, toddlers, most preschoolers	13 Fr	Short semirigid ureteroscope (15 cm) OD: 7.7 Fr Channel: 5.4 Fr	Digital ureteroscope OD: 8.5 Fr Channel: 3.6 Fr	Holmium laser
School-aged children	16 Fr	Semirigid nephroscope OD: 11 Fr Channel: 7 Fr	Digital ureteroscope OD: 8.5 Fr Channel: 3.6 Fr	5.5 Fr ultrasonic/mechanical system with suction ± holmium laser
Adolescents and young adults	24 Fr	Rigid nephroscope OD 19.5 Fr Channel: 12.4 Fr	Fiberoptic cystoscope, ± digital ureteroscope OD: 15.5 Fr Channel: 7 Fr	10.2 Fr ultrasonic/mechanical system with suction ± holmium laser

All measurements are manufacturer's reported dimensions
OD Outer diameter (nominal)
Flexible cystoscope: Storz 11,272 CU
Flexible ureteroscope: Storz 11,278 VUK
Semirigid nephroscope: Olympus A37025A
Semirigid (short) ureteroscope: Olympus MRO-715A (not in production)
Rigid nephroscope: Storz 27,840 KA
Ultrasounic/Mechanic lithotripter: EGSPL-SR. Larger probe: EGSPL-PDBX340. Smaller probe: EGSPL-PDBX183

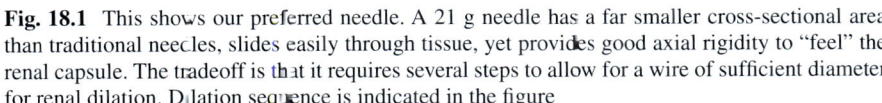

Mini puncture technique with 21g needle

Needle properties
Standard puncture needle   18g needle = 1.27 mm width = 1.27 mm²
Mini puncture needle: 21g needle = 0.82 mm width = 0.54 mm²

Mini puncture procedure sequence
access collecting system →
pass 0.018 inch wire →
pass 6Fr coaxial introducer with dilator →
remove dilator, *leaving* initial wire and introducer →
place additional wires through introducer up to 0.038" and proceed with standard dilation

Fig. 18.1 This shows our preferred needle. A 21 g needle has a far smaller cross-sectional area than traditional needles, slides easily through tissue, yet provides good axial rigidity to "feel" the renal capsule. The tradeoff is that it requires several steps to allow for a wire of sufficient diameter for renal dilation. Dilation sequence is indicated in the figure

promoted in company materials as allowing "use of rigid standard instruments and large lithotripsy probes up to 11.5 Fr" [111]; in our experience gravity-fed saline flow is inadequate for visualization with a 11.3Fr probe (Silver, ShockPulse-SE Probe, Olympus Corporation of the Americas, Center Valley, PA) but excellent with a 10.2 Fr probe (Blue, ShockPulse-SE).

When we place antegrade ureteral stents they will require a second procedure to extract. Many of our patients have experience with stents, and part of their desire to proceed with PCNL is the desire to avoid their previous stent-related discomfort. Our standard drainage is a 10.2Fr nephrostomy tube (8.5Fr for children and infants), and bladder drainage overnight. We remove the tubes the following morning and the patients are dismissed. We do not treat the tract with topical agents, but do apply gentle pressure and close the skin with subcuticular suture around the nephrostomy tube.

Future

We expect to see continued innovation in PCNL, accompanied by broadening of indications for the procedure. A newly developed ClearPetra® nephrostomy tube system creates a closed circuit with controlled outflow; the fragments exit passively through the sheath without need for direct extraction [112]. Similarly, Thulium Fiber laser lithotripters may offer true dusting with improved irrigation, as the fiber is so small and occludes little of the lumen [85]. These are but two examples in a rapidly evolving field. We expect that fluoroscopy use and dose will decrease, sheath sizes will decrease, as will the frequency at which we use stents and nephrostomy tubes.

References

1. Wang HH, Wiener JS, Ferrandino MN, Lipkin ME, Routh JC. Complications of surgical management of upper tract calculi in spina bifida patients: analysis of nationwide data. J Urol. 2015;193(4):1270–4.
2. Mitchell S, Gurung PMS, Choong S, Morris T, Smith D, Woodhouse C, et al. Percutaneous nephrolithotomy and spina bifida: complex major stone surgery? J Endourol. 2018;32(3):205–12.
3. Sancaktutar AA, Bozkurt Y, Tufek A, Soylemez H, Onder H, Atar M, et al. Radiation-free percutaneous nephrostomy performed on neonates, infants, and preschool-age children. J Pediatr Urol. 2013;9(4):464–71.
4. Barnacle A, Wilkinson A, Roebuck D. Paediatric interventional uroradiology. Cardiovasc Intervent Radiol. 2011;34:227–40.
5. Costa K. Hematology. In: The Harriet Lane handbook: a manual for pediatric house officers. Philadelphia: Elsevier; 2018.
6. Raes A, Van Aken S, Craen M, Donckerwolcke R, Vande WJ. A reference frame for blood volume in children and adolescents. BMC Pediatr. 2006;6:3.
7. Thomas K, Smith NC, Hegarty N, Glass JM. The Guy's stone score--grading the complexity of percutaneous nephrolithotomy procedures. Urology. 2011;78(2):277–81.
8. Okhunov Z, Friedlander JI, George AK, Duty BD, Moreira DM, Srinivasan AK, et al. S.T.O.N.E. nephrolithometry: novel surgical classification system for kidney calculi. Urology. 2013;81(6):1154–9.
9. Smith A, Averch TD, Shahrour K, Opondo D, Daels FP, Labate G, et al. A nephrolithometric nomogram to predict treatment success of percutaneous nephrolithotomy. J Urol. 2013;190(1):149–56.

10. Kumar U, Tomar V, Yadav SS, Priyadarshi S, Vyas N, Agarwal N, et al. STONE score versus Guy's stone score – prospective comparative evaluation for success rate and complications in percutaneous nephrolithotomy. Urol Ann. 2018;10(1):76–81.
11. Jiang K, Sun F, Zhu J, Luo G, Zhang P, Ban Y, et al. Evaluation of three stone-scoring systems for predicting SFR and complications after percutaneous nephrolithotomy: a systematic review and meta-analysis. BMC Urol. 2019;19(1):57.
12. Aldaqadossi HA, Khairy Salem H, Kotb Y, Hussein HA, Shaker H, Dikaios N. Prediction of pediatric percutaneous nephrolithotomy outcomes using contemporary scoring systems. J Urol. 2017;198(5):1146–52.
13. Agah M, Ghasemi M, Roodneshin F, Radpay B, Moradian S. Prone position in percutaneous nephrolithotomy and postoperative visual loss. Urol J. 2011;8(3):191–6.
14. Patel RM, Okhunov Z, Clayman RV, Landman J. Prone versus supine percutaneous nephrolithotomy: what is your position? Curr Urol Rep. 2017;18(4):26.
15. Liu L, Zheng S, Xu Y, Wei Q. Systematic review and meta-analysis of percutaneous nephrolithotomy for patients in the supine versus prone position. J Endourol. 2010;24(12):1941–6.
16. Zhan HL, Li ZC, Zhou XF, Yang F, Huang JF, Lu MH. Supine lithotomy versus prone position in minimally invasive percutaneous nephrolithotomy for upper urinary tract calculi. Urol Int. 2013;91(3):320–5.
17. Valdivia Uria JG, Valle Gerhold J, Lopez Lopez JA, Villarroya Rodriguez S, Ambroj Navarro C, Ramirez Fabian M, et al. Technique and complications of percutaneous nephroscopy: experience with 557 patients in the supine position. J Urol. 1998;160(6 Pt 1):1975–8.
18. Astroza G, Lipkin M, Neisius A, Preminger G, De Sio M, Sodha H, et al. Effect of supine vs prone position on outcomes of percutaneous nephrolithotomy in staghorn calculi: results from the Clinical Research Office of the Endourology Society Study. Urology. 2013;82(6):1240–4.
19. Gamal W, Moursy E, Hussein M, Mmdouh A, Hammady A, Aldahshoury M. Supine pediatric percutaneous nephrolithotomy (PCNL). J Pediatr Urol. 2015;11(2):78 e1–5.
20. Desoky EAE, ElSayed ER, Eliwa A, Sleem M, Shabana W, Dawood T, et al. Flank-free modified supine percutaneous nephrolithotomy in pediatric age group. Urology. 2015;85(5):1162–5.
21. Ibarluzea G, Scoffone CM, Cracco CM, Poggio M, Porpiglia F, Terrone C, et al. Supine Valdivia and modified lithotomy position for simultaneous anterograde and retrograde endourological access. BJU Int. 2007;100(1):233–6.
22. Caione P, De Dominicis M, Collura G, Matarazzo E, Nappo SG, Capozza N. Microperc for pediatric nephrolithiasis: technique in valdivia-modified position. Eur J Pediatr Surg. 2015;25(1):94–9
23. Proietti S, Rodriguez-Socarras ME, Eisner B, De Coninck V, Sofer M, Saitta G, et al. Supine percutaneous nephrolithotomy: tips and tricks. Transl Androl Urol. 2019;8(Suppl 4):S381–S8.
24. Wei Gan JJ, Lia Gan JJ, Hsien Gan JJ, Lee KT. Lateral percutaneous nephrolithotomy: a safe and effective surgical approach. Indian J Urol. 2018;34(1):45–50.
25. Miller NL, Matlaga BR, Lingeman JE. Techniques for fluoroscopic percutaneous renal access. J Urol. 2007;178(1):15–23.
26. Munver R, Delvecchio FC, Newman GE, Preminger GM. Critical analysis of supracostal access for percutaneous renal surgery. J Urol. 2001;166(4):1242–6.
27. Budak S, Yucel C, Kisa E, Kozacioglu Z. Comparison of two different renal access techniques in one-stage percutaneous nephrolithotomy: triangulation versus eye of the needle. Ann Saudi Med. 2018;38(3):189–93.
28. Patel U, Anson KM. Percutaneous nephrolithotomy made easier: a practical guide, tips and tricks. BJU Int. 2008;102(9):1178.
29. Sharma GR, Maheshwari PN, Sharma AG, Maheshwari RP, Heda RS, Maheshwari SP. Fluoroscopy guided percutaneous renal access in prone position. World J Clin Cases. 2015;3(3):245–64.
30. Chu C, Masic S, Usawachintachit M, Hu W, Yang W, Stoller M, et al. Ultrasound-guided renal access for percutaneous nephrolithotomy: a description of three novel ultrasound-guided needle techniques. J Endourol. 2016;30(2):153–8.

31. Tzou DT, Metzler IS, Usawachintachit M, Stoller ML, Chi T. Ultrasound-guided access and dilation for percutaneous nephrolithotomy in the supine position: a step-by-step approach. Urology. 2019;133:245–6.
32. Ritter M, Rassweiler MC, Michel MS. The Uro Dyna-CT enables three-dimensional planned laser-guided complex punctures. Eur Urol. 2015;68(5):880–4.
33. Vicentini FC, Botelho LAA, Braz JLM, Almeida ES, Hisano M. Use of the Uro Dyna-CT in endourology - the new frontier. Int Braz J Urol. 2017;43(4):762–5.
34. Majidpour HS. Risk of radiation exposure during PCNL. Urol J. 2010;7(2):87–9.
35. Kumari G, Kumar P, Wadhwa P, Aron M, Gupta NP, Dogra PN. Radiation exposure to the patient and operating room personnel during percutaneous nephrolithotomy. Int Urol Nephrol. 2006;38(2):207–10.
36. Wenzler DL, Abbott JE, Su JJ, Shi W, Slater R, Miller D, et al. Predictors of radiation exposure to providers during percutaneous nephrolithotomy. Urol Ann. 2017;9(1):55–60.
37. Pasciak AS, Jones AK. Time to take the gloves off: the use of radiation reduction gloves can greatly increase patient dose. J Appl Clin Med Phys. 2014;15(6):5002.
38. Miller DL, Vano E, Bartal G, Balter S, Dixon R, Padovani R, et al. Occupational radiation protection in interventional radiology: a joint guideline of the Cardiovascular and Interventional Radiology Society of Europe and the Society of Interventional Radiology. J Vasc Interv Radiol. 2010;21(5):607–15.
39. Arnstein PM, Richards AM, Putney R. The risk from radiation exposure during operative X-ray screening in hand surgery. J Hand Surg Br. 1994;19(3):393–6.
40. Kurtz M, Cilento B, Demers M, MacDougall R, McCarthy I, Venna A, et al. Flat panel detector c-arms are associated with a dramatic reduction in absorbed radiation dose during ureteroscopy. Pediatric Urology Fall Congress, 2019.
41. American Association of Physicists in Medicine. AAPM position statement on radiation risks from medical imaging procedures (PP 25-C), 2018.
42. Ganpule AP, Vijayakumar M, Malpani A, Desai MR. Percutaneous nephrolithotomy (PCNL) a critical review. Int J Surg. 2016;36(Pt D):660–4.
43. Wright A, Rukin N, Smith D, De la Rosette J, Somani BK. 'Mini, ultra, micro' – nomenclature and cost of these new minimally invasive percutaneous nephrolithotomy (PCNL) techniques. Ther Adv Urol. 2016;8(2):142–6.
44. Haghighi R, Zeraati H, Ghorban ZM. Ultra-mini-percutaneous nephrolithotomy (PCNL) versus standard PCNL: a randomised clinical trial. Arab J Urol. 2017;15(4):294–8.
45. Girisha TD, Dev P, Vijaykumar R, Dharwadkar S, Madappa KM. Single-step dilatation in percutaneous nephrolithotomy, its safety and efficacy: a prospective, single-center study. Urol Ann. 2019;11(2):171–4.
46. Jackman SV, Hedican SP, Peters CA, Docimo SG. Percutaneous nephrolithotomy in infants and preschool age children: experience with a new technique. Urology. 1998;52(4):697–701.
47. Handa RK, Matlaga BR, Connors BA, Ying J, Paterson RF, Kuo RL, et al. Acute effects of percutaneous tract dilation on renal function and structure. J Endourol. 2006;20(12):1030–40.
48. Davidoff R, Bellman GC. Influence of technique of percutaneous tract creation on incidence of renal hemorrhage. J Urol. 1997;157(4):1229–31.
49. Frattini A, Barbieri A, Salsi P, Sebastio N, Ferretti S, Bergamaschi E, et al. One shot: a novel method to dilate the nephrostomy access for percutaneous lithotripsy. J Endourol. 2001;15(9):919–23.
50. Pugh JW, Canales BK. New instrumentation in percutaneous nephrolithotomy. Indian J Urol. 2010;26(3):389–94.
51. Helal M, Black T, Lockhart J, Figueroa TE. The Hickman peel-away sheath: alternative for pediatric percutaneous nephrolithotomy. J Endourol. 1997;11(3):171–2.
52. Zhong W, Zeng G, Wu W, Chen W, Wu K. Minimally invasive percutaneous nephrolithotomy with multiple mini tracts in a single session in treating staghorn calculi. Urol Res. 2011;39(2):117–22.
53. Cheng F, Yu W, Zhang X, Yang S, Xia Y, Ruan Y. Minimally invasive tract in percutaneous nephrolithotomy for renal stones. J Endourol. 2010;24(10):1579–82.

54. Desai MR, Kukreja RA, Patel SH, Bapat SD. Percutaneous nephrolithotomy for complex pediatric renal calculus disease. J Endourol. 2004;18(1):23–7.
55. Jackman SV, Docimo SG, Cadeddu JA, Bishoff JT, Kavoussi LR, Jarrett TW. The "miniperc" technique: a less invasive alternative to percutaneous nephrolithotomy. World J Urol. 1998;16(6):371–4.
56. Bilen CY, Kocak B, Kitirci G, Ozkaya O, Sarikaya S. Percutaneous nephrolithotomy in children: lessons learned in 5 years at a single institution. J Urol. 2007;177(5):1867–71.
57. Li LY, Gao X, Yang M, Li JF, Zhang HB, Xu WF, et al. Does a smaller tract in percutaneous nephrolithotomy contribute to less invasiveness? A prospective comparative study. Urology. 2010;75(1):56–61.
58. Traxer O, Smith TG 3rd, Pearle MS, Corwin TS, Saboorian H, Cadeddu JA. Renal parenchymal injury after standard and mini percutaneous nephrostolithotomy. J Urol. 2001;165(5):1693–5.
59. Zeng G, Zhu W, Lam W. Miniaturised percutaneous nephrolithotomy: its role in the treatment of urolithiasis and our experience. Asian J Urol. 2018;5(4):295–302.
60. Mishra S, Sharma R, Garg C, Kurien A, Sabnis R, Desai M. Prospective comparative study of miniperc and standard PNL for treatment of 1 to 2 cm size renal stone. BJU Int. 2011;108(6):896–9; discussion 9–900.
61. Celik H, Camtosun A, Dede O, Dagguli M, Altintas R, Tasdemir C. Comparison of the results of pediatric percutaneous nephrolithotomy with different sized instruments. Urolithiasis. 2017;45(2):203–8.
62. Knoll T, Wezel F, Michel MS, Honeck P, Wendt-Nordahl G. Do patients benefit from miniaturized tubeless percutaneous nephrolithotomy? A comparative prospective study. J Endourol. 2010;24(7):1075–9.
63. Giusti G, Piccinelli A, Taverna G, Benetti A, Pasini L, Corinti M, et al. Miniperc? No, thank you! Eur Urol. 2007;51(3):310–4; discussion 5.
64. Ferakis N, Stavropoulos M. Mini percutaneous nephrolithotomy in the treatment of renal and upper ureteral stones: lessons learned from a review of the literature. Urol Ann. 2015;7(2):141–8.
65. Zanetti SP, Talso M, Palmisano F, Longo F, Gallioli A, Fontana M, et al. Comparison among the available stone treatment techniques from the first European Association of Urology Section of Urolithiasis (EULIS) Survey: do we have a queen? PLoS One. 2018;13(11):e0205159.
66. Desai MR, Sharma R, Mishra S, Sabnis RB, Stief C, Bader M. Single-step percutaneous nephrolithotomy (microperc): the initial clinical report. J Urol. 2011;186(1):140–5.
67. Hatipoglu NK, Tepeler A, Buldu I, Atis G, Bodakci MN, Sancaktutar AA, et al. Initial experience of micro-percutaneous nephrolithotomy in the treatment of renal calculi in 140 renal units. Urolithiasis. 2014;42(2):159–64.
68. Akman T, Binbay M, Yuruk E, Sari E, Seyrek M, Kaba M, et al. Tubeless procedure is most important factor in reducing length of hospitalization after percutaneous nephrolithotomy: results of univariable and multivariable models. Urology. 2011;77(2):299–304.
69. Cho CO, Yu JH, Sung LH, Chung JY, Noh CH. Comparison of percutaneous nephrolithotomy using pneumatic lithotripsy (lithoclast(R)) alone or in combination with ultrasonic lithotripsy. Korean J Urol. 2010;51(11):783–7.
70. Hofbauer J, Hobarth K, Marberger M. Electrohydraulic versus pneumatic disintegration in the treatment of ureteral stones: a randomized, prospective trial. J Urol. 1995;153(3 Pt 1):623–5.
71. Willscher MK, Conway JF Jr, Babayan RK, Morrisseau P, Sant GR, Bertagnoll A. Safety and efficacy of electrohydraulic lithotripsy by ureteroscopy. J Urol. 1988;140(5):957–8.
72. Fuchs GJ. Ultrasonic lithotripsy in the ureter. Urol Clin North Am. 1988;15(3):347–59.
73. Begun FP. Modes of intracorporeal lithotripsy: ultrasound versus electrohydraulic lithotripsy versus laser lithotripsy. Semin Urol. 1994;12(1):39–50.
74. Kim SC, Matlaga BR, Tinmouth WW, Kuo RL, Evan AP, McAteer JA, et al. In vitro assessment of a novel dual probe ultrasonic intracorporeal lithotriptor. J Urol. 2007;177(4):1363–5.

75. Piergiovanni M, Desgrandchamps F, Cochand-Priollet B, Janssen T, Colomer S, Teillac P, et al. Ureteral and bladder lesions after ballistic, ultrasonic, electrohydraulic, or laser lithotripsy. J Endourol. 1994;8(4):293–9.
76. Hofmann R, Olbert P, Weber J, Wille S, Varga Z. Clinical experience with a new ultrasonic and LithoClast combination for percutaneous litholapaxy. BJU Int. 2002;90(1):16–9.
77. Hofmann R, Weber J, Heidenreich A, Varga Z, Olbert P. Experimental studies and first clinical experience with a new Lithoclast and ultrasound combination for lithotripsy. Eur Urol. 2002;42(4):376–81.
78. Auge BK, Lallas CD, Pietrow PK, Zhong P, Preminger GM. In vitro comparison of standard ultrasound and pneumatic lithotrites with a new combination intracorporeal lithotripsy device. Urology. 2002;60(1):28–32.
79. Jou YC, Shen CH, Cheng MC, Lin CT, Chen PC. High-power holmium:yttrium-aluminum-garnet laser for percutaneous treatment of large renal stones. Urology. 2007;69(1):22–5; discussion 5–6.
80. Yiu MK, Liu PL, Yiu TF, Chan AY. Clinical experience with holmium:YAG laser lithotripsy of ureteral calculi. Lasers Surg Med. 1996;19(1):103–6.
81. Teichman JM, Vassar GJ, Bishoff JT, Bellman GC. Holmium:YAG lithotripsy yields smaller fragments than lithoclast, pulsed dye laser or electrohydraulic lithotripsy. J Urol. 1998;159(1):17–23.
82. Blackmon RL, Irby PB, Fried NM. Comparison of holmium:YAG and thulium fiber laser lithotripsy: ablation thresholds, ablation rates, and retropulsion effects. J Biomed Opt. 2011;16(7):071403.
83. Hardy LA, Vinnichenko V, Fried NM. High power holmium:YAG versus thulium fiber laser treatment of kidney stones in dusting mode: ablation rate and fragment size studies. Lasers Surg Med. 2019;51(6):522–30.
84. Andreeva V, Vinarov A, Yaroslavsky I, Kovalenko A, Vybornov A, Rapoport L, et al. Preclinical comparison of superpulse thulium fiber laser and a holmium:YAG laser for lithotripsy. World J Urol. 2019;38:497–503.
85. Kronenberg P, Traxer O. The laser of the future: reality and expectations about the new thulium fiber laser-a systematic review. Transl Androl Urol. 2019;8(Suppl 4):S398–417.
86. Traxer O, Keller EX. Thulium fiber laser: the new player for kidney stone treatment? A comparison with Holmium:YAG laser. World J Urol. 2020;38(8):1883–94.
87. Ganpule AP, Mishra S, Desai MR. Percutaneous nephrolithotomy for pediatric urolithiasis. Indian J Urol. 2010;26(4):549–54.
88. Song G, Guo X, Niu G, Wang Y. Advantages of tubeless mini-percutaneous nephrolithotomy in the treatment of preschool children under 3 years old. J Pediatr Surg. 2015;50(4):655–8.
89. Wickham JE, Miller RA, Kellett MJ, Payne SR. Percutaneous nephrolithotomy: one stage or two? Br J Urol. 1984;56(6):582–5.
90. Aghamir SM, Salavati A, Aloosh M, Farahmand H, Meysamie A, Pourmand G. Feasibility of totally tubeless percutaneous nephrolithotomy under the age of 14 years: a randomized clinical trial. J Endourol. 2012;26(6):621–4.
91. Ozturk A, Guven S, Kilinc M, Topbas E, Piskin M, Arslan M. Totally tubeless percutaneous nephrolithotomy: is it safe and effective in preschool children? J Endourol. 2010;24(12):1935–9.
92. Nagele U, Schilling D, Anastasiadis AG, Corvin S, Seibold J, Kuczyk M, et al. Closing the tract of mini-percutaneous nephrolithotomy with gelatine matrix hemostatic sealant can replace nephrostomy tube placement. Urology. 2006;68(3):489–93; discussion 93–4.
93. Mikhail AA, Kaptein JS, Bellman GC. Use of fibrin glue in percutaneous nephrolithotomy. Urology. 2003;61(5):910–4; discussion 4.
94. Jou YC, Cheng MC, Sheen JH, Lin CT, Chen PC. Cauterization of access tract for nephrostomy tube-free percutaneous nephrolithotomy. J Endourol. 2004;18(6):547–9.
95. Caione P, Collura G, Innocenzi M, De Dominicis M, Gerocarni Nappo S, Capozza N. Percutaneous endoscopic treatment for urinary stones in pediatric patients: where we are now. Transl Pediatr. 2016;5(4):266–74.

96. Brodie KE, Lane VA, Lee TW, Roberts JP, Raghavan A, Hughes D, et al. Outcomes following 'mini' percutaneous nephrolithotomy for renal calculi in children. A single-centre study. J Pediatr Urol. 2015;11(3):120 e1–5.
97. de la Rosette J, Assimos D, Desai M, Gutierrez J, Lingeman J, Scarpa R, et al. The clinical research Office of the Endourological Society Percutaneous Nephrolithotomy Global Study: indications, complications, and outcomes in 5803 patients. J Endourol. 2011;25(1):11–7.
98. Kyriazis I, Panagopoulos V, Kallidonis P, Ozsoy M, Vasilas M, Liatsikos E. Complications in percutaneous nephrolithotomy. World J Urol. 2015;33(8):1069–77.
99. Lee JK, Kim BS, Park YK. Predictive factors for bleeding during percutaneous nephrolithotomy. Korean J Urol. 2013;54(7):448–53.
100. Ibrahim A, Wollin D, Preminger G, Andonian S. Technique of percutaneous nephrolithotomy. J Endourol. 2018;32(S1):S17–27.
101. Tefekli A, Ali Karadag M, Tepeler K, Sari E, Berberoglu Y, Baykal M, et al. Classification of percutaneous nephrolithotomy complications using the modified clavien grading system: looking for a standard. Eur Urol. 2008;53(1):184–90.
102. Michel MS, Trojan L, Rassweiler JJ. Complications in percutaneous nephrolithotomy. Eur Urol. 2007;51(4):899–906; discussion.
103. Shin TS, Cho HJ, Hong SH, Lee JY, Kim SW, Hwang TK. Complications of percutaneous nephrolithotomy classified by the modified Clavien grading system: a single center's experience over 16 years. Korean J Urol. 2011;52(11):769–75.
104. Kreydin EI, Eisner BH. Risk factors for sepsis after percutaneous renal stone surgery. Nat Rev Urol. 2013;10(10):598–605.
105. Karakoc O, Karakeci A, Ozan T, Firdolas F, Tektas C, Ozkaratas SE, et al. Comparison of retrograde intrarenal surgery and percutaneous nephrolithotomy for the treatment of renal stones greater than 2 cm. Turk J Urol. 2015;41(2):73–7.
106. Malhotra SK, Khaitan A, Goswami AK, Gill KD, Dutta A. Monitoring of irrigation fluid absorption during percutaneous nephrolithotripsy: the use of 1% ethanol as a marker. Anaesthesia. 2001;56(11):1103–6.
107. Nikic P, Durutovic O, Kajmakovic B, Nale D, Bumbasirevic U, Radovanovic M, et al. Complications associated with percutaneous nephrolitholapaxy (PCNL)--our experience and literature review. Acta Chir Iugosl. 2014;61(1):51–6.
108. El-Nahas AR, Shokeir AA, El-Assmy AM, Shoma AM, Eraky I, El-Kenawy MR, et al. Colonic perforation during percutaneous nephrolithotomy: study of risk factors. Urology. 2006;67(5):937–41.
109. Yadav R, Aron M, Gupta NP, Hemal AK, Seth A, Kolla SB. Safety of supracostal punctures for percutaneous renal surgery. Int J Urol. 2006;13(10):1267–70.
110. Lee WJ, Smith AD, Cubelli V, Badlani GH, Lewin B, Vernace F, et al. Complications of percutaneous nephrolithotomy. AJR Am J Roentgenol. 1987;148(1):177–80.
111. Karl Storz SE & Co. KG Urology, 10th edition 4/2015 US. Available from: https://www.karlstorz.com/cps/rde/xbcr/karlstorz_assets/ASSETS/3343855.pdf.
112. Lievore E, Zanetti SP, Fontana M, Turetti M, Gallioli A, Longo F, et al. Preliminary results of vacuum-assisted mini-percutaneous nephrolithotomy in a tertiary academic referral center: our first 103 cases. Eur Urol Suppl. 2019;18(7):e2783–e5.

Part V
Other Procedures and Miscellaneous Topics

Chapter 19
Laparoscopic Orchiopexy

Niccolo M. Passoni and Micah A. Jacobs

Introduction

Cryptorchidism is the most common genitourinary malformation affecting newborn boys. Aside from aesthetic considerations, surgical correction of undescended testes is aimed at reducing the risk of malignancy and aiding in its surveillance, infertility, torsion and associated hernia [1].

The choice of surgical management for cryptorchidism depends most importantly whether or not the testicle is palpable on exam. If a testicle is felt on exam, then the preferred surgical approach is either scrotal or inguinal, while if the testicle is not found on exam, current guidelines recommend a laparoscopic approach [1, 2].

Among all children born with cryptorchidism, 20–30% of them will have non-palpable testes [3]. 20–40% of testicles that elude exam are absent or "vanished", 15–35% will be in the inguinal canal or canalicular, 20–50% will be in the abdominal cavity and 2–9% will be ectopic [4–10].

Since its introduction in 1976, laparoscopy has been the gold standard for diagnosis of non-palpable gonads [11]. Despite being an invasive procedure, physical exam and imaging modalities fall short in: (1) Identifying whether or not the non-palpable testis is present; (2) determining whether the testis is intra-abdominal or in the inguinal canal [12].

Ultrasound is a readily available, low cost and minimally invasive diagnostic instrument, but according to a recent meta-analysis, the performance of ultrasound is poor, with a sensitivity and specificity in detecting a non-palpable testis of 45% and 78% respectively [13]. Magnetic resonance imaging outperform ultrasound, with improved sensitivity and specificity, ranging respectively between 85–96% and 79–100% [12], however it is hindered by its cost and the need for the child to be sedated.

N. M. Passoni · M. A. Jacobs (✉)
University of Texas Southwestern Medical Center, Department of Urology, Dallas, TX, USA
e-mail: NiccoloMaria.Passoni@UTSouthwestern.edu; MICAH.JACOBS@childrens.com

The other advantage of laparoscopy is that other than being a diagnostic tool it also functions as a therapeutic one. Indeed, early reports of laparoscopy in non-palpable testes were focused mainly on its diagnostic nature, as a gateway to either abdominal or inguinal exploration. The first-stage Fowler-Stephens approach was first described in 1991 at a time when pelvic laparoscopy was becoming more common [14]. Two years later, use of laparoscopy had been extended to orchiectomies of dystrophic testes as well as for the second stage of a Fowler-Stephens [15]. Since then, laparoscopic orchiopexy has become a well-established approach to the abdominal testis.

In this chapter we will describe the main surgical technique as well as variations of laparoscopic orchiopexy, troubleshooting and complications, and briefly outcomes.

Surgical Technique

Positioning and Trocar Placement

The patient is positioned supine on the operating table. Once the child is anesthetized, a careful exam under anesthesia is conducted. If the testicle is felt, an inguinal or scrotal approach is chosen over laparoscopy.

In order to facilitate surgical ergonomics, the anesthesiology team is preferably positioned at the side of the bed (Fig. 19.1). This allows for the surgeon to operate at the head of the bed, "looking down" toward the pelvis.

The patient's bladder is emptied at the beginning of the case and the bed is placed in a mild Trendelenburg position. The 5-mm camera port is inserted in an umbilical position and pneumoperitoneum is established with CO_2 to 8–10 mmHg, to visualize the operative field.

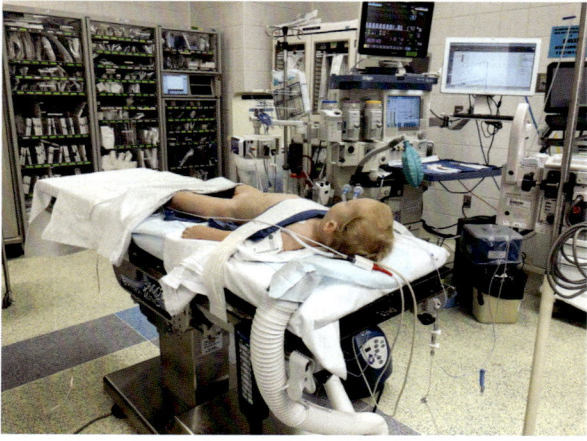

Fig. 19.1 Positioning of surgical bed with regards to anesthesia cart

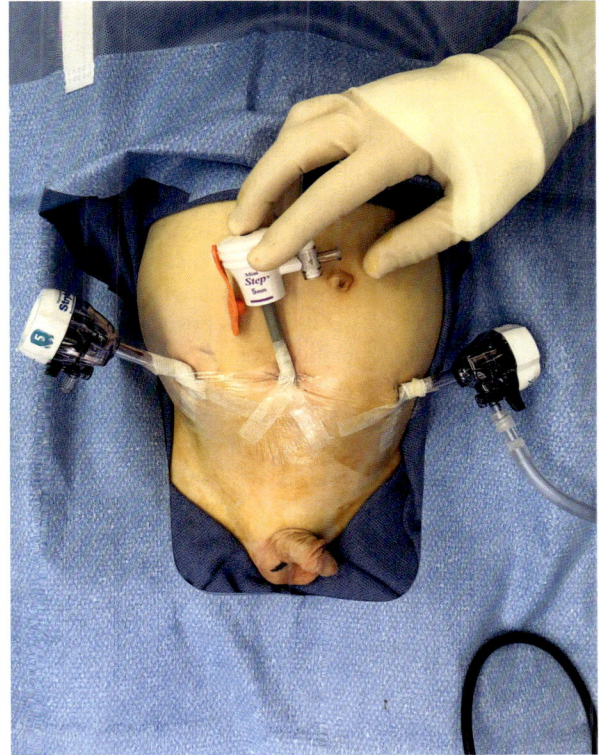

Fig. 19.2 Placement of laparoscopic ports. The midline camera port is placed at the umbilicus (the patient in the picture has a prior gastrostomy scar). The working ports are placed lateral to the rectus muscle at the same height of the umbilicus

The abdominal cavity is carefully explored to identify the testicle and its blood supply.

If working ports are needed, these can be placed under direct visualization. Usually 3- or 5-mm ports are used, based on the surgeon's preference and size of instruments (e.g., a laparoscopic clip applier will require a 5-mm port). Working ports are usually placed lateral to the rectus muscle on either side at the level of the umbilicus or below. The ipsilateral port can be placed higher depending on the position of the testis (Fig. 19.2).

Introduction of 3 mm instruments directly into the abdomen via a skin puncture without trocars has been described as well. This approach does not seem to prolong operative times and has been shown to be cost-effective [16]. These incisions are small enough that they do not require fascial closure.

Single-Site Surgery

To further reduce invasiveness and improve the cosmetic results of laparoscopic orchiopexy, several authors have described single-site techniques [17–20]. These approaches utilize a single umbilical incision.

De Lima and coworkers relied on a single incision above the umbilicus, from the 3 to 9 o'clock. The placed a 5- of 10-mm trocar in the midline, using the traditional Hasson technique, and subsequently placed two other 3- or 5-mm ports on each side. These additional ports are placed through the same skin incision but enter the fascia at a different location than the camera port, making this a single-incision multiport technique. All fascial defects are closed at the end of the case [17]. In a similar manner, Li and colleagues described a multi-incision trans-umbilical approach. Instead of using a single incision for multiple ports, which would limit the range of motions of the instruments, they performed an infraumbilical incision from 4 to 8 o'clock for the 5-mm camera port as well as a second 5 mm working port which is placed at the 4 o'clock position of the same incision. Another incision, at the 10–11 o'clock position is used for the third trocar [18]. Noh et al. reported using a multichannel port through the umbilicus, aided by a flexible tip laparoscope and curved instruments [19]. However, this approach is burdened by the increase costs of specialized equipment. Finally, Mahdi and colleagues used a glove port to perform laparoscopic orchiopexy. This port is low cost and "home-made" alternative to a multiport channel. This technique used standard rigid instruments which must be crossed, making this a more technically demanding approach [20].

Laparoscopic Findings

At preliminary laparoscopy it is important to identify the location of the undescended testicle to plan the following surgical steps. If no testicle is seen upon initial evaluation, there are three possible scenarios: (a) testicular vessels are seen terminating before reaching a closed internal inguinal ring (i.e., "blind-ending" vessels); (b) testicular vessels enter the ring; (c) no vessels are visualized.

In the first case, the testicle has presumably atrophied from torsion, and is a "vanishing" testis, while in the second case, the testicular remnants or "nubbins" can be found in the inguinal canal or scrotum. If no vessels are seen, one must explore higher as testicles can be found as high as the kidney when not immediately identifiable down in the pelvis.

For a true vanishing testis no further treatment is recommended, while inguinal exploration for excision of testicular remnants has been debated. However, large series have shown that these nubbins harbor viable germ cells in 5.3–11% of the cases and seminiferous tubules in 10.7–24% [21–23].. Therefore, in case a vas and vessels are seen entering the inguinal canal in the setting of a non-palpable testis, inguinal exploration is recommended.

If a testicle is seen, it should first be assessed. In case of a dysmorphic testicle, an orchiectomy should be considered, while in the presence of a healthy appearing gonad, other findings will help determine the next step.

If the testis is found near the inguinal ring, careful inspection of the vas should be carried out, to assess whether it is looping into the inguinal canal or not. When a gonad localized at the internal inguinal ring or in a "peeping" position (moving into and out of the inguinal canal), usually a one-stage laparoscopic orchiopexy, with sparing of the testicular vessels, can be performed successfully.

However, if the testicle is in a high position, usually considered greater than 2 cm from the internal ring [24], ligation and division of the testicular vessels, whether with a one stage or two-stage Fowler-Stephens approach, is necessary.

Vascular Supply

The arterial blood supply to the testicle is three-fold: the testicular artery originating from the abdominal aorta or renal artery; the deferential artery originating from the superior or inferior vesical artery; the cremasteric artery, originating from the inferior epigastric artery. The fetal testis is always supplied by at least 2 of these arterial systems (usually the testicular and deferential arteries) [25, 26].

During a Fowler-Stephens procedure, ligation of the testicular artery stimulates growth of the collateral arterial supply. Studies have shown arterial connections between the cremasteric artery, located in the gubernaculum, and the testicular and deferential ones [27, 28]. Collateral circulation tends to predominate from either the cremasteric or the deferential vessels, but never from both; 60% of the time it originates from the gubernaculum, and 40% around the vas deferens [28]. These collaterals were noted as early as 6 weeks after ligation of the vessels. Hence, in the setting of a short instead of long gubernaculum, if a staged Fowler-Stephens procedure is planned, it has been suggested that transection of the gubernaculum at the time of vessel ligation, might stimulate development of the deferential circulation.

One-Stage Orchiopexy

If a viable intra-abdominal testis has been found, the first consideration is whether or not it will be possible to perform an orchiopexy without division of the gonadal vessels during the same surgery. The limiting factor that would require a staged procedure is the length of the gonadal vessels. It can be difficult to determine if the length of these vessels will be adequate to reach the scrotum. If the testicle is found to be >2 cm from the internal inguinal ring, the vessels are often too short to allow proper positioning of the testicle in the scrotum [24]. In this setting, ligation of the vessels followed by a second stage surgery is recommended. One-stage Fowler-Stephens procedures (ligation of the vessels and orchiopexy in the same setting) are associated with lower testis survival rates (74% vs 88% for a staged procedure) [4].

We begin by incising the peritoneum along the lateral aspect of the gonadal vessels up to the internal ring. The peritoneum is also incised along the vas deferens towards the internal ring to create a triangle of peritoneum between the vas deferens and gonadal vessels which will be mobilized. Any structures, namely the epididymis and vas deferens, that might be extending distally into the inguinal canal are carefully mobilized into the abdomen. The gubernaculum is then transected and used as a safe handle for further mobilization of the testis.

The testis is then mobilized on the resulting peritoneal flap until it can easily reach the contralateral internal ring. Once this has been accomplished typically there is typically enough length on the gonadal vessels to deliver the testis in the scrotum. Once adequate length is achieved, the testicle is ready to be brought down to the scrotum. Prentiss and colleagues were the first to describe the importance of delivering the testis in the scrotum without excessive tension, to prevent ischemic injury. In doing so, they reported that the shortest distance between the abdominal cavity to the scrotum is via a neo-canal that passes medial to the epigastric vessels and above the pubic bone [29]. To do so, first, a transverse skin incision is made onto the ipsilateral mid-scrotum. A sub-dartos pouch is created to harbor the testicle. Then, using a laparoscopic grasper from inside the abdominal cavity, a new tract is created by applying gentle pressure medial to the epigastric vessels. Externally, the tips of the grasper can be guided to make sure they pass over the pubic tubercle. The grasper is pushed until the tips exit at the level of the scrotal incision. A 12-mm port is inserted into the abdomen through the scrotal incision via the newly created channel. This is assisted by using the previously passed laparoscopic grasper to pull the end of the sheath of a Step Bladeless trocar (Medtronic, Minneapolis, USA) into the abdomen from scrotal incision (Fig. 19.3a, b). Once the port has been placed, a Maryland grasper can be introduced to grab the gubernaculum. The testis is then delivered into the scrotum via the port, and subsequently the port is removed under vision, ensuring that the cord is neither twisted nor under too much tension. Once in the scrotum, the testis is secured in the usual manner. Prior to removal of ports, the abdominal cavity is inspected and ports are removed under direct vision. All fascial defects are reapproximated once the pneumoperitoneum has been evacuated, and the skin is closed in the preferred manner.

Kahiri and coworkers have described inserting the scrotal trocar right after gubernacular dissection to aid with dissection of the vascular pedicle. Addition of this port early on allows for use of the dissecting instruments from below while the testis is lifted from one of the abdominal ports [30].

Two-Stage Orchiopexy

Fowler and Stephens were the first to describe ligation of testicular vessels in order to salvage high intra-abdominal testes [31].

During the first stage, the vessels are ligated close to the testis. This can be done with either clips or electrocautery. A study conducted by AbouZeid and coworkers did not show any differences in outcomes or testicular histology assess with biopsies between children who had their vessels controlled with clips or electrocautery, although the latter did provide an economical advantage [32].

Once the vessels have been transected, it is preferred to wait 6 months after the first stage, to allow adequate collaterals to develop. A vascularized peritoneal flap is

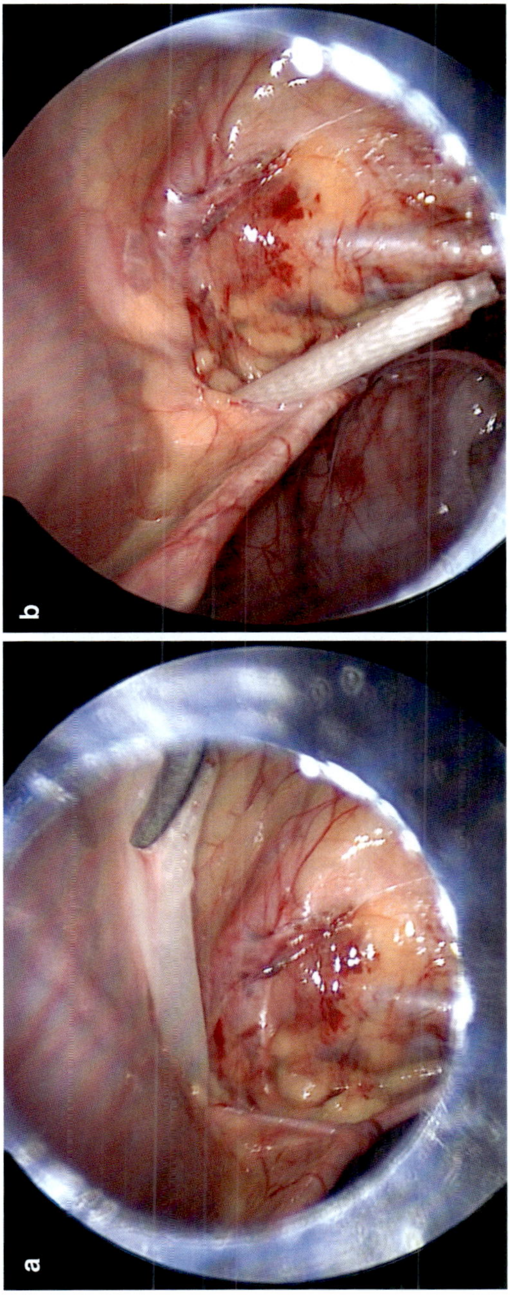

Fig. 19.3 (a) The outer sheath of a Step Bladeless trocar is pulled inside the abdominal cavity with the help of laparoscopic graspers. (b) Final position of the trocar sheath medial to the external epigastric vessels, lateral to the umbilical vessels and above the pubic bone

then created very carefully, maintaining the collateral blood supply that developed from the deferential artery. To do so, the peritoneum is incised sharply lateral and above the internal inguinal ring. The incision is then continued medially ensuring that enough peritoneum is left covering the vas. This will create a V-shaped flap that should cover the vas and testis. At this point, the testicle is then brought down to the scrotum in the same manner as one would do during a one stage orchiopexy. Due to evidence of collateral blood flow developing through the gubernaculum via the cremasteric artery, some surgeons have developed gubernaculum-sparing approaches.

To do so, the dissection of the peritoneum starts as usual lateral to the internal inguinal ring and is carried out medially along the superior margin of the ring. Then, more dissection of the peritoneum is performed proximally at the bifurcation of the iliac vessels. Finally, a laparoscopic grasper is advanced through the internal inguinal ring alongside the gubernaculum, if the ring was open. If the ring is closed, a 5-mm trocar is advanced intra-abdominally through the usual scrotal incision, via the inguinal canal. The testis is then brought down with the preserved gubernaculum. If the testis is under tension, more proximal peritoneal dissection is performed [33, 34]. This technique has shown significantly lower atrophy rates compared to classic laparoscopic orchiopexy (0.6% vs 28.3%, respectively) [33].

Another group described a gubernacular-sparing approach involving a first laparoscopic stage, for vessel ligation, followed by a second stage that combines laparoscopic peritoneal dissection with a groin approach during which the testicle is externalized by gentle traction on gubernacular attachments and blunt dissection [35].

A similar concept of sparing the gubernaculum should be considered when the testis is found high in the abdomen. In this scenario a two stage Fowler Stephens approach can be utilized. The vessels are clipped as done with an ordinary Fowler Stephens approach. The second stage is undertaken 6 months later. At this stage the testis is mobilized on a peritoneal flap whose boarders are the vas deferens and the long gubernacular structures which can be found extending up from the internal ring to the testis. The gubernaculum is spared and passed with the testis through the tunnel created in a similar fashion as is described above.

Surgical Considerations and Debated Topics

Bilateral Laparoscopic Orchiopexy

In the presence of bilateral undescended and non-palpable testicles, in whom disorders of sexual differentiation have been ruled out, judgment should be used when decided to perform orchiopexy at the same time, especially in the setting of high testicles both requiring vessel ligation. If vessel ligation is required for both gonads, then it is prudent to ligate one vessel at the time. In case one testicle can be brought down in the scrotum in one setting and the other requires ligation, it is recommended to first perform the orchiopexy prior to ligating vessels. If both testicles are low intra-abdominally, then bilateral orchiopexy can be performed in the same setting. Kaye and colleagues have reported outcomes of bilateral laparoscopic orchiopexy in 21 patients [36]. Out of 42 gonads, a Fowler-Stephens approach was required in only 4 testicles. Only 2 gonads eventually atrophied, one of which underwent a one-stage Fowler-Stephens and another that underwent a primary laparoscopic orchiopexy. Out of 21 children, 16 underwent only one surgery.

Long-Looping Vas

Occasionally a long vas is noted departing from the intra-abdominal test, entering the inguinal canal via the internal ring and looping back into the abdominal cavity. The looping vas can be gently brought back into the abdominal cavity by careful blunt dissection and indirect grasping. To facilitate handling of long looping limbs, Shalaby and coworkers described wrapping the vas in a fascial sheath to use for traction. In case they weren't able to safely dissect the looping vas, an inguinal incision was required to complete the dissection [37].

On the other hand, Dave and colleagues noted in their series that among children who underwent staged orchiopexy, those with a long-looping vas had significantly lower rates of atrophic gonads at follow up if their second stage was performed with an open approach versus a laparoscopic one (0% vs 83% 5 patients in each group, respectively) [38]. These results could be explained that during laparoscopic dissection of a looping vas, the collateral vessels around the vas might be accidentally injured by traction.

Closure of the Internal Inguinal Ring

The need to close the internal inguinal ring to prevent hernias has been debated. There are only anecdotal reports in the literature reporting cases of inguinal hernia [39].

In the largest series assessing this issue, Kahiri and coworkers assessed 388 boys who underwent laparoscopic orchiopexy. In 46% of them, the right was closed, and in the remaining 54% it was left open. No hernia developed at a mean follow up of 41 months [40].

Traction Orchiopexy

Data from open series where the testicle was placed in the dependent portion of the scrotum under traction with skin puckering have shown good results, with healthy testis in the expected location [41, 42]. Hence, to reduce the number of cases of intra-abdominal testis for which vessel ligation is required, Shehata and colleagues proposed a new staged laparoscopic technique involving application of tension on the testicle to allow for gradual stretching [43]. The patient is not a candidate for this technique if the testicle is >4 cm away from the internal inguinal ring (hence a Fowler-Stephens procedure was recommended) or if the testicle was able to reach the contralateral internal inguinal ring (hence a one-stage laparoscopic orchiopexy was performed).

During the first the gubernaculum was transected and the peritoneum lateral to the vessels was incised. Then, the testicle was fixed with a transcutaneous Ethibond stitch one inch superior and medial the contralateral anterior superior iliac spine.

The second stage was performed 12 weeks after the first one, the stitch was released and the testicle was delivered into the scrotum. If the stitch was noted to have come loose, a new stitch was placed and a third stage was planned.

In their series they were able to document a mean gain of 4.7 cm on vessel length. The success rate with regards to viable testes was 84%. The highest success was in boys younger than 2 years of age (90.3%) as well as in patients with a testis <2 cm from the ipsilateral internal ring (93% vs 78% for testes between 2 and 4 cm). The authors do not recommend this procedure if the testicle is more than 4 cm from the internal inguinal ring.

In theory, the traction is slowly and gently applied by the weight of the intestines. In addition, the testicle is fixed to the anterior abdominal wall, which is mobile and indents, hence not causing too much traction. In all cases, during the second stage, the bowels were seen overlying the vessels. However, no cases of internal hernias were noted in 124 patients.

In a smaller series, Elsherbeny and coworkers replicated similar results [44]. However, when they performed this procedure on two gonads in the same child, they found adhesions between the two vessels where they crossed over each other. Similarly, they were unable to gain enough length on the vessels despite traction for patients with testicles located more than 2 cm from the internal inguinal ring.

Complications

Complications during laparoscopic orchiopexy are relatively rare. The most common complications involved pre-peritoneal insufflation, which limits visibility.

Since the first trocar is placed with the Hasson technique and subsequent trocars are placed under direct vision, viscera and vascular injuries are theoretical and have not been described.

Rough handling of the vessels could lead to vascular injury and subsequent atrophy. Accidental grasping of the vas, apart from potentially damaging the collateral blood supply, could cause long-term blockage of the vas deferens.

Finally, the bladder can be injured when creating a neo-inguinal canal. Hsieh and coworkers reported on 3 bladder injuries in their institution [45]. In all instances, the tunnel towards the scrotum was created medial to the medial umbilical ligament. Furthermore, in one case, the bladder was not emptied at the beginning of the case.

Two patients had injuries recognized intra-operatively due to hematuria: one patient had a cystoscopy at time of surgery that showed the cord traversing the bladder dome. Another patient had irrigation fluid extravasating into the abdomen when the bladder was filled. The third patient had a delayed diagnosis when he developed abdominal bloating and pain on the first post-operative day. Interestingly a cystogram was negative but the bladder was under distended. Eventually he underwent cystoscopy which identified the defect. Two of the boys had an open repair and one had a laparoscopic repair. In order to avoid bladder injuries, it is recommended first, to empty the bladder at the beginning of the case, second to create the tunnel lateral to the medial umbilical ligament and medial to the epigastric vessels or to utilize the native inguinal canal.

Outcomes

Overall success of laparoscopic orchiopexy in a large multi-centric cohort has been reported to be 92.8% [4]. Success was defined as a viable testicle in a dependent scrotal location. When broken down by approach, the highest success rate was seen in primary laparoscopic orchiopexy (97.2%), the lowest was in one-stage Fowler-Stephens (74.1%) while staged Fowler-Stephens had intermediate results (87.9%).

Atrophy was more common in the one-stage Fowler-Stephens (22.2%), followed by the staged approach (10.3%) and the one-stage classic orchiopexy (2.2%). With regards to testicular retraction, once again the one-stage Fowler-Stephens had higher rates (7.4%) followed by the one stage approach (1.7%) and the classic orchiopexy (0.6%). Interestingly, while the outcome differences were statistically significant between classic laparoscopic orchiopexy and the Fowler-Stephens approaches but were not statistically different between the two Fowler-Stephens groups. To date, only one randomized trial assessing differences in outcomes between one- versus two-staged laparoscopic Fowler-Stephens has been published. This small trial, including 27 patients did not show any differences in atrophy rates between one- and two-stages (7% and 8%, respectively) [46].

Long-term outcomes for patients undergoing laparoscopic staged Fowler-Stephens who were followed for >10 years have shown an 83% success rate. The operated testicle was viable but always slightly smaller than the contralateral one, suggesting long term success of this procedure [47].

References

1. Kolon TF, Herndon CD, Baker LA, Baskin LS, Baxter CG, Cheng EY, et al. Evaluation and treatment of cryptorchidism: AUA guideline. J Urol. 2014;192(2):337–45.
2. Radmayr C, Dogan HS, Hoebeke P, Kocvara R, Nijman R, Silay S, et al. Management of undescended testes: European Association of Urology/European Society for Paediatric Urology Guidelines. J Pediatr Urol. 2016;12(6):335–43.

3. Cendron M, Huff DS, Keating MA, Snyder HM 3rd, Duckett JW. Anatomical, morphological and volumetric analysis: a review of 759 cases of testicular maldescent. J Urol. 1993;149(3):570–3.
4. Baker LA, Docimo SG, Surer I, Peters C, Cisek L, Diamond DA, et al. A multi-institutional analysis of laparoscopic orchidopexy. BJU Int. 2001;87(6):484–9.
5. Denes FT, Saito FJ, Silva FA, Giron AM, Machado M, Srougi M. Laparoscopic diagnosis and treatment of nonpalpable testis. Int Braz J Urol. 2008;34(3):329–34; discussion 35.
6. Ferro F, Lais A, Bagolan P, Talamo M, Caterino S. Impact of primary surgical approach in the management of the impalpable testis. Eur Urol. 1992;22(2):142–6.
7. Ferro F, Lais A, Gonzalez-Serva L. Benefits and afterthoughts of laparoscopy for the nonpalpable testis. J Urol. 1996;156(2 Pt 2):795–8; discussion 8.
8. Froeling FM, Sorber MJ, de la Rosette JJ, de Vries JD. The nonpalpable testis and the changing role of laparoscopy. Urology. 1994;43(2):222–7.
9. Kirsch AJ, Escala J, Duckett JW, Smith GH, Zderic SA, Canning DA, et al. Surgical management of the nonpalpable testis: the Children's Hospital of Philadelphia experience. J Urol. 1998;159(4):1340–3.
10. Merguerian PA, Mevorach RA, Shortliffe LD, Cendron M. Laparoscopy for the evaluation and management of the nonpalpable testicle. Urology. 1998;51(5A Suppl):3–6.
11. Cortesi N, Ferrari P, Zambarda E, Manenti A, Baldini A, Morano FP. Diagnosis of bilateral abdominal cryptorchidism by laparoscopy. Endoscopy. 1976;8(1):33–4.
12. Tasian GE, Copp HL, Baskin LS. Diagnostic imaging in cryptorchidism: utility, indications, and effectiveness. J Pediatr Surg. 2011;46(12):2406–13.
13. Tasian GE, Copp HL. Diagnostic performance of ultrasound in nonpalpable cryptorchidism: a systematic review and meta-analysis. Pediatrics. 2011;127(1):119–28.
14. Bloom DA. Two-step orchiopexy with pelviscopic clip ligation of the spermatic vessels. J Urol. 1991;145(5):1030–3.
15. Bogaert GA, Kogan BA, Mevorach RA. Therapeutic laparoscopy for intra-abdominal testes. Urology. 1993;42(2):182–8.
16. Noh PH, Kalyanaraman B. Single trocar skin puncture laparoscopic orchidopexy. Urology. 2012;80(3):695–7.
17. de Lima GR, da Silveira RA, de Cerqueira JB, de Abreu AC, de Abreu Filho AC, Rocha MF, et al. Single-incision multiport laparoscopic orchidopexy: initial report. J Pediatr Surg. 2009;44(10):2054–6.
18. Li N, Zhang W, Yuan J, Zhou X, Wu X, Chai C. Multi-incisional transumbilical laparoscopic surgery for nonpalpable undescended testes: a report of 126 cases. J Pediatr Surg. 2012;47(12):2298–301.
19. Noh PH, Vinson MA, Bansal D. LaparoEndoscopic Single Site orchidopexy for intra-abdominal testes in the pediatric population with a multichannel single port and flexible tip laparoscope. J Endourol. 2013;27(11):1381–3.
20. Mahdi BD, Rahma C, Mohamed J, Hayet Z, Riadh M. Single port laparoscopic orchidopexy in children using surgical glove port and conventional rigid instruments. Korean J Urol. 2015;56(11):781–4.
21. Bader MI, Peeraully R, Ba'ath M, McPartland J, Baillie C. The testicular regression syndrome--do remnants require routine excision? J Pediatr Surg. 2011;46(2):384–6.
22. Nataraja RM, Asher CM, Nash R, Murphy FL. Is routine excision of testicular remnants in testicular regression syndrome indicated? J Pediatr Urol. 2015;11(3):151 e1–5.
23. Nataraja RM, Yeap E, Healy CJ, Nandhra IS, Murphy FL, Hutson JM, et al. Presence of viable germ cells in testicular regression syndrome remnants: is routine excision indicated? A systematic review. Pediatr Surg Int. 2018;34(3):353–61.
24. Yucel S, Ziada A, Harrison C, Wilcox D, Baker L, Snodgrass W. Decision making during laparoscopic orchiopexy for intra-abdominal testes near the internal ring. J Urol. 2007;178(4 Pt 1):1447–50; discussion 50.

25. Sampaio FJ, Favorito LA, Freitas MA, Damiao R, Gouveia E. Arterial supply of the human fetal testis during its migration. J Urol. 1999;161(5):1603–5.
26. Yalcin B, Komesli GH, Ozgok Y, Ozan H. Vascular anatomy of normal and undescended testes: surgical assessment of anastomotic channels between testicular and deferential arteries. Urology. 2005;66(4):854–7.
27. Ellis R, Lahiri R, Mahomed A. Mapping testicular blood supply in gubernaculum-sparing second-stage Fowler-Stephens procedure. Surg Endosc. 2014;28(11):3158–61.
28. Hay SA. Collateral circulation after spermatic vessel ligation for abdominal testis and its impact on staged laparoscopically assisted orchiopexy. J Laparoendosc Adv Surg Tech A. 2007;17(1):124–7.
29. Prentiss RJ, Weickgenant CJ, Moses JJ, Frazier DB. Undescended testis: surgical anatomy of spermatic vessels, spermatic surgical triangles and lateral spermatic ligament. J Urol. 1960;83:686–92.
30. Khairi A, El-Kholi N, Shehata S. Early insertion of trans-scrotal port during laparoscopic orchidopexy: a new concept. J Pediatr Urol. 2011;7(5):548–51.
31. Fowler R, Stephens FD. The role of testicular vascular anatomy in the salvage of high undescended testes. Aust N Z J Surg. 1959;29:92–106.
32. AbouZeid AA, Moussa MH, Shalaby MS, Safoury HS, El-naggar O, Hay S. Feasibility and safety of monopolar diathermy as an alternative to clip ligation in laparoscopic Fowler-Stephens orchiopexy. J Pediatr Surg. 2012;47(10):1907–12.
33. Braga LH, Farrokhyar F, McGrath M, Lorenzo AJ. Gubernaculum testis and cremasteric vessel preservation during laparoscopic orchiopexy for intra-abdominal testes: effect on testicular atrophy rates. J Urol. 2019;201(2):378–85.
34. Robertson SA, Munro FD, Mackinlay GA. Two-stage Fowler-Stephens orchidopexy preserving the gubernacular vessels and a purely laparoscopic second stage. J Laparoendosc Adv Surg Tech A. 2007;17(1):101–7.
35. Mahomed A, Adams S, Islam S. Initial success with gubernacular-sparing laparoscopic-assisted Fowler-Stephens orchidopexy for intra-abdominal testes. J Laparoendosc Adv Surg Tech A. 2012;22(2):192–4.
36. Kaye JD, Palmer LS. Single setting bilateral laparoscopic orchiopexy for bilateral intra-abdominal testicles. J Urol. 2008;180(4 Suppl):1795–9; discussion 9.
37. Shalaby MM, Shoma AM, Elanany FG, Elganainy EO, El-Akkad MA. Management of the looping vas deferens during laparoscopic orchiopexy. J Urol. 2011;185(6 Suppl):2455–7.
38. Dave S, Manaboriboon N, Braga LH, Lorenzo AJ, Farhat WA, Bagli DJ, et al. Open versus laparoscopic staged Fowler-Stephens orchiopexy: impact of long loop vas. J Urol. 2009;182(5):2435–9.
39. Metwalli AR, Cheng EY. Inguinal hernia after laparoscopic orchiopexy. J Urol. 2002;168(5):2163.
40. Khairi A, Shehata S, El-Kholi N. Is it necessary to close the peritoneum over the deep inguinal ring during laparoscopic orchidopexy? J Pediatr Urol. 2013;9(2):157–60.
41. Daher P, Nabbout P, Feghali J, Riachy E. Is the Fowler-Stephens procedure still indicated for the treatment of nonpalpable intraabdominal testis? J Pediatr Surg. 2009;44(10):1999–2003.
42. Dessanti A, Falchetti D, Iannuccelli M, Milianti S, Altana C, Tanca AR, et al. Cryptorchidism with short spermatic vessels: staged orchiopexy preserving spermatic vessels. J Urol. 2009;182(3):1163–7.
43. Shehata S, Shalaby R, Ismail M, Abouheba M, Elrouby A. Staged laparoscopic traction-orchiopexy for intraabdominal testis (Shehata technique): stretching the limits for preservation of testicular vasculature. J Pediatr Surg. 2016;51(2):211–5.
44. Elsherbeny M, Abdallah A, Abouzeid A, Ghanem W, Zaki A. Staged laparoscopic traction orchiopexy for intra-abdominal testis: is it always feasible? J Pediatr Urol. 2018;14(3):267 e1–4.

45. Hsieh MH, Bayne A, Cisek LJ, Jones EA, Roth DR. Bladder injuries during laparoscopic orchiopexy: incidence and lessons learned. J Urol. 2009;182(1):280–4; discussion 4–5.
46. Ostlie DJ, Leys CM, Fraser JD, Snyder CL, St Peter SD. Laparoscopic orchiopexy requiring vascular division: a randomized study comparing the primary and two-stage approaches. J Laparoendosc Adv Surg Tech A. 2015;25(6):536–9.
47. Esposito C, Vallone G, Savanelli A, Settimi A. Long-term outcome of laparoscopic Fowler-Stephens orchiopexy in boys with intra-abdominal testis. J Urol. 2009;181(4):1851–6.

Chapter 20
Laparoscopic Varicocelectomy

Christina P. Carpenter and Dana W. Giel

Introduction

Varicoceles occur in approximately 15% of children and adolescent males [1–3]. They can be associated with changes in the ipsilateral testicle's consistency, growth, and function [4, 5], and are identified in up to 40% of infertile men [6]. The literature is conflicted about the necessity of treating the entity as some argue that intervention does not affect fertility rates, sperm quality, or testicular growth [6–8], while others cite evidence supporting the opposite [4, 5, 9, 10]. If one decides to proceed with intervention, the controversy continues, as there are several options for treatment, all based on the technique and principles first described by Palomo in 1949 [11]. The laparoscopic approach was first described by Aaberg et al. in 1991 [12], and Pastuszak et al. found this approach to be most popular among pediatric urologists [6]. It is also the preference of the authors as it has similar complication rates as open and microsurgical techniques with significantly less operative time [7, 13, 14].

C. P. Carpenter (✉)
Columbia University Irving Medical Center, New York-Presbyterian Morgan Stanley Children's Hospital, Department of Urology, Division of Pediatric Urology, New York, NY, USA
e-mail: cpc2161@curnc.columbia.edu

D. W. Giel (✉)
LeBonheur Children's Hospital, University of Tennessee Health Science Center, Department of Pediatric Urology, Memphis, TN, USA
e-mail: danagiel@uthsc.edu

Patient Selection/Indications

Patients are often referred to a pediatric urologist after a routine visit to a pediatrician raises concern for a varicocele either found routinely on physical exam or incidentally on a scrotal ultrasound. Affected boys are generally asymptomatic, and thus, indication for surgery is based on testicular size difference, which is determined most accurately by applying the dimensions measured on ultrasound to the formula $L \times W \times H \times 0.71$ [15]. The percent differential of the testicles can then be determined by (volume of unaffected testis − volume of affected testis) ÷ volume of unaffected testis × 100. A differential of 20% or greater has been found to be associated with potentially abnormal semen parameters; and, thus, this is used routinely as an indication for intervention [16]. However, the difference in volumes can be transient [17, 18], so it is recommended to intervene only if the discrepancy persists over a year of observation [19].

If a varicocele is present without hypotrophy, however, the appropriateness of surgical intervention is less concrete. Mehta and Sigman postulate that in these scenarios, as in adults, abnormal semen analysis should be used an indication for repair [20]. Further, Nork et al. demonstrated in their meta-analysis that adolescent varicoceles significantly negatively affect semen parameters and that intervening can improve sperm density and motility [21]. This modality, therefore, though not common practice for most pediatric urologists [22], can certainly aid in surgical decision-making if the patient and his guardian agree to evaluation. Nevertheless, just as one abnormal ultrasound should not be indicative of repair, neither should one abnormal analysis, as the majority of boys with initial abnormal results will normalize on subsequent studies [8, 23].

Surgical Technique

After induction of anesthesia, the bladder is drained via straight catheterization. Supraumbilical laparoscopic access using a 5 mm trocar is obtained in standard open or closed fashion (steps detailed in Tables 20.1 and 20.2, respectively). A 30-degree lens camera is used to survey the abdomen and to identify the location of the left spermatic cord. (Note: As 90% of varicoceles occur on the left side [19], "left side/testicle" will be synonymous with "affected side/testicle" for ease of description.) The bed is positioned into slight Trendelenburg position and rotated to raise the patient's left side. Two additional 5 mm trocars are placed as detailed in Table 20.3. Figure 20.1 depicts the configuration of the trocars.

The peritoneum overlying the spermatic cord is opened sharply using laparoscopic scissors. Dissection is continued until the spermatic cord is isolated well enough to allow for placement of surgical clips (two distally and two proximally) before the cord is ligated, as depicted in Figs. 20.2 and 20.3. Alternatively, the cord can be cauterized using a bipolar device. Cautery should be used sparingly, and care

Table 20.1 Open camera trocar placement (Hasson technique)

Pass 2-0 Vicryl stay stich through umbilical stalk
Make a supraumbilical curvilinear incision using a #15 blade scalpel
Dissect down to fascia and around umbilical stalk
Grasp umbilical stalk with Kocher clamp
Incise fascia
Pass second 2-0 Vicryl stay stich through fascia
Open peritoneum sharply
Place blunt-ended trocar through the incision
Insufflate abdomen with carbon dioxide to 12 mm Hg
Pass camera with 30-degree lens and inspect to ensure that no injury occurred while gaining access

Table 20.2 Closed camera trocar placement (Veress needle)

Pass 2-0 Vicryl stay stich through umbilical stalk
Make a supraumbilical curvilinear incision using a #15 blade scalpel
Dissect down to fascia and around umbilical stalk
Pass second 2-0 Vicryl stay stich through fascia
Use tenotomy scissors to make a small incision in the fascia and peritoneum
Pass Veress needle into opening
Confirm placement with saline drop test
Insufflate abdomen with carbon dioxide to 12 mm Hg
While holding upward traction on stay stiches, pass 5 mm trocar into abdomen with obturator in place
Pass camera with 30-degree lens and inspect to ensure that no injury occurred while gaining access

Table 20.3 Working port placement (under direct vision)

Infiltrate skin and underlying tissue with 1% lidocaine with 1:100,000 epinephrine
Use a #15 blade to make a 5 mm incision
Dissect down to facia
Use an #11 blade scalpel to pierce the fascia and peritoneum
Pass trocar with obturator in place into abdomen

should be taken to preserve a wide swath of peritoneum over the vas in order to preserve the associated blood supply, as demonstrated in Fig. 20.2. Of note for completeness, variations on this standard procedure exist, including artery- and/or lymphatic-sparing techniques; however, neither are the authors' standard practice, and thus, are not described in detail here, but will be discussed below. Insufflation pressure is then decreased, and hemostasis assessed. Once this is adequate, the instruments are removed, followed by the trocars under direct vision. The fascia at the trocar sites is closed with interrupted or figure-of-eight sutures, and the skin is reapproximated in a subcuticular fashion.

Fig. 20.1 Placement of 5 mm trocars. A = supraumbilical camera site; B = scissors, bipolar cautery device, clip applier; C = Maryland dissecting forceps; X = location of spermatic cord

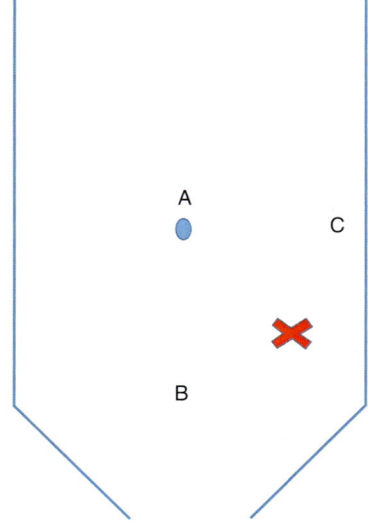

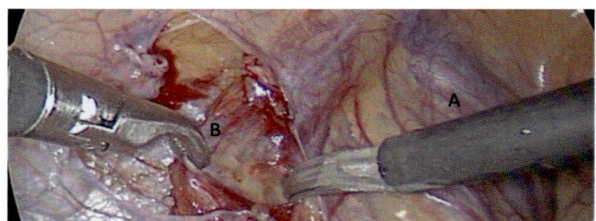

Fig. 20.2 Spermatic cord (B) is well isolated while maintaining a wide swath of peritoneum around the vas (A)

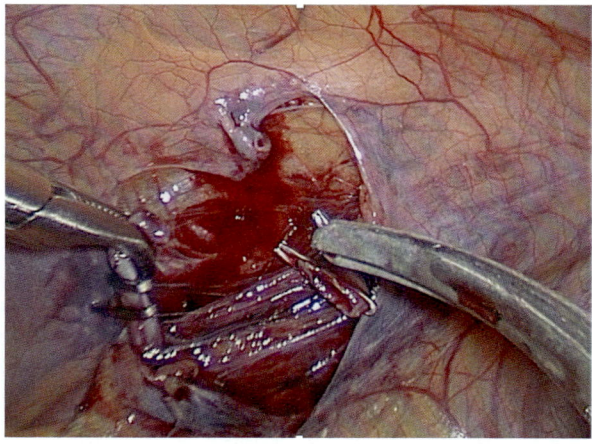

Fig. 20.3 Ligated cord vessels with two proximal and two distal clips in place

Outcomes/Complications/Follow-Up

For all varicocelectomy approaches, the main complications are recurrence and hydrocele formation. In their meta-analysis of 11 studies published between 2000 and 2009, Borruto et al. found these to occur at rates of 5% and 10%, respectively [24]. Comparing laparoscopic and open approaches, hydrocele is slightly more common with the former technique while the reverse is true for recurrence; however, the differences in rates have not been shown to be statistically significant [13, 24]. Specific to laparoscopy, injury to the genitofemoral nerve is cited in some studies as occurring in approximately 2% of patients [13, 25]. This, however, can easily be avoided with careful attention during dissection, as rates have been shown to decrease as surgeons gain experience [13].

The artery-sparing technique was first compared to the standard procedure by Kass and Marcol in 1992 [5]. They found this method to have a significantly higher rate of persistent/recurrent varicocele when compared to high retroperitoneal ligation of the spermatic vessels. This finding has been echoed in several other studies [26, 27], but the appropriateness and efficacy of this modification continues to be a topic of discussion due to concern for testicular atrophy or hypotrophy without it.

This concern, however, is not supported by data in the literature nor by understanding of the anatomy. In a study by Esposito et al., none of the 189 boys who underwent ligation of the testicular veins and artery during varicocelectomy suffered testicular hypotrophy postoperatively. The authors explain that this is to be expected because of the existing collateral blood supply to the testis from the gubernaculum, the anterior and posterior scrotal vessels, and the deferential vessels [26]. Further, in their review of pathologic specimens of vessels ligated during open varicocelectomy, Cuda et al. found that men who had inadvertently had arterial segments ligated during their procedures had no clinical testicular hypotrophy [28]. Lastly, in their separate series comparing patients treated with and without artery-sparing varicocelectomies, McManus et al. and Atassi et al. both concluded that the former approach increased surgical time without providing any clinical benefit [27, 29].

With regards to hydrocele formation, the slightly higher occurrence associated with laparoscopic intervention can be decreased with application of the lymphatic-sparing technique first described by Oswald et al. in 2001 [30]. In their series of 28 boys, isosulphan blue injected "under the tunica dartos near to the parietal wall of the tunica vaginalis" 15 minutes prior to starting the operation was used to identify and spare the lymphatic channels. None of their 28 patients developed reactive hydroceles, but four underwent traditional Palomo varicocelectomy due to failure of mapping [30]. Several published series have echoed the success of this method, and its applicability to both open and laparoscopic approaches [31–33].

Nevertheless, Esposito et al. were dismayed that mapping was unsuccessful in up to 30% of cases, and sought to standardize the technique in order to delineate the lymphatics in every patient [34]. In 2014, they described their approach of injecting 2 ml of 2.5% isosulfan blue into the intra-dartos space and 0.5 ml into the testicular parenchyma 5 minutes prior to surgical start. This provided effective mapping in all cases, and none of the patients developed reactive hydroceles. This modification, therefore, can be reproducibly applied to decrease hydroceles formation when using a laparoscopic approach.

Summary

Laparoscopic varicocelectomy is a safe and cost-effective procedure for treating pediatric varicoceles. Use of an artery-sparing modification is not advised as it increases operative time and risk of recurrence without any clear benefit. Though not significantly different from the rate associated with an approach, hydrocele formation is the main complication during laparoscopic intervention. This commonly does not require intervention [27]; however, it can potentially be avoided by sparing the lymphatic vessels.

References

1. Akbay E, Çayan S, Doruk E, et al. The prevalence of varicocele and varicocele-related testicular atrophy in Turkish children and adolescents. BJU Int. 2000;86:490–3.
2. Kumanov P, Robeva RN, Tomova A. Adolescent varicocele: who is at risk? Pediatrics. 2008;121:e53–7.
3. Skoog SJ, Roberts KP, Goldstein M, et al. The adolescent varicocele: what's new with an old problem in young patients? Pediatrics. 1997;100(1):112–21.
4. Li F, Chiba K, Yamaguchi K, et al. Effect of varicocelectomy on testicular volume in children and adolescents: a meta-analysis. Urology. 2012;79:1340–5.
5. Kass EJ, Belman AB. Reversal of testicular growth failure by varicocele ligation. J Urol. 1987;137:475–6.
6. Pastuszak AW, Kumar V, Shah A, et al. Diagnostic and management approaches to pediatric and adolescent varicocele: a survey of pediatric urologists. Urology. 2014;84:450–6.
7. Locke JA, Noparast M, Afshar K. Treatment of varicocele in children and adolescents: a systematic review and meta-analysis of randomized controlled trials. J Pediatr Urol. 2017;13:437–45.
8. Chu DI, Zderic SA, Shukla AR, et al. The natural history of semen parameters in untreated asymptomatic adolescent varicocele patients: a retrospective cohort study. J Pediatr Urol. 2017;13:77.e1–5.
9. Okuyama A, Nakamura M, Namiki M, et al. Surgical repair of varicocele at puberty: preventive treatment for fertility improvement. J Urol. 1988;139:562–4.
10. Lipshultz LI, Corriere JN. Progressive testicular atrophy in the varicocele patient. J Urol. 1977;117:175–6.
11. Palomo A. Radical cure of varicocele by a new technique: preliminary report. J Urol. 1949;61:604–7.
12. Aaberg RA, Vancaillie TG, Schuessler WW. Laparoscopic varicocele ligation: a new technique. Fertil Steril. 1991;56:776–7.
13. Podkamenev VV, Stalmakhovich VN, Urkov PS, et al. Laparoscopic surgery for pediatric varicoceles: randomized controlled trial. J Pediatr Surg. 2002;37:727–9.

14. Parrilli A, Roberti A, Escolino M, et al. Surgical approaches for varicocele in pediatric patient. Transl Pediatr. 2016 5:227–32.
15. Sakamoto H, Saito K, Oohta M, et al. Testicular volume measurement: comparison of ultrasonography, orchidometry, and water displacement. Urology. 2007;69:152–7.
16. Diamond DA, Zurakowski D, Bauer SB, et al. Relationship of varicocele grade and testicular hypotrophy to semen parameters in adolescents. J Urol. 2007;178:1584–8.
17. Kolon TF, Clement MR, Cartwright L, et al. Transient asynchronous testicular growth in adolescent males with a varicocele. J Urol. 2008;180:1111–5.
18. Spinelli C, Di Giacomo M, Lo Piccolo R, et al. The role of testicular volume in adolescents with varicocele: the better way and time of surgical treatment. J Urol. 2010;184:1722–6.
19. Diamond DA, Gargollo PC, Caldamone AA. Current management principles for adolescent varicocele. Fertil Steril. 2011;96:1294–8.
20. Mehta A, Sigman M. The adult urologist's perspective on management of varicoceles in the pediatric population. Dialogues Pediatr Urol. 2008;30:2–4.
21. Nork JJ, Berger JH, Crain DS, et al. Youth varicocele and varicocele treatment: a meta-analysis of semen outcomes. Fertil Steril. 2014;102:381–387.e6.
22. Fine RG, Gitlin J, Reda EF, et al. Barriers to use of semen analysis in the adolescent with a varicocele: survey of patient, parental, and practitioner attitudes. J Pediatr Urol. 2016;12:41.e1–6.
23. Moursy EES, ElDahshoury MZ, Hussein MM, et al. Dilemma of adolescent varicocele: long-term outcome in patients managed surgically and in patients managed expectantly. J Pediatr Urol. 2013;9:1018–22.
24. Borruto FA, Impellizzeri P, Antonuccio P, et al. Laparoscopic vs open varicocelectomy in children and adolescents: review of the recent literature and meta-analysis. J Pediatr Surg. 2010;45:2464–9.
25. Jarow JP, Assimos DG, Pittaway DE. Effectiveness of laparoscopic varicocelectomy. Urology. 1993;42:544–7.
26. Esposito C, Monguzzi G, Gonzalez-Sabin MA, et al. Results and complications of laparoscopic surgery for pediatric varicocele. J Pediatr Surg. 2001;36:767–9.
27. McManus MC, Barqawi A, Meacham RB, et al. Laparoscopic varicocele ligation: are there advantages compared with the microscopic subinguinal approach? Urology. 2004;64:357–60.
28. Cuda SP, Musser JE, Belnap CM, et al. Incidence and clinical significance of arterial injury in varicocele repair: arterial injury in varicocele repair. BJU Int. 2011;107:1635–7.
29. Atassi O, Kass EJ, Steinert BW. Testicular growth after successful varicocele correction in adolescents: comparison of artery sparing techniques with the Palomo procedure. J Urol. 1995;153:482–3.
30. Oswald J, Körner I, Riccabona M. The use of isosulphan blue to identify lymphatic vessels in high retroperitoneal ligation of adolescent varicocele – avoiding postoperative hydrocele. BJU Int. 2001;87:502–4.
31. Capolicchio J-P, El-Sherbiny M, Brzezinski A, et al. Dye-assisted lymphatic-sparing laparoscopic varicocelectomy in children. J Pediatr Urol. 2013;9:33–7.
32. D'Alessio A, Piro E, Beretta F, et al. Lymphatic preservation using methylene blue dye during varicocele surgery: a single-center retrospective study. J Pediatr Urol. 2008;4:138–40.
33. Ishibashi H, Mori H, Yada K, et al. Indigo carmine dye-assisted lymphatic-sparing laparoscopic Palomo varicocelectomy in children. J Med Investig. 2014;61:151–5.
34. Esposito C, Iaquinto M, Escolino M, et al. Technical standardization of laparoscopic lymphatic sparing varicocelectomy in children using isosulfan blue. J Pediatr Surg. 2014;49:660–3.

Chapter 21
Special Considerations in Infants

Natalia Ballesteros and Miguel Alfredo Castellan

Advancements in minimally invasive surgery (MIS), specifically in laparoscopic and robotic surgery in adults and subsequently children, have allowed these modalities to become part of the standard of interventions for many conditions. Drawbacks of laparoscopy include the significant skills and dexterity needed for dissection and suturing. Utilization of the robotic platform allows for improved ergonomics and visualization (magnified, three-dimensional) as well as ease of instrument dexterity which most closely imitates the open technique, while maintaining the advantages of minimally invasive surgery [1]. This is especially helpful when operating in small working spaces such as that of infants. National trends over the last decade, for example in pyeloplasties, have shown that the number of open cases are decreasing as robotic cases increase, while pure laparoscopy has plateaued [2]. This same study showed adolescents were 40 times more likely to undergo robotic pyeloplasty as compared to infants. Significant debate remains among surgeons as to the benefits of robot-assisted laparoscopic surgery (RALS) in infants when considering longer operative and anesthetic time as compared to open surgery [3]. Regarding cosmesis, although it has been shown that children and parents prefer robotic/laparoscopic surgical scars compared to incisions from open urologic surgery [4], this has not been evaluated in the infant population, in which open surgeries frequently entitle very small incisions. Additionally, surgeons may feel that the standard robotic trocars and instruments are too large to use in small children. For example, the intra-abdominal space of a 1-year-old child is about 1 L, while that of an adult is up to 6 L in volume [5]. Although there are no dedicated fine pediatric robotic instruments and trocars, with the release of the 5-mm trocars and instruments, in 2003–2004 as well as lessons learned over the last couple of decades, multiple studies have documented the ease and feasibility of performing RALS in children using 8 mm and smaller instruments and across multiple specialties [1, 6]. In pediatric urology, the

N. Ballesteros (✉) · M. A. Castellan
Nicklaus Children's Hospital, Department of Pediatric Urology, Miami, FL, USA

increased experience and expertise with performing RALS has allowed expansion of the scope into the infant population. With careful operative planning, port placement, and adjustments for smaller patients, this can be accomplished in a safe and effective manner. In this chapter, we will highlight the current advances in the field of RALS in infants, defined as patients younger than 12 months of age.

RALS in Infants

In 2006, Kutikov et al. published their initial experience performing robot assisted laparoscopic pyeloplasties (RALP) in nine infants ranging from 3 to 8 months of age (5.1–8.3 kg) [7]. They reported a mean operative time of 122.8 minutes (console time 72.1 minutes), which is shorter than RALP in older children. They attributed this to the lack of crossing vessels in their series, thus avoiding further dissection time, the nature of the tissues in infants such as a more translucent mesentery and clearer view of the renal collecting system, and the expertise of the attending surgeon with prior infant pure-laparoscopic pyeloplasties. Since then, several studies have demonstrated the safety and feasibility of performing RALS in infants weighing 10 kg or less [1, 3, 5, 8–11]. The latter was on a solitary kidney, a previously considered contraindication to RALP. The small size of the pediatric patient compared to the adult presents unique challenges which must be considered when choosing between surgical approaches. For example, while traditional open pyeloplasty is typically performed retroperitoneally, RALP is typically performed with a transperitoneal approach, allowing for utilization of increased working space provided by abdominal insufflation. Other RALS in infants have been performed and deemed safe: ureteroureterostomies (UU) [12], extravesical [13] and intravesical ureteral reimplantations [14]. For the latter, the bladder size (bladder capacity of 130 mL) limits the ability to perform the procedure effectively [14]. Additionally, Srougi et al. described performing partial and total nephrectomies, and even excision of a retrovesical Mullerian remnant in children as young as 8 months of age [5]. Wiestma et al. also described a robotic lower-pole partial nephrectomy on an 11-month old weighing 10.7 kg [15].

In terms of operative time (OT), Bansal et al. in 2014 compared their experience with previously published conventional laparoscopic and robot-assisted urologic reconstructive studies in infants, showing RALS to be comparable or better than laparoscopy with mean/median OTs ranging from 103 to 278 minutes for all studies [12]. This OT is not that much longer when compared to open techniques. One study found a mean total OT for open pyeloplasty to range from 131 to 242 minutes [9]. Another study revealed that the longer operative time in children weighing less than 15 kg resulted from the robotic set-up [6]. At our institution, we performed RALP and UUs on nine infants with a mean weight of 10.1 kg, mean operative time of 181.5 minutes (console time 106 minutes), three postoperative Clavien I–III complications, and surgical success as evidenced by postoperative imaging [16].

RALS in infants has been shown to have comparable, or even lower, postoperative narcotic analgesic use and length of hospitalization [8, 10, 12]. In comparison to laparoscopy, one author hypothesized that despite the trocars and incisions being larger, improved pain control may be due to the shorter OT and therefore shorter duration of abdominal distention [12].

Cosmesis and wound healing are frequently debated when comparing surgical approaches in infants, as many open surgeries can be accomplished with incisions 1.5–2 cm long [17, 18]. However, wound tension is reduced in smaller incisions, so it is inaccurate to "sum up" the 3–4 MIS incisions to that of an open case [19]. Furthermore, it has been shown that wound healing and inflammation are also improved with the delicate suturing and tissue manipulation provided by robot-assisted surgery, as in pyeloplasty anastomoses [18, 20].

Lastly, the associated cost of performing RALS has been debated as a limitation. However, direct costs such as operation and hospitalization expenses have been shown to be comparable to open surgery [21]. One study performed a cost analysis which showed that infant RALP was about US$500 more expensive than that of open pyeloplasty [9]. Analysis included hospitalization expenses, which being longer in open procedures, contributes to cost leveling. Indirect costs, such as the robot and console, annual servicing fees, and operating room accommodations, have been shown to be significantly increased as compared to open procedures in both pediatric general and urologic surgeries [22]; however, with increased experience and use, these can be offset in the long run.

Anesthetic and Physiologic Considerations in the Infant Patient

The pediatric anesthesia team performs induction of anesthetic, appropriate IV access, tracheal intubation, placement of esophageal temperature probe, and orogastric tube placement when indicated. Lines, ventilator tubing, electrodes, and others should be placed away from the surgical field and robot system. The anesthesia team should be acquainted with the robotic platform and performing anesthesia during these cases. Close communication between all teams is crucial before, during, and after surgery. Limited access to the patient during the procedure requires advanced preparation and special monitoring. Likewise, quick undocking and removal of the robot from the vicinity during an airway or cardiac emergency is imperative to allow proper resuscitation.

Physiologic differences in children as compared to adults increase the complexity of MIS, with greater implications in the infant population including rate dependent cardiac output, higher right to left cardiac shunting, high chest wall compliance, and increased diaphragmatic respiration [23]. Prolonged intraperitoneal insufflation with CO_2 has physiologic effects that must be closely monitored such as decreased lung volumes and diaphragmatic mobility, impaired ventilation, increased CO_2

absorption, decreased venous return, and reduction of cardiac index [24]. Patient positioning such as reverse Trendelenburg or lateral decubitus can further exaggerate these effects [25]. Arterial blood gas monitoring, correction of acidosis, avoidance of excessive IV fluids and monitoring for peripheral edema, are all crucial. Potential oliguria should be closely monitored as the known renal effects of increased intra-abdominal pressure are exacerbated in infants [10]. Although robotic retroperitoneoscopic pyeloplasty has been reported successfully in older children [26], the even smaller infant retroperitoneal space pose an additional respiratory challenge. For example, increased intrathoracic pressure leads to decreased chest wall compliance and increased dead space. This results in a significant increase in respiratory rate, peek airway pressure, and end-tidal CO_2 [25]. At present, robot-assisted retroperitoneoscopic surgery in infants has not been performed.

Complications

Complication rates in infant RALS are comparable to those described in older children for open, laparoscopic, and robotic surgeries. None of the reported complications were intraoperative or directly related to use of the robot [3, 5, 8, 12]. In 2013, Bansal et al. evaluated the complications of RALS in pediatric urology [8]. This study reported an overall complication rate of 8.1%, with 27.3% of these occurring in infants. However, the infant population was small and underpowered, and all complications were Clavien III or less, including urinary retention due to bowel dysfunction, UTI, and ureteral stent migration. Avery et al. described the results from a multi-institution study which aimed to assess the success of RALP in infants [3]. The authors reported a 91% surgical success rate and the complication rate was 11% (complication rate for open pyeloplasty is reported between 0% and 24%). Complications included port-side hernias, urinary leak, UTI, postoperative ileus, and retained ureteral stents. More recently, Neheman et al. [10] compared RALP to the laparoscopic approach with a complication rate (Clavien I–III) of 23.8% and 30.8%, respectively. For these studies, the Clavien III complications were usually related to placement or replacement of stents due to urinary leaks or migrations, respectively.

Troubleshooting Robotic Surgery in Infants

Patient Selection

As previously mentioned, RALS has been successfully performed in infants weighing 10 kg or less. Limitations to using the robot have been related to patient and trocar/instrument size. It has been previously shown that robotic tasks cannot be performed in a 40-mm edge cube due to severe external arm collisions [27]. Major technical difficulties have been reported with infants weighing 3–5 kg or less due to the very small working space [1, 6]. In 2015, Finkelstein et al. sought to investigate which infants were amenable for RALS [28]. They performed robotic urologic interventions on 45 infants ages 3–12 months and correlated surgical feasibility with the patient's weight and abdominal surface area. In addition to age or weight relationship, an inverse relationship was demonstrated between abdominal surface area and the number of arm collisions and console time. For this reason, small infants weighing 3–5 kg and with small abdominal surface areas (puboxyphoid distance <15 cm and/or <13 cm in between each anterior superior iliac spine) are not ideal candidates for RALS.

Special Considerations

Typically, bowel preparation is not performed in advance although some have described the use of a single enema [11]. As with older children, infants normally undergo bowel and bladder decompression with an orogastric tube and urethral catheter, respectively [5, 9]. In some cases, decompression of colonic gas may be accomplished by placement of a flatus tube [9].

Infants lose more heat in comparison to older children. The Bair Hugger® system, along with plastic covering which excludes the operative field, allows for proper temperature management. Room temperature control and an insufflation warmer are indispensable.

Although a pneumoperitoneum of 4–6 mm Hg has been described [11], pneumoperitoneum is usually maintained at 8–12 mm Hg with a flow rate of 0.6 L/min. Technology used in adults to maintain a proper pneumoperitoneal space at 8 mm Hg is currently under development for the pediatric population.

Patient and Robot Positioning

Advanced planning should be performed to ensure patient safety throughout the case. Positioning is aided with egg crate, gel rolls, and/or blanket support depending on the specific case with the goal of padding pressure points and protecting the face, eyes, and limbs (Fig. 21.1). Regardless, one should aim to minimize external clutter. One consideration to avoid collision of the robotic arms with the OR table during the procedure is to elevate the patient a few inches using egg crate so that the ports can be placed more laterally [1]. Additionally, the patient should be as close to the edge of the bed as possible. If tape is used to secure the infant, care should be taken to avoid skin contact (Fig. 21.2). For transperitoneal renal RALS, consider placing the patient in lateral decubitus position at a 90° angle, rather than the traditional 45–65°, to facilitate exposure of the working space by adequately displacing the intestines from the working field [5]. When draping, it is useful to have a drape with

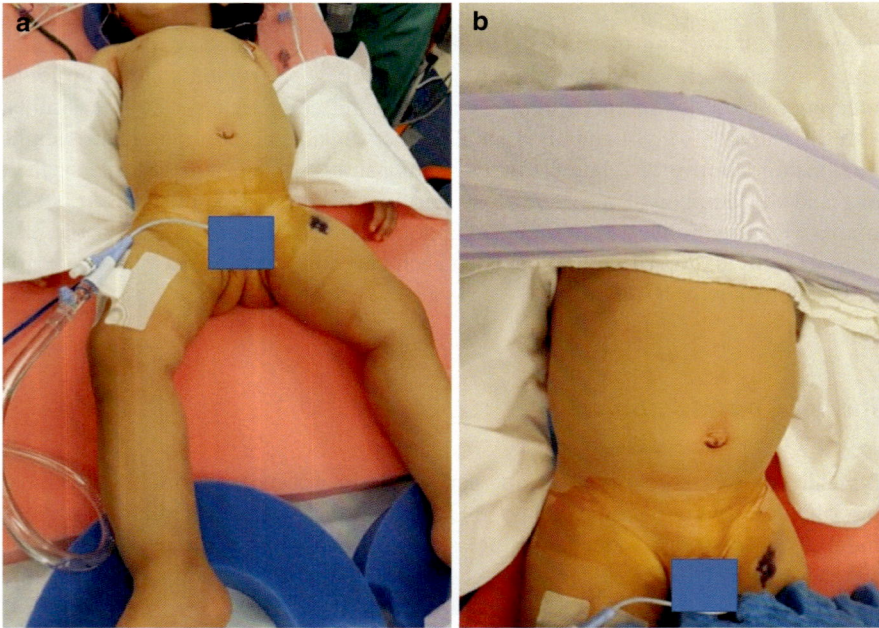

Fig. 21.1 (**a**, **b**) Patient padding is accomplished with egg crate, foam and blankets, with care to support all pressure points

clear plastic covering over the head, or when one is unavailable, drawing a face on the drape where the head lays to allow adequate visualization. The robot should be positioned in a manner which allows proper access for both the surgical and anesthesia teams. One author recommends placing the robot at a 5–10° angle to the patient's main axis and positioning the anesthesia team on a line between the robot cart and the patient's head [6]. At our institution, due to the room configuration, the robot cart is placed in the same manner for all procedures regardless of type of case, patient size, or laterality: midway towards the lower end to the left side of the operating bed, with the anesthesia team at the head of the patient. The robotic boom and arms are then rotated and triangulated depending on the particular case (Fig. 21.3). We should note that we use the DaVinci Xi platform (Intuitive Surgical Inc., Sunnyvale, CA, USA).

Trocar Placement and Instrumentation

In general, children have increased bowel distention, due to rapid gastric emptying times, which can limit visualization and may compromise access and lead to bowel or vascular injury. Open Hasson technique (Fig. 21.4) or trocar intussusception allows for direct visualization of the initial peritoneal access [21].

Fig. 21.2 When securing the patient, avoid tape from contacting with the delicate infant's skin

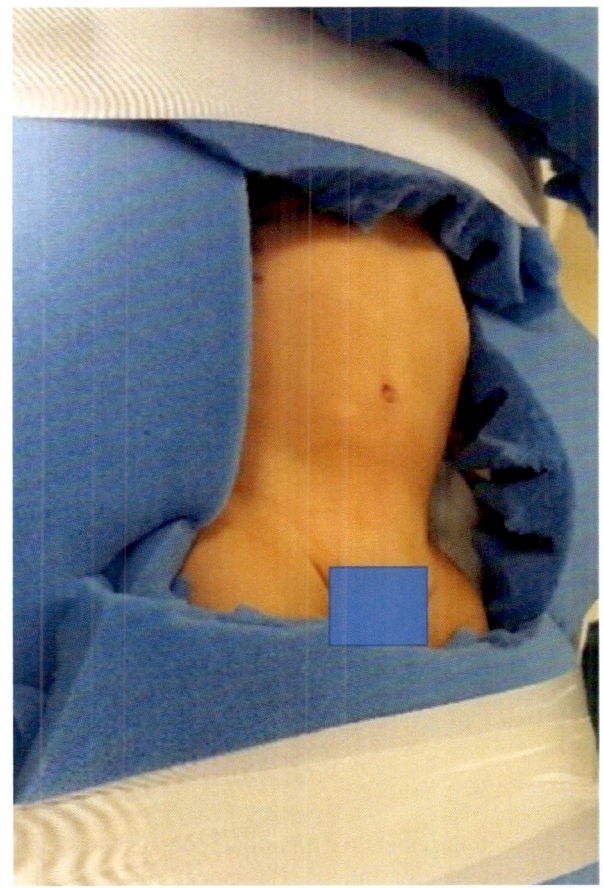

Fig. 21.3 Docked robot configuration: the robotic cart is brought in on the left side midway towards the end of the bed, the boom is deployed as far as possible and aligned with the target organ, and the arms are triangulated and docked. (© 2020 Intuitive Surgical, Inc. https://www.intuitive.com/en-us/about-us/press/press-resources)

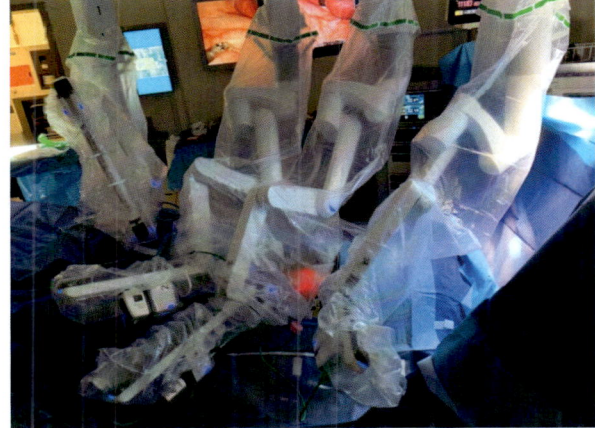

Fig. 21.4 Transumbilical access using an open Hasson technique

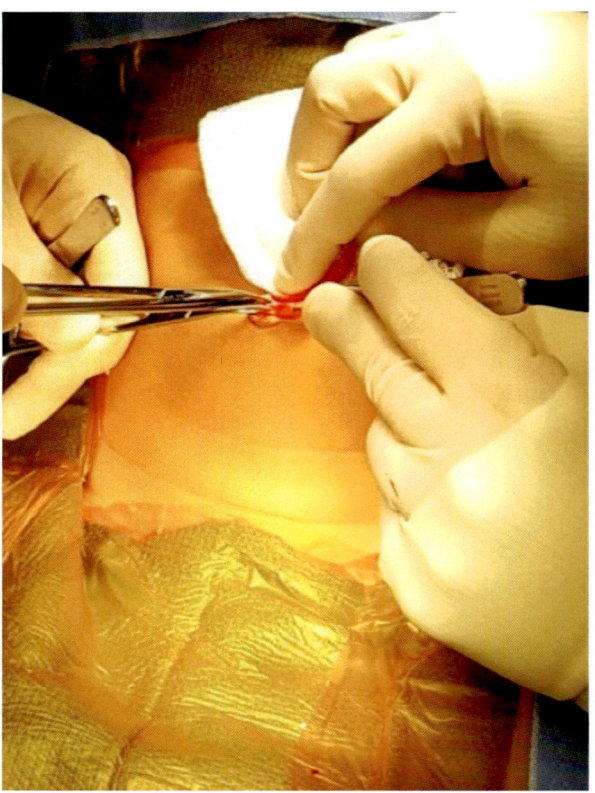

The port placement for traditional robotic cases in older children and adults may not be optimal for infants. Placement should be individualized for each case. However, placing the trocars slightly more caudally and laterally than the traditional position, with respect to the camera position, may aid to prevent instrument collision outside while maximizing working space and view inside the abdominal cavity [1, 29]. One disadvantage of the instruments is the depth in which they need to be within the abdominal cavity to function properly, which in small patients, decreases the available working space. The manufacturer recommends placing the remote center (the black thick line) of the cannula just below the skin level. In adults and older children with thicker abdominal walls, this allows for minimal trauma to the skin and fascia. One way to maneuver around the long instruments is to decrease the trocar depth so that the remote center is just outside of the skin edge. This can allow an extra centimeter of workspace without placing harmful torque at the skin level since infants have much thinner abdominal walls [1]. Trocar positioning should be carefully planned as the smaller the patient, the greater risk of internal and external instrument and robot arm collisions. Placing the trocars in an in-line, less triangulated, configuration and with a 4–5 cm separation of each trocar, when possible, also allows for easier manipulation of the instruments [3, 5, 6]. For upper tract surgery, they should be placed vertically along the midline. For pelvic cases, trocars should be placed horizontally as with older children, but slightly more cephalad (either parallel to the camera port or slightly behind it) [5]. On the other hand, port placement in the arrangement of the hidden incision endoscopic surgery (HIdES) technique, initially described by Gargollo in 2011 [30], has also been used for infant surgery [12]. The trocars should be anchored to the abdominal wall to decrease the risk of loss of access and pneumoperitoneum. First, the skin incision should fit for the trocar size only [6] and then the anchoring can be accomplished with a box suture, fascial anchoring, and/or adhesive tape from the skin that is then wrapped around the trocar.

Small 5- and 3-mm assistant ports can be used [6], although one should consider omitting placement [28]. To pass suture, one can briefly remove an instrument and pass the suture through the robotic trocar or this can be done percutaneously [7]. Furthermore, one should be very cautious with the handling of needles laparoscopically in an infant as traditional sutures come with large needles where manipulation can pose a risk of injury to the bowel or another organ. At our institution, we often use a 6-0 monofilament suture on a TF needle for easier handling. When an antegrade ureteral stent placement is needed, as for pyeloplasties, this can be introduced into the abdominal cavity by placing a subcostal percutaneous 18-gauge angiocatheter directly in line with the renal pelvis [8].

Before 2004, the only available size of the robotic camera was 12 mm. With the release of the 5 mm instruments and camera (2-dimensional) in 2004, concerns about large incisions decreased. The use of 5 mm instruments have been reported by some to be comparable, and of more advantage for infant use, to their 8 mm counterparts [29, 31]. However, other authors prefer the 8.5 mm camera and 8 mm instruments because the gooseneck-type joint of the 5 mm instruments has a relatively large radius of movement and requires greater clearance from the tissue, limiting articulation and the available functional space [3, 6, 9, 12].

Due to the limited space in the infant cavity, heat dissipation from cautery is limited. Accordingly, cautery settings should be reduced, and active cautery should be performed a few seconds at a time [3].

Conclusions

RALS has evolved from adult surgery to include the pediatric population and is pushing the envelope expanding applications to smaller children. Although mainly used for pyeloplasties, other applications have been performed successfully in infants. Despite the lack of dedicated pediatric robotic platform and instruments, intrabdominal infant robotic surgery has been shown to be safe and feasible in patients as small as 3–5 kg. Concerns regarding smaller work space, cosmesis and wound healing, and for cost implications have been addressed showing comparable or, in some cases, superior results. Infant RALS is accomplished with careful planning, preparation and communication among all involved teams, and a few technical modifications. Nonetheless, success is dependent on surgeon experience and on first achieving the robotic learning curve on older patients and in a variety of procedures.

References

1. Meehan JJ. Robotic surgery in small children: is there room for this? J Laparoendosc Adv Surg Tech A. 2009;19(5):707–12.
2. Varda BK, Johnson EK, Clark C, Chung BI, Nelson CP, Chang SL. National trends of perioperative outcomes and costs for open, laparoscopic and robotic pediatric pyeloplasty. J Urol. 2014;191(4):1090–5.
3. Avery DI, Herbst KW, Lendvay TS, Noh PH, Dangle P, Gundeti MS, et al. Robot-assisted laparoscopic pyeloplasty: multi-institutional experience in infants. J Pediatr Urol. 2015;11(3):139.e1–5.
4. Barbosa JA, Barayan G, Gridley CM, Sanchez DC, Passerotti CC, Houck CS, et al. Parent and patient perceptions of robotic vs open urological surgery scars in children. J Urol. 2013;190(1):244–50.
5. Srougi V, Yorioka M, Sanchez DC, Onal B, Houck CS, Nguyen HT. The feasibility of robotic urologic surgery in infants and toddlers. J Pediatr Urol. 2013;9(6 Pt B):1198–203.
6. Ballouhey Q, Villemagne T, Cros J, Szwarc C, Braik K, Longis B, et al. A comparison of robotic surgery in children weighing above and below 15.0 kg: size does not affect surgery success. Surg Endosc. 2015;29(9):2643–50.
7. Kutikov A, Nguyen M, Guzzo T, Canter D, Casale P. Robot assisted pyeloplasty in the infant-lessons learned. J Urol. 2006;176(5):2237–9; discussion 9–40.
8. Bansal D, Defoor WR Jr, Reddy PP, Minevich EA, Noh PH. Complications of robotic surgery in pediatric urology: a single institution experience. Urology. 2013;82(4):917–20.
9. Dangle PP, Kearns J, Anderson B, Gundeti MS. Outcomes of infants undergoing robot-assisted laparoscopic pyeloplasty compared to open repair. J Urol. 2013;190(6):2221–6.
10. Neheman A, Kord E, Zisman A, Darawsha AE, Noh PH. Comparison of robotic pyeloplasty and standard laparoscopic pyeloplasty in infants: a bi-institutional study. J Laparoendosc Adv Surg Tech A. 2018;28(4):467–70.
11. Pelizzo G, Nakib G, Goruppi I, Avolio L, Romano P, Raffaele A, et al. Pediatric robotic pyeloplasty in patients weighing less than 10 kg initial experience. Surg Laparosc Endosc Percutan Tech. 2014;24(1):e29–31.
12. Bansal D, Cost NG, Bean CM, Vanderbrink BA, Schulte M, Noh PH. Infant robot-assisted laparoscopic upper urinary tract reconstructive surgery. J Pediatr Urol. 2014;10(5):869–74.
13. Smith RP, Oliver JL, Peters CA. Pediatric robotic extravesical ureteral reimplantation: comparison with open surgery. J Urol. 2011;185(5):1876–81.
14. Kutikov A, Guzzo TJ, Canter DJ, Casale P. Initial experience with laparoscopic transvesical ureteral reimplantation at the Children's Hospital of Philadelphia. J Urol. 2006;176(5):2222–5; discussion 5–6.
15. Wiestma AC, Cho PS, Hollis MV, Badway J, Yu RN. Robot-assisted laparoscopic lower pole partial nephrectomy in the pediatric patient. J Pediatr Urol. 2016;12(6):428–9.
16. Moscardi P, Alam A, Blachman-Braun R, Ballesteros N, Salvitti M, Kozakowski K, et al. Robot-assisted laparoscopic urological surgery for infants and children under 15 kg: a single-center experience. Paper presented at 2nd annual meeting of the North American robotic urologic symposium, Las Vegas, NV, Feb 16–17, 2019.
17. Koyle MA. Minimally invasive survey in infants CON. J Urol. 2012;188(5):1664–5.
18. Casale P. Minimally invasive survey in infants. Pro. J Urol. 2012;188(5):1665–6.

19. Blinman T. Incisions do not simply sum. Surg Endosc. 2010;24(7):1746–51.
20. Passerotti CC, Passerotti AM, Dall'Oglio MF, Leite KR, Nunes RL, Srougi M, et al. Comparing the quality of the suture anastomosis and the learning curves associated with performing open, freehand, and robotic-assisted laparoscopic pyeloplasty in a swine animal model. J Am Coll Surg. 2009;208(4):576–86.
21. Howe A, Kozel Z, Palmer L. Robotic surgery in pediatric urology. Asian J Urol. 2017;4(1):55–67.
22. Mahida JB, Cooper JN, Herz D, Diefenbach KA, Deans KJ, Minneci PC, et al. Utilization and costs associated with robotic surgery in children. J Surg Res. 2015;199(1):169–76.
23. Wedgewood J, Doyle E. Anaesthesia and laparoscopic surgery in children. Paediatr Anaesth. 2001;11(4):391–9.
24. Mariano ER, Furukawa L, Woo RK, Albanese CT, Brock-Utne JG. Anesthetic concerns for robot-assisted laparoscopy in an infant. Anesth Analg. 2004;99(6):1665–7, table of contents.
25. Halachmi S, El-Ghoreimi A, Bissonnette B, Zaarour C, Bagli DJ, McLorie GA, et al. Hemodynamic and respiratory effect of pediatric urological laparoscopic surgery: a retrospective study. J Urol. 2003;170(4 Pt 2):1651–4; discussion 4.
26. Olsen LH, Rawashdeh YF, Jorgensen TM. Pediatric robotic assisted retroperitoneoscopic pyeloplasty: a 5-year experience. J Urol. 2007;178(5):2137–41; discussion 41.
27. Thakre AA, Bailly Y, Sun LW, Van Meer F, Yeung CK. Is smaller workspace a limitation for robot performance in laparoscopy? J Urol. 2008;179(3):1138–42; discussion 42–3.
28. Finkelstein JB, Levy AC, Silva MV, Murray L, Delaney C, Casale P. How to decide which infant can have robotic surgery? Just do the math. J Pediatr Urol. 2015;11(4):170.e1–4.
29. Pelizzo G, Nakib G, Romano P, Avolio L, Mencherini S, Zambaiti E, et al. Five millimetre-instruments in paediatric robotic surgery: advantages and shortcomings. Minim Invasive Ther Allied Technol. 2015;24(3):148–53.
30. Gargollo PC. Hidden incision endoscopic surgery: description of technique, parental satisfaction and applications. J Urol. 2011;185(4):1425–31.
31. Baek M, Silay MS, Au JK, Huang GO, Elizondo RA, Puttmann KT, et al. Does the use of 5 mm instruments affect the outcomes of robot-assisted laparoscopic pyeloplasty in smaller working spaces? A comparative analysis of infants and older children. J Pediatr Urol. 2018;14(6):537.e1–6.

Chapter 22
Minimally Invasive Pediatric Oncology for Renal Malignancies

Rohit Tejwani and Jonathan C. Routh

Introduction

Minimally invasive surgery (MIS) is increasingly used in adult tumor resections. MIS has been shown to be associated with reduced pain and reduced length of stay, with similar oncologic and long-term survival outcomes [1–4]. However, the use of MIS in pediatric cancer cases has been adopted slowly, due in part to concerns about oncologic outcomes including tumor spillage, ability to achieve negative margins, and nodal harvest, in addition to technical concerns due to tumor size in relatively small abdominal compartments [5]. A recent survey indicated that 88% of pediatric surgeons favor laparoscopic appendectomy, 90% favor laparoscopic fundoplication, but only 13% favor laparoscopic Wilms tumor (WT) resection [6]. However this group opinion is not exactly based on an overabundance of data; a recent Cochrane review found no published clinical trials comparing MIS to open surgery in pediatric abdominal malignancies [7].

A recently presented analysis of the National Inpatient Sample (NIS) database observed that children underwent MIS for resection of renal tumors at an overall low rate compared to open resections, and that MIS utilization varied by patient age. Children and adolescents had overall MIS proportions of 1% and 10%, respectively. However, after adjusting for covariates, there was no evidence of a significant association between surgery type and postoperative complications, inpatient LOS or cost [8]. A previous NIS analysis investigating MIS trends in pediatric urology patients found an MIS rate of 5.7% for both benign and oncologic urology surgeries. When stratified by surgical procedures, nephrectomy accounted for 30% of MIS procedures; however, these rates are likely conservative because hospitals

---

R. Tejwani · J. C. Routh (✉)
Duke University Medical Center, Division of Urologic Surgery, Department of Surgery, Durham, NC, USA
e-mail: rohit.tejwani@duke.edu; jonathan.routh@duke.edu

performing <5 MIS procedures per year were excluded [9]. Similarly, an analysis of the National Cancer Database compared MIS versus open surgery in children with neuroblastoma or WT. That analysis noted MIS rates for WT to be 5%, with MIS being more frequently used in older children (>5 years old) with smaller tumors (<10 cm) [5]. Overall, these large database studies strongly suggest an overall low utilization of MIS in pediatric patients with renal tumors; whether this low rate is appropriate is an open question, however.

One reported advantage of MIS for treatment of renal tumors is postoperative complication rate [10–12]. In adult patients, Semerjian et al. utilized the National Surgical Quality Improvement Program to examine 30-day outcomes between MIS and open kidney procedures. They found that MIS procedures had lower surgical site infections, sepsis, pneumonia, transfusion, and return to operating room rates events when adjusting for operative time [11]. This trend of improved postoperative outcomes is also seen in pediatric patients [7, 9]. The same study found that MIS had significantly lower odds of a post-operative complication compared to open surgery (OR 0.70) [9].

Other studies have found that MIS for renal tumors was associated with a shorter LOS. Phelps et al. found that MIS resection was associated with decreased blood loss, decreased operating time, and shorter hospital stays. The authors suggested that MIS may promote a sooner initiation of adjuvant chemotherapy [13]. Romao et al. compared laparoscopic to open radical nephrectomy in children with renal tumors and found that mean LOS was significantly shorter for the laparoscopic patients (3 vs 6 days) [14]. Of note, renal tumors undergoing laparoscopic nephrectomy in this study were significantly smaller than open (6.6 vs. 11.0 cm), potentially predisposing the latter group to a prolonged postoperative stay.

Another common issue with MIS use is its historically higher cost [15, 16]. However, with surgeon experience, improved laparoscopic instrumentation, and similar complication rates, cost associated with MIS procedures is declining and appears in more recent analyses to be comparable to open procedures [17–19].

Overall, the management of renal neoplasms is multifaceted and has evolved considerably over the past two decades as new operative techniques and medical therapies have come to the fore. Surgical intervention remains a foundational cornerstone of management strategies for most renal cancers, and is associated with relatively high cure rates for localized disease as well as oncologic benefits for those with metastatic disease and good performance status [20–22]. The surgical armamentarium has grown over time with the proliferation of MIS and paradigm shifts among patients and physicians favoring less-traumatic, less-invasive approaches when possible given improvements in cosmesis, postoperative pain, and recovery times without oncologic detriment when used appropriately [22]. Open, traditional laparoscopic, and – increasingly – robot-assisted laparoscopic approaches are commonly utilized at many centers today. The choice of operative modality as well as general procedure steps for each are explored here in greater detail.

Indications for MIS Nephrectomy or Partial Nephrectomy

In general, radiographic presence of a solid or complex cystic renal mass on imaging (Figs. 22.1 and 22.2) should prompt further evaluation and consideration for possible surgical intervention [20, 23]. Redemonstration of an enhancing mass on contrasted imaging, presence of symptoms, associated risk factors, and overall patient health may further influence the decision to pursue surgery. Biopsy-proven malignancy is not necessarily required prior to surgery barring suspicion for alternate etiologies for a mass (e.g. hematologic malignancy, infectious/ inflammatory processes, or concern for an alternate primary malignancy) [20]. As with most invasive procedures, surgical intervention may be less desirable in those with limited

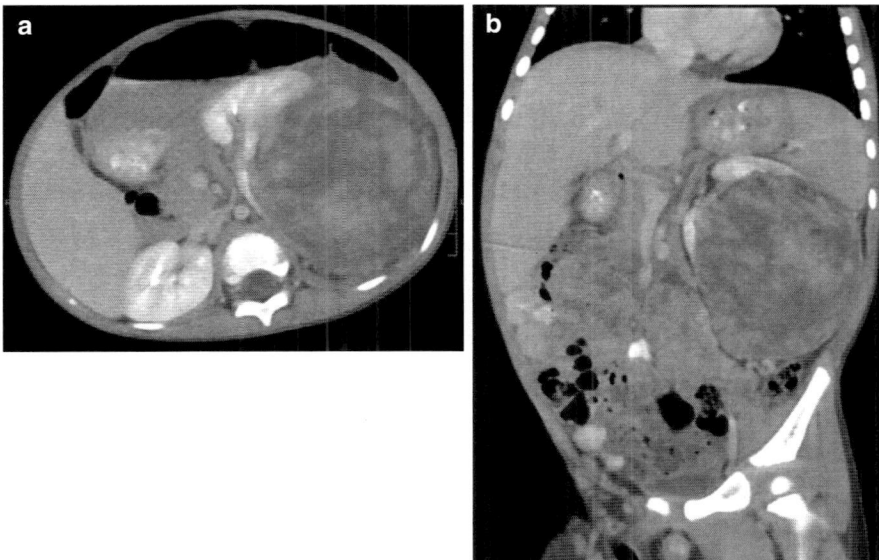

Fig. 22.1 Axial (**a**) and coronal (**b**) images of a left renal tumor, later found to be a clear cell sarcoma of the kidney

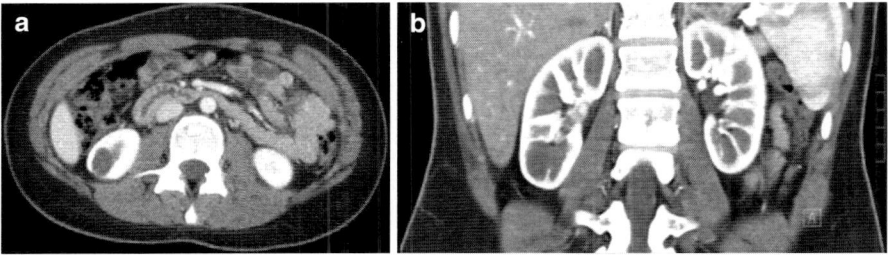

Fig. 22.2 Axial (**a**) and coronal (**b**) image of a right renal tumor, later found to be a cystic nephroma

life expectancy, who (when adequately informed of risks of oncologic progression) prefer not to undergo surgery, and for whom the risk of surgery itself far outweighs potential benefit (e.g. a highly comorbid individual for whom general anesthesia or surgical strain may be far riskier than potentially cancer-related mortality, or a diagnosis such as medullary renal cell carcinoma with a very grim prognosis). A small subset of individuals – mainly those with small, localized renal masses <2 cm for whom the risks of active treatment outweigh the oncologic benefit of treatment, may instead be actively monitored, although in children this strategy is rather more controversial than in adults [20]. Conversely, patients with widely metastatic disease and multiple comorbidities may benefit from transitioning to medical management immediately rather than surgical intervention.

Modality Selection

Radical Versus Partial Nephrectomy

The use of radical nephrectomy for the purposes of oncologic management dates back to the nineteenth century in the United States and remains the benchmark standard of treatment for many renal masses – particularly for larger tumors (>7 cm), those without clear radiographic or physical demarcation within the renal parenchyma (potentially suggestive of more aggressive disease-types), those with spread beyond the kidney (e.g. cT3 tumors or higher), and for masses which are in high-risk locations within the kidney (e.g. primarily endophytic masses, those closely associated with major vessels, etc.) [24]. Radical nephrectomy for a localized mass further provides more definitive oncologic control [21, 25]. However, this occurs at the expense of presumably functional renal tissue in most individuals, with potential long-term consequences for overall renal function and risk for development of chronic kidney disease (CKD) [25, 26].

Partial nephrectomy, initially also primitively pioneered in the nineteenth century (primarily for benign renal pathologies), remained limited in use until the latter part of the twentieth century as better imaging modalities helped more clearly define small, localized tumors combined with advances in understanding of the need for nephron preservation and comparable oncologic outcomes in carefully selected patients [27]. Today, partial nephrectomy is the preferred treatment modality for small (cT1a–cT2) localized renal masses, cases with bilateral renal involvement (e.g. hereditary syndromes), in individuals with compromised baseline renal function, and in individuals with either functional or anatomical solitary kidneys [20, 21, 28, 29].

Clinical decision tools such as the R.E.N.A.L. Nephrometry Score by Kutikov et al., the PADUA classification system by Ficarra et al., and the C-Index method by Simmons et al. have been developed to aid surgeons in determining the appropriateness of radical versus partial nephrectomy based on tumor characteristics and potential tumor proximity to critical renal structures such as the collecting system and renal vasculature [30–32].

Open Versus Laparoscopic Versus Robotic Approaches

Pioneered in the 1990s, the use of laparoscopy in radical nephrectomy sparked a significant shift in practice toward MIS approaches for many patients with renal masses [33]. Whereas open-approach nephrectomies frequently require large, often painful abdominal or flank incisions, both traditional "straight" laparoscopy as well as single-incision and robot-assisted approaches allow for comparable oncologic outcomes with improved postoperative outcomes in terms of hospital length of stay, cosmesis, analgesic demand, and speed of return to normal physical functioning [34]. Patients with localized disease without evidence of vascular involvement, extracapsular invasion/locoregional spread, and for whom laparoscopy would not otherwise be unsafe are more suitable for MIS approaches [20, 22]. Conversely, patients with very large tumors, bilateral involvement requiring simultaneous intervention, concern for/evidence of tumor thrombus, vascular or other local spread, or those with complex or altered anatomy (e.g. those with multiple prior intraabdominal surgeries) may instead benefit from the improved exposure and options for tissue dissection and quick vascular control afforded by open approaches [20, 31].

Straight laparoscopy is challenging, in part, due to the rigidity of traditional laparoscopic instruments. For partial nephrectomy, where operative speed to minimize warm ischemia time and precision to Consequently, robotic approaches have become more popular for MIS partial nephrectomy (RPN), given the articulating instruments and multiple arms of modern robotic systems which provide a significant benefit to surgeons in terms of dexterity [35, 36]. Indeed, several analyses have found improved outcomes vis-à-vis intra- and post-operative complications for RPN versus LPN [37, 38]. Similar to radical nephrectomy, patients with larger, more endophytic tumors, those with concern for vascular For partial nephrectomy, where operative speed to minimize warm ischemia time and precision to involvement, or those with complex anatomy may instead benefit from pursuit of open PN rather than an MIS approach. Additionally, use of robotic approaches have been associated with increased procedural costs and operative times [38, 39].

Pre-procedural Care

During initial evaluation, a thorough history and physical should be collected – including a complete past surgical history, past medical history, and social history. Young patients, those with multifocal or bilateral tumors, or with a strong family history of renal malignancy should undergo genetic counseling [20]. Lab evaluation should include an assessment of the patient's baseline kidney function and determination of CKD stage if present. Patients for whom CKD is found should be referred to nephrology prior to surgery [20]. Multiphase cross-sectional abdominal imaging should also be obtained to thoroughly characterize any suspicious mass(es), as well as the patient's renovascular anatomy which may influence surgical planning.

Shared decision-making along with frank assessments of surgeon proficiency should guide surgical modality choice when otherwise equivocal options are present. Patients should be informed of, and understand, common postoperative complications and the surgeon's experience with a particular surgical modality. Precautions to reduce the risk of such complications, such as careful intraoperative positioning, minimizing surgical and anesthesia time, and the use of routine prophylactic measures (e.g. compression boots to prevent DVT, intravenous antibiosis to reduce the risk of surgical infection) should be utilized.

Intraoperative Details

General Principles

Access to the kidney may be obtained either transperitoneally or extraperitoneally depending on the patient's anatomy, surgical history, and tumor location. Transperitoneal approaches tend to be more commonly utilized for most situations; this is particularly true for pediatric and adolescent tumors, where working space is often limited [40, 41]. Regardless of modality choice, each entails careful dissection of the kidney away from surrounding structures and excellent control of the renal hilum to prevent potentially catastrophic vascular injury. Radical nephrectomy entails the removal of the entire kidney, including Gerota's fascia, along with (frequently) the proximal ureter. Partial nephrectomy is limited to resection of a mass (or masses) with as little excess parenchymal tissue removed as needed to obtain negative margins. Automatic adrenalectomy in the absence of tumor involvement, as well as lymphadenectomy in the absence of clinically-concerning abnormalities may not be necessary [20, 42].

Each procedure below assumes the following steps have already been completed: induction of anesthesia, intubation, initial DVT and antibiotic prophylaxis measures, Foley catheter placement and bladder decompression, and orogastric/nasogastric tube placement and gastric decompression.

Laparoscopic Radical Nephrectomy (LRN)

The patient is placed in a modified flank position with the target kidney facing the ceiling. The patient should be positioned in such a way so as to align their pelvis with the table break if present. All pressure points should be extensively padded, with particular attention to the ipsilateral arm, and contralateral shoulder and axilla to prevent plexopathy. Once adequately padded and secured, the table may be flexed; if positioned appropriately, this should increase available working space for trocar placement [41]. The patient's abdomen and flank should then be prepped and draped widely. Pneumoperitoneum can then be established using the Varess or Hasson techniques [40]. Multiple trocar templates may be used depending on surgeon preference and the patient's anatomy. Frequently, surgeons employ a single camera port (located at or slightly lateral to the umbilicus), 1–2 working ports, and 1–2 assistant ports [40]. Following surveillance of the abdomen, additional trocars may be added as needed. A hand port for hand-assisted nephrectomy may also be placed, particularly for larger tumors or if concerned for vascular involvement. For single-incision laparoscopic surgery (SILS), we typically employ a 4 cm Pfannenstiel incision gel port with or without an umbilical assistant or camera port (Fig. 22.3).

After surveillance of the abdomen for trocar insertion injuries, the colon is mobilized via dissection along the white line of Toldt using judicious electrocautery cranially to the hepatic flexure (right) and splenic flexure (left) and toward the iliac vessels caudally (Fig. 22.4). The colon is then gently rolled medially to expose the anterior aspect of Gerota's fascia. Additional sub-xiphoid or sub-costal 5 mm port placements to facilitate cephalad retraction of the liver or spleen may be useful [40]. On the right, the duodenum is then gently mobilized and rolled medially (Kocher maneuver), exposing the inferior vena cava (IVC).

Caudally, the ureter and gonadal vein are identified coursing along the medial aspect of the psoas muscle. The ureter is freed by gentle dissection in the plane between it and the gonadal vein so as to prevent injury to the latter and allow for elevation of the former. This dissection continues cranially, leading to the lower pole of the kidney which should be mobilized, and eventually, to the renal hilum.

The renal artery and vein should be gently skeletonized, clipped or stapled, and transected. The remaining attachments along the superior aspect of the kidney are subsequently dissected. The adrenal gland may be mobilized away from the kidney if uninvolved. The ureter may then be clipped or stapled and transected, liberating

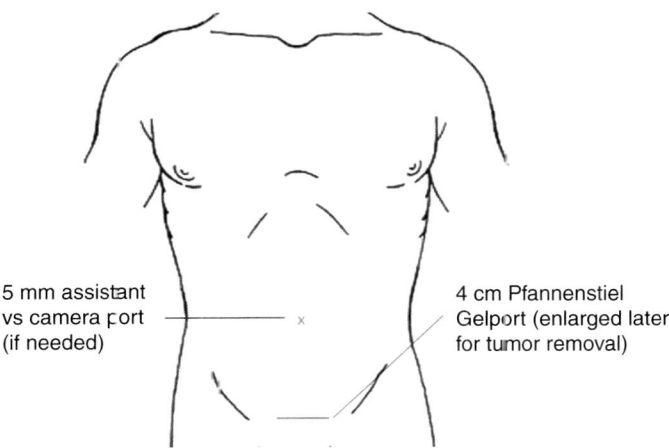

Fig. 22.3 Example port placement for a laparoscopic-assisted single incision (SILS) radical nephrectomy

Fig. 22.4 Representative intraoperative image of a laparoscopic-assisted radical nephrectomy via a single Pfannenstiel incision (SILS nephrectomy)

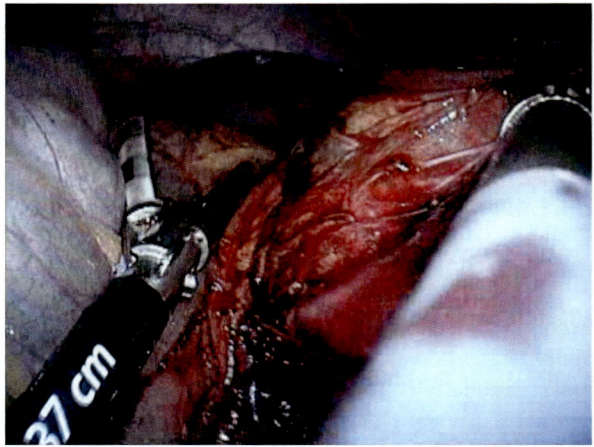

the kidney from any remaining attachments [41]. The kidney is then placed in an endoscopic retrieval bag, and extracted via an expanded port site or Pfannenstiel incision (Fig. 22.3) [33, 41]. After ensuring hemostasis and absence of surrounding organ injury, pneumoperitoneum is released, trocars removed, and fascia and skin closed.

Robotic Radical Nephrectomy (RRN)

In the robotic approach to radical nephrectomy (RRN), the patient is similarly positioned on the contralateral flank to the target kidney. A camera port is placed lateral to the umbilicus, and additional robotic ports placed in the anterior axillary line superior to the iliac crest and inferior the costal margin under vision, taking care to ensure each port is spaced appropriately to prevent robotic arm clashing (usually 8 cm or more apart). A 12 mm bedside assistant port may be placed medially during this time as well (Fig. 22.5) [40]. The robot is then docked, and dissection proceeds as above.

Laparoscopic (LPN) and Robotic (RPN) Partial Nephrectomy

The patient is positioned in a similar modified flank position as described above. Once pneumoperitoneum is established, trocar placement occurs in a similar fashion to LRN and RRN. Caution should be taken to ensure assistant ports are of sufficient caliber (12–15 mm) to accommodate vascular clamps, bolsters, and other instruments which may be required intraoperatively [43, 44].

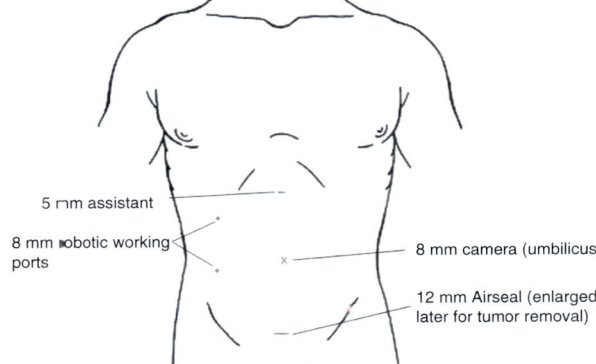

Fig. 22.5 Example port placement for a robotic-assisted radical nephrectomy, in this case for a right renal lesion using a Si robot

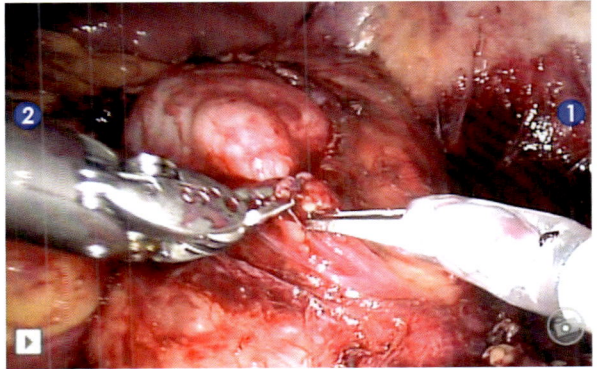

Fig. 22.6 Representative intraoperative image of a robotic-assisted radical nephrectomy

For both LPN and RFN, dissection and mobilization of the kidney proceeds similarly to the technique described for LRN and RRN. The colon is reflected off the kidney, liver and spleen retracted, and the ureter and gonadal vessel identified and traced back to their origins. The renal hilum is thoroughly dissected, ensuring adequate exposure of the main renal artery and vein. Extreme caution must be taken to identify any accessory or aberrant renal vasculature, which should also be dissected free [44]. In the absence of adrenal involvement, the adrenal vasculature should also be identified and the adrenal gland mobilized off of the kidney. The kidney should be mobilized to the extent needed to both adequately control the renal vasculature, and to access and completely excise the mass in question [40].

Gerota's fascia is then entered away from the mass and the perirenal fat gently dissected free except overlying the mass itself (Fig. 22.6). Intraoperative ultrasound may be used to better delineate the boundaries of the lesion, and the mass may be demarcated using an electrocautery hook (LPN) or monopolar scissor tips (RPN) circumferentially [40, 41, 44]. Prior to clamping the renal vasculature, the surgeon should pause to confirm the presence of critical personnel and equipment in the operating room.

Once the kidney is mobilized and defatted, mass demarcated, and hilum isolated, bulldog or Satinsky clamps may then be placed around both the renal artery, vein, and any accessory renal vasculature [40, 43, 44]. Intravenous mannitol may be administered shortly before this time for the theoretical prevention of free-radical injury to the ischemic kidney, though data on the efficacy of this remains mixed [45]. The mass is then excised sharply to prevent thermal injury from electrocautery to surrounding parenchyma. Margin samples may be sent for intraoperative pathology review if available. Collecting system injuries, if present, should be repaired intraoperatively followed by renorrhaphy and capsulotomy repair. Multiple techniques to do this have been described, most commonly involving oversewing the resection bed with 2-0 to 4-0 V-lock suture, and further closing the capsular defect with binding-like 0-absorbable suture with or without the use of hemostatic bolsters [46, 47]. Vascular clamps should subsequently be removed, and warm ischemia time noted.

Once resection bed hemostasis is confirmed, the specimen may be extracted using an endoscopic bag and extracted via an enlarged port site. The abdomen is again surveilled for bleeding or surrounding organ injury. Pneumoperitoneum is subsequently released, trocars removed, and port sites closed.

Conclusion

In conclusion, management of renal neoplasms is multifaceted and has evolved considerably over the past two decades as new operative techniques and medical therapies have come to the fore. MIS is a viable albeit rarely used option for renal malignancies in children, with similar outcomes as compared to open procedures across multiple analyses of multiple data sources.

References

1. Elfenbein DM, Scarborough JE, Speicher PJ, Scheri RP. Comparison of laparoscopic versus open adrenalectomy: results from American College of Surgeons-National Surgery Quality Improvement Project. J Surg Res. 2013;184(1):216–20.
2. Miller DC, Taub DA, Dunn RL, Wei JT, Hollenbeck BK. Laparoscopy for renal cell carcinoma: diffusion versus regionalization? J Urol. 2006;176(3):1102–6; discussion 1106–1107.
3. Veldkamp R, Kuhry E, Hop WC, et al. Laparoscopic surgery versus open surgery for colon cancer: short-term outcomes of a randomised trial. Lancet Oncol. 2005;6(7):477–84.
4. Hu JC, Gu X, Lipsitz SR, Barry MJ, D'Amico AV, Weinberg AC, Keating NL. Comparative effectiveness of minimally invasive vs open radical prostatectomy. JAMA. 2009;302(14):1557–64.
5. Ezekian B, Englum BR, Gulack BC, et al. Comparing oncologic outcomes after minimally invasive and open surgery for pediatric neuroblastoma and Wilms tumor. Pediatr Blood Cancer. 2018;65(1) https://doi.org/10.1002/pbc.26755.
6. Jones VS, Cohen RC. Two decades of minimally invasive pediatric surgery-taking stock. J Pediatr Surg. 2008;43(9):1653–9.

7. Eriksen KO, Johal NS, Mushtaq I. Minimally invasive surgery in management of renal tumours in children. Transl Pediatr. 2016 5(4):305–14.
8. Simmons K, Chandrapal J, Wolf S, et al. Open versus minimally-invasive surgical techniques in pediatric renal tumors: a population-level analysis. Paper presented at: Annual Meeting of the Southeastern Section of the American Urological Association, New Orleans, LA, 2020.
9. Tejwani R, Young BJ Wang HS, et al. Open versus minimally invasive surgical approaches in pediatric urology: trends in utilization and complications. J Pediatr Urol. 2017;13(3):283 e281–9.
10. Liu JJ, Leppert JT, Maxwell BG, Panousis P, Chung BI. Trends and perioperative outcomes for laparoscopic and robotic nephrectomy using the National Surgical Quality Improvement Program (NSQIP) database. Urol Oncol. 2014;32(4):473–9.
11. Semerjian A, Zettervall SL, Amdur R, Jarrett TW, Vaziri K. 30-day morbidity and mortality outcomes of prolonged minimally invasive kidney procedures compared with shorter open procedures: National Surgical Quality Improvement Program Analysis. J Endourol. 2015;29(7):830–7.
12. Xia L, Wang X, Xu T, Guzzo TJ. Systematic review and meta-analysis of comparative studies reporting perioperative outcomes of robot-assisted partial nephrectomy versus open partial nephrectomy. J Endourol. 2017;31(9):893–909.
13. Phelps HM, Lovvorn HN 3rd. Minimally invasive surgery in pediatric surgical oncology. Children (Basel). 2018;5(12):158.
14. Romao RL, Weber B, Gerstle JT, et al. Comparison between laparoscopic and open radical nephrectomy for the treatment of primary renal tumors in children: single-center experience over a 5-year period. J Pediatr Urol. 2014;10(3):488–94.
15. Springer C, Inferrera A, Pini G, Mohammed N, Fornara P, Greco F. Costs analysis of laparoendoscopic, single-site laparoscopic and open surgery for cT1 renal masses in a European high-volume centre. World J Urol. 2014;32(6):1501–10.
16. Mahida JB, Cooper JN, Herz D, et al. Utilization and costs associated with robotic surgery in children. J Surg Res. 2015;199(1):169–76.
17. Jacobs BL, Seelam R, Lai JC, et al. Cost analysis of treatments for ureteropelvic junction obstruction. J Endourol. 2017;31(2):204–9.
18. Fitch K, Engel T, Bochner A. Cost differences between open and minimally invasive surgery. Manag Care. 2015;24:40–8.
19. Mahomed AA, McLean V. Cost analysis of minimally invasive surgery in a pediatric setting. J Laparoendosc Adv Surg Tech A. 2007;17(3):375–9.
20. Campbell S, Uzzo RG, Allaf ME, et al. Renal mass and localized renal cancer: AUA guideline. J Urol. 2017;198(3):520–9.
21. Van Poppel H, Da Pozzo L, Albrecht W, et al. A prospective, randomised EORTC intergroup phase 3 study comparing the oncologic outcome of elective nephron-sparing surgery and radical nephrectomy for low-stage renal cell carcinoma. Eur Urol. 2011;59(4):543–52.
22. MacLennan S, Imamura M, Lapitan MC, et al. Systematic review of perioperative and quality-of-life outcomes following surgical management of localised renal cancer. Eur Urol. 2012;62(6):1097–117.
23. Escudier B, Porta C, Schmidinger M, et al. Renal cell carcinoma: ESMO Clinical Practice Guidelines for diagnosis, treatment and follow-up††Approved by the ESMO Guidelines Committee: September 2008, last update January 2019. This publication supersedes the previously published version—Ann Oncol. 2016;27(Suppl 5):v58–v68. Ann Oncol. 2019;30(5):706–20.
24. Wotkowicz C, Libertino JA. Renal cell cancer: radical nephrectomy. BJU Int. 2007;99(5b):1231–8.
25. Colombo JR Jr, Haber GP, Jelovsek JE, Lane B, Novick AC, Gill IS. Seven years after laparoscopic radical nephrectomy: oncologic and renal functional outcomes. Urology. 2008;71(6):1149–54.
26. Huang WC, Levey AS, Serio AM, et al. Chronic kidney disease after nephrectomy in patients with renal cortical tumours: a retrospective cohort study. Lancet Oncol. 2006;7(9):735–40.

27. Herr HW. A history of partial nephrectomy for renal tumors. J Urol. 2005;173(3):705–8.
28. Crépel M, Jeldres C, Perrotte P, et al. Nephron-sparing surgery is equally effective to radical nephrectomy for T1BN0M0 renal cell carcinoma: a population-based assessment. Urology. 2010;75(2):271–5.
29. Volpe A, Amparore D, Mottrie A. Treatment outcomes of partial nephrectomy for T1b tumours. Curr Opin Urol. 2013;23(5):403–10.
30. Simhan J, Smaldone MC, Tsai KJ, et al. Objective measures of renal mass anatomic complexity predict rates of major complications following partial nephrectomy. Eur Urol. 2011;60(4):724–30.
31. Kutikov A, Uzzo RG. The R.E.N.A.L. nephrometry score: a comprehensive standardized system for quantitating renal tumor size, location and depth. J Urol. 2009;182(3):844–53.
32. Simmons MN, Ching CB, Samplaski MK, Park CH, Gill IS. Kidney tumor location measurement using the C index method. J Urol. 2010;183(5):1708–13.
33. Clayman RV, Kavoussi LR, Soper NJ, et al. Laparoscopic nephrectomy. N Engl J Med. 1991;324(19):1370–1.
34. Wilson CH, Sanni A, Rix DA, Soomro NA. Laparoscopic versus open nephrectomy for live kidney donors. Cochrane Database Syst Rev. 2011;(11):CD006124.
35. Camarillo DB, Krummel TM, Salisbury JK Jr. Robotic technology in surgery: past, present, and future. Am J Surg. 2004;188(4A Suppl):2S–15S.
36. Wang HS, Tejwani R, Cannon GM Jr, Gargollo PC, Wiener JS, Routh JC. Open versus minimally invasive ureteroneocystostomy: a population-level analysis. J Pediatr Urol. 2016;12(4):232.e1–6.
37. Benway BM, Bhayani SB, Rogers CG, et al. Robot assisted partial nephrectomy versus laparoscopic partial nephrectomy for renal tumors: a multi-institutional analysis of perioperative outcomes. J Urol. 2009;182(3):866–72.
38. Jeong IG, Khandwala YS, Kim JH, et al. Association of robotic-assisted vs laparoscopic radical nephrectomy with perioperative outcomes and health care costs, 2003 to 2015. JAMA. 2017;318(16):1561–8.
39. Asimakopoulos AD, Miano R, Annino F, et al. Robotic radical nephrectomy for renal cell carcinoma: a systematic review. BMC Urol. 2014;14:75.
40. Smith JA, Howards SS, Preminger GM, Hinman F. Hinman's atlas of urologic surgery. 3rd ed. Philadelphia: Elsevier/Saunders; 2012.
41. Wein AJ, Kavoussi LR, Campbell MF. Campbell-Walsh urology/editor-in-chief, Alan J. Wein; [editors, Louis R. Kavoussi … et al.]. 10th ed. Philadelphia: Elsevier Saunders; 2012.
42. O'Malley RL, Godoy G, Kanofsky JA, Taneja SS. The necessity of adrenalectomy at the time of radical nephrectomy: a systematic review. J Urol. 2009;181(5):2009–17.
43. Ho H, Schwentner C, Neururer R, Steiner H, Bartsch G, Peschel R. Robotic-assisted laparoscopic partial nephrectomy: surgical technique and clinical outcomes at 1 year. BJU Int. 2009;103(5):663–8.
44. Sukumar S, Rogers CG. Robotic partial nephrectomy: surgical technique. BJU Int. 2011;108(6b):942–7.
45. Spaliviero M, Power NE, Murray KS, et al. Intravenous mannitol versus placebo during partial nephrectomy in patients with Normal kidney function: a double-blind, clinically-integrated, randomized trial. Eur Urol. 2018;73(1):53–9.
46. Benway BM, Wang AJ, Cabello JM, Bhayani SB. Robotic partial nephrectomy with sliding-clip renorrhaphy: technique and outcomes. Eur Urol. 2009;55(3):592–9.
47. Shikanov S, Wille M, Large M, et al. Knotless closure of the collecting system and renal parenchyma with a novel barbed suture during laparoscopic porcine partial nephrectomy. J Endourol. 2009;23(7):1157–60.

Chapter 23
The Use of Minimally Invasive RPLND in the Treatment of Para-Testicular Rhabdomyosarcoma in the Pediatric Population

Stephen W. Reese, Emily Ji, Venkat M. Ramakrishnan, Andrew A. Wagner, and Richard S. Lee

Introduction

Tumors of the para-testis are tumors that arise from the spermatic cord, epididymis, tunica vaginalis, and any vestigial remnants. Para-testicular rhabdomyosarcoma (PT-RMS), a tumor of mesenchymal origin, is the most common malignant tumor of the para-testis, accounting for 7% of all rhabdomyosarcomas and approximately 12% of all pediatric scrotal tumors [1]. Age at presentation is bimodal, with peak incidence occurring at 5 years of age and again at 16 years of age [1]. The most common PT-RMS, the embryonal histologic subtype, carries a favorable prognosis and commonly presents with a palpable, painless scrotal mass that is often detected early [2, 3]. Metastases occur primarily via the lymphatics, although local and hematogenous spread are also possible [4, 5]. At time of presentation, 25% to 40% of patients with PT-RMS will have lymph node involvement [6–8].

PT-RMS patients are sorted into low, medium, and high risk categories based on TNM stage, tumor histology, and post-surgical resection margins [9]. Nodal involvement increases the stage and risk categories of the disease, and is necessary for determining radiation and adjuvant chemotherapy regimens [9, 10]. Retroperitoneal

S. W. Reese (✉) · E. Ji · V. M. Ramakrishnan
Brigham and Women's Hospital, Harvard Medical School, Department of Urology, Division of Urological Surgery, Boston, MA, USA
e-mail: emily_ji@hms.harvard.edu; vramakrishnan@bwh.harvard.edu

A. A. Wagner
Beth Israel Deaconess Medical Center, Harvard Medical School, Department of Urology, Boston, MA, USA
e-mail: awagner@bidmc.harvard.edu

R. S. Lee
Boston Children's Hospital, Harvard Medical School, Department of Urology, Boston, MA, USA
e-mail: richard.lee@childrens.harvard.edu

© Springer Nature Switzerland AG 2020
P. C. Gargollo (ed.), *Minimally Invasive and Robotic-Assisted Surgery in Pediatric Urology*, https://doi.org/10.1007/978-3-030-57219-8_23

lymph node dissection (RPLND) has historically been utilized to accurately stage these patients, as radiographic imaging of the retroperitoneum has been shown to be suboptimal in identifying patients with micro-metastatic disease [11].

Multi-modal approaches are employed in the treatment of these malignancies, including chemotherapy, radiation, and surgery. The mainstay of surgical treatment is primary excision of the tumor via an inguinal incision. RPLND is utilized as a diagnostic step to determine the degree of involvement of the regional lymphatic drainage of the testicle. The role of surgery in the treatment of testicular and paratesticular malignancies continues to evolve with advancements in chemo-radiation therapies, imaging technologies, and surgical innovation.

The traditional approach to RPLND in the treatment of these tumors and primary germ cell malignancies of the testicle has been via an open transabdominal or thoracoabdominal approach. This was considered to be a morbid surgery requiring an extensive dissection. With the advent of minimally invasive surgery in the 1990s, there has been a growing interest in applying these techniques to RPLND. With appropriate experience and expertise, the utilization of laparoscopic RPLND (L-RPLND) and robotic-assisted RLPND (RA-RPLND) offer a potential alternative to the open approach with potential for decreased peri-operative morbidity and enhanced surgical recovery.

As in the adult population, the application of minimally invasive techniques to the pediatric population must be undertaken by experienced surgeons well-versed in these techniques without any compromise in oncologic care. Indeed, while minimally invasive techniques offer the possibility for enhanced recovery, the open surgical approach with sound oncologic principals continues to remain the standard of care and should be utilized if appropriate experience is not available.

This chapter summarizes the use of RPLND in the pediatric population, with specific emphasis on the evolution and adoption of minimally invasive approaches. We discuss minimally invasive surgical techniques, associated complications, and oncologic outcomes. While we focus our discussion in the context of PT-RMS, the most common pediatric indication for RPLND, the techniques described here apply to other indications for RPLND such as patients with testicular germ cell tumors.

RPLND

Indications for RPLND

In the pediatric patient, the primary indication for undergoing RPLND is in the setting of PT-RMS. Based on the work from the Intergroup Rhabdomyosarcoma Study Group (IRSG), current recommendations for the use of RPLND by the Children's Oncology Group (COG) are for (1) patients younger than 10 years of age who have evidence of enlarged nodes on CT scan and (2) patients greater than 10 years of age regardless of radiographic imaging findings [12].

These recommendations are primarily derived from historical antecedents. The IRSG conducted a series of studies from 1973 to 1991 (IRS I, II, III) that required patients to undergo RPLND for staging and to guide treatment. However, due to RPLND morbidity and concern for overtreatment, routine RPLND was not recommended during the IRSG IV study (1991 to 1997) and was only reserved for patients with radiographic evidence of retroperitoneal involvement [13]. Unfortunately, those patients were noted to have a higher incidence of retroperitoneal nodal relapse, particularly in children over 10 years of age, and worse outcomes [6, 14]. As a result, since 2003, the COG has advocated for the use of RPLND in the circumstances listed above in order to achieve better staging and oncologic outcomes [12].

However, despite COG recommendations and multiple studies demonstrating improved overall and evidence free survival [15–17], surgical compliance with these recommendations is poor and RPLND continues to be underutilized within the pediatric population. Multiple studies of PT-RMS patients have found that the 2003 COG recommendation have not significantly changed clinical practice and nearly one-third to up to one-half of adolescent patients with PT-RMS do not receive RPLND [15, 17].

Anatomic Considerations

The theoretical rationale for utilizing RPLND to treat PT-RMS and germ cell tumors arises from the consistent and predictable anatomy of the lymphatic drainage of the testis (Fig. 23.1). Lymphatic drainage occurs via the para-aortic pathway, with lymphatic channels originating in the spermatic cord moving cephalad along the retroperitoneal nodal chain. The sentinel nodes of the right testicle are the interaortocaval nodes located at the level of the second lumbar vertebral body. In contrast, the sentinel nodes of the left testicle are the left para-aortic nodal group, which lies inferior to the renal vein. Lymphatic drainage also proceeds in a right-to-left direction, as lymphatic drainage from the aortocaval nodes travels via the cisterna chyli and ultimately into the thoracic duct. For this reason, contralateral tumor involvement is appreciated more often in right-sided tumors, following the natural flow of lymphatic fluid. Involvement of the iliac nodes may occur in bulky retroperitoneal disease via retrograde flow, tumor invasion into the scrotum, or as a result of a scrotal incision as opposed to an inguinal approach during orchiectomy [18].

Defining the neuroanatomy of the retroperitoneum was paramount in preventing ejaculatory dysfunction from RPLND [19]. The nerve-sparing RPLND technique pioneered by Donohue and colleagues significantly reduced the risk of ejaculatory dysfunction after RPLND without compromising oncologic outcomes [20]. Antegrade movement of semen through the urethra requires the coordinated events of emission and ejaculation [21]. Emission starts with the closure of the bladder neck (mediated via the sympathetic nervous system) followed by deposition of semen and secretions into the posterior urethra by way of contractions of the seminal vesicles, vas deferens, Cowper's glands, and prostate. Ejaculation is the

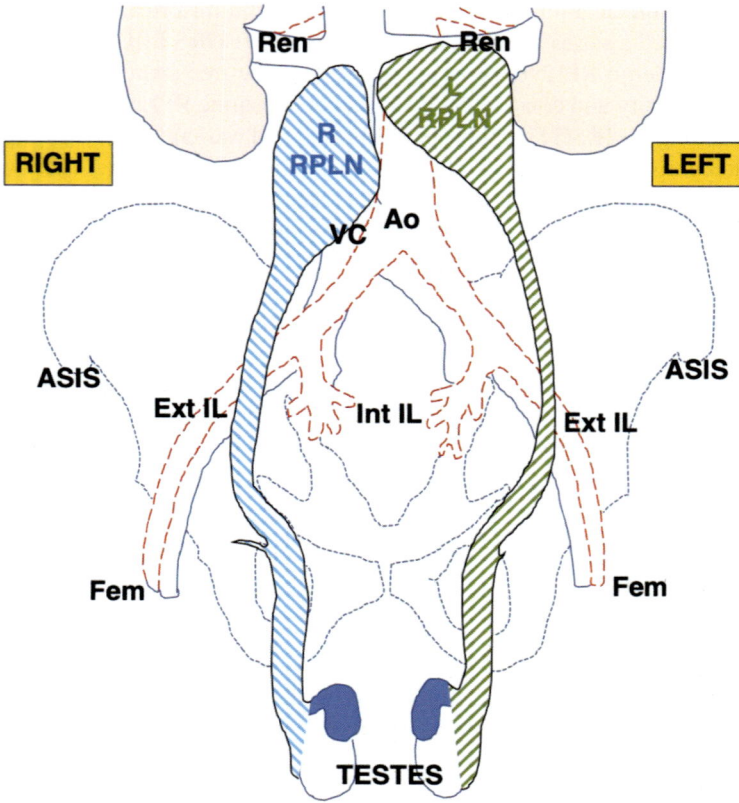

Fig. 23.1 Lymphatic drainage of the testes. The testes are drained via the para-aortic pathway. Lymphatic channels originating in the spermatic cord proceed in a cephalad direction. Note that lymph drainage proceeds from right to left, and therefore right-sided tumors are more likely to have contralateral involvement. Also note that the inter-aortocaval nodes are located at L2

expulsion of semen distally through the urethra and is mediated via a parasympathetic reflex along with contraction of the bulbocavernosus muscle, which is somatically innervated by the pudendal nerve.

The sympathetic nervous system is responsible for emission and closure of the bladder neck and mediated by nerves exiting the ventral roots of T12 through L3. These nerves form the sympathetic chain and are found medial to the vena cava on the right and aorta on the left [18]. Caudally, these nerve fibers converge to create the hypogastric plexus at the bifurcation of the abdominal aorta. Traveling along the right and left hypogastric nerves, these fibers ultimately form the pelvic plexus. The nerves terminate by draping the peri-rectum, seminal vesicles, bladder, and prostate. Therefore, disruption of this nervous system complex may lead to ejaculatory dysfunction. However, with careful nerve-sparing technique, antegrade ejaculation can be preserved in over 90% of patients without oncologic compromise [20, 22, 23].

Surgical Approach

Theoretical Benefits of a Minimally Invasive Approach

With the advent of minimally invasive techniques in the 1990s, there has been broad interest in applying such techniques to reduce the morbidity of open RPLND. In the treatment of germ cell tumors, conventional laparoscopy (L-RPLND) was the first attempt at a minimally invasive approach. Early laparoscopic efforts were performed primarily for staging. Attempts at complete dissection were noted to be technically challenging given the rigid arms of laparoscopic instruments, making dissection of the retrocaval and retroaortic nodes difficult. As such, the laparoscopic approach has not been widely adopted. Nevertheless, in patients with germ cell tumors, laparoscopy contributed to less blood loss, a shorter hospital stay, and shorter convalescence [24, 25].

The robotic-assisted RPLND (RA-RPLND) combined the benefits of a minimally invasive approach with the ability to articulate the wrists for finer, more precise movements, and visualize previously inaccessible tight spaces. RA-RPLND is also benefitted by a faster learning curve compared to traditional laparoscopy in various other procedures within the surgical literature [26, 27].

Recent multi-institutional data in the adult germ-cell literature have demonstrated that minimally invasive approaches are associated with enhanced peri-operative outcomes [28–30] while maintaining oncologic equivalency [31]. There is also the possibility of enhanced recovery in experienced hands. In the pediatric literature, various case series have demonstrated that RA-RPLND is technically feasible, safe, and associated with improved peri-operative outcomes [32, 33].

In patients with PT-RMS, the primary goal of lymph node harvesting is to appropriately stage the disease and guide treatment. While there is no definitive data that RPLND is therapeutically beneficial for PT-RMS, studies using modern RPLND techniques have yet to be conducted to address this question. For current purposes, the utilization of a robotic approach can provide adequate exposure and similar oncologic surgical principles with the additional benefit of shorter convalescence and shorter time to chemotherapy commencement.

Operative Planning

Surgically, RA-RPLND can be approached in either a transperitoneal or extraperitoneal fashion, with most surgeons preferring the former as it provides a familiar working environment, more expansive operative space, and ease of bilateral dissection if necessary. Patients may also be positioned supine or in the flank position. With the patient positioned on his flank, the bowel can be pushed medially to expose the retroperitoneum. Patients can be placed in the supine position and rotated left/right if properly secured to the bed.

Another technique described in the supine position requires a "bottom-up dissection". The patient is placed in Trendelenberg position and the peritoneum is tacked along the cephalad anterior abdominal wall, creating a "hammock." The robotic system can be docked over the shoulders and the dissection proceed from inferior to superior. This approach allows for better exposure for a bilateral dissection but has less working space and the potential for unfamiliar angles. Notably, concerns for bilateral approaches are decreased with new robotic systems that allow for easier docking and bed repositioning during surgery.

Patient Positioning and Port Placement for RPLND

After the patient is intubated, an orogastric tube and Foley catheter are inserted. The patient is then positioned in either the supine or modified flank position (45 degrees), with the side of the dissection elevated off the bed. In general, particularly when using the *Intuitive Surgical daVinci Si Robot,* we prefer to approach the dissection with the patient in the modified flank position. Great care is taken to appropriately pad the patient, especially over bony prominences, to prevent nerve injury, pressure sores, and rhabdomyolysis. Intraperitoneal access is achieved via a Veress needle at the umbilicus and the abdomen is insufflated to a pressure of 12 mmHg. An alternative access point is via Palmer's point. See Fig. 23.2 for placement of robotic ports and set-up.

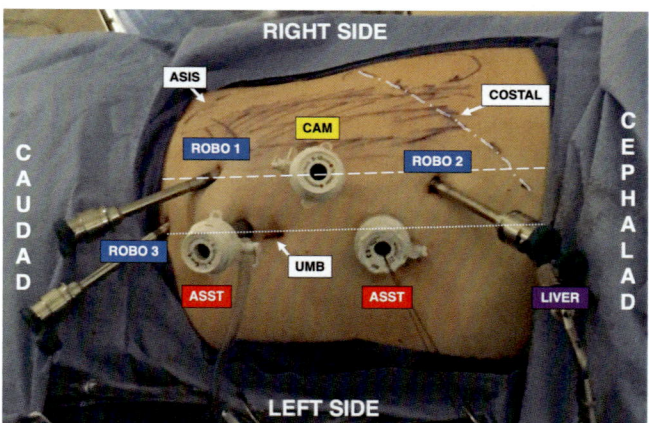

Fig. 23.2 Robotic port placement for RPLND. Pictured here is robotic port placement for a right-sided template RPLND, with the patient in right lateral decubitus position, and the caudad and cephalad positions identified. The trocar for robotic arm 1 (ROBO 1, 8 mm), robotic arm 2 (ROBO 2, 8 mm), and the camera port (CAM, 12 mm) are all placed along the mid-clavicular line (wide dashed line) ipsilaterally. The trocar for robotic arm 3 (ROBO 3, 8 mm), both assistant ports (ASST, 12 mm), and the liver retractor (LIVER, 5 mm) are all placed along the umbilical midline (narrow dashed line). For anatomic reference, the costal margin (COSTAL; curved dashed line), umbilicus (UMB), and anterior superior iliac spine (ASIS) are also identified

Spermatic Cord Dissection

Depending on the side of the primary lesion, the surgical dissection should begin by dissecting the spermatic vessels proximally and clipping near the IVC or renal vein. The dissection is carried distally into the internal inguinal ring and every effort is made to identify and resect the spermatic cord stump suture placed during the initial orchiectomy. Gentle traction on the vessels is used to aid during this distal dissection. This initial step is sometimes performed using conventional laparoscopy if the robotic system being utilized is found to be cumbersome. As a reminder, excision of the primary tumor should always be via an inguinal incision to prevent violation of the lymphatics to the scrotum. Moreover, a non-absorbable suture should be used to ligate the spermatic cord for future identification. This cord specimen is then passed off the table.

Right-Sided Dissection

The right-sided template extends from the right ureter laterally, the infra-renal abdominal aorta medially, the crossing of the right ureter and common iliac artery inferiorly, and the renal hilum superiorly.

The ascending colon is mobilized by excising the white line of Toldt to the level of the hepatic flexure. With the colon mobilized, the duodenum is then kocherized, exposing the ureter approximately at the level where it crosses over the common iliac. This delineates the lowest aspect of the dissection border. The duodenal mobilization is then carried cephalad to the renal vein, exposing the paracaval space and IVC. For right sided tumors, in general, we attempt to perform a bilateral procedure by removing the lymph node packets of the right common iliac, para-caval, inter-aortocaval, pre-aortic, and para-aortic lymph nodes. It is important to note that the most distal extent of the dissection along the aorta is the origin of the inferior mesenteric artery during a nerve-sparing approach.

Lymphatic channels are clipped using Weck® Hem-o-Lck® clips to reduce the risk of lymphocele formation and chylous ascites. Alternatively, 10 mm metal clips can be used. Using a split and roll technique, lymphatic tissue is cleanly dissected away from the IVC at the anterior position. The termination of the right gonadal vein is divided. Care must be taken to identify any precaval right-sided lower pole renal arteries. If the paracaval dissection is performed first, the tissue between the right ureter, IVC, and right common iliac artery are mobilized until they cross under the IVC prior to the renal hilum cephalad. The split tissue along the IVC is then rolled medially. Care must be taken to identify lumbar veins emanating off the IVC and along with any accessory renal vessels. Lumbar veins are clipped, ligated, and divided during the dissection. Attention is paid to identify the sympathetic chain and post-ganglionic nerve fibers emanating from the medial aspect of the IVC. These fibers are preserved during this dissection. The dissection is considered complete when all of the lymphatic tissue has been removed from beneath the IVC, such that the interaortocaval tissue is appreciated and harvested from the anterior spinous ligament.

Dissection over the aorta is started anteriorly at the right renal artery. If needed, the dissection can be taken in a cephalad direction, but great care must be taken near the superior mesenteric artery. The dissection is then extended distally and the lymphatic tissue is rolled medially. This is taken to the level of the inferior mesenteric artery (IMA). Great care must be taken at the IMA as the sympathetic plexus can coalesce just below the IMA. Lumbar arteries are identified and can be ligated and divided to provide adequate exposure posteriorly to the aorta to remove the lymphatic tissue in the interaortocaval space down to the anterior spinous ligament in conjunction with the tissue mobilized medial from the IVC. We typically do not ligate all of the lumbar arteries for fear of postoperative claudication. The left post-ganglionic fibers should be lateral to the aorta. These fibers are often much more delicate in this location.

Left-Sided Dissection

The left-sided template is demarcated by the left ureter laterally, the medial aspect of the infra-renal inferior vena cava medially, the crossing of the ureter at the common iliac inferiorly and the renal hilum superiorly (Fig. 23.3).

For left sided dissections, the case begins with mobilization of the descending colon along the splenic flexure to expose the left renal vein and aorta. The lateral attachments of the spleen are excised. With care, the tail of the pancreas is gently reflected to maximize exposure to the retroperitoneum.

The left-sided dissection proceeds in a similar manner as described above for the right dissection. Care is taken to prospectively identify the sympathetic chain and post-ganglionic fibers, lymph node packets are excised and clipped to prevent formation of lymphoceles, and lumbar vessels are ligated.

Bilateral Dissection

In cases where bilateral dissection is necessary, the patient is repositioned to the alternate flank. We prefer to begin our dissection on the right side and then move to the left side. In general, we find it necessary to reposition the patient when using the *daVinci Si* system in order to safely and thoroughly perform a complete bilateral dissection. This is often the case with right-sided tumors. However with the introduction of the *daVinci Xi* system, in which the table and robotic arms move harmoniously, there is less need to reposition and redock the patient. Typically, the patient will remain supine while the table is rotated (tilted from left to right), in turn

23 The Use of Minimally Invasive RPLND in the Treatment of Para-Testicular...

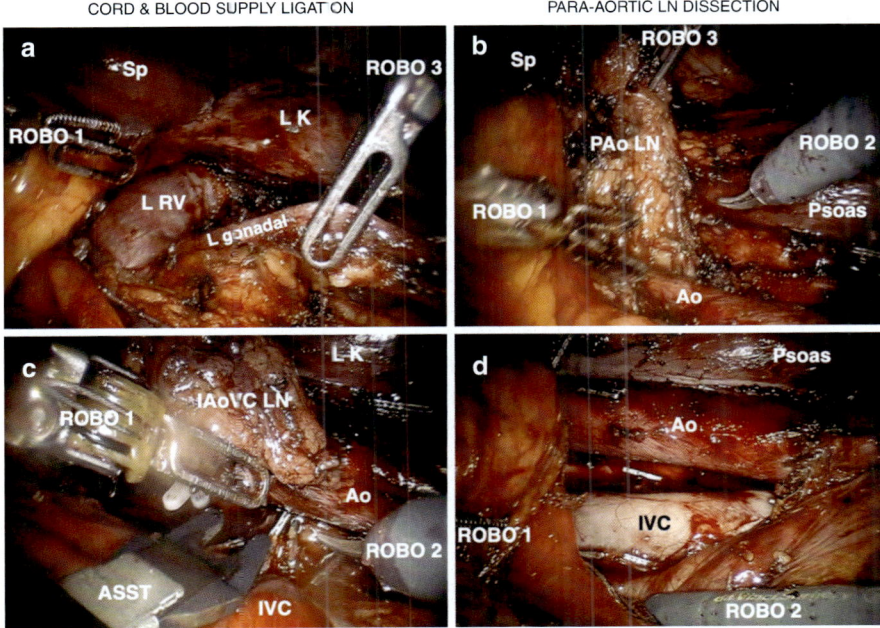

Fig. 23.3 Left-sided RPLND sequence. The descending colon is mobilized medially until the renal vein, aorta and edge of the IVC are exposed. (**a**) The left gonadal vessels are mobilized and ligated. The remainder of the spermatic cord is dissected distally until the stump is identified (not shown). The left kidney (L K) is shown for spatial reference. (**b**) The lymph nodes (PAo LN) surrounding the aorta (Ao) are dissected out and mobilized. A classic split and role technique is performed. The Pao LN are mobilized laterally to the ureter and medially under the Ao. Note the relation of the PAo LN packet to the Ao, and psoas muscle. Cephalad margin of the PAo LN packet generally terminates inferior and posterior to the left renal vein (not shown). (**c**) To mobilize the Ao, lumbar vessels are identified and appropriately ligated to provide mobilization of the Ao. The allows for complete removal of the PAo LN packet. With the aorta mobilized, the inter-aortocaval lymph nodes (IAoVC LN) are dissected and mobilized. Again a split and role technique is used to permit a nerve sparing technique. During the meticulous dissection of the IAoVC LN, identification of the nerve bundles is important. Lumbar veins are then mobilized and ligated to allow for complete mobilization of the IVC. Complete mobilization is critical for complete dissection and for appropriate nerve sparing. (**d**) The completed dissection is seen, with the aorta (Ao) and inferior vena cava (IVC) cleanly identified relative to the psoas muscle and spinous ligament

providing an appropriate degree of bowel retraction. It is mandatory to adequately secure the patient to the table when rotating the patient in the supine position as this often requires a significant degree of table tilt. If using tape to secure the patient, the tape should be wrapped completely around the patient and table at three separate locations to avoid patient slipping off the bed. The right side is typically approached first. Once completed, the table can be rotated to the left to expose the left colon. The *Xi* boom would then be turned and redocked in order to facilitate left-sided dissection.

Nerve Sparing and Prevention of Nerve Injury

The goal of nerve sparing is to preserve antegrade ejaculation in patients undergoing RPLND. Ejaculatory dysfunction is a known complication of this surgery. As noted earlier, ejaculatory function primarily occurs with disruption of the post-ganglionic fibers of the para-aortic lumbar sympathetic nerves. While this was reported with higher frequency in older series [34, 35], new advances in surgical technique and approach have made this side effect quite rare [20, 22, 23].

Two approaches have been formulated to prevent injury to the para-aortic sympathetic nerves. The first approach utilizes modified templates that spare the contralateral sympathetic nerves by primarily limiting the surgical dissection to the ipsilateral side and to above the inferior mesenteric artery on the contralateral side of the primary tumor. The nerve-sparing technique preserves nerves within the area of dissection. Fibers of the sympathetic chain, hypogastric, and hypogastric plexus are prospectively identified and preserved. A split-and-roll technique is used to achieve this end, whereby lymph nodes are grasped and rolled away from sympathetic fibers. The use of these techniques has led to excellent preservation of antegrade ejaculation. Indeed, case series from the pediatric and germ testicular cell tumor literature have demonstrated preservation of ejaculatory function at rates of >90% [20, 22, 23].

Post-operative Considerations

After completion of the case, patients are extubated and transferred to the post-anesthesia care unit. Given minimal manipulation of bowel, patients are advanced to a liquid diet early in recovery. Nasogastric tubes are rarely used postoperatively. Post-operative tachycardia secondary to manipulation and stimulation of sympathetic nerves can occur but resolves with time, usually over the span of several weeks. Some physicians advocate for the consumption of a low-fat diet for a few weeks after surgery to reduce the risk of developing lymphoceles, though this has not been conclusively shown to reduce the risk of this complication [36].

Benefits, Outcomes, Complications

The benefits of a minimally invasive approach are (1) enhanced surgical recovery and (2) shorter convalesce. In patients undergoing this procedure for oncologic reasons, an added benefit is the shorter time to commencement of radiation or chemotherapy. Limited case studies in the pediatric population have reported lower EBL (100 cc vs. 400 cc), shorter length of stay (2d vs. 4–8d), and faster return to normal activity compared to the traditional open approach [32]. However, minimally invasive approaches often call for longer operative times. Given the rarity of PT-RMS, there is a paucity of data formally comparing lymph node yield or oncologic outcomes in open vs. robotic approaches. Nevertheless, extrapolating from the germ-cell tumor literature, lymph node yield and oncologic outcomes are equivalent independent of the approach utilized [31, 37–40]. These results should be interpreted in the context of highly skilled minimally invasive surgeons at relatively high-volume centers and may not be applicable to the national experience or the experience of a non-expert. Moreover, teaming up with adult urologic oncology colleagues with robotic RPLND familiarity can provide additional experience in the room during these rare cases.

With respect to complications, a recent systematic review of RA-RPLND in adult testicular cancer patients reported an overall complication rate of 8%, with 4% major and 4% minor complications [40]. However, reports have been as high as 17% for minor complications (when including post-chemotherapy patients) [41]. A few series from the pediatric literature have demonstrated favorable morbidity with this procedure and the use of minimally invasive approaches have demonstrated a favorable complication profile [32, 33].

Conversion to an open approach remains a possibility and vascular injury is cited as the most common reason for conversion, with reported rates up to 5.5% [40]. Complication profiles unique to RPLND are the development of ejaculatory dysfunction and chylous ascites. With respect to antegrade ejaculatory dysfunction, with the advent of nerve-sparing techniques, even with bilateral dissections, the risk is quite low at 4.5% [40]. Pre-operative counseling should include this as a potential consequence of the surgery and discussion surrounding pre-operative sperm-banking should also be considered if the patient has reached sexual maturity. The development of chylous ascites has been reported to be less than 2% [37, 40, 42] bydd experienced teams. Other reported complications include ileus, small bowel obstruction, lymphocele, retroperitoneal hematoma, and ureteral injury, however these are reported in the single digits [40, 42].

Diagnostic or Therapeutic?

The benefits of RPLND in patients with PT-RMS has historically been viewed as primarily for staging purposes. However, there may be therapeutic benefits to performing RPLND for at-risk patients with PT-RMS. Patients who underwent RPLND had better survival advantage compared to those patients who did not in IRS-III vs. IRS-IV [12]. Multiple studies have also confirmed improved overall survival and evidence free survival in patients who receive RPLND [15–17]. While this was largely attributed to more precise identification of patients with micro-metastatic disease, extrapolating from the germ-cell tumor literature, RPLND likely has both a diagnostic and therapeutic benefit. Indeed, in patients with Stage I NSGCT, RPLND is curative as a mono-therapy [37].

This is particularly relevant in pediatric populations where early exposure to chemotherapy and radiation has non-trivial long-term consequences of secondary malignancies, nephrotoxicity and cardiopulmonary toxicity [43, 44]. Thus, surgical treatment modalities may serve the benefit of (1) enhancing overall survival from both staging and therapeutic perspectives and (2) open the door to treatment protocols with reduced exposure to chemoradiation, thereby reducing long-term sequelae and toxicity.

Summary

RPLND for PT-RMS and pediatric germ cell tumors is an evolving procedure that has made great strides within the past 20 years. Despite these advances, surgical adoption of RPLND within the pediatric population has been poor, likely due to long-held beliefs that the surgery is excessively morbid. However, modified templates, nerve-sparing techniques, and minimally invasive approaches have greatly decreased the morbidity associated with this procedure. Robotic RPLND is a viable and oncologically sound alternative to open RPLND and should be offered by experienced surgeons and centers that are familiar with the procedure. While currently viewed as purely diagnostic, the lower morbidity of modern techniques combined with promising literature from germ cell cancer management may change this trajectory. A paradigm shift could be on the horizon, with RPLND as a potential therapeutic tool for PT-RMS that increases overall survival and reduces the need for chemoradiation and associated long-term toxicities.

References

1. Ahmed HU, Arya M, Muneer A, Mushtaq I, Sebire NJ. Testicular and paratesticular tumours in the prepubertal population. Lancet Oncol. 2010;11(5):476–83. https://doi.org/10.1016/S1470-2045(10)70012-7.
2. Stewart RJ, Martelli H. Treatment of children with nonmetastatic paratesticular rhabdomyosarcoma: results of the Malignant Mesenchymal Tumors studies (MMT 84 and MMT 89) of the International Society of Pediatric Oncology. J Clin Oncol. 2003;21(5):793–8. https://doi.org/10.1200/JCO.2003.06.040.
3. Ferrari A, Bisogno G, Casanova M, et al. Paratesticular rhabdomyosarcoma: report from the Italian and German Cooperative Group. J Clin Oncol. 2002;20(2):449–55. https://doi.org/10.1200/JCO.20.2.449.
4. Elsässer E. Tumors of the epididymis. Recent results. Cancer Res. 1977;60:163–75.
5. Ferrari A, Casanova M, Massimino M, Luksch R, Piva L, Fossati-Bellani F. The management of paratesticular rhabdomyosarcoma: a single institutional experience with 44 consecutive children. J Urol. 1998;159(3):1031–4.
6. Crist BWM, Anderson JR, Meza JL, et al. Intergroup rhabdomyosarcoma study-IV : results for patients with nonmetastatic disease. J Clin Oncol. 2001;19(12):3091–102.
7. Wiener ES, Lawrence W, Hays D, et al. Retroperitoneal node biopsy in paratesticular rhabdomyosarcoma. J Pediatr Surg. 1994;29(2):171–8. https://doi.org/10.1016/0022-3468(94)90313-1.

8. Hays DM, Heyn RM, Newton WA, et al. Paratesticular sarcoma in childhood and adolescence. Cancer. 1983;58:446–50.
9. Harel M, Ferrer FA, Shapiro LH, Makari JH. Future directions in risk stratification and therapy for advanced pediatric genitourinary rhabdomyosarcoma. Urol Oncol. 2016;34(2):103–15. https://doi.org/10.1016/J.UROLONC.2015.09.013.
10. Dagher R, Helman L. Rhabdomyosarcoma: an overview. Oncologist. 1999;4(1):34–44.
11. Sung T, Riedlinger WFJ, Diamond DA, Chow JS. Solid extratesticular masses in children: radiographic and pathologic correlation. Am J Roentgenol. 2006;186(2):483–90. https://doi.org/10.2214/AJR.04.1895.
12. Wiener ES, Anderson JR, Ojimba JI, et al. Controversies in the management of paratesticular rhabdomyosarcoma: is staging retroperitoneal lymph node dissection necessary for adolescents with resected paratesticular rhabdomyosarcoma? Semin Pediatr Surg. 2001;10(3):146–52.
13. Beverly Raney R, Maurer HM, Anderson JR, et al. The intergroup Rhabdomyosarcoma Study Group (IRSG): major lessons from the IRS-I through IRS-IV studies as background for the current IRS-V treatment protocols. Sarcoma. 2001;5(1):9–15. https://doi.org/10.1080/13577140120048890.
14. Crist W, Gehan EA, Ragab AH, et al. The third intergroup rhabdomyosarcoma study. J Clin Oncol. 1995;13(3):610–30. https://doi.org/10.1200/JCO.1995.13.3.610.
15. Hamilton EC, Miller CC, Joseph M, Huh WW, Hayes-Jordan AA, Austin MT. Retroperitoneal lymph node staging in paratesticular rhabdomyosarcoma—are we meeting expectations? J Surg Res. 2018;224:44–9.
16. Dang ND, Dang P-T, Samuelian J, Paulino AC. Lymph node management in patients with paratesticular rhabdomyosarcoma. Cancer. 2013;119(17):3228–33. https://doi.org/10.1002/cncr.28198.
17. Lobeck I, Dupree P, Karns R, Rodeberg D, von Allmen D, Dasgupta R. Quality assessment of lymph node sampling in rhabdomyosarcoma: a surveillance, epidemiology, and end results (SEER) program study. J Pediatr Surg. 2017;52(4):614–7. https://doi.org/10.1016/j.jpedsurg.2016.08.024.
18. Beveridge TS, Allman BL, Johnson M, Power A, Sheinfeld J, Power NE. Retroperitoneal lymph node dissection: anatomical and technical considerations from a cadaveric study. J Urol. 2016;196(6):1764–71. https://doi.org/10.1016/j.juro.2016.06.091.
19. Donohue JP, Rowland RG. Complications of retroperitoneal lymph node dissection. J Urol. 1981;125(3):338–40.
20. Donohue JP, Foster RS, Rowland RG, Bihrle R, Jones J, Geier G. Nerve-sparing retroperitoneal lymphadenectomy with preservation of ejaculation. J Urol. 1990;144(2 Pt 1):287–91; discussion 291–2.
21. Revenig L, Leung A, Hsiao W. Ejaculatory physiology and pathophysiology: assessment and treatment in male infertility. Transl Androl Urol. 2014;3(1):41–9. https://doi.org/10.3978/j.issn.2223-4683.2014.02.02.
22. Jewett MA, Kong YS, Goldberg SD, et al. Retroperitoneal lymphadenectomy for testis tumor with nerve sparing for ejaculation. J Urol. 1988;139(6):1220–4.
23. Donohue JP, Thornhill JA, Foster RS, Rowland RG, Bihrle R. Retroperitoneal lymphadenectomy for clinical stage a testis cancer (1965 to 1989): modifications of technique and impact on ejaculation. J Urol. 1993;149(2):237–43.
24. Bhayani SB, Allaf ME, Kavoussi LR. Laparoscopic RPLND for clinical stage I nonseminomatous germ cell testicular cancer: current status. Urol Oncol. 2004;22:145–8. https://doi.org/10.1016/j.urolonc.2004.01.005.
25. Faria EF, Neves HS, Dauster B, et al. Laparoscopic retroperitoneal lymph node dissection as a safe procedure for postchemotherapy residual mass in testicular cancer. J Laparoendosc Adv Surg Tech A. 2018;28(2):168–73. https://doi.org/10.1089/lap.2017.0381.
26. Hanzly M, Frederick A, Creighton T, et al. Learning curves for robot-assisted and laparoscopic partial nephrectomy. J Endourol. 2015;29(3):297–303. https://doi.org/10.1089/end.2014.0303.

27. Pilka R, Gágyor D, Študentová M, Neubert D, Dzvinčuk P. Laparoscopic and robotic sacropexy: retrospective review of learning curve experiences and follow-up. Ceska Gynekol. 2017;82(4):261–7.
28. Abdel-Aziz KF, Anderson JK, Svatek R, Margulis V, Sagalowsky AI, Cadeddu JA. Laparoscopic and open retroperitoneal lymph-node dissection for clinical stage I nonseminomatous germ-cell testis tumors. J Endourol. 2006;20(9):627–31. https://doi.org/10.1089/end.2006.20.627.
29. Poulakis V, Skriapas K, de Vries R, et al. Quality of life after laparoscopic and open retroperitoneal lymph node dissection in clinical stage I nonseminomatous germ cell tumor: a comparison study. Urology. 2006;68(1):154–60. https://doi.org/10.1016/j.urology.2006.01.023.
30. Janetschek G, Hobisch A, Höltl L, Bartsch G. Retroperitoneal lymphadenectomy for clinical stage I nonseminomatous testicular tumor: laparoscopy versus open surgery and impact of learning curve. J Urol. 1996;156(1):89–93; discussion 94.
31. Nicolai N, Tarabelloni N, Gasperoni F, et al. Laparoscopic retroperitoneal lymph node dissection for clinical stage I nonseminomatous germ cell tumors of the testis: safety and efficacy analyses at a high volume center. J Urol. 2018;199(3):741–7. https://doi.org/10.1016/j.juro.2017.09.088.
32. Cost NG, DaJusta DG, Granberg CF, et al. Robot-assisted laparoscopic retroperitoneal lymph node dissection in an adolescent population. J Endourol. 2012;26(6):635–40. https://doi.org/10.1089/end.2011.0214.
33. Glaser AP, Bowen DK, Lindgren BW, Meeks JJ. Robot-assisted retroperitoneal lymph node dissection (RA-RPLND) in the adolescent population. J Pediatr Urol. 2017;13(2):223–4. https://doi.org/10.1016/j.jpurol.2017.01.007.
34. Mosharafa AA, Foster RS, Koch MO, Bihrle R, Donohue JP. Complications of post-chemotherapy retroperitoneal lymph node dissection for testis cancer. J Urol. 2004;171(5):1839–41. https://doi.org/10.1097/01.ju.0000120141.89737.90.
35. Narayan P, Lange PH, Fraley EE. Ejaculation and fertility after extended retroperitoneal lymph node dissection for testicular cancer. J Urol. 1982;127(4):685–8.
36. Lv S, Wang Q, Zhao W, et al. A review of the postoperative lymphatic leakage. Oncotarget. 2017;8(40):69062–75. https://doi.org/10.18632/oncotarget.17297.
37. Pearce SM, Golan S, Gorin MA, et al. Safety and early oncologic effectiveness of primary robotic retroperitoneal lymph node dissection for nonseminomatous germ cell testicular cancer. Eur Urol. 2017;71(3):476–82.
38. Harris KT, Gorin MA, Ball MW, Pierorazio PM, Allaf ME. A comparative analysis of robotic vs laparoscopic retroperitoneal lymph node dissection for testicular cancer. BJU Int. 2015;116(6):920–3. https://doi.org/10.1111/bju.13121.
39. Abdul-Muhsin HM, L'esperance JO, Fischer K, Woods ME, Porter JR, Castle EP. Robot-assisted retroperitoneal lymph node dissection in testicular cancer. J Surg Oncol. 2015;112(7):736–40. https://doi.org/10.1002/jso.24018.
40. Tselos A, Moris D, Tsilimigras DI, et al. Robot-assisted retroperitoneal lymphadenectomy in testicular cancer treatment: a systematic review. J Laparoendosc Adv Surg Tech A. 2018;28(6):682–9. https://doi.org/10.1089/lap.2017.0672.
41. Cheney SM, Andrews PE, Leibovich BC, Castle EP. Robot-assisted retroperitoneal lymph node dissection: technique and initial case series of 18 patients. BJU Int. 2015;115(1):114–20. https://doi.org/10.1111/bju.12804.
42. Subramanian VS, Nguyen CT, Stephenson AJ, Klein EA. Complications of open primary and post-chemotherapy retroperitoneal lymph node dissection for testicular cancer. Urol Oncol. 2010;28(5):504–9.
43. Haugnes HS, Bosl GJ, Boer H, et al. Long-term and late effects of germ cell testicular cancer treatment and implications for follow-up. J Clin Oncol. 2012;30(30):3752–63. https://doi.org/10.1200/JCO.2012.43.4431.
44. Fosså SD, Oldenburg J, Dahl AA. Short- and long-term morbidity after treatment for testicular cancer. BJU Int. 2009;104(9 B):1418–22. https://doi.org/10.1111/j.1464-410X.2009.08869.x.

Chapter 24
Laparoendoscopic Single-Site Surgery

Laura B. Cornwell and George Chiang

Abbreviations

CL	Conventional laparoscopy
LESS	Laparoendoscopic single site surgery
MIS	Minimally Invasive Surgery
OPUS	One-port umbilical surgery
RA	Robotic-assisted

Introduction

Minimally invasive surgical techniques continue to be pushed throughout pediatric urology. A badge of honor for today's surgeon is the diminutive size or appearance of an incision rather than the usual metrics of speed and efficacy which are considered more of a required competency. Laparoendoscopic single site surgery (LESS) offers perhaps the greatest advantage in terms of cosmesis compared to other techniques [1, 2] which may be especially important to the pediatric population who have a lifetime in front of them in regards to perception of body image and associated self-esteem. Although LESS poses its own set of challenges and limitations, it is a valuable approach and technique that can be used for multiple procedures.

L. B. Cornwell · G. Chiang (✉)
University of California San Diego, Rady Children's Hospital, Department of Urology, San Diego, CA, USA
e-mail: Lcornwell@rchsd.org; GChiang@rchsd.org

© Springer Nature Switzerland AG 2020
P. C. Gargollo (ed.), *Minimally Invasive and Robotic-Assisted Surgery in Pediatric Urology*, https://doi.org/10.1007/978-3-030-57219-8_24

Background

The nomenclature of LESS has been controversial and varied. It has been called single access/port/site/incision/trocar surgery, one-port umbilical surgery (OPUS), and embryonic natural orifice transluminal endoscopic surgery [3]. The Urologic NOTES working group has recommended that LESS be designated the terminology of choice to define laparoendoscopic procedures performed through a single port, multiple port, and single multiport platform used via a single incision or location anywhere in the abdomen, flank or the back [4].

The first form of laparoendoscopic single site surgery was done in the late 1960s for tubal ligations. Electrocauterization and excision of a portion of each fallopian tube was performed through a fiberoptic laparoscope (Fig. 24.1) [5]. Single-port laparoscopic surgery had been reported for cholecystectomy and appendectomy since 1998; however, the approach did not gain momentum because of technical challenges. The initial report of a single port nephrectomy in an adult occurred in 2007 [6]. Although a multitude of pediatric cases soon followed, it could be argued that the first form of pediatric urological LESS surgery was the retroperitoneal single site surgery that was described by Lima in 2005 where a single flank 12 mm incision was located 1 cm under the XII rib. A balloon 12 mm Hasson trocar was then inserted; After the creation of the working space with a peanut, using a 10 mm coaxial operative telescope, the renal pelvis and the proximal ureter were inspected, isolated and then exteriorized at skin level with a vessel loop for performance of the pyeloplasty [7].

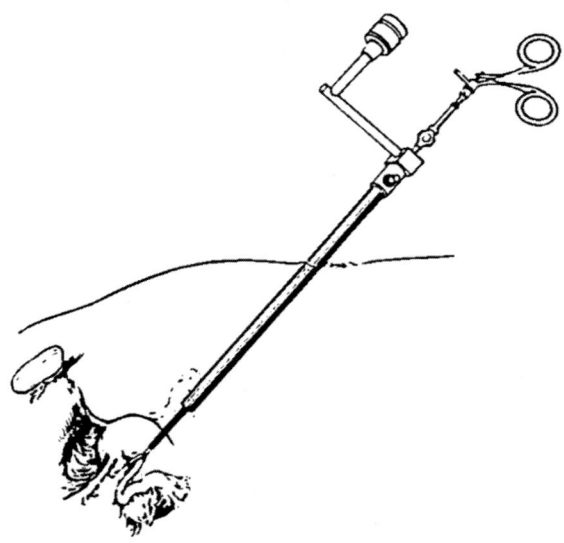

Fig. 24.1 Operating laparoscope for tubal ligation. (*Used with permission of Wolters Kluwer Health, Inc.*)

Overview

The relevant background for pediatric laparoscopy including physiological considerations, anesthesia, and relevant anatomy are covered in prior chapters. However as a general rule to LESS, patient positioning is slightly altered for upper tract surgery. Port placement is radically different and counterintuitive to the hallmark of conventional laparoscopy which stresses triangulation on the target area. For flank transabdominal approaches to renal surgery including nephrectomies, heminephrectomies or pyeloplasties, the patient is positioned as close to the edge of the bed to help minimize clashing of instruments extracorporally [8]. For pelvic transperitoneal surgery, the patient is positioned supine, often with slight trendelenberg, and the dissecting surgeon would stand on the side of the bed allowing better dexterity of their dominant operating hand [9].

LESS can be considered more difficult for multiple reasons including: (1) Instrument clashing (2) Lack of triangulation, (3) Difficulty in visualization with parallel instrumentation/optics, (4) Reduced operating space. The cause of this difficulty, when compared to conventional laparoscopy, is placement of all instruments and trocars through a single incision or port.

There is a great variety of multi-trocar single ports as well as adapted devices or approaches. The shown multi-trocar single ports are not exhaustive (Figs. 24.2, 24.3, and 24.4). Adapted devices include use of an abdominal wound protector with a glove port (Fig. 24.5) [10–14]. Incisional adaptive approaches include (1) making an extended skin incision of approximately 2–3 cm in a transverse or longitudinal direction through the umbilicus or peri-umbilically with subsequent placement of multiple trocars via separate stab incisions through the underlying fascia (Fig. 24.6) [15] or (2) making a longitudinal or transverse 2.5 cm incision through the umbilicus, disarticulating the umbilical stalk and then placing one trocar via the open umbilical ring and the lens and additional instruments directly through adjacent

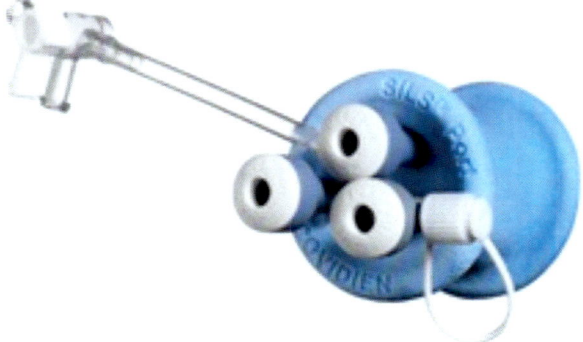

Fig. 24.2 Covidien SILS™. (©2019 Medtronic. All rights reserved. Used with permission of Medtronic)

Fig. 24.3 Olympus Triport+™. (*Image Courtesy of Olympus America Inc.*)

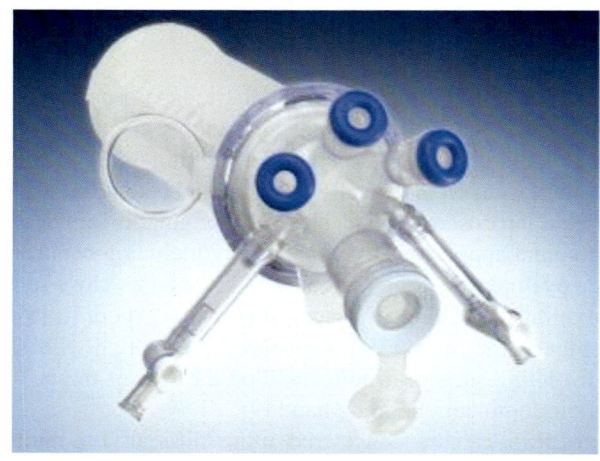

Fig. 24.4 Applied medical GelPOINT™ advanced access platform. (*©2019 Applied Medical Resources. All rights reserved. Used with permission of Applied Medical*)

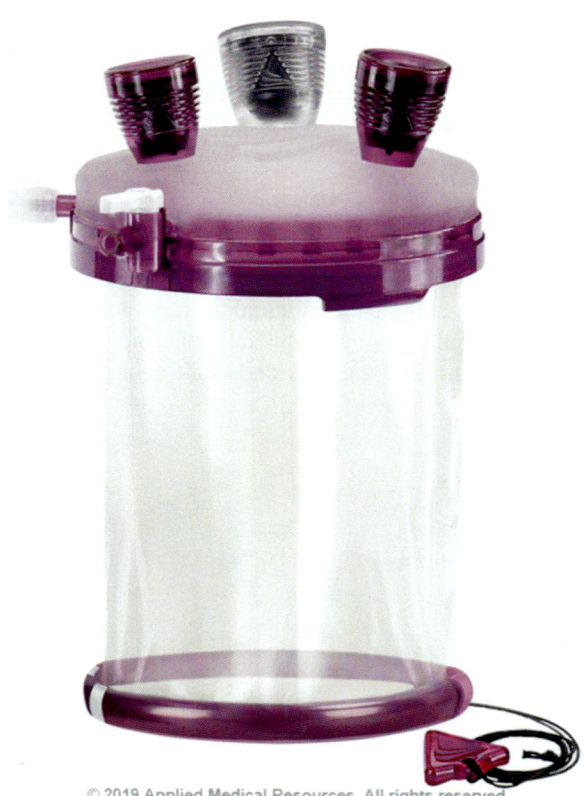

24 Laparoendoscopic Single-Site Surgery

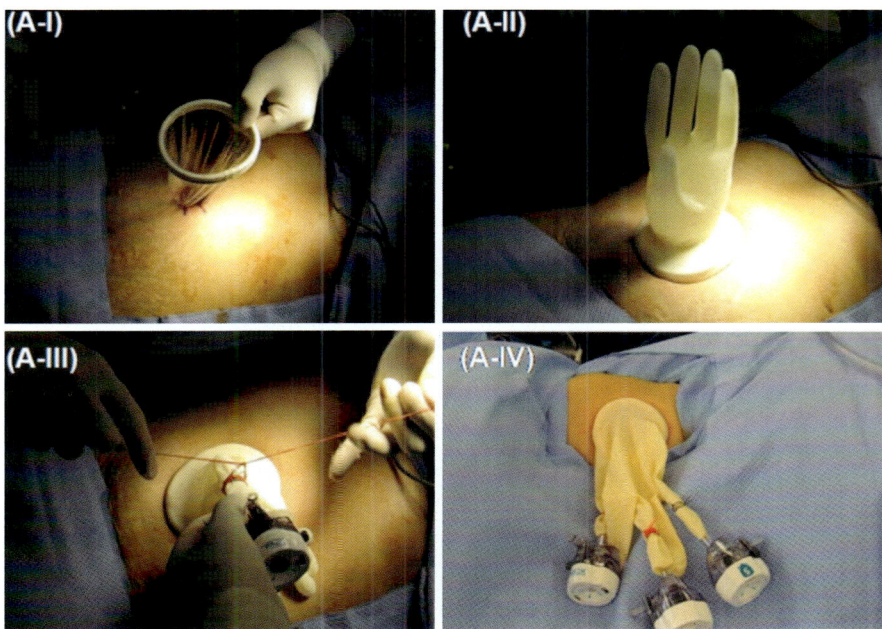

Fig. 24.5 (**AI-IV**) A self-constructed glove port, created from a wound protector and glove, for single-incision laparoscopic surgery (*Used with permission of Elsevier*)

Fig. 24.6 Single incision technique with one 10-mm and 2 5-mm trocars. (*Used with permission of Elsevier*)

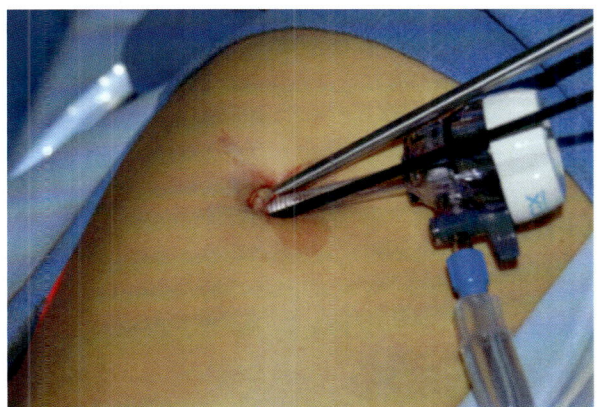

fascial stab incisions, without additional trocars (Fig. 24.7) [16]. This approach is cheaper since less trocars are used but can be difficult since exchange of instruments is limited to the one trocar; a lens and a grasper are generally kept intracorporeal for the duration of the procedure on either side of the trocar. Additional needlescopic instruments can often be used such as a percutaneous alligator grasper (Fig. 24.8) through any percutaneous location desired for technical feasibility.

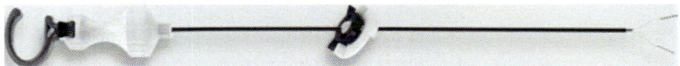

Fig. 24.7 Single 2 cm longitudinal incision with working trocar via umbilical ring and telescope/grasper placed through adjacent stab incisions. (*Used with permission of Elsevier*)

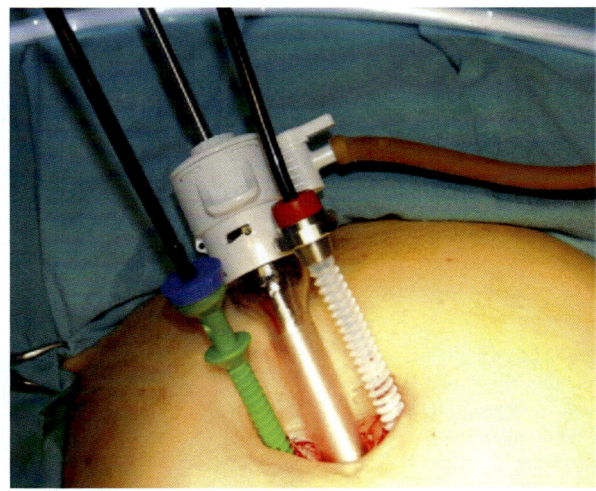

Fig. 24.8. Teleflex Minilap™ Alligator Grasper using a 2.3 mm sheath. (*Image courtesy of Teleflex Incorporated. ©2010 Teleflex Incorporated. All rights reserved*)

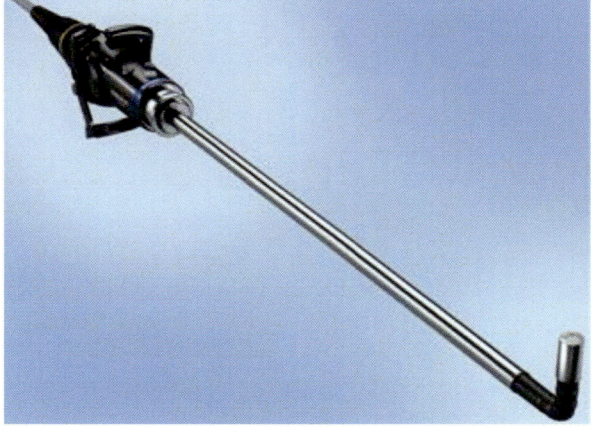

Fig. 24.9 Flexible 5 mm telescope with charged couple device chip at the tip (Olympus EndoEye). (*Image Courtesy of Olympus America Inc.*)

Fig. 24.10 Bariatric length telescope with right angled light connector

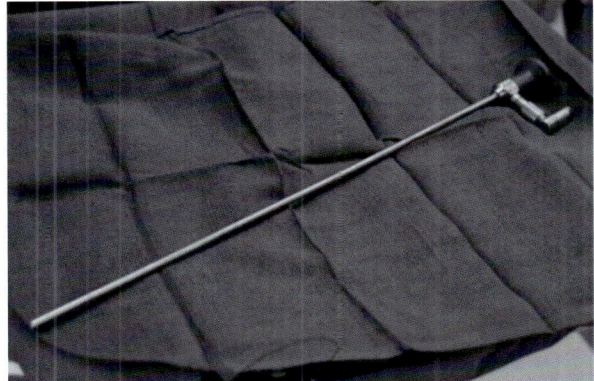

Fig. 24.11 5 mm articulating dissector (Covidien SILS™ Dissect). (©*2019 Medtronic. All rights reserved. Used with permission of Medtronic*)

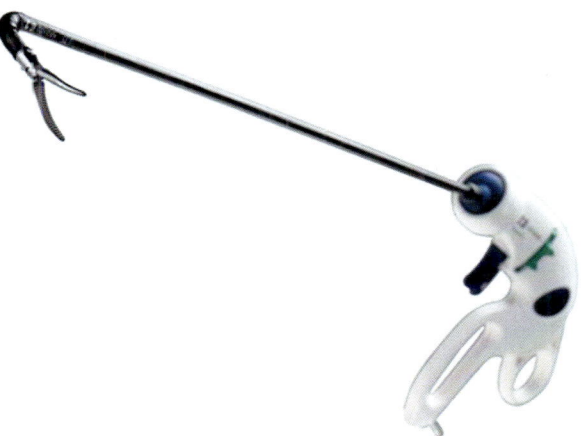

There is no one optimal approach or port, and preference is certainly related to surgeon experience. However, when using an adaptive incisional technique, the direction of the umbilical incision must take into account the area of interest whether that is the pelvis (transverse incision) or lateral structures (longitudinal incision).

Multiple technological advancements have arisen to overcome the inherent limitations of LESS. Better optics and specialized instrumentation have been used in all specialties. Flexible tip laparoscopes were created where the tip can be angled towards the operative site (Fig. 24.9) [4, 17]. This allows for appropriate visualization during the procedure while remaining outside of crowded port space and internal laparoscopic instruments. In our experience, utilizing a bariatric length telescope with a right-angled light connector is sufficient (Fig. 24.10). Multiple articulating instruments have been created as well in the forms of dissectors, graspers, scissors or a hook (Fig. 24.11). However, we have found that aside from a multi-port and a bariatric length telescope, specialized instrumentation is not necessary for the overwhelming number of procedures specific to pediatric urology [18]. Perhaps more

Fig. 24.12 5 mm articulating needle driver (Flexdex™). (*Used with permission of FlexDex, Inc. All rights reserved*)

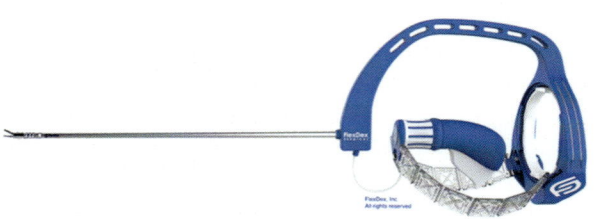

complex reconstructive procedures which require intracorporeal suturing may require advanced tools (Fig. 24.12) but extirpative procedures do not, based on multiple case series [19].

When considering financial aspects of LESS, some authors have commented on the cost of LESS as compared to conventional laparoscopy, open procedures, or robotics [20, 21]. For nephrectomy, the robotic approach has been noted to be the most expensive while open the least expensive in comparison to LESS; further details are summarized in upcoming paragraphs.

Noh et al. summarized supply costs in 2013 using orchiopexy as an example: a 5 mm Covidien Step™ trocar for diagnostic laparoscopy costs $92, followed by an Olympus Triport at a cost of $395, bringing to a total of $487 in access supply costs for a single LESS procedure. This would compare to $276 if three 5-mm ports were used. If two 3 mm trocars at $54 each were used, the cost would be $238. Although many authors do not rely on the use of a flexible-tip laparoscope, in that publication Noh et al. reported that the cost to invest in the purchase of two scopes was $41,722, in addition to $17,712 for the required video system, and $3842 for sterilization trays [22].

Technical Considerations

Overall LESS requires a greater deal of dexterity, patience and persistence. There are slight alterations in technique including (1) Crossing of instruments may be required, (2) Setting grasper retraction followed by the insertion of other working instrumentation may be required to minimize clashing (3) Energy devices such as scissors or the harmonic scalpel must be used by either hand since the angles of approach are limited (4) Placement of the telescope is variable but usually the inferior position of a multi-port is preferable. Additional technical considerations will be described as they apply to separate procedures on the following pages.

Applications and Outcomes

Retrospective studies comparing LESS to other surgical approaches are summarized in Table 24.1.

Table 24.1 Retrospective series comparing LESS approach to others

First author	Year	Where	Case matched	# in series	OR time (min)	LOS (days)	Analgesia	Other	f/u amt	Outcome
Nephrectomy/nephroureterectomy										
Woldrich [21]	2011	USA	No	LESS – 7 CL – 11 Open – 8	192 219 127	2 1 1	Narcotics equivalent *Open got more toradol*	Included multiple concomitant procedures *Hospital costs: LESS 96.8% of CL, open 54.4%*	–	1 LESS converted to open 2/2 bleeding (excluded from analysis)
Kocherov [33]	2011	Israel	Yes	LESS – 4 CL – 4	72.5? 	*1.1* *1.9*	*0 mg/kg* *0.46*	–	–	–
Kim	2012	USA	No	LESS – 11 CL – 11 RA – 11 Open – 39	*133* *162* *188* *94*	*1.3* *1.4* *1.8* *3.2*	*0.18 mg/kg* *0.10* *0.23* *0.63*	–		
Tam [35]	2013	China	Yes	LESS – 8 CL – 12	*156* *99*	2.9 2.6	0.08 mg/kg 0.28		"3 mo – 3 yr"	1 wound infection in CL
Bansal [20]	2014	USA	No	LESS – 8 RA – 24	*174* *221*	1 2	LESS had more blocks Comparable narcotics, toradol	*RA hospital charges cost 30% more*	18.8 22	1 abscess needed outpatient antibiotics in LESS. 1 retention, 1 stump leak in RAL

(continued)

Table 24.1 (continued)

First author	Year	Where	Case matched	# in series	OR time (min)	LOS (days)	Analgesia	Other	f/u amt	Outcome
Heminephroureterectomy										
Neheman [37]	2019	USA + Israel	No	LESS – 10 CL – 7 RA – 18 Open – 24	*140* 190 256 154	*1* 1 2 3	*Toradol only used in MIS* *Open needed more morphine and acetaminophen*	More MIS cases over study period. Epidural for all open, local for all MIS. 8 concomitant procedures.	–	1 LESS patient had ipsilateral moiety atrophy
Pyeloplasty										
Naitoh [41]	2014	Japan	Yes	LESS – 14 CL – 14	243 229	–	*Pain score lower for LESS on POD3, 4*	–	–	No issues
Khambati [42]	2015	Canada	Yes	LESS – 7 CL – 28	233 210	2.2 2.8	–	No cost difference	15.7 –	1 LESS conversion to open due to dissection issue 1 LESS near loss of renal function
Varicocelectomy										
Bansal	2014	USA	No	LESS – 11 CL – 32	46 55	0	*81.8% received narcotics* *31.2% received narcotics*		*15* 22	1 LESS got hydrocele 1 CL got hydrocele
Khambati [42]	2015	Canada	Yes	LESS – 5 CL – ?	54 48	0				No issues

Legend: Summary of series that compare the LESS approach for multiple procedures to conventional laparoscopy (CL), Robotic-assisted laparoscopy (RA), or open surgery. Variables highlighted in italics had significant differences between groups, as summarized in the text

Upper Urinary Tract Surgery

Nephrectomy

A number of case reports, case series, and retrospective chart reviews have been published describing the techniques and feasibility of using a LESS approach in pediatric patients undergoing unilateral simple nephrectomy, single-system nephroureterectomy, as well as bilateral simple nephrectomies. The first case reports were published in 2009 following the first reports in the adult literature [12, 23, 24], and a number of retrospective reviews comparing the LESS approach to conventional laparoscopy, robotic assistance, and open have followed [20, 21, 25].

Techniques described are relatively consistent with the use of transperitoneal, umbilical access and incisions are consistently reported at 1–2.5 cm. Most authors describe the use of commercially available ports, with Coviden SILS© and Olympus Triport© being common choices, and less commonly Karl Storz X-CONE, Advanced Surgical Concepts R-port, Applied Medical GelPOINT®, and the OCTO™ port. One series specifies that a 2.5 cm incision could be used for a SILS© port while 1.5 cm for TriPort© [26]. Adaptive ports were commonly reported to be preferred by Korean urologists [12–14], which used Alexis® retractors and modified sterile gloves. Of the series that used an incisional approach, one used it due to the lack of an available LESS port at the time of surgery [23], and the other used it for patients <10 kg without an appropriately sized LESS port [27]. Most authors described using a combination of both flexible and straight instruments, oftentimes preferring a flexible endoscopic camera with straight instruments vs a straight camera, 0 vs 30 degrees, and a flexible grasper. One exception to this was the use of an end-on light source or a 45-degree bariatric lens with routine straight laparoscopic instruments [8, 18, 19, 28]. Both LigaSure™ and Harmonic® tools were described for assisting with dissection. Hilar control was accomplished with Hem-o-lok® clips in a number of series, and another specified the use of an Endo GIA™ stapler [19].

There was almost no reporting of a need to extend incision sizes for extraction. Some publications described using aspiration or morcellation to assist with extraction [19, 24, 26, 29, 30]. Other series describe using EndoBags™ for retrieval, with one series specifically describing that the larger specimens were removed in a piecemeal fashion within the EndoBag™ [31].

Other technical considerations include that a number of series described using percutaneous retraction sutures to assist with hilar mobilization [20, 27], as well as the use of a percutaneous 2.3 mm alligator liver retractor [8], where needed. The series that included bilateral nephrectomies describe using an Ioban™ to protect the incision then repositioning the patient lateral decubitus contralaterally [8].

There are also a small number of series describing single-incision retroperitoneal approaches for nephrectomy. Incisions sizes are described at 1.1–2.5 cm, with about 50% port and 50% incisional techniques used. One series describe using only 1 instrument with their camera using a 1.1 cm incision [32]. Reported mean operative times are 60–63 min, length of stay 1–1.5 days. Reviewed series do not describe experience with post-operative pain or aesthetic results [31, 32].

Demographics and perioperative outcomes were broad in the pediatric literature, with mean ages reported from 2 to 13 years old. The series with bilateral nephrectomies included the oldest of patients, consistent with age-appropriate pathologies. Most OR times ranged between 70–192 min, with nephroureterectomy 116–174 min, and bilateral cases ranging 128–342 min [8, 19, 28]. Definitions of OR time were not often specified. One series commented on a notable improvement in operative times over the study period, with the first half of cases averaging 102 min and the second half measuring 70, suggesting a learning curve can be expected [19]. Blood loss was consistently negligible or less than 50 cc, and length of stay was also consistent with most discharges on postoperative day 1, however one series did describe that they found nephroureterectomy discharges were slightly longer (1.5 day) and multiple papers including bilateral cases had longer LOS at 1–4.5 day mean stays reported, with medical/dialysis needs accounting for the longer stays [8, 19]. Many series looked at postoperative pain medication requirements and of those, about half report no postoperative narcotic requirement with the use of non-narcotics only [23, 27, 33, 34].

Reported complications associated with LESS are uncommon and not shown to be significantly different from open or laparoscopic approaches where they were compared. Reported complications out of the >250 cases described include 1 conversion to open for bleeding, two port site infections requiring outpatient antibiotics, 1 ileus requiring PICC placement [18, 20]. Follow up information is limited with many publications having no postoperative follow up specified, and of those that do, the time frame is only 1–18 months [20].

Only a few retrospective case-matched cohort reviews are available to compare LESS nephrectomy vs open or other minimally invasive approaches, and findings do vary from series to series [20, 21, 25, 33]. Patients undergoing LESS have been found to have either equivalent or less narcotic requirements, equivalent or shorter length of stay, and longer operative times than open cases. Compared to conventional laparoscopy, both equivalent and shorter operative times have been reported, as well as shorter hospital stay for LESS patients [33]. As for the robotic approach, LESS has shorter operative time reported. Lastly, open cases have been found to have significantly lower hospitalization charges than LESS by about 56% [21], while robotic-assisted approaches have 30% higher charges than LESS procedures [20].

Hemi-Nephrectomy

The role of LESS has also been well-described in performing hemi-nephroureterectomies of upper or lower duplicated systems [30, 35–38]. Consistent with pathological incidences, upper pole moieties are more commonly removed than lower pole moieties. The technique has also been described for partial nephrectomy of a mass as well [11]. Approaches to surgery mirror those described above for single-system nephrectomy, however the partial nephrectomy case report did use a larger fascial incision for extraction at 3 cm.

In the available literature, most patients were infants or a mean of 1–2 years old, consistent with the expected pathologies for this procedure. Mean operative times were similar to LESS single system nephrectomies at 58–140 min, EBL was minimal, and length of stay was 1 day. Regarding outcomes, one series had 11 months of mean follow up with no reported complications and normal postoperative imaging [36]. A multi-institutional chart review series reported one case (out of 10) that developed an ipsilateral moiety atrophy, at unspecified mean follow up [37]. Another series reported that a LESS hemi-nephroureterectomy attempted on a lower pole moiety was converted to open due to difficulty with dissection [35]. Another series reported one ipsilateral renal artery spasm as well as a transient urine leak [30].

Neheman's 2019 multi-institutional retrospective chart review compared LESS hemi-nephroureterectomy to the open approach as well as conventional laparoscopic and robotic-assisted approaches over the same time period (2007–2017) [37]. The LESS approach had a significantly shorter operative time than both conventional laparoscopy and robotics, and was found to have comparable EBL, LOS, narcotic requirements, and acetaminophen requirements to the other MIS approaches which all were superior to the open approach.

Pyeloplasty

LESS pyeloplasty is very well described with numerous series, mostly outside of the USA with most publications from China and Japan [26, 34, 39–45]. Techniques again mirror the approach to nephrectomy with 1.5–2.5 cm incisions, a dominance of commercial port usage with SILS©, TriPort ©, and GelPOINT® being commonly described. Of authors reporting on the use of port devices, both flexible and straight instruments were preferred. The largest series by far was published in 2017 by Liu et al. where 704 patients underwent a LESS approach for dismembered pyeloplasty and this series as well as one other by Bi et al. 2011 also used an incisional approach and both of these groups preferred straight laparoscopic instruments only [44, 45].

Unique technical considerations include again the use of percutaneous sutures to assist with retraction as well needlescopic ports for retraction and later drain placement [26, 34, 39, 41]. Drains were also placed via the port site [39], when used. Stent placement was accomplished by the use of a percutaneous angiocatheter vs a retrograde placement using pre-procedural cystoscopic ureteral access [39, 42].

OR times were reported at means of 110–243 min, with the largest series by Liu et al. describing a OR time of 110 min that did not include instrument placement or closures. This series did report a significant learning curve for LESS pyeloplasty with improvements from 175 min in 2010 procedures to 100 min in 2015. EBL was consistently reported at less than 100 cc, and length of stay from 2–7 days. Postoperative pain control spanned from no narcotics [34] to multiple days with a routine pain pump [43]. Complications as described by the Liu series which had

25 months of mean follow up included 8.1% minor complications requiring medication or observation (most commonly UTI > flank pain > ileus > urine leakage), and 2.0% major complications needing minimal invasive procedures (stenosis > stent block > urinoma, stent migration, serosal tear, bleeding requiring additional trocars). Success rates were reported at over 95% with most patients reportedly being evaluated with postoperative renal drainage nuclear studies [44]. Other series described similar outcomes except one article which did report a conversion to open for difficult dissection and another patient who had a near loss of renal function in the operated kidney [42].

A few series have been published comparing the LESS approach to pyeloplasty with conventional laparoscopy in a case-matched cohort. OR times were comparable as were length of stay. One series found lower pain scores on POD3 and 4 for patients in the LESS groups, but otherwise equivalent postoperative pain reports.

Other

Additional renal procedures accomplished with a LESS approach include a number of reports for renal cyst decortication or ablation, reports of pyelolithotomy, and one on a calyceal diverticulectomy. Surgical materials, techniques and outcomes again mirror those described for the above procedures [19, 38, 42, 46].

Pelvic Surgery

Varicocelectomy

A number of small series and case-matched retrospective reviews have been described from authors around the world regarding LESS experiences with laparoscopic varicocelectomy, with the earliest report published in 2008 [18, 26, 30, 33, 34, 38, 42, 47, 48]. The largest series described included only 11 patients [47, 48]. Both unilateral and bilateral procedures have been described.

The most common techniques utilized Olympus TriPort©, GelPOINT®, or SILS©, and two series used an incisional approach. One series only used an incisional approach for patients under 10 kg while another preferred the technique for all pelvic procedures [18, 30]. Incisions were 1.5–2.5 cm. Flexible and straight instrumentation was preferred in all series except with the incisional approach in Patel's 2016 series, only using straight instruments with an offset 45-degree endoscopic camera [18]. Dissection technique was not described by most series but one did describe that the testicular artery was only spared if technically easy to complete [42].

Reported mean operative times were 26–85 min, EBL was minimal and most patients were discharged the same day. Most series reported no narcotic requirements postoperatively except Bansal 2014 that found 81.8% of patients required some narcotics postoperatively [48]. Most series did not describe the duration of follow up but up to 15 months was available in the largest series with 11 patients that reported one hydrocele development as the only adverse outcome. One report of varicocele persistence was described, 2 hydroceles, 1 conversion from port to incisional technique secondary to pneumo leak, and 1 problematic postoperative pain experience were reported [18, 30, 48].

Series that retrospectively compared the LESS approach to a case-matched group of patients who had a conventional laparoscopic approach found the LESS patients either needed less *or more* postoperative narcotics and had shorter or equivalent operative time. Complication rates were not significantly different [48].

Orchiopexy

The use of LESS for laparoscopic orchiopexy has been described in case series including up to 18 patients [18, 22, 26, 30, 34, 47, 49], including both unilateral and bilateral, staged and non-staged procedures from multiple countries of publications. As would be expected, the technique would be initiated with a single trocar placement to perform diagnostic laparoscopy before proceeding with the LESS procedure.

Similar to the varicocelectomy procedures, a port device is most popular with TriPort being utilized the most in the literature, and two series preferring an incisional approach. Again the incisional approach was preferred in one series for patients under 10 kg while the other preferred an incisional approach for all gonadal/inguinal procedures [18, 30]. Also mirroring the techniques described for varicocelectomy, most surgeons preferred a combination of flexible and straight instrumentation while one series had comparable results with only straight instrument usage with a 45 degree offset laparoscopic camera.

Mean operative times were 37–89 min including bilateral procedures where performed, the majority of patients were discharged the same day, and almost no narcotic usage was required. Six series including 49 patients reported no adverse outcomes or complications with up to 12 months of follow up. One series which was the largest identified, including 18 patients, did report one vas deferens injury intraoperatively, and one scrotal cellulitis postoperative infection requiring outpatient antibiotic therapy [47].

Gonadectomy

Numerous small series have described the experience of LESS with gonadectomy, both unilateral and bilateral, including one with concomitant hysterectomy for a DSD condition [18, 19, 33, 34, 47, 50]. On similar trajectory, another case report described the technique in use for an ovarian detorsion and cystectomy [19].

Again, most published surgeons describe a preference to use a commercially available port and flexible and straight instruments for each procedure as described previously, however one series does endorse the use of an incisional approach with an end-on 45-degree lens camera with straight instruments [18].

Mean operative times are reported at about 60 min for unilateral gonadectomy cases and from 37.5 to 82 min for bilateral gonadectomy, and 189 min for the case report that included the hysterectomy as well [34]. One series reported the procedure to be done outpatient while others reported 1–2 day mean length of stays. Where described, no narcotics were required. Almost no follow up data was available, but no complications or adverse outcomes were reported.

Inguinal hernia or Hydrocele Repair

A technique that predates most LESS experience and literature, single-site laparoscopic percutaneous extra-peritoneal closure (SLPEC) of hernia sac/processus vaginalis has been widely performed for repair of inguinal hernia/hydrocele in children for the past few decades, with procedures dating as early as 2006 [9, 51–53]. The technique is most popularized in Eurasian countries, with one series by Chen et al. from 2017 reporting a systematic review that includes 11,815 surgeries done in Eurasian countries [52].

The technique's main similarity to LESS is the use of a transumbilical transperitoneal approach to groin surgery, where only a 5–10 mm incision for camera trocar placement is required at the umbilicus while percutaneous needles at the site of the inguinal hernia are used to hydrodissect, tunnel, and purse-string the patent processus vaginalis closed. Permanent suture is usually required. A similar approach, modified transumbilical two-port laparoscopic suturing (M-TTLS), utilizes two rather than one umbilical port placement to assist with suturing of the repair. This technique was compared to the SLPEC approach in a retrospective review by Wang et al. 2019 and found no significant differences in outcomes but did find M-TTLS to have longer operative times (13.3 min vs 10.8 min). No flexible instrumentation is described as a routine part of this procedure [53].

Mean operative times for SLPEC were reported from 11 to 18.3 min, and the 18.3 min operative time was specified as time from incision to dressings. Learning curve improvements in operative time were found to stabilize after 31 cases in another series by Wang et al. [9] Length of stay was reported from 1–2 days and no outcomes regarding postoperative narcotic requirements were describes.

Summarizing the largest systematic review by Chen which included 49 studies with up to 40 months of follow up, 0.70% of patients experienced a recurrence, 0.33% had a suture knot reaction, 0.32% had vessel injury, most commonly inferior epigastrics, 0.23% developed a hydrocele, 0.05% required a conversion. No testicular atrophy reported [52].

Lower Urinary Tract Surgery

Reports of the use of LESS in the lower urinary tract are rare, but procedures described include utricle excision, ureterolithotomy, distal ureterectomy, and urachal cyst excision [18, 47]. Only urachal cyst excision was reported in more than one patient, so generalizable technique, outcomes on the other procedures cannot be well described. However, success rates in the available reports are poor compared to renal, inguinal or gonadal surgery with the utricle excision requiring additional port placement for dissection, the ureterolithotomy converting to open for failure to progress, and the distal ureterectomy having a febrile UTI and ileus requiring prolonged admission and IV antibiotics [47]. Of three patients described to have a LESS assisted urachal remnant excision, 1 required a redo excision at 10 months postoperatively [18].

Miscellaneous Reconstruction

ACE

A small collection of series have been published describing the use of LESS for Malone antegrade continence enema creation [16, 18, 19]. An incisional approach is more commonly described, as well as a predominance of only straight instrument usage. Mean operative times range from 67 to 119 min, length of stay 1–2 days, and narcotic usage from none to needing narcotic only on POD1. Of 6 patients in these series, complications reported included 1 wound infection requiring outpatient antibiotic and 1 stenosis requiring anesthesia for Chait tube placement at unspecified follow up. No series comparing the technique to the open or conventional laparoscopic approach were identified.

Conclusion

LESS can performed for a variety of procedures, albeit with its technical challenges and learning curves. Multiple technological advances have ushered in greater opportunities to use LESS, including various multi-ports, articulating instruments, or needlescopic instruments. No technical approaches or instrumentation have yet been proven to be superior. There is no apparent increase in complications when comparing LESS to conventional laparoscopy or robotic surgery in current series. Depending on the technique or supplies used, it may reduce material costs, lead to less narcotic needs, and lead to either decreased, equivalent, or increased operative time. Aesthetic benefits are known to be significant.

We feel extirpative or minor reconstructive procedures are ideal for most surgeons as complex reconstructive procedures require a greater deal of flexibility. Authors reporting on the more complex procedures described above deserve merit for their achievements in LESS. In both procedure selection and technical considerations, surgeon familiarity and experience will take precedence.

References

1. Park SK, Olweny EO, Best SL, Tracy CR, Mir SA, Cadeddu JA. Patient-reported body image and cosmesis outcomes following kidney surgery: comparison of laparoendoscopic single-site, laparoscopic, and open surgery. Eur Urol. 2011;60(5):1097–104. https://doi.org/10.1016/j.eururo.2011.08.007. Epub 2011 Aug 12.
2. Reibetanz J, Ickrath P, Hain J, Germer CT, Krajinovic K. Single-port laparoscopic cholecystectomy versus standard multiport laparoscopic cholecystectomy: a case-control study comparing the long-term quality of life and body image. Surg Today. 2013;43(9):1025–30. https://doi.org/10.1007/s00595-012-0393-4. Epub 2012 Nov 2.
3. Box G, Averch T, Cadeddu J, Cherullo E, Clayman R, Desai M. Nomenclature of natural orifice translumenal endoscopic surgery (NOTES) and laparoendoscopic single-site surgery (LESS) procedures in urology. J Endourol. 2008;22(11):2575–81. https://doi.org/10.1089/end.2008.0471.
4. Chittawar PB, Magon N, Bhandari S. Laparoendoscopic single-site surgery in gynecology: LESS is actually how much less? J Midlife Health. 2013;4(1):46–51. https://doi.org/10.4103/0976-7800.109638.
5. Wheeless CR, Thompson BH. Laparoscopic sterilization: review of 3600 cases. Obstet Gynecol. 1973;42(5):751–8.
6. Gill IS, Canes D, Aron M, Haber GP, Goldfarb DA, Flechner S. Single port transumbilical (E-NOTES) donor nephrectomy. J Urol. 2008;180(2):637–41; discussion 641. https://doi.org/10.1016/j.juro.2008.04.028. Epub 2008 Jun 12.
7. Lima M, Ruggeri G, Tursini S. One trocar assisted pyeloplasty (OTAP): initial experience and codification of a technique. Paper presented at Annual Congress for Endosurgery in Children, Venice Lido, Italy, June 1–4, 2005.
8. Marietti S, Holmes N, Chiang G. Laparoendoscopic single-site (LESS) bilateral nephrectomy in the pretransplant pediatric population. Pediatr Transplant. 2011;15(4):396–9. https://doi.org/10.1111/j.1399-3046.2011.01504.
9. Wang F, Shou T, Zhong H. Is two-port laparoendoscopic single-site surgery (T-LESS) feasible for pediatric hydroceles? Single-center experience with the initial 59 cases. J Pediatr Urol. 2018;14(1):67.e1–6. https://doi.org/10.1016/j.jpurol.2017.09.016. Epub 2017 Oct 16.
10. Chue KM, Goh GH, Kow AWC. Right adrenal gland pseudocyst masquerading as a large symptomatic hepatic cyst: single incision laparoscopic (SILS) resection and a review of current literature. Ann Hepatobiliary Pancreat Surg. 2018;22(1):75–8. https://doi.org/10.14701/ahbps.2018.22.1.75. Epub 2018 Feb 26.
11. Jeon HG, Kim DS, Jeoung HB, Han SW, Hong CH, Im YJ. Pediatric laparoendoscopic single-site partial nephrectomy: initial report. Urology. 2010;76(1):138–41. https://doi.org/10.1016/j.urology.2010.01.088. Epub 2010 May 2.
12. Park YH, Kang MY, Jeong MS, Choi H, Kim HH. Laparoendoscopic single-site nephrectomy using a homemade single-port device for single-system ectopic ureter in a child: initial case report. J Endourol. 2009;23(5):833–5. https://doi.org/10.1089/end.2009.0025.
13. Lee DG, Baek M, Ju SH, Jeong BC, Han DH. Laparoendoscopic single-site nephrectomy for single-system ectopic ureters with dysplastic kidneys in children: early experience. J

Laparoendosc Adv Surg Tech A. 2011;21(5):461–5. https://doi.org/10.1089/lap.2010.0429. Epub 2011 Apr 27.
14. Ham WS, Im YJ, Jung HJ, Hong CH, Han WK, Han SW. Initial experience with laparoendoscopic single-site nephrectomy and nephroureterectomy in children. Urology. 2011;77(5):1204–8. https://doi.org/10.1016/j.urology.2010.07.535. Epub 2010 Dec 4.
15. Ferreres AR, Asbun HJ. Technical aspects of cholecystectomy. Surg Clin North Am. 2014;94(2):427–54. https://doi.org/10.1016/j.suc.2014.01.007.
16. Chiang G. Fairbanks T Initial use of LESS for the ACE Malone procedure in children. Urology. 2012;80(3):717–8. https://doi.org/10.1016/j.urology.2012.01.031. Epub 2012 Apr 1.
17. Ramesh B, Sharma P. Laparoendoscopic single-site surgery in gynecology: dawn of a new era. J Midlife Health. 2013;4(1):52–3.
18. Patel N, Santomauro M, Marietti S, Chiang G. Laparoendoscopic single site surgery in pediatric urology: does it require specialized tools? Int Braz J Urol. 2016;42(2):277–83.
19. Gor RA, Long CJ, Shukla AR, Kirsch AJ, Perez-Brayfield M, Srinivasan AK. Multi-institutional experience in laparoendoscopic single-site surgery (LESS): for major extirpative and reconstructive procedures in pediatric urology. Urology. 2016;88:173–8. https://doi.org/10.1016/j.urology.2015.11.012. Epub 2015 Nov 17.
20. Bansal D, Cost NG, Bean CM, Riachy E, Defoor WR Jr, Reddy PP. Comparison of pediatric robotic-assisted laparoscopic nephroureterectomy and laparoendoscopic single-site nephroureterectomy. Urology. 2014;83(2):438–42. https://doi.org/10.1016/j.urology.2013.08.066. Epub 2013 Nov 6.
21. Woldrich JM, Holmes N, Palazzi-Churas K, Alagiri M, DeCambre M, Kaplan G. Comparison of laparoendoscopic single-site, conventional laparoscopic, and open nephrectomy in a pediatric population. Urology. 2011;78(1):74–7. https://doi.org/10.1016/j.urology.2010.11.030. Epub 2011 Feb 18.
22. Noh PH, Vinson MA, Bansal D. Laparoendoscopic single site orchidopexy for intra-abdominal testes in the pediatric population with a multichannel single port and flexible tip laparoscope. J Endourol. 2013;27(11):1381–3. https://doi.org/10.1089/end.2013.0182. Epub 2013 Aug 2.
23. Bayazit Y, Aridogan IA, Abat D, Satar N, Doran S. Pediatric transumbilical laparoendoscopic single-site nephroureterectomy: initial report. Urology. 2009;74(5):1116–9. https://doi.org/10.1016/j.urology.2009.05.096. Epub 2009 Sep 20.
24. Johnson KC, Cha DY, DaJusta DG, Barone JG, Ankem MK. Pediatric single-port-access nephrectomy for a multicystic, dysplastic kidney. J Pediatr Urol. 2009;5(5):402–4. https://doi.org/10.1016/j.jpurol.2009.03.011. Epub 2009 Apr 29.
25. Kim PH, Patil MB, Kim SS, Dorey F, De Filippo RE, Chang AY. Early comparison of nephrectomy options in children (open, transperitoneal laparoscopic, laparo-endoscopic single site(LESS), and robotic surgery). BJU Int. 2012;109(6):910–5. https://doi.org/10.1111/j.1464-410X.2011.10524.x. Epub 2011 Aug 23.
26. Abdel-Karim AM, Elmissery M, Elsalmy S, Moussa A, Aboelfotoh A. Laparoendoscopic single-site surgery (LESS) for the treatment of different urologic pathologies in pediatrics: single-center single-surgeon experience. J Pediatr Urol. 2015;11(1):33.e1–7. https://doi.org/10.1016/j.jpurol.2014.08.012. Epub 2014 Oct 2.
27. Luithle T, Szavay P, Fuchs J. Single-incision laparoscopic nephroureterectomy in children of all age groups. J Pediatr Surg. 2013;48(5):1142–6. https://doi.org/10.1016/j.jpedsurg.2013.01.040.
28. Vricella GJ, Ross JH, Vourganti S, Cherullo EE. Laparoendoscopic single-site nephrectomy: initial clinical experience in children. J Endourol. 2010;24(12):1957–61. https://doi.org/10.1089/end.2010.0034. Epub 2010 Sep 16.
29. Till H, Basharkhah A, Hock A. What's the best minimal invasive approach to pediatric nephrectomy and heminephrectomy: conventional laparoscopy (CL), single-site (LESS) or robotics (RAS)? Transl Pediatr. 2016;5(4):240–4. Review.
30. Szavay PO, Luithle T, Nagel C, Fuchs J. Weight-adapted surgical approach for laparoendoscopic single-site surgery in pediatric patients using low-cost reusable instrumentation:

a prospective analysis. J Laparoendosc Adv Surg Tech A. 2013;23(3):281–6. https://doi.org/10.1089/lap.2012.0466. Epub 2013 Feb 12.
31. Featherstone NC, De Win G, Undre S, Cherian A. Single incision prone retroperitoneoscopic paediatric nephrectomy. J Pediatr Urol. 2015;11(5):283–4. https://doi.org/10.1016/j.jpurol.2015.04.010. Epub 2015 May 29.
32. Liem NT, Mai Thuy NT, Viet ND, Dung le A. Single trocar retroperitoneoscopic nephrectomy for dysplastic poorly functioning kidney with ectopic ureter in children. J Pediatr Urol. 2013;9(4):424–6. https://doi.org/10.1016/j.jpurol.2012.10.007. Epub 2012 Oct 25.
33. Kocherov S, Lev G, Shenfeld OZ, Chertin B. Laparoscopic single site surgery: initial experience and description of techniques in the pediatric population. J Urol. 2011;186(4 Suppl):1653–7. https://doi.org/10.1016/j.juro.2011.03.100. Epub 2011 Aug 19.
34. Yamada Y, Naitoh Y, Kobayashi K, Fujihara A, Johnin K, Hongo F. Laparoendoscopic single-site surgery for pediatric urologic disease. J Endourol. 2016;30(1):24–7. https://doi.org/10.1089/end.2015.0130. Epub 2015 Oct 27.
35. Tam YH, Pang KK, Tsui SY, Wong YS, Wong HY, Mou JW. Laparoendoscopic single-site nephrectomy and heminephroureterectomy in children using standard laparoscopic setup versus conventional laparoscopy. Urology. 2013;82(2):430–5. https://doi.org/10.1016/j.urology.2013.02.057. Epub 2013 May.
36. Bansal D, Cost NG, Bean CM, Noh PH. Pediatric laparo-endoscopic single site partial nephrectomy: feasibility in infants and small children for upper urinary tract duplication anomalies. J Pediatr Urol. 2014;10(5):859–63. https://doi.org/10.1016/j.jpurol.2014.01.025. Epub 2014 Feb 19.
37. Neheman A, Kord E, Strine AC, VanderBrink BA, Minevich EA, DeFoor WR. Pediatric partial nephrectomy for upper urinary tract duplication anomalies: a comparison between different surgical approaches and techniques. Urology. 2019;125:196–201. https://doi.org/10.1016/j.urology.2018.11.026. Epub 2018 Nov 24.
38. Soto-Aviles OE, Escudero-Chu K, Perez-Brayfield MR. Laparoscopic single-site surgery in pediatric urology: where do we stand today? Curr Urol Rep. 2015;16(10):68. https://doi.org/10.1007/s11934-015-0542-6.
39. Tugcu V, Ilbey YO, Polat H, Tasci AI. Early experience with laparoendoscopic single-site pyeloplasty in children. J Pediatr Urol. 2011;7(2):187–91. https://doi.org/10.1016/j.jpurol.2010.10.014. Epub 2010 Dec 4.
40. Zhou H, Sun N, Zhang X, Xie H, Ma L, Shen Z, Zhou X, Tao T. Transumbilical laparoendoscopic single-site pyeloplasty in infants and children: initial experience and short-term outcome. Pediatr Surg Int. 2012;28(3):321–5. https://doi.org/10.1007/s00383-011-3040-z. Epub 2011 Dec 29.
41. Naitoh Y, Kawauchi A, Yamada Y, Fujihara A, Hongo F, Kamoi K. Laparoendoscopic single-site versus conventional laparoscopic pyeloplasty: a matched pair analysis. Int J Urol. 2014;21(8):793–6. https://doi.org/10.1111/iju.12427. Epub 2014 Mar 25.
42. Khambati A, Wehbi E, Farhat WA. Laparo-endoscopic single site surgery in pediatrics: feasibility and surgical outcomes from a preliminary prospective Canadian experience. Can Urol Assoc J. 2015;9(1–2):48–52. https://doi.org/10.5489/cuaj.2379.
43. Liu D, Zhou H, Ma L, Xie H, Tao T, Cao H. Transumbilical multi-port laparoscopic pyeloplasty versus transumbilical single-site laparoscopic pyeloplasty for ureteropelvic junction obstruction in children: a retrospectively comparative study. J Pediatr Urol. 2017;13(6):618.e1–5. https://doi.org/10.1016/j.jpurol.2017.05.009. Epub 2017 Jun 3.
44. Liu D, Zhou H, Chao M, Qi J, Wei H, An N. Transumbilical single-site multiport laparoscopic pyeloplasty for children with Ureteropelvic junction obstruction in China: a multicenter study. J Laparoendosc Adv Surg Tech A. 2017;27(6):655–9. https://doi.org/10.1089/lap.2016.0306. Epub 2017 Mar 28.
45. Bi Y, Lu L, Ruan S. Using conventional 3- and 5-mm straight instruments in laparoendoscopic single-site pyeloplasty in children. J Laparoendosc Adv Surg Tech A. 2011;21(10):969–72. https://doi.org/10.1089/lap.2011.0103. Epub 2011 Nov 14.

46. Uygun I, Okur MH, Aydogdu B, Arslan MS, Cimen H, Otcu S. Transumbilical scarless surgery with thoracic trocar easy and low-cost. J Korean Surg Soc. 2013;84(6):360–6. https://doi.org/10.4174/jkss.2013.84.6.360 Epub 2013 May 28.
47. Bansal D, Cost NG, Bean CM, Minevich EA, Noh PH. Pediatric urological laparoendoscopic single site surgery: single surgeon experience. J Pediatr Urol. 2014;10(6):1170–5. https://doi.org/10.1016/j.jpurol.2014.04.020. Epub 2014 Jun 19.
48. Bansal D, Riachy E, Defoor WR Jr, Reddy PP, Minevich EA, Alam S. Pediatric varicocelectomy: a comparative study of conventional laparoscopic and laparoendoscopic single-site approaches. J Endourol. 2014;28(5):513–6. https://doi.org/10.1089/end.2013.0125. Epub 2013 Dec 11.
49. Sultan RC, Johnson KC, Ankem MK, Barone JG. Laparoendoscopic single site orchiopexy. J Pediatr Surg. 2011;46(2):421–3. https://doi.org/10.1016/j.jpedsurg.2010.06.037.
50. Mizuno K, Kojima Y, Nishio H, Tozawa K, Mizuno H, Kohri K. Transumbilical laparoendoscopic single-site gonadectomy for Turner's syndrome with Y-chromosome mosaicism. J Pediatr Urol. 2012;8(4):e39–42. https://doi.org/10.1016/j.jpurol.2012.02.010. Epub 2012 Mar 13.
51. Wang F, Zhong H, Chen Y, Zhao J, Li Y, Chen J, Dong S. Single-site laparoscopic percutaneous extraperitoneal closure of the internal ring using an epidural and spinal needle: excellent results in 1464 children with inguinal hernia/hydrocele. Surg Endosc. 2017;31(7):2932–8. https://doi.org/10.1007/s00464-016-5309-8. Epub 2016 Nov 4.
52. Chen Y, Wang F, Zhong H, Zhao J, Li Y, Shi Z. A systematic review and meta-analysis concerning single-site laparoscopic percutaneous extraperitoneal closure for pediatric inguinal hernia and hydrocele. Surg Endosc. 2017;31(12):4888–901. https://doi.org/10.1007/s00464-017-5491-3. Epub 2017 Apr 7.
53. Wang F, Zhong H, Shou T, Chen Y, Zhao J. Single-site laparoscopic percutaneous extraperitoneal closure versus modified transumbilical two-port laparoscopic suturing of the hernia sac for the treatment of pediatric inguinal hernia: comparison of the outcomes of two different approaches. J Laparoendosc Adv Surg Tech A. 2019;29(1):103–8. https://doi.org/10.1089/lap.2018.0405. Epub 2018 Sep 14.

Chapter 25
Robotic Fetal Surgery: The Next Frontier?

Timothy C. Boswell, Edward S. Ahn, Rodrigo Ruano, and Patricio C. Gargollo

Introduction

In the modern era, surgeons have pursued minimally invasive techniques through smaller incisions wherever possible due to myriad benefits in patient recovery. Robotic assistance also dramatically improved surgeon dexterity, visualization, and magnification. As a result, we are not only doing procedures robotically that were once performed open or laparoscopically, but **robotic surgery is poised for application to new or blossoming surgical frontiers, including fetal surgery.**

Major developments have been made in fetal surgery since the first attempts at fetal intervention in the 1960s, with a growing focus on the field especially at the turn of the twenty-first century. Robotic surgical platforms are particularly well suited for addressing prenatally diagnosed conditions because of the inherent requirement for small incisions, minimal tissue trauma, and exquisite dexterity, not to mention further advancements under development such as new energy devices and even telesurgery.

In this chapter, we will discuss the history of fetal surgery, its unique considerations, specific conditions targeted for fetal surgical treatment, robotic surgical technique considerations, and major areas of ongoing development.

T. C. Boswell · P. C. Gargollo (✉)
Mayo Clinic, Department of Urology, Rochester, MN, USA
e-mail: Boswell.Timothy@mayo.edu; Gargollo.Patricio@mayo.edu

E. S. Ahn
Mayo Clinic, Department of Neurological Surgery, Rochester, MN, USA
e-mail: Ahn.Edward@mayo.edu

R. Ruano
Mayo Clinic, Department of Obstetrics and Gynecology, Rochester, MN, USA
e-mail: Ruano.Rodrigo@mayo.edu

History of Fetal Surgery

While operations on fetuses in the setting of fetal demise date back to antiquity, procedural interventions on the living fetus required means of accurate prenatal diagnosis, which did not come about until the mid twentieth century (Fig. 25.1). In the 1960s, the first modern attempts at fetal procedural intervention focused on treating erythoblastosis fetalis caused by Rh incompatibility. Various groups around the world pursued percutaneous and open fetal transfusion to address this lethal condition, made possible by detection of markers in amniotic fluid predicting fetal demise. Championed by Sir William Liley of New Zealand, who was then considered the father of fetal therapy [1], these efforts demonstrated the feasibility of fetal intervention, but also were the world's first view of the complications including fetal injury, amniotic leak, premature labor, chorioamnionitis, and maternal sepsis.

Prenatal ultrasound, which became increasingly available in the 1970s and 1980s, propelled further antenatal interventions through detection of other life-threatening conditions, which remained the focus of fetal interventions. Hydrocephalus, obstructive uropathy, congenital diaphragmatic hernia, twin-twin transfusion syndrome, sacrococcygeal teratoma, and pulmonary malformations were several of these ultrasound-detectable conditions targeted for interventions [2]. Animal models were developed to resemble the human pathophysiology of each condition and then used to test *in utero* correction. Anesthetic and tocolytic techniques had to be developed and tested in animals as well to ensure feasibility and safety for mother and fetus. Interventions initially centered on placement of shunts (ventriculo-peritoneal shunt for hydrocephalus, vesico-amniotic shunt for obstructive uropathy, etc.) and other predominantly percutaneous measures in the early periods. Ongoing developments led to open procedures via maternal incision and hysterotomy, for surgical access to the fetus. The common thread through all of

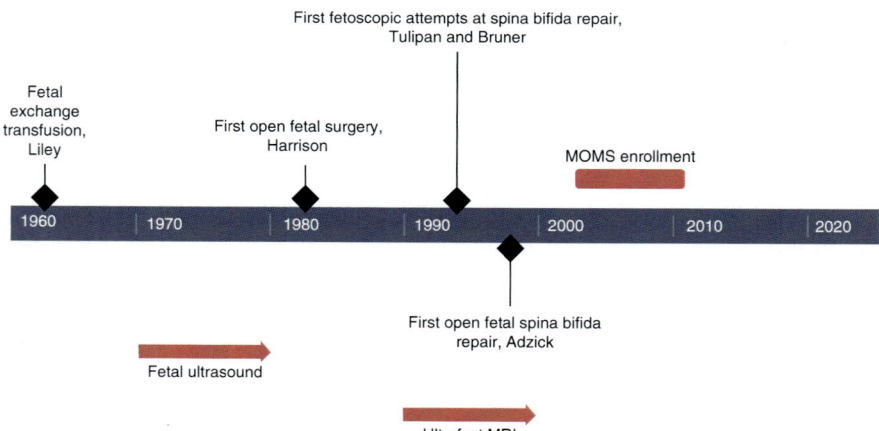

Fig. 25.1 Timeline of key milestones in fetal surgery

these procedures was the focus on conditions that are lethal or life-threatening to the fetus, given the attendant risks of intervention to both mother and baby.

A major paradigm shift occurred when the thought leaders of fetal surgery started pursuing prenatal surgery for myelomeningocele (MMC), because this is typically not a life-threatening disorder, and so the goals of surgery were improved quality of life rather than saving life. This focus came about in the 1990s, in concert with the development of ultrafast MRI which served to more accurately characterize these and other fetal anomalies. Furthermore, myelomeningocele was significantly more prevalent (and in more healthy fetuses overall) than the other conditions pursued via fetal surgery, and so this opened the door to a significantly increased volume in fetal surgery.

Notably the first attempts at spina bifida closure, led at Vanderbilt by Noel Tulipan and Joseph Bruner, were performed *fetoscopically* in the mid-1990s [3]. Poor results in the four index patients (two expired, two required neonatal repairs) led to abandoning the fetoscopic approach and pursuit of open surgery, which became the focus of ongoing efforts. The thought leaders eventually developed the well-designed randomized controlled trial, the Prenatal vs. Postnatal Repair of Myelomeningocele (MOMS) trial, which dominated the fetal surgery field pertaining to MMC between 2003 and 2010. This study showed that prenatal closure of spina bifida caused lower ventriculoperitoneal shunt rates as well as improved composite scores for mental development and motor function [4]. Importantly, during this time, all patients undergoing prenatal spina bifida closure in the US were done at one of the three study centers (Vanderbilt, University of California at San Francisco, and Children's Hospital of Philadelphia) as a part of the MOMS protocol, and no other centers in the United States were permitted to pursue MMC fetal surgery during this period. Meanwhile, Europe and the rest of world were free to experiment and develop new surgical techniques, outside of the MOMS protocol. Providers in Europe and South America were further developing and perfecting their percutaneous/fetoscopic techniques.

After the MOMS trial, the number of fetal surgery programs rapidly increased across the world, with increasing volumes of fetal surgery performed and an ever-growing interest in improved and new applications.

Major Prerequisite Considerations for Fetal Surgery

Diagnosis

Successful prenatal intervention depends on accurate diagnosis of index conditions as well as imaging to guide procedure planning and execution. The development and improvement of **prenatal ultrasound** was the centerpiece of prenatal diagnosis. Its low cost and relative ease of performance have permitted its use to become ubiquitous and, in fact, standard of care for prenatal evaluation and pregnancy monitoring. Key improvements including high-frequency transducers, Doppler flow evaluations, and multi-dimensional reconstructions have been further applied to improve sensitivity of detection as well as to better define disease severity. Both preoperatively and real-time intraoperatively, ultrasound is also facile for identification of placental location, amniotic fluid volume, fetal positioning, and cardiac parameters. This information is essential to guide percutaneous procedures as well as open surgeries, especially the site of hysterotomy, and serves as the core means for intraoperative fetal monitoring.

However, ultrasound has its limitations including limited visibility in situations of oligohydramnios, excessive maternal adiposity, or wave attenuation by maternal pelvic bones. When ultrasound is limited or further resolution is required, fetal MRI delivers even better imaging. This opportunity was brought about by the development of **ultrafast MRI**, as MRI acquisition was previously limited in fetal application by the deleterious combination of long image acquisition time and fetal movement. Complex malformations can now be exquisitely defined and mapped via MRI for diagnosis and planning of intervention [5].

Maternal-Fetal Anatomy and Physiology

The early efforts at fetal surgery demonstrated the key maternal-fetal considerations in antenatal surgery: **tocolysis is essential, premature delivery is likely, and the amniotic sac never truly heals leading to a high risk of amniotic leak.**

Fetal surgery depends on a robust knowledge of uterine, placental, and fetal anatomy. Surgical access to the fetus requires incision through the uterine wall and fetal membranes. The chorion (outer membrane) and amnion (inner membrane) are typically fused by 14–16 weeks gestation. Uterine bleeding that dissects along the chorion can cause placental separation from the uterine wall (see complications below). Furthermore, the amniotic sac is a balloon-like structure with delicate membranes prone to leakage after intervention.

The timing of prenatal surgery is a delicate balance: the fetus needs to be advanced enough in size and structural development to permit intervention, but should not be close to anticipated delivery due to the diminished benefit of prenatal versus postnatal surgery. As such, most fetal surgeries occur at mid-gestation. For example, the MOMS trial specified that a fetus must be less than 26 weeks gestation at time of surgery for inclusion.

Team Approach

Fetal surgery is a unique overlap of multiple disciplines encompassing obstetrics, maternal-fetal medicine, surgery and its subspecialties, anesthesiology, radiology, neonatal intensivists, and more. Given the complexity of each discipline, pursuing fetal surgery requires a strong grasp of all these areas, ideally as part of a dedicated multidisciplinary team. **Having a well-established multidisciplinary team in place is likely the most important prerequisite for fetal surgery success.**

Fetal Surgery Techniques

Anesthesia and Monitoring

Aspects of obstetric anesthesia have been thoroughly described elsewhere given its frequency for use in cesarean section and other procedures. **Tocolysis is the unique necessity for fetal surgery, as an essential goal is to prevent uterine contractions and precipitation of premature labor.** In general, the mother is typically induced under a combination of regional (epidural) anesthesia and inhaled general anesthesia. Common tocolytic protocols include indomethacin, desflurane (with increasing MAC at time of uterine incision), oxygen and nitrous oxide, vecuronium, and magnesium sulfate continuing postoperatively with addition of oral and/or rectal suppository indomethacin [6].

One of the key challenges of fetal surgery is fetal monitoring. In open surgery, fetal intravenous access for sampling, monitoring, and infusion can be obtained but can be difficult and prone to dislodgement. Access to fetal chorionic plate vessels has been performed as well and is an alternative. Pulse oximetry has been shown to be both non-invasive and sensitive, as well as applicable to both open and fetoscopic fetal surgery [7, 8]. Furthermore, monitoring intrauterine pressure and temperature in fetoscopic cases can be done with intrauterine probes.

The most valuable fetal monitoring tool both perioperatively and intraoperatively is ultrasound. Periodic ultrasonography permits monitoring of fetal heart rate and cardiac contractility, fetal positioning, amniotic fluid volume, and Doppler assessment of fetoplacental circulation [9]. Open fetal surgery can cause varying degrees of heart rate variability, decreased cardiac output with fetal manipulation, ventricular and valvular dysfunction, and acute constriction of the ductus arteriosus. All of these occur in patients undergoing procedures involving the cardiopulmonary system and even in unrelated systems including in MMC repair [6, 10].

Setup and Positioning

For positioning, the mother is typically placed in low lithotomy which allows a provider to stand between abducted legs with the other surgeons and assistants standing at each side. The maternal right side is typically partially bumped to minimize reduction of cardiac return by caval compression from the gravid uterus.

Open Surgery

The techniques of open surgery will continue to inform fetoscopic approaches, and remain essential to know in case of fetoscopic complications. For open surgery, a laparotomy incision is used to exteriorize the uterus. Preoperative and intraoperative ultrasound can be performed to determine placental location and fetal lie, which are essential for planning the site of hysterotomy. Hysterotomy is likely the most dangerous portion of the procedure and is typically performed in stapled fashion. Initial uterine access to facilitate stapler placement is obtained with a trocar or by electrocautery, taking care to avoid membrane injury [4, 11]. Bleeding with hysterotomy can lead to subchorionic hematoma which can be a devastating complication to the fetus. Placement of absorbable sutures at the apices of hysterotomy is a key step to minimize this risk of disastrous bleeding (Fig. 25.2).

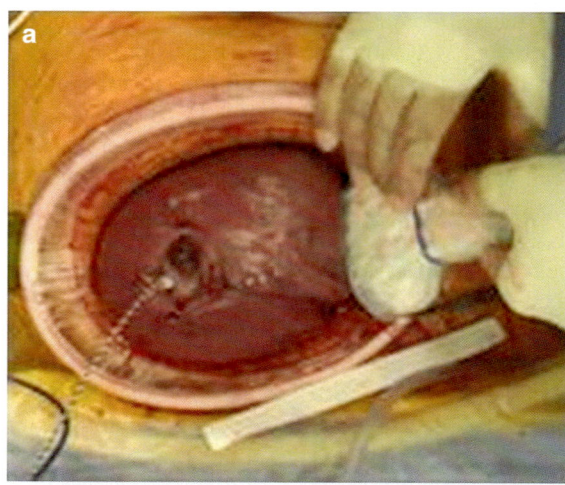
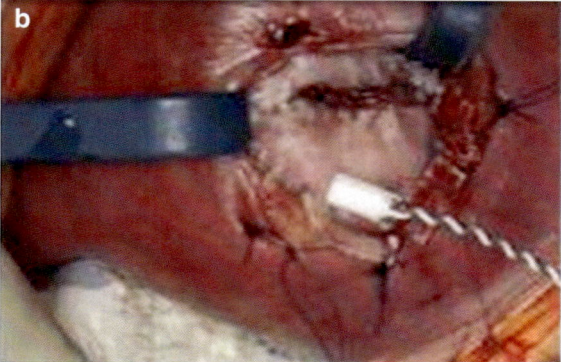

Fig. 25.2 Open fetal surgery for myelomeningocele using uterine staplers with continuous fetal heart monitoring in a fetus at 24 weeks: (**a**) exposure of the myelomeningocele (**b**) final closure of the myelomeningocele

Fetoscopic Access

Fetoscopic access (Fig. 25.3) can be obtained percutaneously or after maternal laparotomy and exposure of the gravid uterus, depending classically on placental location (with anterior placentas often requiring laparotomy and direct access to the uterus for port placement). However, Thomas Kohl has suggested that percutaneous access specifically for spina bifida surgery can almost always be safely performed irrespective of placental location [12]. For port placement, preference has been for radially dilating ports ideally in the 1–5 mm size range. Radial expansion can help

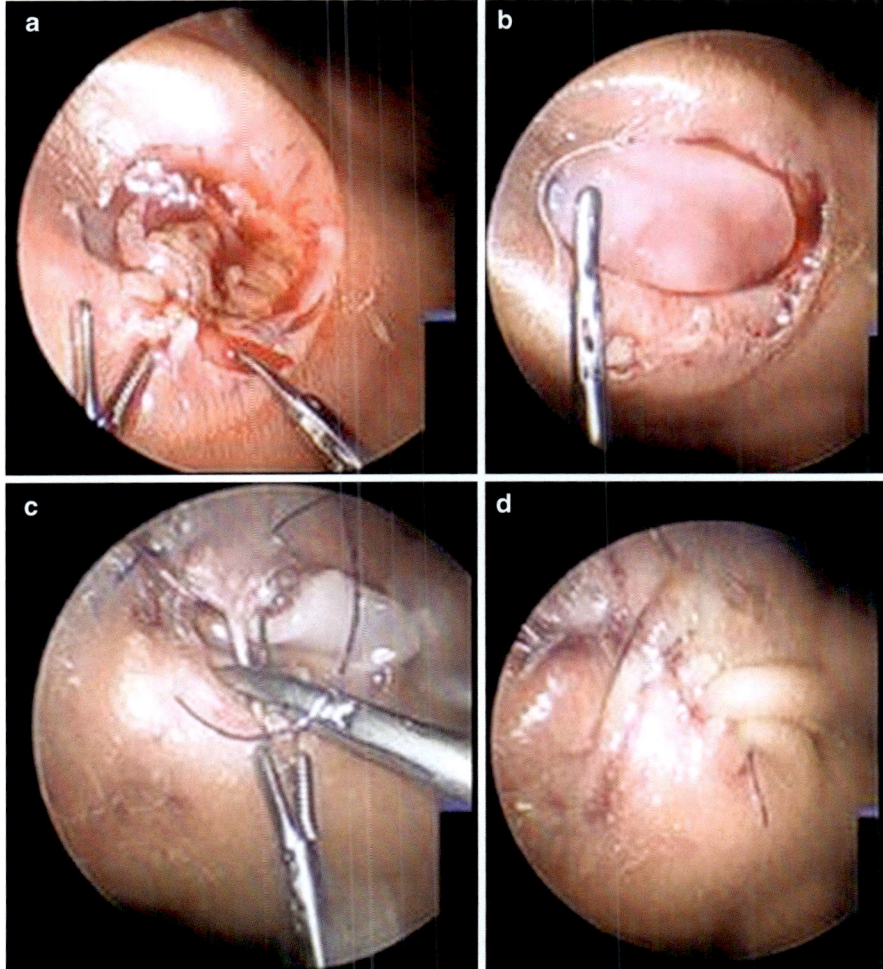

Fig. 25.3 Fetoscopic views of fetal spina bifida dissection (**a**), dura patch (**b**), skin closure (**c**), and final closure (**d**) at 25 weeks

to minimize uterine bleeding [13]. These are typically placed under ultrasound guidance (with ideally at least 3 cm clearance from the placental edge) and via Seldinger technique. Balloon-tipped trochars can help to prevent port dislodgement as well [14, 15], or ports can be sutured directly to the skin or uterine wall to minimize the risk of dislodgement. Trocar dislodgement can occur due to sudden changes in intrauterine volume, uterine contractions, uterine collapse due to amniotic or gas leak, or traction between abdominal or uterine walls. For port site closure, instillation of fibrin glue and ligature with suture is preferred when there is access to the uterus; completely percutaneous procedures have no means for port site closure, which may elevate the risk for amniotic leak [12, 13, 16].

Insufflation and Amnioinfusion

After establishing transuterine access, amniotic fluid removal and gas insufflation are typically performed in fetoscopic surgery. Historically, initial attempts at the use of carbon dioxide insufflation were limited due to concerns for fetal hypercarbia and acidosis, requiring maternal hyperventilation to help manage this effect [17]. As such, attempts at liquid media instillation including amniotic fluid, lactated ringers, or glycine [18] were performed but were plagued by limited visibility due to fluid cloudiness or turbidity from blood, despite efforts at fluid cycling [13]. Kohl later demonstrated the safety and efficacy of partial amniotic CO_2 insufflation (PACI) in both animal studies and human reports [12, 19]. Amniotic volume is periodically measured with ultrasound and adjusted by changing insufflation pressure settings or by addition or removal of intra-amniotic fluid.

Most providers instill antibiotic solution at the conclusion of the procedure when replacing lost amniotic fluid volume to decrease the risk of chorioamnionitis, although this practice has not been studied in comparative fashion.

Complications

Fetal surgery is a calculated effort balancing the risks of intervention (to both fetus and mother) with the potential benefit of treatment in the fetus. The risks of intervention are high, which is why initial fetal surgeries were limited to lethal fetal conditions but have since expanded to quality of life indications with growing experience.

Maternal Risks

Fetal interventions pose a variety of risks to the mother, ranging in magnitude for minimally invasive, fetoscopic, and open procedures. The predominant maternal risk through all procedural techniques is infection, including chorioamnionitis potentially leading to maternal sepsis, which fortunately is quite rare. Chorioamnionitis occurs in approximately 2–3% of laser treatments for twin-twin transfusion syndrome (TTTS) and in 6% of open spina bifida repairs. Bleeding leading to intraoperative or postoperative transfusion in the mother occurs in about 9–13% of open spina bifida repairs.

Hysterotomy results in uterine scar formation. This brings the attendant risk for subsequent scar dehiscence and uterine rupture in the index pregnancy or subsequent pregnancies. Dehiscence of scar at delivery occurs in about 7–11% of mothers after open spina bifida repair. Due to this risk, women who have undergone open fetal surgery deliver by elective cesarean section to prevent scar rupture in the index and all subsequent pregnancies. In subsequent pregnancies after open prenatal surgery, uterine dehiscence and uterine rupture both have been reported to occur in about 14% of pregnancies.

Finally, maternal anesthesia, tocolysis, and particularly large open or prolonged procedures have been noted to cause maternal pulmonary edema in some instances. This has been found to be associated with volume overloading, general anesthesia (hence the effort to perform these procedures under regional anesthesia, or combined general/regional anesthesia), combination tocolytics, and fluid absorption from the surgical field. It has been reported ranging in up to 30% of open surgeries, but with improvement over time due to provider experience and the learning curve [20].

Fetal Risks

The predominant fetal risks with prenatal intervention are premature rupture of membranes and prematurity, with all of its attendant complications. Rates of prematurity are about 40–100% depending on fetal pathology and type of intervention. After open MMC repair, the average delivery is at 34 weeks; fetuses with more severe conditions often experience earlier prematurity. Consequences of prematurity occur on a spectrum depending on the severity, but can include pulmonary issues (respiratory distress syndrome, bronchopulmonary dysplasia, apnea of prematurity), intraventricular hemorrhage, necrotizing enterocolitis, and retinopathy of prematurity. Long-term disabilities such as developmental delay, ADHD, asthma, and hearing impairment have been associated with prematurity.

Fetal surgeons often report that the single most dangerous part of open fetal surgery is the creation of the hysterotomy, because this can cause a subchorionic venous injury leading to a subchorionic hematoma which dissects the fetal membranes, subsequently causing membrane collapse. If significant bleeding occurs after hysterotomy, digital pressure should be applied followed by full-thickness mattress sutures. Clearly, this risk is highest with open hysterotomy but could occur with ports in fetoscopy as well [16].

The other primary problem with fetal intervention is the unrelenting fact that the amniotic sac never truly heals; as such, amniotic leak is a frequent complication. If severe enough, resultant oligohydramnios or anhydramnios can cause pulmonary hypoplasia and associated complications, and this too can contribute to premature delivery.

Specific Conditions Amenable to Robotic Fetal Surgery

Myelomeningocele

Spina bifida is a severe neurologic birth defect resulting from the incomplete closure of the spinal canal in early development (4–6 weeks gestation), which results in exposure of meninges and spinal cord to the amniotic environment. It typically results in significant morbidity including varying degrees of hydrocephalus, lower extremity neurologic impairments, bowel and bladder dysfunction, and mental impairment. While folic acid supplementation in pregnancy has drastically curbed the incidence, it still occurs at a rate of about 3.5 in 10,000 live births [21] and is the cause of a significant number of pregnancy terminations each year [22]. Standard of care has been operative closure after birth, but patients still require lifelong medical care for the ongoing sequelae.

As described above, a significant portion of what we know about fetal surgery comes from the efforts to pursue prenatal closure of myelomeningocele with the hopes to improve the subsequent condition of the child. Fetal myelomeningocele closure is based on the theory that ongoing exposure of the spinal contents to the intraamniotic environment promotes progressive neural destruction, and that this can be reduced by adding neural coverage. In addition, the continuous exit of cerebrospinal fluid through the open defect leads to herniation of the hindbrain into the spinal canal, which contributes to a Chiari II malformation. Early closure of the spinal defect could lessen this effect on the brain.

Almost concurrently with validation of the concept in multiple animal models, particularly sheep [23, 24], MMC repair in humans was pursued. The initial attempts at human fetal MMC closure were performed fetoscopically [3], but difficulty with this led to a focus on open repair in the United States. After several initial series were published showing the feasibility of the technique (Fig. 25.4) and likelihood of improved outcomes [25–27], the multi-institutional MOMS trial was developed.

The MOMS randomized controlled trial was the keystone trial of fetal surgery, occupying the first decade of the twenty-first century [4]. This trial was thoroughly designed and executed such that all potential enrollees were evaluated by a single institution, and then assigned to either Children's Hospital of Philadelphia, Vanderbilt, or University of California at San Francisco for protocolized treatment. Enrollment was ended early at 183 patients (of goal 200) after initial results showed that prenatal surgery resulted in a reduced need for ventriculoperitoneal shunting by 12 months of age (40% in the prenatal surgery group vs. 82% in the postnatal surgery group, $p < 0.01$) and further improved motor function by 30 months when compared to standard postnatal surgery. These improved outcomes came at the anticipated costs of higher rates of pregnancy complications and preterm delivery in the prenatal surgery group. Based on this trial, fetal MMC closure is now regularly offered to pregnant mothers, and fetal surgery programs dramatically increased in number and productivity across the country. Subsequent trials have confirmed the MOMS results [28–30] and added to what we know about the benefits of prenatal

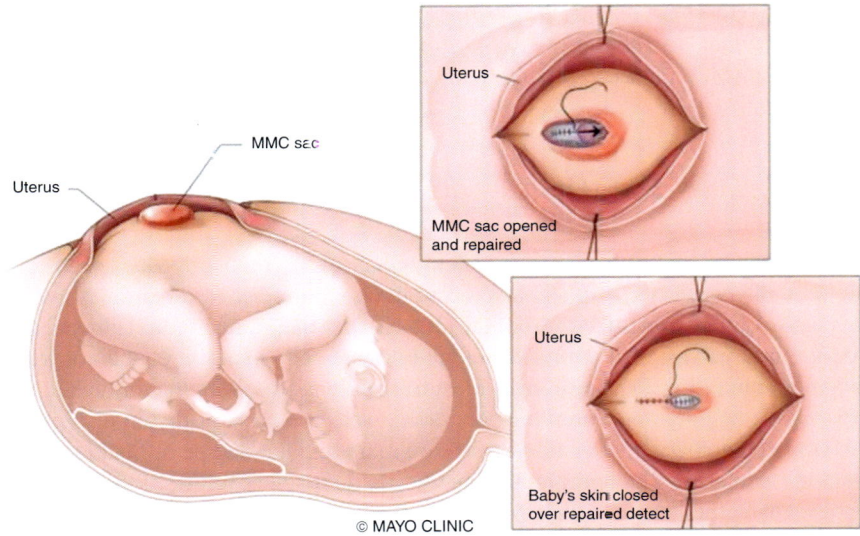

Fig. 25.4 Open fetal myelomeningocele repair is performed via maternal abdominal and uterine incisions. (*Used with permission of Mayo Foundation for Medical Education and Research, all rights reserved*)

closure. Serial fetal MRIs have shown that the reversal in hindbrain herniation occurs as early as 3–6 weeks after fetal repair [31, 32]. Long-term MOMS follow-up also showed that prenatal repair improves volitional voiding and lowers the rate of clean intermittent catheterization in school-aged children [33]. While the evidence for fetal benefit improves, a focus on efforts to minimize the drawbacks is underway, including pursuits of fetoscopic techniques.

Fetoscopic MMC closure was most thoroughly explored outside of the US (especially in Germany and Brazil), largely due to the restrictions during the MOMS period. However, since the MOMS trial, efforts at fetoscopic repair have grown. A systematic review of the post-MOMS studies involving open and fetoscopic repairs was performed to assess their comparative success. This review encompassed 5 fetoscopic and 6 open studies and found no significant difference in fetal mortality or the need for ventriculoperitoneal shunt in the first year of life. However, fetoscopic repairs were associated with higher rates of repair dehiscence or leak requiring postnatal repeat surgery (30% vs. 7%, $p < 0.01$) and premature rupture of membranes (79 vs. 36%, $p = 0.04$). Uterine dehiscence was higher with open repair (11% vs 0%, $p < 0.01$) [34]. This corroborates the main debate: while fetoscopic repair is less invasive, is it good enough to be performed safely and to create a watertight repair?

As such, myelomeningocele may be the ideal condition to target for fetal robotic surgery. Spina bifida coverage and closure requires precise dissection and intra-amniotic suturing. Open surgery has validated the benefit of closure through the MOMS randomized controlled trial and there are several groups working at mastering fetoscopic repairs. Just as many adult procedures progressed from open, to laparoscopic, to robotic, MMC closure may indeed be the ideal frontier for robotic application in this growing field of fetal surgery.

Lower Urinary Tract Obstruction

Lower urinary tract obstruction (LUTO) occurs most frequently due to posterior urethral valves (PUVs), but can also occur due to a number of other abnormalities that cause outflow obstruction from the fetal bladder including urethral atresia, anterior urethral valves, obstructing ureterocele, prune belly syndrome, and congenital megalourethra [35]. Furthermore, it must be differentiated from the mimicker, non-obstructive megacystis. The ultrasonographic variables best at distinguishing true LUTO from non-obstructive megacystis are male sex, the degree of bladder distention, ureteral size, oligohydramnios, and gestational age at referral [36]. These are better than the classic ultrasound triad of megacystis, keyhole sign, and hydronephrosis.

Because the degree of obstruction can vary by patient, selection of patients most likely to benefit from an antenatal intervention is essential. On the one hand, patients with mild partial obstruction will likely survive to delivery with minimal sequela and can undergo treatment in the postnatal period. By contrast, those patients with severe obstruction and associated severe renal dysplasia, oligohydramnios, and/or pulmonary hypoplasia may stand little to benefit from establishing urinary tract drainage in utero. There are ongoing efforts to establish predictive LUTO staging and prognostication factors, relying on both ultrasound findings and fetal urine chemistries. Ultrasound aspects associated with eventual renal replacement therapy or mortality include early gestational age at first oligohydramnios detection, larger bladder volume, and evidence of renal disease such as cysts, hyperechogenicity, and dysplasia [37, 38]. Fetal urine analytes including electrolytes, beta-2 microglobulin, and proteomic markers, while initially debated in their value [39], are now being shown to have increasing value for predicting renal prognosis in LUTO [40, 41]. Thought leaders have been working to develop the best staging systems to guide intervention [42, 43], with the most recent coming from the 2016 Society of Fetal Urology panel discussion [44]. This group proposed the staging and intervention criteria in Table 25.1.

Interestingly, the first fetal surgery for LUTO in the literature was bilateral cutaneous ureterostomies in a 21 week fetus with PUVs and functional bilateral uretero-vesical junction obstruction [45]. **Modern intervention for LUTO has been performed by both vesicoamniotic shunting (VAS)** (Fig. 25.5) **and fetal cystoscopy** (Fig. 25.6). VAS has been plagued by shunt dislodgement or malfunction which were seen in up to 60% [46], lack of physiologic bladder cycling [47], and questionable efficacy. The PLUTO trial (2013) was a randomized controlled trial of vesicoamniotic shunting versus conservative therapy which closed early due to poor recruitment. This showed no clear benefit to VAS over conservative therapy [48]. A

Table 25.1 Staging criteria based on the 2016 SFU panel discussion

	Stage I (mild LUTO)	Stage II (severe LUTO, with prenatal findings suggestive of preserved renal function)	Stage III (severe LUTO, with prenatal findings suggestive of fetal abnormal renal function)
Amount of amniotic fluid	Normal	Oligohydramnios or anhydramnios	Oligohydramnios, but usually anhydramnios
Echogenicity of fetal kidneys	Normal	Hyperechogenic	Hyperechogenic
Renal cortical cysts	Absent	Absent	Can be present
Renal dysplasia	Absent	Absent	Can be present
Fetal urinary biochemistry	Favorable	Favorable within three consecutive evaluations	Not favorable after three consecutive evaluations
Fetal intervention	Not indicated	Indicated to prevent pulmonary hypoplasia and severe renal impairment	May be indicated to prevent pulmonary hypoplasia but not postnatal renal impairment; further studies are necessary

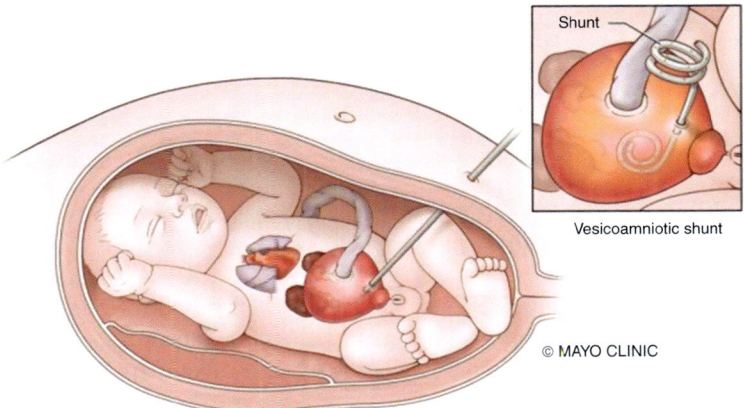

Fig. 25.5 Vesicoamniotic shunt procedure for fetal lower urinary tract obstruction. (*Used with permission of Mayo Foundation for Medical Education and Research, all rights reserved*)

subsequent systematic review and meta-analysis of the literature has suggested that VAS may be associated with improved perinatal mortality but no difference in 6–24 month mortality or renal function [49]. Fetal cystoscopy has the added benefit of evaluating the urethra and differentiating posterior urethral valves from other less common (and often worse prognosticating) conditions such as urethral atresia. With fetal cystoscopy, valve ablation is therapeutic [50, 51]. Retrospective data comparing vesicoamniotic shunting and fetal cystoscopy suggests that both are associated with improved survival over conservative management in PUV patients, and that fetal cystoscopy is associated with an improved survival rate and renal function at 6 months [52].

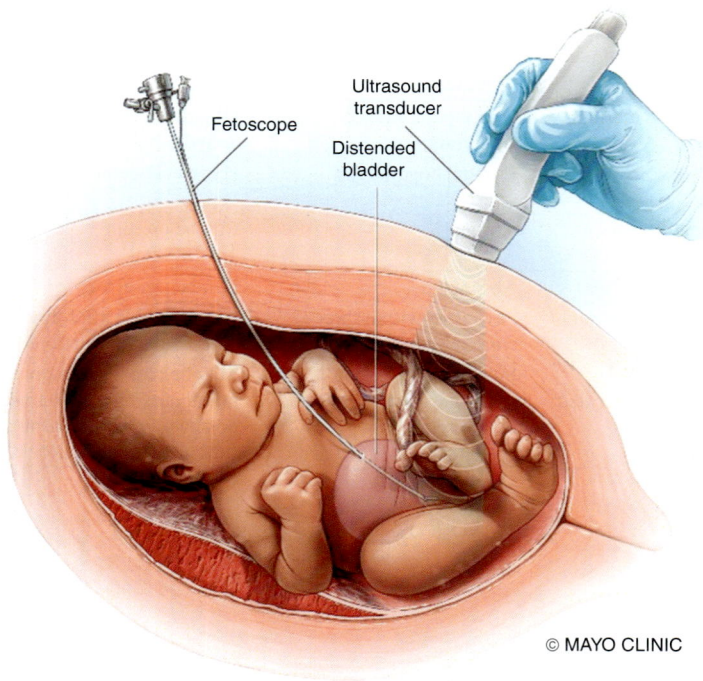

Fig. 25.6 Fetal cystoscopy procedure for lower urinary tract obstruction. (*Used with permission of Mayo Foundation for Medical Education and Research, all rights reserved*)

For future interventions, PUVs appears to be well-suited for fetal cystoscopy. However, granted that the original treatment started as bilateral cutaneous ureterostomies, one could imagine unique scenarios when a robotic application could be beneficial.

Others

Fetal surgery has been pursued in a variety of additional conditions. Brief review of several of these will serve to highlight several prenatal surgical principles and may shed light on additional conditions which could benefit from similar prenatal intervention.

Congenital diaphragmatic hernia (CDH) occurs due to a defect within the diaphragm, permitting herniation of intraabdominal contents into the chest. The deleterious effect is maldevelopment of the compressed lung and is often lethal. Postnatal surgery previously required extracorporeal membrane oxygenation (ECMO) due to poor pulmonary function, often plagued by poor results, which prompted a focus on prenatal intervention because of the dependence of fetal oxygenation on the placenta, rather than the lungs. Early attempts at prenatal open repair showed no improvement in survival when compared to patients treated postnatally [53]. Subsequent attempts at prenatal interventions for CDH focused on tracheal occlusion to promote lung growth, initially by tracheal ligation and subsequently by balloon occlusion. Initial studies showed limited improvement compared to postnatal repairs [54]. However, fetal endoscopic advancements were further pursued to include development of trials suggesting benefit [55] and more recently a multinational randomized controlled trial, Tracheal Occlusion to Accelerate Lung Growth (TOTAL), which has recently completed enrollment with results forthcoming. Overall, CDH treatment shows the hope that fetal surgery may not only permit repair of fetal anomalies, but also may permit improved organ development as a result of the intervention [56].

Likewise, interventions for congenital pulmonary airway malformations focused on open resections of these lesions, often requiring fetal lobectomy. Cardiopulmonary problems like congenital diaphragmatic hernia and congenital pulmonary airway malformations prompted the development of another unique approach to fetal surgery. Instead of operating on these patients at mid-gestation, or postpartum with the patient on ECMO, these conditions could be corrected at the time of caesarean section through the development of ex utero intrapartum therapy (EXIT), also called operation on placental support (OOPS), by leaving the placenta attached for fetal placental bypass while operating on these essential organs [57, 58].

Twin-twin transfusion syndrome has been largely amenable to fetoscopy with laser ablation of the vascular anastomoses, demonstrating the value of fetoscopic intervention as well as therapeutic energy applications.

Some interest has been directed to the potential role of fetal surgery for the treatment of gastroschisis. The main morbidity is believed to occur due to bowel exposure to amniotic fluid due to the periumbilical defect [59], lending thought to the potential benefit of organ coverage. An attempt at surgical repair in sheep models demonstrated significant difficulty in reducing the bowel contents back into the abdomen by a fetoscopic approach. Furthermore, doing so resulted in hemodynamic compromise due to pressure on the fetal umbilical vessels. Instead, this study showed that the gastroschisis defect could be widened, which could serve as a potential application in fetuses at risk for bowel strangulation through the defect [60]. The potential efforts to address abdominal wall defects such as gastroschisis bring to mind whether fetal surgery could be used to address the main urologic abdominal wall defect, bladder exstrophy, although no reports of attempted fetal repair in this area have been published.

Ongoing Research and Future Directions

As the field of robotic fetal surgery is still in its infancy, its maturity will be brought about by **development of better robots with smaller instruments and new capabilities: an ideal vision at present is a tiny single-port fetoscopic robot, operated even by a telesurgeon.**

To date, there are few truly robotic fetal surgery studies in the literature, all limited to animal models. One study demonstrated the feasibility of using the Da Vinci robot (Intuitive Surgical, Sunnyvale, CA) for MMC repair in fetal sheep [61]. This was performed by the group at Vanderbilt led by Tulipan who initially tried and abandoned endoscopic MMC repair, ultimately choosing to focus on the open repair. Two other studies employed the Zeus robot (Computer Motion Inc., Goleta, CA), both in sheep as well. The first compared robotic and fetoscopic approaches wherein the authors felt there was no benefit of robotics for straightforward repairs but it could become beneficial in complex repairs [62]. Another evaluated fetal robotic surgery via uterus exteriorization versus a completely percutaneous approach, and noted an overall better surgical experience with the percutaneous approach [63]. Further robotic platform, instrument, and technique developments are ongoing.

Robot and Instrument Development

There is a flurry of activity in development of better surgical robots [64]. While the Da Vinci robot has dominated the robotic surgical market since FDA approval in 2000, multiple companies world-wide are developing new robotic designs.

Small instrument size is a necessity for fetal robotic surgery, in order to minimize maternal/uterine trauma and the risks of amniotic leak or premature labor. The vast majority of robotic surgeries worldwide have been performed on adult patients, with a less rigid requirement for smaller instruments, and there are no dedicated pediatric or fetal surgical robots to date. Also, most robotic surgeries have been applied to body cavities (laparoscopic) or orifices (endoscopic) with minimal performed on the surface such as for plastic or reconstructive microsurgery [65]. These things have minimized the pressure to pursue smaller instruments and to develop microsurgical techniques in robotic surgery. However, a key consideration in robotic fetal surgery is the need for smaller instruments and even microsurgical techniques. Current studies suggest that, even in small working spaces, the surgeons operating with the larger instruments (8 mm Da Vinci vs. 5 mm Da Vinci) perform more accurately and efficiently, further suggesting the need for ongoing improvement in small instrument design [66].

Single port instrumentation limits the number of incisions to one for the robot plus any additional assistant ports. The Da Vinci Single-Port (SP) has been shown to be feasible for application to a variety of adult and pediatric surgeries. Furthermore, for fetal application, single-port fetal tracheoscopic surgery has been successfully performed in a fetal lamb [67]. Having a single access site into the uterus would seem to dramatically limit the risks associated with fetal surgery and represents an exciting area of new potential application to human fetal surgery.

Beyond standard robotic surgery, researchers are working to develop deployable robots. These are small devices that are not tethered but instead have battery-derived energy, mobility, therapeutic energy options, and remote control [64].

Telesurgery

Because a robotic surgeon does not necessarily have to be at the immediate bedside of the patient undergoing robotic surgery, this opens the opportunity for **increasing patient access to robotic surgical procedures through telesurgery**. The Lindberg procedure, a cholecystectomy performed on a patient in France by a surgeon in New York in 2001, was the first documented transatlantic robotic surgery [68]. Likewise, the feasibility and safety of telestenting in acute coronary syndrome patients has been demonstrated [69]. Clearly, programs such as this require a skilled on-site team. However, given the high complexity of fetal surgeries, it would be feasible to have trained local fetal surgery support teams directed by a remote expert fetal surgeon, which could allow dramatic increase in patient access to care, not to mention growing expertise of the operating surgeon through increased volume of experience.

Simulation and Training

As alluded to above, conditions amenable to fetal surgeries are relatively uncommon, which limits surgical experience. Likewise, robotic surgeries are typically performed by a single surgeon at the robotic console, in contrast to classic open surgery which has a primary surgeon, often co-surgeons, and several assistants (often trainees) involved in the case. Having a single robotic surgeon limits the experience of the training surgeon, and suggests the need for a formal training program, ideally supplemented by robotic simulation. This begs the development and oversight of such simulation to create surgical training experiences in fetal robotic surgeries. Models made possible by three-dimensional printing may contribute to this realm of procedural simulation and even to patient-specific surgical planning (Fig. 25.7).

Conclusion

Fetal surgery is a growing field for the treatment of prenatally detected anomalies. The current capabilities and future advancements of robotic surgery suggest that it has significant potential for application to fetal surgery, and it behooves providers addressing these fetal conditions to study and explore robotic application to this growing field.

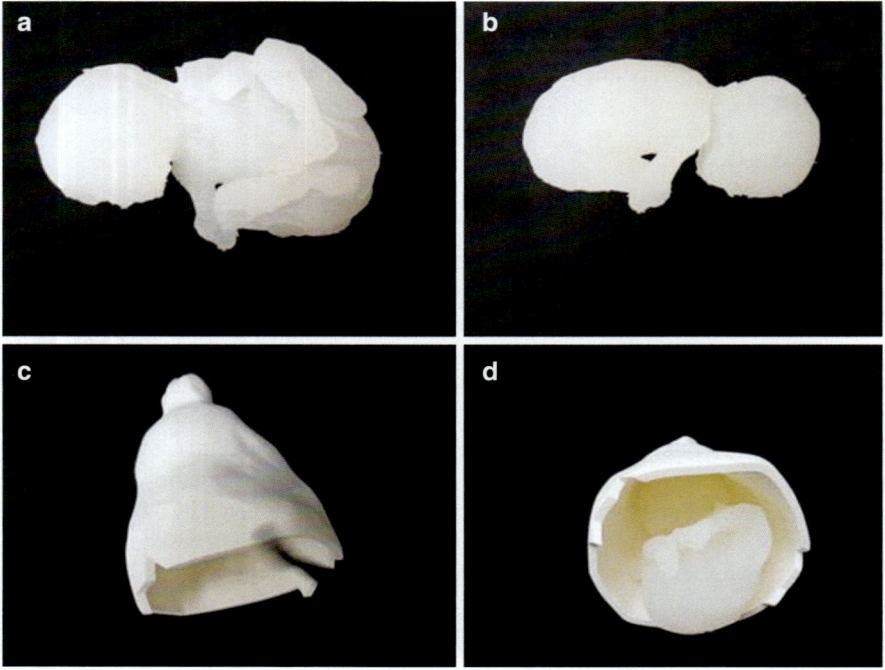

Fig. 25.7 Three-dimensional printed model of a 22-week fetus and uterus to be used for robotic simulation in MMC closure and LUTO vesicostomy creation: (**a**, **b**) fetus from two different angles, (**c**) uterus, (**d**) fetus inside uterus

References

1. Liley A, Intrauterine W. Transfusion of foetus in haemolytic disease. Br Med J. 1963;2:1107–9.
2. Flake AW. Surgery in the human fetus: the future. J Physiol. 2003;547:45–51.
3. Bruner JP, Richards WO, Tulipan NB, Arney TL. Endoscopic coverage of fetal myelomeningocele in utero. Am J Obstet Gynecol. 1999;180:153–8.
4. Adzick NS, et al. A randomized trial of prenatal versus postnatal repair of myelomeningocele. N Engl J Med. 2011;364:993–1004.
5. Hubbard AM. Ultrafast fetal MRI and prenatal diagnosis. Semin Pediatr Surg. 2003;12:143–53.
6. Jack R, et al. Acute cardiovascular effects of fetal surgery in the human. Circulation. 2004;110:1549–56.
7. Luks FI, Deprest JA, Vandenberghe K, Brosens IA, Lerut T. A model for fetal surgery through intrauterine endoscopy. J Pediatr Surg. 1994;29:1007–9.
8. Luks FI, Johnson BD, Papadakis K, Traore M, Piasecki GJ. Predictive value of monitoring parameters in fetal surgery. J Pediatr Surg. 1998;33:1297–301.
9. Warner LL, Arendt KW, Ruano R, Qureshi MY, Segura LG. A call for innovation in fetal monitoring during fetal surgery. J Matern Fetal Neonatal Med. 2020:1–7. https://doi.org/10.1080/14767058.2020.1767575.
10. Santana EFM, et al. Fetal modified left myocardial performance index monitoring during open surgery for myelomeningocele repair. Echocardiogr (Mount Kisco NY). 2018;35:1664–70.

11. Bennett KA, et al. Reducing perinatal complications and preterm delivery for patients undergoing in utero closure of fetal myelomeningocele: further modifications to the multidisciplinary surgical technique: clinical article. J Neurosurg Pediatr. 2014;14:108–14.
12. Kohl T. Percutaneous minimally invasive fetoscopic surgery for spina bifida aperta. Part I: surgical technique and perioperative outcome. Ultrasound Obstet Gynecol. 2014;44:515–24.
13. Sydorak RM, Albanese CT. Minimal access techniques for fetal surgery. World J Surg. 2003;27:95–102.
14. Kohl T, et al. Analysis of the stepwise clinical introduction of experimental percutaneous fetoscopic surgical techniques for upcoming minimally invasive fetal cardiac interventions. Surg Endosc. 2006;20:1134.
15. Kohl T, et al. Percutaneous fetal access and uterine closure for fetoscopic surgery. Surg Endosc. 1997;11:819–24.
16. Bruner JP. Intrauterine surgery in myelomeningocele. Semin Fetal Neonatal Med. 2007;12:471–6.
17. Saiki Y, et al. Reducing the deleterious effects of intrauterine CO_2 during fetoscopic surgery. J Surg Res. 1997;69:51–4.
18. Ford WDA, Cool JC, Byard R, Allanson M. Glycine as a potential window for minimal access fetal surgery. Fetal Diagn Ther. 1997;12:145–8.
19. Kohl T, et al. Partial amniotic carbon dioxide insufflation (PACI) during minimally invasive fetoscopic surgery: early clinical experience in humans. Surg Endosc. 2010;24:432–44.
20. Al-Refai A, Ryan G, Van Mieghem T. Maternal risks of fetal therapy. Curr Opin Obstet Gynecol. 2017;29:80–4.
21. Parker SE, et al. Updated National Birth Prevalence estimates for selected birth defects in the United States, 2004-2006. Birth Defects Res A. 2010;88:1008–16.
22. Johnson CY, et al. Pregnancy termination following prenatal diagnosis of anencephaly or spina bifida: a systematic review of the literature. Birth Defects Res A. 2012;94:857–63.
23. Adzick NS. Prospects for fetal surgery. Early Hum Dev. 2013;89:881–6.
24. Bouchard S, et al. Correction of hindbrain herniation and anatomy of the vermis after in utero repair of myelomeningocele in sheep. J Pediatr Surg. 2003;38:451–8.
25. Bruner JP, et al. Fetal surgery for myelomeningocele and the incidence of shunt-dependent hydrocephalus. JAMA. 1999;282:1819–25.
26. Tulipan N, Hernanz-Schulman M, Bruner JP. Reduced hindbrain herniation after intrauterine myelomeningocele repair: a report of four cases. Pediatr Neurosurg. 1998;29:274–8.
27. Tulipan N, et al. The effect of intrauterine myelomeningocele repair on the incidence of shunt-dependent hydrocephalus. Pediatr Neurosurg. 2003;38:27–33.
28. Moldenhauer JS, et al. Fetal myelomeningocele repair: the post-MOMS experience at the Children's Hospital of Philadelphia. Fetal Diagn Ther. 2015;37:235–40.
29. Zamłyński J, et al. Comparison of prenatal and postnatal treatments of spina bifida in Poland--a non-randomized, single-center study. J Mater. 2014;27:1409–17.
30. Elbabaa SK, Gildehaus AM, Pierson MJ, Albers JA, Vlastos EJ. First 60 fetal in-utero myelomeningocele repairs at Saint Louis fetal care institute in the post-MOMS trial era: hydrocephalus treatment outcomes (endoscopic third ventriculostomy versus ventriculo-peritoneal shunt). Childs Nerv Syst. 2017;33:1157–68.
31. Sutton LN, et al. Improvement in hindbrain herniation demonstrated by serial fetal magnetic resonance imaging following fetal surgery for myelomeningocele. JAMA. 1999;282:1826–31.
32. Ruano R, et al. In utero restoration of hindbrain herniation in fetal myelomeningocele as part of prenatal regenerative therapy program at Mayo Clinic. Mayo Clin Proc. 2020;95:738–46.
33. Brock JW, et al. Effect of prenatal repair of myelomeningocele on urological outcomes at school age. J Urol. 2019;202:812–8.
34. Kabagambe SK, Jensen GW, Chen YJ, Vanover MA, Farmer DL. Fetal surgery for myelomeningocele: a systematic review and meta-analysis of outcomes in fetoscopic versus open repair. Fetal Diagn Ther. 2018;43:161–74.

35. Clayton DB, Brock JW. Lower urinary tract obstruction in the fetus and neonate. Clin Perinatol. 2014;41:643–59.
36. Fontanella F, et al. Prenatal diagnosis of LUTO: improving diagnostic accuracy. Ultrasound Obstet Gynecol. 2018;52:739–43.
37. Johnson MP, et al. Natural history of fetal lower urinary tract obstruction with normal amniotic fluid volume at initial diagnosis. Fetal Diagn Ther. 2018;44:10–7.
38. Fontanella F, et al. Antenatal staging of congenital lower urinary tract obstruction. Ultrasound Obstet Gynecol. 2019;53:520–4.
39. Morris RK, Quinlan-Jones E, Kilby MD, Khan KS. Systematic review of accuracy of fetal urine analysis to predict poor postnatal renal function in cases of congenital urinary tract obstruction. Prenat Diagn. 2007;27:900–11.
40. Abdennadher W, et al. Fetal urine biochemistry at 13–23 weeks of gestation in lower urinary tract obstruction: criteria for in-utero treatment. Ultrasound Obstet Gynecol. 2015;46:306–11.
41. Dreux S, et al. Urine biochemistry to predict long-term outcomes in fetuses with posterior urethral valves. Prenat Diagn. 2018;38:964–70.
42. Ruano R, et al. Fetal lower urinary tract obstruction: proposal for standardized multidisciplinary prenatal management based on disease severity. Ultrasound Obstet Gynecol. 2016;48:476–82.
43. Ruano R, Dunn T, Braun MC, Angelo JR, Safdar A. Lower urinary tract obstruction: fetal intervention based on prenatal staging. Pediatr Nephrol. 2017;32:1871–8.
44. Farrugia MK, Braun MC, Peters CA, Ruano R, Herndon CD. Report on the Society for Fetal Urology panel discussion on the selection criteria and intervention for fetal bladder outlet obstruction. J Pediatr Urol. 2017;13:345–51.
45. Harrison MR, et al. Fetal surgery for congenital hydronephrosis. N Engl J Med. 1982;306:591–3.
46. Quintero RA, Gomez Castro LA, Bermudez C, Chmait RH, Kontopoulos EV. In utero management of fetal lower urinary tract obstruction with a novel shunt: a landmark development in fetal therapy. J Mater. 2010;23:806–12.
47. Kitagawa H, et al. Valved shunt as a treatment for obstructive uropathy: does pressure make a difference? Pediatr Surg Int. 2013;29:381–6.
48. Morris RK, et al. Percutaneous vesicoamniotic shunting versus conservative management for fetal lower urinary tract obstruction (PLUTO): a randomised trial. Lancet. 2013;382:1496–506.
49. Nassr AA, et al. Effectiveness of vesicoamniotic shunt in fetuses with congenital lower urinary tract obstruction: an updated systematic review and meta-analysis. Ultrasound Obstet Gynecol. 2017;49:696–703.
50. Quintero RA, et al. Percutaneous fetal cystoscopy and endoscopic fulguration of posterior urethral valves. Am J Obstet Gynecol. 1995;172:206–9.
51. Welsh A, Agarwal S, Kumar S, Smith RP, Fisk NM. Fetal cystoscopy in the management of fetal obstructive uropathy: experience in a single European centre. Prenat Diagn. 2003;23:1033–41.
52. Ruano R, et al. Fetal intervention for severe lower urinary tract obstruction: a multicenter case–control study comparing fetal cystoscopy with vesicoamniotic shunting. Ultrasound Obstet Gynecol. 2015;45:452–8.
53. Harrison MR, et al. Correction of congenital diaphragmatic hernia in utero VII: a prospective trial. J Pediatr Surg. 1997;32:1637–42.
54. Harrison MR, et al. A randomized trial of fetal endoscopic tracheal occlusion for severe fetal congenital diaphragmatic hernia. N Engl J Med. 2003;349:1916–24.
55. Ruano R, et al. A randomized controlled trial of fetal endoscopic tracheal occlusion versus postnatal management of severe isolated congenital diaphragmatic hernia. Ultrasound Obstet Gynecol. 2012;39:20–7.
56. Ruano R, et al. Fetoscopic therapy for severe pulmonary hypoplasia in congenital diaphragmatic hernia: a first in prenatal regenerative medicine at Mayo Clinic. Mayo Clin Proc. 2018;93:693–700.
57. Mychaliska GB, et al. Operating on placental support: the ex utero intrapartum treatment procedure. J Pediatr Surg. 1997;32:227–31.

58. Skarsgard ED, et al. The OOPS procedure (operation on placental support): in utero airway management of the fetus with prenatally diagnosed tracheal obstruction. J Pediatr Surg. 1996;31:826–8.
59. Luton D, Guibourdenche J, Vuillard E, Bruner J, de Lagausie P. Prenatal management of gastroschisis: the place of the amnioexchange procedure. Clin Perinatol. 2003;30:551–72.
60. Kohl T, Tchatcheva K, Stressig R, Gembruch U, Kahl P. Is there a therapeutic role for fetoscopic surgery in the prenatal treatment of gastroschisis? A feasibility study in sheep. Surg Endosc. 2009;23:1499–505.
61. Aaronson OS, et al. Robot-assisted endoscopic intrauterine myelomeningocele repair: a feasibility study. Pediatr Neurosurg. 2002;36:85–9.
62. Kohl T, et al. Percutaneous fetoscopic patch coverage of experimental lumbosacral full-thickness skin lesions in sheep. Surg Endosc. 2003;17:1218–23.
63. Knight CG, et al. Robot-enhanced fetoscopic surgery. J Pediatr Surg. 2004;39:1463–5.
64. Khandalavala K, Shimon T, Flores L, Armijo PR, Oleynikov D. Emerging surgical robotic technology: a progression toward microbots. Ann Laparosc Endosc Surg. 2020;5:3.
65. Tan YPA, Liverneaux P, Wong KF. Current limitations of surgical robotics in reconstructive plastic microsurgery. Front Surg. 2018;5:22.
66. Ballouhey Q, et al. Comparison of 8 and 5 mm robotic instruments in small cavities. Surg Endosc. 2018;32:1027–34.
67. Papadakis K, et al. Single-port tracheoscopic surgery in the fetal lamb. J Pediatr Surg. 1998;33:918–20.
68. Brower V. The cutting edge in surgery. EMBO Rep. 2002;3:300–1.
69. Patel TM, Shah SC, Pancholy SB. Long distance tele-robotic-assisted percutaneous coronary intervention: a report of first-in-human experience. EClinicalMedicine. 2019;14:53–8.

Chapter 26
Complications in Pediatric Urology Minimally Invasive Surgery

Christina Kim

Abbreviations

CHD	Congenital Heart Disease
LESS	Laparoendoscopic Single Site Surgery
LP	Laparoscopic Pyeloplasty
MIS	Minimally invasive surgery
NSQIP	National Surgical Quality Improvement Program
OPN	Open Pyeloplasty
RALMA	Robotic Assisted Laparoscopic Mitrofanoff Appendicovesicostomy
RALP	Robotic Assisted Laparoscopic Pyeloplasty
UPJO	Ureteropelvic Junction Obstruction
UTI	Urinary Tract Infection

Introduction

Minimally invasive surgery (MIS) continues to evolve in pediatric urology. Initially MIS started as a diagnostic procedure with standard laparoscopy and later expanded to robotic surgery. Over the years, MIS has evolved into a preferable approach for many urologic extirpative and reconstructive cases. The use of MIS has progressed slower in pediatrics than in adults for a variety of reasons. Many providers are hesitant despite multiple reports of MIS in children with lower pain scales, shorter hospitalizations, and improved cosmesis [1, 2]. Its acceptance in pediatrics have been hampered by longer operative times, smaller working space, and limited fine surgical instruments. Also, MIS carries the burden of more expenses and resources.

C. Kim (✉)
University of Wisconsin-Madison, Department of Urology, Madison, WI, USA
e-mail: ckim@urology.wisc.edu

© Springer Nature Switzerland AG 2020
P. C. Gargollo (ed.), *Minimally Invasive and Robotic-Assisted Surgery in Pediatric Urology*, https://doi.org/10.1007/978-3-030-57219-8_26

Table 26.1 Clavien-Dindo classification [3]

Grade	Definition
Grade I	Any deviation from the normal post-operative course not requiring surgical, endoscopic, or radiological intervention. This includes the need for certain drugs (e.g., antiemetics, antipyretics, analgesics, diuretics, and electrolytes), treatment with physiotherapy and wound infections that are opened at the bedside
Grade II	Complications requiring drug treatments other than those allowed for grade I complications; this includes blood transfusions and total parenteral nutrition (TPN)
Grade III	Complications requiring surgical, endoscopic, or radiological intervention
Grade IIIa	Intervention not under general anesthesia
Grade IIIb	Intervention under general anesthesia
Grade IV	Life-threatening complications; this includes CNS complications (e.g., brain hemorrhage, ischemic stroke, subarachnoid hemorrhage) which require intensive care, but excludes transient ischemic attacks (TIAs)
Grade IVa	Single-organ dysfunction (including dialysis)
Grade IVb	Multi-organ dysfunction
Grade V	Death of the patient

This is from an open access article distributed under the terms of the Creative Commons Attribution 4.0 International License. From Bolliger et al. [3]

Multiple reports have shown low complication rates of robotic surgery in children. When complications have occurred, they are usually Clavien Grade I and II (Table 26.1) [3]. Often the complications are not from the robotic technique, but are linked to the ureteral stents [4–6].

A wide variety of laparoscopic and robotic procedures have been described in children. Pyeloplasty is the most commonly performed MIS performed by pediatric urologists. This approach has had comparable safety and efficacy when compared to open surgery. This has been supported by large multi-centric studies [7]. Also, this has been supported by the European Association of Urology Pediatric guidelines. The guidelines recognize the benefits of minimally invasive surgery by stating that "in experienced hands, laparoscopic or retroperitoneoscopic techniques and robot-assisted techniques have the same success rates as standard open procedures." Also, they state that "Robotic-assisted laparoscopic pyeloplasty has all the same advantages as laparoscopic pyeloplasty plus better maneuverability, improved vision, ease in suturing and increased ergonomics but higher costs" [8].

Laparoscopic and robotic ureteral reimplantation have not been widely accepted due to longer operative times and varied success rates. Many reports show success rates with robotic reimplantation lower than open repairs [9–11]. This experience continues to evolve but is a surgical option for correction of vesicoureteral reflux.

Robotic total and partial nephrectomy has been described in children. Some find the dexterity and visualization of vascularity superior with robotics. When needed, many find suturing more efficient with robotics. This is pertinent when buttressing sutures are placed in the remaining healthy renal tissue. Also, suturing may be required in the collecting system.

Given the increased dexterity, robotics can be helpful when performing complex reconstruction (e.g. bladder augmentation, Mitrofanoff creation, bladder neck reconstruction). Laparoscopic and robotic appendicovesicostomies have evolved since its first description in 1993 [12]. Minimally invasive bladder augmentation have longer operative times than open surgery, but also has been associated with lower blood loss and shorter hospital stays [13, 14]. However, these complex reconstructive cases represent a small part of the existing literature in pediatric robotic surgery [15–17].

The potential benefits of MIS need to be considered in the context of potential complications associated with the approach. Many reported complications of MIS in pediatric urology have been limited to small case series and case reports. But some larger multi-center experiences have been reported. This chapter will summarize reported complications of various pediatric urologic surgery performed with laparoscopy and robotic techniques.

Experience and Results with Laparoscopy

Initially, urologic interest in minimally invasive surgery was demonstrated in the adult population. In 1993, Kavoussi and Peters described laparoscopic pyeloplasty as an alternative to the open technique. This case was in a 24 year old female [18]. Experience with technique continued to grow with more results in the adult population. Moore et al. reported their institution's first 30 adult laparoscopic pyeloplasties. Mean operative time was 4.5 h. At the time, their postoperative morbidity was low with convalescence of 3 weeks and a mean hospital stay of 3.5 days. Mean follow up of 16.3 months demonstrated radiographic improvement in 97% of the patients [19]. In the adult populations, initial complication rates were as high as 11.5–12.7%. The most common complications were bowel injury or bleeding. Other reported complications include hematomas, hernias, anastomotic stricture, stent migration, urinary leakage, pulmonary embolus, thrombophlebitis, urinoma, pyelonephritis, thrombophlebitis, ileus, and ureteral edema. Although reported complication rates in children is still limited when compared to the adult experience, the overall rate of complications is still fairly low [20–23].

Initially MIS was performed with standard laparoscopy. In 1996, Peters sent a survey to 251 pediatric urologists inquiring about their experience with laparoscopy. 153 responded. The survey included more than 5400 laparoscopic cases with ages ranging from newborn to 20 years old. Complications were reported in 5.3% of cases. But the majority of these complications were preperitoneal insufflation and subcutaneous emphysema. When these two complications were excluded, the complication rate was only 1.18%. Complications requiring surgery occurred in 0.39% of cases. The greatest predictor for complications was the surgeon experience. The technique for access was notable. Specifically, complications occurred in 2.6% of patients when using a Veress needle, but complications only occurred in 1.2% of patients when using an open technique [24].

Esposito et al. reported on 4350 laparoscopic procedures in children. Their complication rate was 2.7%. Six complications required conversion to open surgery. Eight complications were bleeding or dissection problems. Three had hypercapnia, three had peritoneal perforation during retroperitoneoscopy, 1 had injury to the spermatic vessels, and one had injury to the iliac vein. And 3 had technical difficulties [25].

Passerotti et al. reported on 806 laparoscopic procedures between 1995–2005. There were 16 complications (2%). 14 of these complications occurred during access. This included seven Clavien Grade IIIb, one Grade IVa, and one Grade IVb. Complications requiring open conversion were due to preperitoneal insufflation and bleeding, as well as injury to blood vessels, small bowel, vas deferens and the bladder. Seven cases were electively converted to open surgery (0.9%). Surgeon experience was a factor. Specifically, surgeons who performed more than 12 laparoscopic cases annually had a significantly lower complication rate ($p = 0.024$). The authors concluded that laparoscopic procedures are safe but significant injury is still possible. The authors felt that most complications, if not all, are avoidable if surgeons are diligent with proper technique and continue their education in the field of MIS [26].

Luque Mialdea et al. reviewed 106 urologic laparoscopic cases performed over a 5-year period of time. Mean age was 7 years. 65 cases were diagnostic in nature. There were three conversions to open surgery (two were secondary to preperitoneal insufflation and one was secondary to bleeding associated with a renal biopsy). There were no postoperative complications seen [27].

Colaco et al. did a retrospective review of the National Surgical Quality Improvement Program Pediatrics database from 2014. This review revealed 207 nephrectomies, 72 partial nephrectomies, 920 ureteroneocystostomies, and 625 pyeloplasties. The 30-day postoperative complication rates were assessed. Pediatric MIS was associated with longer operative times. Most cases had a shorter hospital stay. Partial nephrectomy was the only surgery with a longer operative hospital stay. There were no differences in postoperative complication rates when comparing open and MIS surgeries. Specifically, the rate of superficial and deep wound infections, urinary tract infections, bleeding requiring transfusion, pneumonia, and readmission within 30 days was <0.1% for all operations queried in this study. This was the rate for both open and MIS approaches [28].

There are some specific patient populations that warrant special consideration. Patients with congenital heart disease (CHD) represent one such population. Chu et al. did a retrospective review of patients with minor and major CHD. They reviewed data from the National Surgical Quality Improvement Projects-Pediatrics between 2013–2015. This allowed a match of 45,012 children who had laparoscopic surgery and an equal number of children who had open surgery. They looked at length of stay, in hospital mortality, 30-day morbidity rates and 30-day mortality rates. When intraabdominal laparoscopic surgery was compared to open surgery, there was lower morbidity in patients with no CHD. Also, laparoscopic surgery had lower morbidity and mortality rates in patients with minor CHD. But there was less benefit noted in the patients with severe CHD. Length of hospital stay was shorter for the laparoscopic approaches, but was associated with higher readmission rates [29].

Overall, multiple series confirm that laparoscopy is a safe option for healthy pediatric patients.

Experience and Results with Robotic Surgery

MIS has expanded from standard laparoscopy to robotic surgery. When robotic surgery was introduced, there was excitement due to three-dimensional imaging, tenfold camera magnification, tremor filtering, and new camera control by the surgeon. Also, there is instrument articulation with full range of motion. Surgeons hoped these enhancements would allow precise suturing, improve tissue handling, and increase ease of doing complex surgical cases. Robotics quickly gained popularity in adult urology for prostate surgery [30, 31]. In 1995, Partin et al. described a variety of robotic procedures in 17 adult patients. They saw three minor complications and no significant difference in operative time. They were encouraged by the feasibility of robotic surgery, but the authors encouraged more data collection to assess safety and efficacy of robotic surgery [32].

Although robotic surgery was originally designed and implemented in adults, there has been favorable results when robotic surgery has been performed in children. Specifically, pediatric robotic surgery has been associated with lower pain scales, less narcotic use, and shorter hospital stays [33]. Shorter hospital stays may lower morbidity relative to pulmonary complications. Prolonged hospital stays may lead to more atelectasis, pneumonia, and upper respiratory infections [34].

Looking more specifically at reported complications of robotic urologic surgery in children, Bansal et al. gave an early report of robotic results from three surgeons at a single pediatric institution. They reviewed their experience after initiating robotic surgery between 2009–2013. They reviewed complication rates with the Clavien system. This included 136 patients with 10 different surgeries. There were 11 total complications (8.1%): 2 were Grade I, 7 were Grade II, and 7 were Grade IIb. Urinary retention did not seem directly related to the techniques of surgery. Retention was seen in two patients with renal surgery. When excluding urinary retention and urinary tract infections, the complication rate was 5.1%. Most complications in their study were managed without operative intervention. Although there was not an even distribution of infant and older patients, there were more complications in infants. Specifically, complications occurred in 3 of 10 infant patients (30%). This was in contrast to the 6.3% complication rate of non-infants (8 of 126 patients). However, the Clavien grade/degree of complication was not higher in infants. None of the complications were intraoperative or directly related to robotic malfunction. There were no visceral injuries or blood transfusions. There were no conversions to open or purely laparoscopic surgery. In this series, the type of surgery did not affect the risk of complication. There was no difference in complication rates between the three surgeons in their series. In their series, surgeon experience was not a factor for complications. The surgeon with the least experience had the lowest complication rate [5].

Barashi et al. reviewed their 10-year experience of postoperative complications with robotic surgery. Their database included 326 patients. 57% underwent upper tract surgery, 30% underwent ureteral surgery, and 13% had bladder reconstructive surgery. They also summarized complications using the Clavien-Dindo scale. They grouped complications into 30, 60 and 90-day time intervals. Multivariable logistic regression analysis was performed to identify predictors of high-grade complications. There were no access related complications. But the most common complications were urinary tract infections and urinary complications (e.g., urine leaks and urolithiasis). The bladder reconstructive procedures had the highest rate of complications (37%). High grade complications occurred in 12% renal and 5% of ureteric procedures. Factors associated with an increased odds of high grade complications were: length of stay, estimated blood loss, and operative time [35].

Dangle et al. did a multi-institutional review of robotic complications from seven participating centers between 2007–2011. This included a cohort of 858 patients with 880 robotic procedures. The most common surgeries performed were pyeloplasty and ureteral reimplantation. There were 171 complications amongst these 880 procedures: 59 were Clavien grade I (6.7%), 70 were Clavien grade II (7.9%), 41 were Clavien Grade III (4.7%), 1 was Clavien grade IVa (0.1%). The patient with a Grade IVa complication had a complete recovery and on postoperative day 1 was recovering on the regular floor. Conversion to open or a purely laparoscopic approach occurred in 14 patients (1.6%). Mean age for the converted cases was 10.6 years. Primary reasons for conversion were mechanical: poor visibility [6], instrument failure [1], robotic malfunction [3]. However, four patients required conversion to open surgery due to injury of adjacent organs: partial transection of renal vein, needle injury to renal parenchyma, injury to hypogastric vein, and traction injury to small bowel. 97% of the Grade I complications resolved during their hospital stay. Most of the Grade II complications had smooth resolution. All surgical infections were successfully treated with antibiotics. Two corneal abrasions were treated conservatively. One patient developed a deep vein thrombosis and was treated with enoxaparin. The overall rate of Clavien Grade IIIa and IIIb complications was 4.7%. When reviewed the two most commonly performed cases, robotic pyeloplasties and ureteral reimplantations. Amongst the pyeloplasties, 20 patients had Clavien Grade IIIA and IIIb complications (4.9%). 12 patients required cystoscopy and stent placement (2.9%). Eight patients required ureteroscopy for a migrated stent (2%). Four patients required nephrostomy tube due to anastomotic leak or stenosis (0.9%). One patient required open conversion to repair a vascular injury to an aberrant vessel (0.2%). In the ureteral reimplantation group, four patients had Clavien Grade IIIa and IIIb complications (1.7%). This included three patients with bilateral repairs who had prolonged catheter drainage after surgery (8.6%). The unilateral reimplantations had a 2.3% rate of Clavien Grade III complications, whereas the bilateral reimplantations had a rate of 12.9%. When looking at the complex reconstructive cases, volume of cases was smaller. 2 of the 34 appendicovesicostomy patients (5.8%) required additional surgery (stoma revision and injection of bulking agent). 2 of the 12 augmentation cystoplasty patients (16%) required additional surgery (stoma stenosis and excision of mucosal granuloma) [36].

Regardless of the technique uses, MIS has become more prevalent in training, as well as practice. However, 60–85% residents have reported inadequate exposure to robotic and laparoscopic surgery during their training [37, 38]. Despite these reports, rates of MIS nephrectomies, ureteroureterostomies, appendicovesicostomies, and bladder neck slings have doubled since 2000 [39]. Urologic surgery accounts for 15% of domestic laparoscopic procedures in children [26, 40]. As volume increases, data regarding surgical results continue to grow.

Pyeloplasties

As stated earlier, the most commonly performed pediatric urologic robotic surgery is a pyeloplasty for a ureteropelvic junction obstruction (UPJO). For many years, open pyeloplasty has been considered the gold standard for therapy [8]. Many early reports on pediatric minimally invasively pyeloplasties were small, single center case series on ten or fewer patients [41–43].

Looking at national trends for pyeloplasties, it appears the overall rate of performing pyeloplasty has gone down. However, when the case is performed, it is more common to perform it robotically. Varda et al. looked the Premier database for open, laparoscopic and robotic pyeloplasties performed between 2003–2015. This database includes information from over 600 hospitals. It represents 20% of all annual inpatient discharges in the United States. All three techniques had low 90-day complication rates with no significant difference amongst the approach used. They conclude that robotics matches open pyeloplasty for safety [44].

In 1999, Bauer et al. compared outcomes of laparoscopic and open pyeloplasties. Specifically, they compared 42 laparoscopic and 35 open cases. Pain relief, improved activity levels, and radiographic improvement were similar in these two groups [45]. Other series continued to show advantages relative to length of stay (LOS), pain, and cosmesis when comparing laparoscopic and open pyeloplasties [45, 46]. Some find visualization in the peritoneum and retroperitoneum superior with MIS. This could potentially lead to more precise tissue manipulation and decrease morbidity of the procedure [47].

In 2006, Lee et al. compared robotic assisted laparoscopic pyeloplasties (RALP) to an age matched cohort of patients undergoing open pyeloplasties (OPN). There were 33 patients in each cohort. In this series RALP was safe and effective. 31 of the 35 RALP had improvement in radiographic follow up and/or symptoms. Their LOS was shorter (2.3 days vs. 3.5 days). RALP patients had higher intraoperative narcotic use. But use of epidurals was vastly different. 18 OPN patients had an epidural and no RALP patients had an epidural. Overall, the RALP patients had lower postoperative and total narcotic use ($p = 0.001$). Also, linear regression analysis showed a longer LOS in the OPN group as age of patient increased. However, there was no difference in LOS for the RALP group. There was similar estimated blood loss (EBL) in both cohorts. And no blood transfusions were required for either group. Mean operative time was higher in the RALP group (219 minutes vs. 181 min). But this was not statistically significant (p = 0.031). There were no complications in the OPN group. One patient from the RALP group required repeat surgery. This patient initially had a retroperitoneal surgery and crossing vessels were not recognized. Due to persistent obstruction, this patient had a temporary percutaneous nephrostomy tube and later had a transperitoneal repair. Follow up in this series was short, with a mean follow up of 10 months for the RALP cohort. Similar to other studies, increased experience correlated with quicker operative times [48].

Riachy et al. compared Laparoscopic pyeloplasty (LP) and RALP at their institution. There were 18 LP and 46 RALP. Mean follow up for LP was 43 months and follow up for RALP was 22 months (RALP). Both groups were comparable in operative time, hospital stay, narcotic use, and complication rates [49].

Surgical approach can be transperitoneal or retroperitoneal. Olsen et al. reported a 5-year experience of retroperitoneal RALP. 67 cases were performed in 65 children. Complications occurred in 12 procedures (17.9%). Complications included urinary tract infection, hematuria, and displaced ureteral stents. Four patients underwent additional surgery (6%) [50].

Favorable results with minimally invasive pyeloplasties have been demonstrated not only in older children, but also in infants. Kafka et al. reviewed pyeloplasties performed on very small children. 15 laparoscopic and open cases were age matched. Median age was 8 months and median weight was 7 kg. There was one Clavien grade I-II complication in both arms. Although limited in volume, this study suggested that a robotic pyeloplasty has similar outcomes, even in the very young patient [51].

Kutikov et al. had one of the earliest reports of robotic surgery in infants. They did a retrospective review of robotic pyeloplasties in 9 infants aged 3–8 months. Mean operative time was 122. 8 min with a mean console time of 72.1 min. The mean hospital stay was 1.4 days. 78% had resolution or improvement in their hydronephrosis. No patient required conversion to open or standard laparoscopic techniques [42].

Kawal et al. looked at their 4-year experience of robotic pyeloplasties in 138 patients. In their series, multivariate and comparative analysis showed lower morphine equivalents in infants. Of note, infants had a higher chance of placing a percutaneous stent. The infant cohort had success rates of 96%. Six patients (4%) required repeat surgery. Although infants had a 29.4% complication rate, this was similar to the older population (30.8%). There were no intraoperative complications and no conversions to open surgery. The postoperative complications were low grade: 60% were Clavien grade I and II (pain, urinary tract infection). 40% were Clavien grade III (stent dislodgement and replacement). The most common complications with both infants and older children were stent related, with evaluation in the emergency room for pain and hematuria [52].

Dangle et al. reviewed their experience with infant pyeloplasties comparing open and robotic approaches. They had 10 patients in each arm. Mean patient age was

3.31 months. Postoperative outcomes were similar in for the open vs. robotic arms: length of stay (2.2 vs. 2.1 days), estimated blood loss (6.5 vs. 7.6 mL), days to regular diet (1 vs. 1.1 days), and time to foley removal (1.3 vs. 1.3 days). However, total operating time was longer in the robotic group (199 vs. 242 min). When excluding amortization, robotic cost, maintenance and depreciation, direct costs were similar ($4410 vs $4979 per case). In regards to surgical success, improvement in hydronephrosis was identical in both groups. These authors recognize the importance of surgeon experience before performing robotic surgery infants. Their senior author had performed 28 pyeloplasties and 60 other complex robotic procedures in older children before forging into robotic surgery in infants [6].

Neheman et al. compared results in infant pyeloplasties performed robotically versus laparoscopically. This was a retrospective review all MIS pyeloplasties performed in infants at two different hospitals between October 2009 and February 2016. 13 patients had standard laparoscopic pyeloplasties (LP) and 21 patients had a robotic pyeloplasty (RP). Although complication rates were similar with both approaches, it was high in both groups with a rate of 30.8% for LP and 23.8% for RP (p = 0.65) [53].

Silay et al. did a retrospective review of 783 pyeloplasties performed at 15 academic centers. Cases were done laparoscopically or robotically. All patients were <18 years old. Mean follow up was 12.8 months for the RALP and 45.2 months for LP. Success rates were comparable (RALP 99.5% and LP 97.3% p = 0.11) Intraoperative complication rates were also comparable (RALP 3.8% and LP 7.4% p = 0.06). However, the postoperative complication rate was higher in the LP group (7.7% vs 3.2% p = 0.02). All complications were Clavien IIIb or lower [54].

Andolfi et al. reviewed 19 original articles and 5 meta-analyses on laparoscopic and robotic pyeloplasties. This review showed that a robotic approach was associated with shorter operative times, shorter lengths of stay, and lower complication rates. The success rate was comparable to laparoscopic repairs. Therefore, cost of robotics continues to be an area of concern [55].

Minimally invasive surgery has evolved into an option for complex pyeloplasties. Jacobsen et al. reported long-term results of robotic repair after a failed pyeloplasty. Specifically, they retrospectively reviewed 36 patients (31 re-do pyeloplasties and 5 ureterocalicostomies). The patients were followed for a mean of 35.4 months. Mean age at time of surgery was 3.7 years. Mean operative time was 285 minutes and mean hospital stay was 1 day. Complications occurred in 6 patients (four with Clavien grade I or II, and six with Clavien grade III-V). Only one patient had worsening hydronephrosis after surgery. The authors felt robotics was a safe, effective and feasible approach even for the complicated, re-do surgeries [56].

Minimally invasive pyeloplasties has comparable outcomes to open repairs. Multiple series confirm a high safety profile with a minimally invasive approach. It has been successfully utilized in older and infant patients. Additionally, it has been used in complex situations (e.g., re-do surgery). When a UPJO required surgical repair, a minimally invasive approach should be considered.

Ureteral Reimplantations

Although laparoscopic and robotic ureteral reimplantations have grown over the past two decades, its use is still limited in many pediatric centers.

Bowen et al. reviewed a 10-year period of open, laparoscopic, and robotic reimplantations recorded in the Kids' Inpatient Database. Before 2009, all laparoscopic and robotic cases were classified as minimally invasive ureteral reimplantations. However, between 2009 and 2012, a detailed analysis was done of open versus robotic ureteral reimplantations. This analysis revealed that the overall rate of reimplantations between 2002–2012 decreased 14.3%, but minimally invasive reimplantations increased from 0.3% to 6.3%. Specifically, robotic reimplantations accounted for 3.8% of all reimplantations in 2009, and accounted for 5.1% of all reimplantations in 2012. In this report, the robotic cases had shorter hospital stays, but higher costs. Although robotic reimplantations are becoming more prevalent, the total volume is still modest and is clustered at a small number of hospitals [57].

Wang et al. reviewed the 1998–2012 Nationwide Inpatient Sample to evaluate the results of ureteroneocystostomies (UNC) performed via open and minimally invasive techniques. They identified 780 MIS and 75,976 UNC admissions. MIS cases had a higher rate of postoperative urinary complications such as UTIs, urinary retention, and renal injury. [58]

Understandably, surgeons want to know efficacy and safety of a new technique before embracing its usage. And the outcomes with robotic ureteral reimplantation continue to evolve. Initial robotic experience entailed an intravesical approach. This approach had varied success rates between 83–100%. And complication rates widely varied between 0–52%. Chan et al. had no complications but it was only a series of three patients [59]. Although the complication rate for Peters et al. was 17%, it was small series of six patients. One patient had a urine leak secondary to incomplete bladder closure [60].

Marchini et al. looked at both intravesical and extravesical ureteral reimplantations. The intravesical robotic group had shorter hospital stays, shorter catheter drainage, and fewer bladder spasms. But they also had a higher complication rate [61].

There is more data with robotically-assisted laparoscopic ureteral reimplantation (RALUR) performed with an extravesical approach. Initially this was described by Peters 2004. In his series there were 24 patients with a complication rate of 13%. The most common complication was bladder leak (eight patients). Four of these patients also had voiding difficulty. Four patients had transient ureteral obstruction [62]. Over time, more series have reported on extravesical ureteral reimplantation. There is a wide range of reported complication rates ranging from 0–40%. Success rates have also varied between 77–100%. Some series have shown very favorable outcomes and safety profiles [63]. Whereas other series, RALUR have not reached the high standards of open reimplantation surgery [9]. Robotic ureteral reimplantation has not become a standard of care for anti-reflux surgery [6, 9, 10, 48, 64–66].

Dangle et al. did see a higher rate of complications in robotic ureteral reimplantations. The rate of Clavien Grade I and II complications was 3.5% for unilateral and 16.2% for bilateral. And the rate of Clavien grade III complications was 2.3% for unilateral and 12.9% for bilateral reimplantations [36].

Esposito et al. reviewed 55 patients who had robotic extravesical ureteral reimplantation surgery. This was an international compilation of patients with a mean age was 4.9 years. There were no intraoperative complications and no conversions to open surgery. There were 3 postoperative complications (5.4%). These complications were Clavien grade II and III. The Clavien IIIb was related to re-do surgery for persistent reflux after surgery [67].

Chalmers et al. reported their experience from a single institution of 16 patients who underwent an extxravesical RALUR. There were no intraoperative or postoperative complications in this series [66].

Silay et al. reported on 72 patients with a 3% complication rate. All of these patients had urinary retention [68].

Dangle et al. did see a higher rate of complications in the bilateral repairs. The rate of Clavien Grade I and II complications was 3.5% for unilateral and 16.2% for bilateral. And the rate of Clavien grade III complications was 2.3% for unilateral and 12.9% for bilateral reimplantations [36].

Grimsby et al. reported the combined experience from two institutions with 93 ureters treated in 61 patients. The mean age was 6.7 years. Their results were concerning in both outcomes and complications. Their success rate was only 72%. Six major complications occurred that included ureteral obstruction and urinary leak. Nine patients under reoperations (11%). They concluded that bilateral RALUR had higher complications, higher reoperation rates, more postoperative UTIs, and more nonsurgical admissions than unilateral RALUR [65].

Akhavan et al. reported on 78 ureteral reimplantations performed at their institution. Success rates were favorable with only 7.7% of patients having persistent reflux. However, there was 10% complication rate including ureteral obstruction, ureteral injury, perinephric fluid collection, febrile UTI, ileus, and urinary retention. The mean age was 6.2 years old with the youngest patient 1.9 years old. The authors felt RALUR was effective and safe treatment for primary vesicoureteral reflux [64].

Many reports come from single institutional experiences. However Boysen et al. led a prospective series amongst 8 institutions. Their goal was evaluation of safety and efficacy of robotic ureteral reimplantation in children. Mean age was 6.6 years. There were 143 patients treated between 2015–2017 with an extravesical reimplantation. At mean follow up of 7.4 months, there were five ureteral complications (2.5%). There was transient urinary retention in four patients (7.1%). All retention was in bilateral repairs. Although follow up was limited, it was encouraging to see low complication rates with a large series of RALUR [69].

Boysen et al. did a multi-institutional review from nine institutions. This included a total of 260 patients (363 ureters). The overall complication rate was 9.6%. There were no Clavien Grade IV or V complications. There were four patients with transient urinary retention (3.9%). Although the radiographic success rates were slightly lower than the results of open surgery, the overall complication rate was consistent with published series of open reimplantation [69].

Deng et al. did a literature search to compare the efficacy and safety of both robotic and open ureteral reimplantation. A total of six studies with 7122 children were included. There were no significant differences in estimated blood loss during the operation or intraoperative complications between the two groups. However, the robotic group had a higher rate of short-term postoperative complications [70].

When looking at specific circumstances, minimally invasive ureteral reimplantations have been reported in infants, duplicated systems, and complex patients.

Most of the reported outcomes of robotic ureteral reimplantations are in older children. But there is some limited data in smaller children that show favorable results as well. In 2011, Smith et al. described an infant extravesical robotic reimplantation on a 3-month old infant [63].

Most other series include a few younger patients in their series. Herz et al. reported their experience with extravesical ureteral reimplantation in 72 ureters (54 patients). They had success in 84.7%, with the youngest patient was 2.5 years old [9]. Dangle et al. reported on 29 patients with a success rate of 87.5% but the youngest patient was 3 years old [71].

Rodriguez et al. looked at results with a common sheath reimplantations. There was a total of 13 patients and 3 had bilateral repairs. Mean follow up was 17.18 months. There were no high-grade complications (Clavien grade III-V). There were two Clavien grade II complications [72].

Arlen et al. looked at ureteral reimplantation in complex situations. They identified complex patients as those who had (a) prior antireflux surgery, (b) tapered or dismembered ureter, or (c) duplicated system or an associated diverticulum. Their series included 17 patients over a 2-year period. This was compared to 41 open ureteral reimplantations done at the same time. There was no significant difference in complications (11.8% in the robotic arm and 12.2% in the open arm). They lacked clear success rates since VCUGs were not performed in all patients. Although this was a small series that lacked randomization, it was encouraging that robotic reimplantation appeared safe for even the complex situations [73].

Historically, extravesical ureteral reimplantation have been associated with postoperative urinary retention. Barrieras et al. reviewed the incidence of urinary retention after bilateral extravesical ureteral reimplantation. This was a chart review of 220 patients between 1991 and 1997. There were two techniques described: the Y detrusorrhaphy and the advancing suture technique. The rate of retention with each technique was 8.4% and 15.2% respectively. This difference was not statistically significant. There were higher retention rates in patients with grades IV and V reflux, in younger patients <3 years, and in male patients (24.6%, 35.6%, and 20.3%) [74].

Specific surgical techniques have not consistently impacted the rate of postoperative retention. However, rates of retention are consistently low in RALUR. Some theorize the low retention rate is due to magnified visualization of the pelvic plexus. Others believe the surgical exposure of MIS lowers traction at the ureterovesical junction which lowers postoperative neuropraxia.

Casale et al. reported their initial experience with a nerve sparing technique in 2008. In this series, there were 41 patients with no reported complications and no voiding issues [75]. In 2012, they had a larger series of 150 patients. There was mean follow up of 2 years. These patients had a nerve sparing reimplantation. There was one postoperative febrile UTI, but there were no voiding complications [76].

In 2005, the American College of Surgeons collaborated with the American Pediatric Surgical association to create the National Surgical Quality Improvement Program (NSQIP) Peds. This is a prospective database of reported cases performed in patients under 18 years. Voluntary input comes from over 100 sites. Data includes preoperative and postoperative data. This allows review of 30-day complication rates from multiple pediatric surgical subspecialties. Wang et al. reviewed NSQIP Peds for ureteral reimplantations performed between 1998–2012. There was a marked difference in volume of open cases compared to MIS. (75,976 open and 780 MIS cases, giving a ratio of 100:1 for open and MIS). This large discrepancy in volume makes comparisons challenging. But MIS was associated with shorter lengths of stay ($p = 0.02$) and higher costs ($p = 0.008$). But MIS had a significantly higher rate of postoperative complications ($p = 0.02$). The most common postoperative complications included urinary tract infections, urinary retention, and renal injury [58].

In summary, there are numerous reports of minimally invasive ureteral reimplantations that show favorable outcomes and low complication rates. However, it has not replaced other options for anti-reflux surgery. But it is an additional technique to offer patients when choosing an anti-reflux surgical approach.

Nephrectomies

When total or partial nephrectomy is indicated, it can be done with an open, laparoscopic, and robotic approach. When a minimally invasive approach is used, it can be transperitoneal or retroperitoneal. All approaches have favorable outcomes and safety profiles.

Nehemen reviewed the results of partial nephrectomy performed with a variety of techniques. This retrospective review included open and minimally invasive techniques. The minimally invasive techniques included laparoscopic, robotic, and laparoscopic single port approaches. Over a 10-year period there were 24 open and 25 minimally invasive cases. The minimally invasive cases had shorter hospital stays, lower blood loss, and lower postoperative analgesic use. The overall safety and efficacy were favorable. There were no intraoperative complications. The six postoperative complications were all Clavien grade II (four urinary tract infections, one fever, and one with respiratory distress requiring medication). There were no reports of postoperative loss of function to the remaining moiety [77].

MacDonald et al. compared outcomes of both total and partial nephrectomies done by a retroperitoneal approach. This included 173 cases over a 10-year period of time (2005–2015). Mean age was 5 years and mean weight was 24.9 kg. There were four conversions to open surgery and 17 postoperative complications. A predictor of postoperative complication was the choice of vessel control [78].

Ballouhey et al. looked at robotic partial nephrectomy in small children. This was a cohort of 28 patients all <15 kg: 15 patients done with a robotic approach and 13 patients done with an open approach. Mean at the time of surgery was 20.2 months for the robotic arm and 18.4 months for the open arm. The mean hospital stay was significantly longer for the open arm (6.3 days vs 3.4 days) $p < 0.001$. Also, the postoperative pain control in total morphine equivalent intake was significantly greater in the open arm (1.08 mg/kg/day vs. 0.52 mg/kg/day) $P < 0.001$. There was no significant difference in terms of operating time, complication rate, or renal outcomes [79].

Esposito et al. compared partial nephrectomies performed with a transperitoneal and retroperitoneal approach. Specifically, they reviewed results in 102 patients over a 5-year period. Mean age at surgery was 4.2 years. 52 patients had a transperitoneal laparoscopic partial nephrectomy (LPN) and 50 patients had a retroperitoneal partial nephrectomy (RPN). Neither group had conversion to open surgery. However, the overall complication rate was higher in the RPN group (30% vs 19%). The complications in the LPN group were: urinoma [4], symptomatic refluxing ureteral stumps [2], urinary leakage [4]. The complications in the RPN group were: urinoma (6), symptomatic refluxing ureteral stumps [8], and open calyx [1]. 2 of the 50 RPN patients underwent additional surgery. Many find a retroperitoneal approach technically more challenging. And this series suggests a transperitoneal approach is faster and safer for performing partial nephrectomies. A transperitoneal approach allows a larger working space and low dissection of the distal ureter [80].

Minimally invasive nephrectomies can be safely performed in infants as well. Bansal et al. reviewed their experience in ten infants who underwent robotic upper tract reconstructive surgery at their institution between March 2009 and February 2013. Eight patients underwent pyeloplasty and two underwent ureteroureterostomy. The mean age was 10 months and mean weight was 7.7 kg. Mean follow up was 10 months. Postoperative ultrasound showed improved in all patients. There were three complications (one Grade 1 and two Grade IIIb). Complications included ileus, urinary tract infection, and one urine leak [81].

Pediatric nephrectomies can be done an open, laparoscopic, or robotic approach. Surgeon experience often guides the technique chosen. Minimally invasive nephrectomies in children have been shown safe and effective.

Bladder Reconstructive Cases

There are limited series on minimally invasive bladder reconstructive surgery. Likely inhibitors to a minimally invasive approach are a lack of standardized training in robotic surgery, the significant learning curve, surgeon preference with open techniques, and smaller working space in pediatric patients. Despite these barriers, minimally invasive surgery has been used in many bladder reconstructive cases.

The first laparoscopic-assisted appendicovesicostomy was described in 1993. [12] Then the first completely laparoscopic appendicovesicostomy was performed in 2004. That same year, a robotic-assisted appendicovesicostomy was described [82]. And the first completely intracorporeal robotic assisted laparoscopic appendicovesicostomy (RALMA) was completed in 2008 [83].

Nerli et al. reported their experience with a purely laparoscopic appendicovesicostomy in six patients. At 33-month follow up, there were no reported stomal stenosis. Although two patients had incontinence they responded to medical therapy [84].

Famakinwa et al. looked at robotic augmentation/Mitrofanoff creation in 20 pediatric patients. Their patients had a mean follow up of 24.2 months. Mean age was 11 years. There were no intraoperative complications. There were three patients (16.7%) with postoperative stomal issues (two stomal stenosis and one parastomal hernia) [85].

Wille et al. reported on 11 patients who underwent RALMA. There were no intraoperative complications. Median follow up was 20 months. Three patients did require a skin flap revision due to stenosis [86].

Nguyen et al. reported their experience on ten patients who had RALMA. One case was converted to open surgery. Median follow up was 14.2 months. One patient required an open revision due to urinary leakage. One patient had Deflux injection due to incontinence [87].

Not surprisingly, more complex reconstructive cases carry a higher risk of complications when compared to minimally invasive pyeloplasties, ureteral reimplantations, and nephrectomies. However, even with higher rates of complications with these reconstructive cases, the overall complication rates are similar to results reported with open reconstructive surgery. Leslie et al. reported on 169 patients who underwent open appendicovesicostomy. Mean follow up was 5.8 years. 39% of their patients had surgical revision. Thomas et al. followed 78 patients who had open appendicovesicostomy. At mean follow up of 28.4 months there were 14% stomal stenosis and 23% channel-related complications. Liard et al. reviewed 20 year follow up in 23 patients who had an open appendicovesicostomy between 1976–1984. There was one death related to infection that involved the ventriculoperitoneal shunt. In the remaining 22 patients, most postoperative complications occurred in the first 10 years. These complications included stomal stenosis or persistent leakage [11] and intestinal occlusion [5]. They did have ten patients with bilateral upper tract deterioration with secondary bladder augmentation. Over time they saw fewer cases of delayed bladder augmentation. This correlated with the evolving knowledge of optimal bladder storage and coordinated bladder augmentation at the time of their appendicovesicostomy [88–90]. Schlomer et al. reviewed the Pediatric Health Information System from 1999 to 2010. 2831 AC patients were identified. A large percentage (40.1%) experienced a high-grade complication or underwent a subsequent procedure within 1 year. Some of the high grade complications were bladder rupture (1.1%), stone formation (3.2%), bowel obstruction (3.6%), stoma surgery (5.6%), bladder neck surgery (2.9%), and re-augmentation (1.8%) [91].

The existing literature with minimally invasive bladder reconstruction is encouraging. But a minimally invasive approach for bladder reconstructive surgery is definitely not a standard of care. However, in experienced hands, it is a reasonable option to consider.

LESS Surgery

Laparoendoscopic Single Site Surgery (LESS) offers potential advantages compared to conventional laparoscopy. Some reports cite lower postoperative pain, fewer port site hernias, better cosmesis, and faster recovery [92]. LESS is more commonly performed in adults.

In 2009, LESS procedures expanded into pediatrics. Initially reports were simple nephrectomies [93, 94]. Lee et al. looked at four LESS nephrectomies performed for dysplastic kidneys with an ectopic ureter. Mean age was 3.2 years. There were no complications in these four patients. There were no additional ports placed and no conversion to open surgery [95]. Overtime, more challenging and reconstructive cases have been performed in children with LESS. For example, Naitoh et al. reviewed outcomes of LESS pyeloplasties from 2008–2013. They retrospectively reviewed 26 cases. Mean age was 20.4 years. 14 patients were pediatric. However, no intraoperative or postoperative complications were seen in the entire cohort. They recognize that a prospective, randomized study would be necessary to solidify conclusions. But their analysis suggest that LESS can be used safely in both adult and pediatric pyeloplasties [96].

Bansal et al. reviewed four patients who had LESS partial nephrectomies for upper tract duplication anomalies. Mean age was 6.2 months and mean weight was 7.7 kg. Mean follow up was 9.9 months. There were no postoperative complications seen [97].

Symeonidis et al. looked at 29 studies reviewing LESS procedures in children. Specifically, they looked at reports of single site surgery in more than one pediatric patient. These included nephrectomy, pyeloplasty, varicocelectomy, nephroureterectomy, and partial nephrectomy. They looked at intraoperative and postoperative complications. Conversion included transition to an open approach as well as addition of working ports. All but one study was retrospective in nature. There were 55 partial nephrectomies with no intraoperative complications. There were 3 postoperative complications (5.45%): two Clavien grade I and one Clavien grade III. There were 174 transperitoneal nephrectomies and nephroureterectomies. There were no intraoperative complications. There were postoperative complications in 5 patients (2.87%): four Clavien grade II and one Clavien grade III. There were 20 retroperitoneal nephrectomies. In this group there were no intraoperative or postoperative complications. 92 pyeloplasties were reviewed. Two cases required either conversion to open or additional port placements. There were ten postoperative complications (10.86%): eight Clavien grade I and two Clavien grade II. 60 varicocelectomies were reviewed. There were no intraoperative complications and only one postoperative complication (1.7%): Clavien grade I [98].

Although limited in volume, the experience with LESS in children has low rates of complications. However, many surgeons are still hesitant to embrace LESS due to lack of resources, inadequate proficiency, and disbelief in the technique [99].

Infant Robotic Surgery

Results of minimally invasive surgery in infants is limited to smaller case series. Smaller patient size can hamper docking of robotic equipment. Infants recover quickly from both open and minimally invasive surgery. Therefore, the interest and experience to perform MIS in infants is smaller in scope. However, many reports of MIS in infants are favorable. Some of these series were reviewed in the pyeloplasty section.

Additionally, Fuchs et al. did a retrospective review of multiple minimally invasive upper tract surgeries performed in infants. A total of 67 patients had surgery: 26 pyeloplasties, 18 heminephrectomies, and 23 nephrectomies. Mean weight was 6.4 kg and mean operative time was 113 min. One pyeloplasty required conversion to open technique. One patient had a missed intraoperative bowel injury. No blood transfusions were required. All of the pyeloplasties had improvement in their drainage time. And the heminephrectomy patients had stable postoperative renal function. This group preferred a transperitoneal approach due to the size limitations in infants [100].

Srougi et al. looked at their institution's experience doing robotic surgery in infants and toddlers. There was a wide range of cases performed (pyeloplasty, nephrectomy, reimplantation, ureteroureterostomy, orchidopexy, excision of Mullerian remnant and pyelolithotomy). Mean hospital stay was 1.3 days. They divided results on patients over and under 10 kg. Mean weight was 11.6 kg and 23 patients under 10 kg (34%). In these smaller patients, there were 12 postoperative complications. Most were Clavien grade I and II. But there was one grade IIIB complication. There was not a higher complication rate in the smaller children. In fact, the patients >10 kg had higher complication rates, but it was not statistically significant [101].

Bansal et al. looked at results by 3 surgeons during the first 4 years of their robotic program. Ten different surgeries were performed in 136 patients. All surgeries were performed transperitoneally. There were no robotic malfunctions or conversions to open surgery. There were no intraoperative complications, but 11 patients experienced a postoperative complication. When comparing infant and older patients, 3 of these 11 complications occurred in infants. Therefore, the complication rate for infants was 30% (3 out of 10) and 8.6% for the other pediatric patients (8 out of 126 noninfants) p = 0.035. There were two Clavien grade I, seven Clavien grade II, and two Clavien grade IIIb. The degree of complications was not higher in the infant patients. And none of the complications were due to intraoperative or due to robotic malfunction [5].

Avery et al. reviewed the experience amongst six surgeons who performed robotic pyeloplasties on children <1 year old between 2006–2012. A total of 62 procedures were performed on 60 patients at 5 different institutions. Mean age was 7.3 months. Two patients had recurrent obstruction and required additional surgery. Seven patients had intraoperative or immediate postoperative complications (11%). (one patient Clavien grade I, two patients with Clavien grade II, four patients with Clavien grade III). The specific complications were port site hernia, urine leak, urinary tract infection, retained stent, renal calculus, and prolonged ileus [4].

Overview of National Experience with Pediatric MIS

Colaco et al. looked at the NSQIP Peds database for all reported urologic cases in 2014. This included 207 nephrectomies (98 open and 109 MIS), 92 partial nephrectomies (48 open and 24 MIS), 920 ureteral reimplantations (803 open and 117 MIS), and 625 pyeloplasties (349 open and 276 MIS). The rate of superficial or deep wound infections, bleeding requiring transfusion, urinary tract infections, pneumonia, and readmission was <0.1% for all queried cases, regardless of the approach used. There were no significant differences in the rate of 30-day complications for any of the surgeries reviewed [28].

Colaco et al. also looked at the short-term complication rates of open versus laparoscopic renal and ureteral surgery. They did a retrospective cross-sectional analysis of the National Surgical Quality Improvement Program database. Specifically, they reviewed all nephrectomies, partial nephrectomies, pyeloplasties, and ureteroneocystotomy performed in 2014. There was no difference in the rate of short-term complications with either approach. Pediatric MIS was associated with longer operative times for nephrectomy, but also associated with shorter length of stay for partial nephrectomy [28].

Tejwani et al. analyzed the 1998–2012 Nationwide Inpatient Sample to review children who had open and minimally invasive inpatient procedures. They looked at postoperative complications that occurred during that postoperative hospitalization. They used propensity score matching and multivariable logistic regression to adjust for confounding factors. They found narrowed 163,838 encounters to 70,273 encounters that occurred at centers where more than five MIS procedures performed in the identified time frame. This specialized cohort consisted of 66,510 open and 3763 MIS cases. Comparing the MIS patients to the open patients, MIS had older patients (7.8 years vs. 4.7 years) with lower comorbidities. And there were more males in the MIS cases (51.6% vs. 43%). They saw an increased use of MIS techniques for multiple procedures, but most markedly for nephrectomy. The overall complication rate for MIS was lower than open surgery (6% vs 11%, $p < 0.001$). Specialized centers had overall lower complications than unspecialized centers (9% vs. 12%, $p < 0.001$). At the specialized centers, MIS had lower complication rates than open surgery (7% vs. 9%, p < 0.001). The authors recognize limitations with their analysis. NIS represents 20% stratified sample of hospital admissions in the United States [39].

Conclusion

Minimally invasive surgery continues to evolve in pediatric urology. There are multiple series demonstrating excellent surgical results. The benefits of shorter hospital stays, less narcotic use, improved cosmesis has been demonstrated in both adult and pediatric populations.

MIS in pediatrics had steadily gained acceptance, but there are many surgeons still hesitant to utilize this technique. Some concerns include the limited operative space, relatively large port sizes, increased operative time, and potential decreased anesthesia access to the patient [62, 102].

Although it has been used for a wide variety of urologic cases, the most common MIS in pediatric urology is a pyeloplasty. National trends in pediatric pyeloplasties have remained fairly stable. However, the volume of robotic repairs has increased and the number of open repairs has decreased [103]. As outlined, many reports demonstrate comparable results of minimally invasive pyeloplasty relative to open surgery.

Minimally invasive ureteral reimplantation has varied results. But many reports cite low complication rates with encouraging surgical results. Minimally invasive nephrectomy has also been shown safe and effective, albeit in modest data. Although minimally invasive bladder reconstruction has more complications, the rates are comparable to existing results with an open technique.

Hesitancy to use MIS in children may be misguided. There are numerous reports that confirm pediatric urologic minimally invasive surgery is safe and has favorable outcomes.

References

1. Reddy MN, Nerli RB. The laparoscopic pyeloplasty: is there a role in the age of robotics? Urol Clin North Am 2015;42(1):43–52.
2. Tasian GE, Wiebe DJ, Casale P. Learning curve of robotic assisted pyeloplasty for pediatric urology fellows. J Urol. 2013;190(4 Suppl):1622–6.
3. Bolliger M, Kroehnert JA, McIineus F, Kandioler D, Schindl M, Riss P. Experiences with the standardized classification of surgical complications (Clavien-Dindo) in general surgery patients. Eur Surg. 2018;50(6):256–61.
4. Avery DI, Herbst KW, Lendvay TS, Noh PH, Dangle P, Gundeti MS, et al. Robot-assisted laparoscopic pyeloplasty: multi-institutional experience in infants. J Pediatr Urol. 2015;11(3):139.e1–5.
5. Bansal D, Defoor WR Jr, Reddy PP, Minevich EA, Noh PH. Complications of robotic surgery in pediatric urology: a single institution experience. Urology. 2013;82(4):917–20.

6. Dangle PP, Kearns J, Anderson B, Gundeti MS. Outcomes of infants undergoing robot-assisted laparoscopic pyeloplasty compared to open repair. J Urol. 2013;190(6):2221–6.
7. Spinoit AF, Nguyen H, Subramaniam R. Role of robotics in children: a brave new world! Eur Urol Focus. 2017;3(2–3):172–80.
8. Riedmiller H, et al. EAU guidelines on paediatric urology. Eur Urol. 2001;40(5):589.
9. Herz D, Fuchs M, Todd A, McLeod D, Smith J. Robot-assisted laparoscopic extravesical ureteral reimplant: a critical look at surgical outcomes. J Pediatr Urol. 2016;12(6):402.e1–9.
10. Schomburg JL, Haberman K, Willihnganz-Lawson KH, Shukla AR. Robot-assisted laparoscopic ureteral reimplantation: a single surgeon comparison to open surgery. J Pediatr Urol. 2014;10(5):875–9.
11. Timberlake MD, Peters CA. Current status of robotic-assisted surgery for the treatment of vesicoureteral reflux in children. Curr Opin Urol. 2017;27(1):20–6.
12. Jordan GH, Winslow BH. Laparoscopically assisted continent catheterizable cutaneous appendicovesicostomy. J Endourol. 1993;7(6):517–20.
13. Grimsby GM, Jacobs MA, Gargollo PC. Comparison of complications of robot-assisted laparoscopic and open appendicovesicostomy in children. J Urol. 2015;194(3):772–6.
14. Snodgrass W. Re: long-term outcomes of bladder neck reconstruction without augmentation cystoplasty in children: G. M. Grimsby, V. Menon, B. J. Schlomer, L. A. Baker, R. Adams, P. C. Gargollo and M. A. Jacobs J Urol. 2016;195:155–161. J Urol. 2016;196(1):286–8.
15. Bagrodia A, Gargollo P. Robot-assisted bladder neck reconstruction, bladder neck sling, and appendicovesicostomy in children: description of technique and initial results. J Endourol. 2011;25(8):1299–305.
16. Murthy P, Cohn JA, Selig RB, Gundeti MS. Robot-assisted laparoscopic augmentation ileocystoplasty and Mitrofanoff appendicovesicostomy in children: updated interim results. Eur Urol. 2015;68(6):1069–75.
17. Thakre AA, Yeung CK, Peters C. Robot-assisted Mitrofanoff and Malone antegrade continence enema reconstruction using divided appendix. J Endourol. 2008;22(10):2393–6; discussion 6.
18. Kavoussi LR, Peters CA. Laparoscopic pyeloplasty. J Urol. 1993;150(6):1891–4.
19. Moore RG, Averch TD, Schulam PG, Adams JB 2nd, Chen RN, Kavoussi LR. Laparoscopic pyeloplasty: experience with the initial 30 cases. J Urol. 1997;157(2):459–62.
20. Jarrett TW, Chan DY, Charambura TC, Fugita O, Kavoussi LR. Laparoscopic pyeloplasty: the first 100 cases. J Urol. 2002;167(3):1253–6.
21. Soulie M, Salomon L, Patard JJ, Mouly P, Manunta A, Antiphon P, et al. Extraperitoneal laparoscopic pyeloplasty: a multicenter study of 55 procedures. J Urol. 2001;166(1):48–50.
22. Soulie M, Thoulouzan M, Seguin P, Mouly P, Vazzoler N, Pontonnier F, et al. Retroperitoneal laparoscopic versus open pyeloplasty with a minimal incision: comparison of two surgical approaches. Urology. 2001;57(3):443–7.
23. Ben Slama MR, Salomon L, Hoznek A, Cicco A, Saint F, Alame W, et al. Extraperitoneal laparoscopic repair of ureteropelvic junction obstruction: initial experience in 15 cases. Urology. 2000;56(1):45–8.
24. Peters CA. Complications in pediatric urological laparoscopy: results of a survey. J Urol. 1996;155(3):1070–3.
25. Esposito C, Lima M, Mattioli G, Mastroianni L, Centonze A, Monguzzi GL, et al. Complications of pediatric urological laparoscopy: mistakes and risks. J Urol. 2003;169(4):1490–2; discussion 2.
26. Passerotti CC, Nguyen HT, Retik AB, Peters CA. Patterns and predictors of laparoscopic complications in pediatric urology: the role of ongoing surgical volume and access techniques. J Urol. 2008;180(2):681–5.
27. Luque Mialdea R, Martin-Crespo Izquierdo R. Laparoscopy in pediatric urology. Arch Esp Urol. 2002;55(6):737–47.
28. Colaco M, Hester A, Visser W, Rasper A, Terlecki R. Relative to open surgery, minimally-invasive renal and ureteral pediatric surgery offers no improvement in 30-day complications,

yet requires longer operative time: data from the National Surgical Quality Improvement Program Pediatrics. Investig Clin Urol. 2018;59(3):200–5.
29. Chu DI, Tan JM, Mattei P, Simpao AF, Costarino AT, Shukla AR, et al. Outcomes of laparoscopic and open surgery in children with and without congenital heart disease. J Pediatr Surg. 2018;53(10):1980–8.
30. Abdelshehid CS, Eichel L, Lee D, Uribe C, Boker J, Basillote J, et al. Current trends in urologic laparoscopic surgery. J Endourol. 2005;19(1):15–20.
31. Eichel L, Ahlering TE, Clayman RV. Role of robotics in laparoscopic urologic surgery. Urol Clin North Am. 2004;31(4):781–92.
32. Partin AW, Adams JB, Moore RG, Kavoussi LR. Complete robot-assisted laparoscopic urologic surgery: a preliminary report. J Am Coll Surg. 1995;181(6):552–7.
33. Harel M, Herbst KW, Silvis R, Makari JH, Ferrer FA, Kim C. Objective pain assessment after ureteral reimplantation: comparison of open versus robotic approach. J Pediatr Urol. 2015;11(2):82.e1–8.
34. Brooks-Brunn JA. Predictors of postoperative pulmonary complications following abdominal surgery. Chest. 1997;111(3):564–71.
35. Barashi NS, Andolfi C, Wallace A, Rodriguez MV, Schadler E, Gundeti MS. Lessons learned from a single-surgeon series of paediatric robot-assisted laparoscopic urological procedures: predictors of high-grade postoperative complications. BJU Int. 2019; https://doi.org/10.1111/bju.14757.
36. Dangle PP, Akhavan A, Odeleye M, Avery D, Lendvay T, Koh CJ, et al. Ninety-day perioperative complications of pediatric robotic urological surgery: a multi-institutional study. J Pediatr Urol. 2016;12(2):102.e1–6.
37. Duchene DA, Moinzadeh A, Gill IS, Clayman RV, Winfield HN. Survey of residency training in laparoscopic and robotic surgery. J Urol. 2006;176(5):2158–66; discussion 67.
38. Wang DS, Winfield HN. Survey of urological laparoscopic practice patterns in the Midwest. J Urol. 2004;172(6 Pt 1):2282–6.
39. Tejwani R, Young BJ, Wang HS, Wolf S, Purves JT, Wiener JS, et al. Open versus minimally invasive surgical approaches in pediatric urology: trends in utilization and complications. J Pediatr Urol. 2017;13(3):283.e1–9.
40. Colodny AH. Laparoscopy in pediatric urology: too much of a good thing? Semin Pediatr Surg. 1996;5(1):23–9.
41. Kozlov Y, Kovalkov K, Nowogilov V. 3D laparoscopy in neonates and infants. J Laparoendosc Adv Surg Tech A. 2016;26(12):1021–7.
42. Kutikov A, Nguyen M, Guzzo T, Canter D, Casale P. Robot assisted pyeloplasty in the infant-lessons learned. J Urol. 2006;176(5):2237–9; discussion 9–40.
43. Yee DS, Shanberg AM, Duel BP, Rodriguez E, Eichel L, Rajpoot D. Initial comparison of robotic-assisted laparoscopic versus open pyeloplasty in children. Urology. 2006;67(3):599–602.
44. Varda BK, Wang Y, Chung BI, Lee RS, Kurtz MP, Nelson CP, et al. Has the robot caught up? National trends in utilization, perioperative outcomes, and cost for open, laparoscopic, and robotic pediatric pyeloplasty in the United States from 2003 to 2015. J Pediatr Urol. 2018;14(4):336.e1–8.
45. Bauer JJ, Bishoff JT, Moore RG, Chen RN, Iverson AJ, Kavoussi LR. Laparoscopic versus open pyeloplasty: assessment of objective and subjective outcome. J Urol. 1999;162(3 Pt 1):692–5.
46. Klingler HC, Remzi M, Janetschek G, Kratzik C, Marberger MJ. Comparison of open versus laparoscopic pyeloplasty techniques in treatment of uretero-pelvic junction obstruction. Eur Urol. 2003;44(3):340–5.
47. Camarillo DB, Krummel TM, Salisbury JK Jr. Robotic technology in surgery: past, present, and future. Am J Surg. 2004;188(4A Suppl):2s–15s.

48. Lee RS, Retik AB, Borer JG, Peters CA. Pediatric robot assisted laparoscopic dismembered pyeloplasty: comparison with a cohort of open surgery. J Urol. 2006;175(2):683–7; discussion 7.
49. Riachy E, Cost NG, Defoor WR, Reddy PP, Minevich EA, Noh PH. Pediatric standard and robot-assisted laparoscopic pyeloplasty: a comparative single institution study. J Urol. 2013;189(1):283–7.
50. Olsen LH, Rawashdeh YF, Jorgensen TM. Pediatric robot assisted retroperitoneoscopic pyeloplasty: a 5-year experience. J Urol. 2007;178(5):2137–41; discussion 41.
51. Kafka IZ, Kocherov S, Jaber J, Chertin B. Pediatric robotic-assisted laparoscopic pyeloplasty (RALP): does weight matter? Pediatr Surg Int. 2019;35(3):391–6.
52. Kawal T, Srinivasan AK, Shrivastava D, Chu DI, Van Batavia J, Weiss D, et al. Pediatric robotic-assisted laparoscopic pyeloplasty: does age matter? J Pediatr Urol. 2018;14:540–e1.
53. Neheman A, Kord E, Zisman A, Darawsha AE, Noh PH. Comparison of robotic pyeloplasty and standard laparoscopic pyeloplasty in infants: a bi-institutional study. J Laparoendosc Adv Surg Tech A. 2018;28(4):467–70.
54. Silay MS, Spinoit AF, Undre S, Fiala V, Tandogdu Z, Garmanova T, et al. Global minimally invasive pyeloplasty study in children: results from the Pediatric Urology Expert Group of the European Association of Urology Young Academic Urologists working party. J Pediatr Urol. 2016;12(4):229.e1–7.
55. Andolfi C, Adamic B, Oommen J, Gundeti MS. Robot-assisted laparoscopic pyeloplasty in infants and children: is it superior to conventional laparoscopy? World J Urol. 2020;38(8):1827–33.
56. Jacobson DL, Shannon R, Johnson EK, Gong EM, Liu DB, Flink CC, et al. Robot-assisted laparoscopic reoperative repair for failed pyeloplasty in children: an updated series. J Urol. 2019;201(5):1005–11.
57. Bowen DK, Faasse MA, Liu DB, Gong EM, Lindgren BW, Johnson EK. Use of pediatric open, laparoscopic and robot-assisted laparoscopic ureteral Reimplantation in the United States: 2000 to 2012. J Urol. 2016;196(1):207–12.
58. Wang HH, Tejwani R, Cannon GM Jr, Gargollo PC, Wiener JS, Routh JC. Open versus minimally invasive ureteroneocystostomy: a population-level analysis. J Pediatr Urol. 2016;12(4):232.e1–6.
59. Chan KW, Lee KH, Tam YH, Sihoe JD. Early experience in robotic-assisted laparoscopic bilateral intravesical ureteral reimplantation for vesicoureteral reflux in children. J Robot Surg. 2012;6(3):259–62.
60. Peters C, Woo R. Intravesical robotically assistend bilateral ureteral reimplantation. J Endourol. 2005;19:618–21.
61. Marchini GS, Hong YK, Minnillo BJ, Diamond DA, Houck CS, Meier PM, et al. Robotic assisted laparoscopic ureteral reimplantation in children: case matched comparative study with open surgical approach. J Urol. 2011;185(5):1870–5.
62. Peters CA. Robotically assisted surgery in pediatric urology. Urol Clin North Am. 2004;31(4):743–52.
63. Smith RP, Oliver JL, Peters CA. Pediatric robotic extravesical ureteral reimplantation: comparison with open surgery. J Urol. 2011;185(5):1876–81.
64. Akhavan A, Avery D, Lendvay TS. Robot-assisted extravesical ureteral reimplantation: outcomes and conclusions from 78 ureters. J Pediatr Urol. 2014;10(5):864–8.
65. Grimsby GM, Dwyer ME, Jacobs MA, Ost MC, Schneck FX, Cannon GM, et al. Multi-institutional review of outcomes of robot-assisted laparoscopic extravesical ureteral reimplantation. J Urol. 2015;193(5 Suppl):1791–5.
66. Chalmers D, Herbst K, Kim C. Robotic-assisted laparoscopic extravesical ureteral reimplantation: an initial experience. J Pediatr Urol. 2012;8(3):268–71.
67. Esposito C, Masieri L, Steyaert H, Escolino M, Cerchione R, La Manna A, et al. Robot-assisted extravesical ureteral reimplantation (revur) for unilateral vesico-ureteral reflux in children: results of a multicentric international survey. World J Urol. 2018;36(3):481–8.

68. Silay MS, Baek M, Koh CJ. Robot-assisted laparoscopic Extravesical ureteral reimplantation in children: top-down suturing technique without stent placement. J Endourol. 2015;29(8):864–6.
69. Boysen WR, Ellison JS, Kim C, Koh CJ, Noh P, Whittam B, et al. Multi-institutional review of outcomes and complications of robot-assisted laparoscopic extravesical ureteral reimplantation for treatment of primary vesicoureteral reflux in children. J Urol. 2017;197(6):1555–61.
70. Deng T, Liu B, Luo L, Duan X, Cai C, Zhao Z, et al. Robot-assisted laparoscopic versus open ureteral reimplantation for pediatric vesicoureteral reflux: a systematic review and meta-analysis. World J Urol. 2018;36(5):819–28.
71. Dangle PP, Shah A, Gundeti MS. Robot-assisted laparoscopic ureteric reimplantation: extravesical technique. BJU Int. 2014;114(4):630–2.
72. Rodriguez MV, Boysen WR, Gundeti MS. Robot-assisted laparoscopic common sheath ureteral reimplantation in duplex ureters: LUAA technique tips for optimal outcomes. J Pediatr Urol. 2018;14(4):353–5.
73. Arlen AM, Broderick KM, Travers C, Smith EA, Elmore JM, Kirsch AJ. Outcomes of complex robot-assisted extravesical ureteral reimplantation in the pediatric population. J Pediatr Urol. 2016;12(3):169.e1–6.
74. Barrieras D, Lapointe S, Reddy PP, Williot P, McLorie GA, Bagli D, et al. Urinary retention after bilateral extravesical ureteral reimplantation: does dissection distal to the ureteral orifice have a role? J Urol. 1999;162(3 Pt 2):1197–200.
75. Casale P, Patel RP, Kolon TF. Nerve sparing robotic extravesical ureteral reimplantation. J Urol. 2008;179(5):1987–9; discussion 90.
76. Kasturi S, Sehgal SS, Christman MS, Lambert SM, Casale P. Prospective long-term analysis of nerve-sparing extravesical robotic-assisted laparoscopic ureteral reimplantation. Urology. 2012;79(3):680–3.
77. Neheman A, Kord E, Strine AC, VanderBrink BA, Minevich EA, DeFoor WR, et al. Pediatric partial nephrectomy for upper urinary tract duplication anomalies: a comparison between different surgical approaches and techniques. Urology. 2019;125:196–201.
78. MacDonald C, Small R, Flett M, Cascio S, O'Toole S. Predictors of complications following retroperitoneoscopic total and partial nephrectomy. J Pediatr Surg. 2019;54(2):331–4.
79. Ballouhey Q, Binet A, Clermidi P, Braik K, Villemagne T, Cros J, et al. Partial nephrectomy for small children: robot-assisted versus open surgery. Int J Urol. 2017;24(12):855–60.
80. Esposito C, Escolino M, Miyano G, Caione P, Chiarenza F, Riccipetitoni G, et al. A comparison between laparoscopic and retroperitoneoscopic approach for partial nephrectomy in children with duplex kidney: a multicentric survey. World J Urol. 2016;34(7):939–48.
81. Bansal D, Cost NG, Bean CM, Vanderbrink BA, Schulte M, Noh PH. Infant robot-assisted laparoscopic upper urinary tract reconstructive surgery. J Pediatr Urol. 2014;10(5):869–74.
82. Pedraza R, Weiser A, Franco I. Laparoscopic appendicovesicostomy (Mitrofanoff procedure) in a child using the da Vinci robotic system. J Urol. 2004;171(4):1652–3.
83. Gundeti MS, Eng MK, Reynolds WS, Zagaja GP. Pediatric robotic-assisted laparoscopic augmentation ileocystoplasty and Mitrofanoff appendicovesicostomy: complete intracorporeal--initial case report. Urology. 2008;72(5):1144–7; discussion 7.
84. Nerli RB, Reddy M, Devraju S, Prabha V, Hiremath MB, Jali S. Laparoscopic mitrofanoff appendicovesicostomy: our experience in children. Indian J Urol. 2012;28(1):28–31.
85. Famakinwa OJ, Rosen AM, Gundeti MS. Robot-assisted laparoscopic Mitrofanoff appendicovesicostomy technique and outcomes of extravesical and intravesical approaches. Eur Urol. 2013;64(5):831–6.
86. Wille MA, Zagaja GP, Shalhav AL, Gundeti MS. Continence outcomes in patients undergoing robotic assisted laparoscopic mitrofanoff appendicovesicostomy. J Urol. 2011;185(4):1438–43.
87. Nguyen HT, Passerotti CC, Penna FJ, Retik AB, Peters CA. Robotic assisted laparoscopic Mitrofanoff appendicovesicostomy: preliminary experience in a pediatric population. J Urol. 2009;182(4):1528–34.

88. Leslie B, Lorenzo AJ, Moore K, Farhat WA, Bagli DJ, Pippi Salle JL. Long-term followup and time to event outcome analysis of continent catheterizable channels. J Urol. 2011;185(6):2298–302.
89. Thomas JC, Dietrich MS, Trusler L, DeMarco RT, Pope JC, Brock JW 3rd, et al. Continent catheterizable channels and the timing of their complications. J Urol. 2006;176(4 Pt 2):1816–20; discussion 20.
90. Liard A, Seguier-Lipszyc E, Mathiot A, Mitrofanoff P. The Mitrofanoff procedure: 20 years later. J Urol. 2001;165(6 Pt 2):2394–8.
91. Schlomer BJ, Copp HL. Cumulative incidence of outcomes and urologic procedures after augmentation cystoplasty. J Pediatr Urol. 2014;10(6):1043–50.
92. Fan X, Lin T, Xu K, Yin Z, Huang H, Dong W, et al. Laparoendoscopic single-site nephrectomy compared with conventional laparoscopic nephrectomy: a systematic review and meta-analysis of comparative studies. Eur Urol. 2012;62(4):601–12.
93. Park YH, Kang MY, Jeong MS, Choi H, Kim HH. Laparoendoscopic single-site nephrectomy using a homemade single-port device for single-system ectopic ureter in a child: initial case report. J Endourol. 2009;23(5):833–5.
94. Johnson KC, Cha DY, DaJusta DG, Barone JG, Ankem MK. Pediatric single-port-access nephrectomy for a multicystic, dysplastic kidney. J Pediatr Urol. 2009;5(5):402–4.
95. Lee DG, Baek M, Ju SH, Jeong BC, Han DH. Laparoendoscopic single-site nephrectomy for single-system ectopic ureters with dysplastic kidneys in children: early experience. J Laparoendosc Adv Surg Tech A. 2011;21(5):461–5.
96. Naitoh Y, Kawauchi A, Yamada Y, Fujihara A, Hongo F, Kamoi K, et al. Laparoendoscopic single-site versus conventional laparoscopic pyeloplasty: a matched pair analysis. Int J Urol. 2014;21(8):793–6.
97. Bansal D, Cost NG, Bean CM, Noh PH. Pediatric laparo-endoscopic single site partial nephrectomy: feasibility in infants and small children for upper urinary tract duplication anomalies. J Pediatr Urol. 2014;10(5):859–63.
98. Symeonidis EN, Nasioudis D, Economopoulos KP. Laparoendoscopic single-site surgery (LESS) for major urological procedures in the pediatric population: a systematic review. Int J Surg (London, England). 2016;29:53–61.
99. Rich BS, Creasy J, Afaneh C, Muensterer OJ. The international experience of single-incision pediatric endosurgery: current state of the art. J Laparoendosc Adv Surg Tech A. 2014;24(1):43–9.
100. Fuchs J, Luithle T, Warmann SW, Haber P, Blumenstock G, Szavay P. Laparoscopic surgery on upper urinary tract in children younger than 1 year: technical aspects and functional outcome. J Urol. 2009;182(4):1561–8.
101. Srougi V, Yorioka M, Sanchez DC, Onal B, Houck CS, Nguyen HT. The feasibility of robotic urologic surgery in infants and toddlers. J Pediatr Urol. 2013;9(6 Pt B):1198–203.
102. Mariano ER, Furukawa L, Woo RK, Albanese CT, Brock-Utne JG. Anesthetic concerns for robot-assisted laparoscopy in an infant. Anesth Analg. 2004;99(6):1665–7, table of contents.
103. Varda BK, Johnson EK, Clark C, Chung BI, Nelson CP, Chang SL. National trends of perioperative outcomes and costs for open, laparoscopic and robotic pediatric pyeloplasty. J Urol. 2014;191(4):1090–5.

Chapter 27
New Robotic Systems

Marianne M. Casilla-Lennon, Adam Benjamin Hittelman, and Jose Murillo B. Netto

Robotic technologies have manifested in many ways in medicine, from assisting in EKG pattern recognition and improving detection of pathology, to transportation of medications, supplies and meals. In surgery, robotics has been contributing to advances in minimally invasive surgical techniques. Despite the widespread acceptance of laparoscopy that touted multiple benefits over conventional open surgery, a void was left in techniques that require delicate tissue dissection and complex movements for intricate suturing. Robotic systems have addressed these limitations, expanding the application of minimally invasive techniques to surgical procedures previously unable to capitalize on the benefits of laparoscopy.

The use of robotic technology in surgery dates back to 1985, when the robot Puma 200 was used to perform stereotactic neurosurgical biopsies [1] and subsequently transurethral prostatic resection [2]. This robotic system was termed PROBOT and together with its successor, the ROBODOC system, it became the precursor to the modern robotic systems [3]. It was only in 2000, when the FDA approved the da Vinci Surgical System that the use of robots in surgery began to intensify. With the addition of robotic assistance, the limitations in degrees of motion, exaggerated tremor and lack of depth perception that hindered conventional laparoscopy, were no longer absolute barriers to intricate soft-tissue, intra-abdominal surgery [3]. Magnification, stereoscopic vision and articulating instruments facilitate deep pelvic surgery during prostatectomies, and delicate wrist

M. M. Casilla-Lennon · A. B. Hittelman (✉)
Yale New Haven Hospital, Yale School of Medicine, Department of Urology, New Haven, CT, USA
e-mail: marianne.casilla-lennon@yale.edu; adam.hittelman@yale.edu

J. M. B. Netto
Hospital Universitario da Universidade Federal de Juiz de Fora e Hospital e Maternidade Therezinha de Jesus da Faculdade de Ciências Médicas e da Saúde de Juiz de Fora, Department of Surgery – Urology. Juiz de Fora, MG, Brazil
e-mail: jose.murillo@ufjf.edu.br

© Springer Nature Switzerland AG 2020
P. C. Gargollo (ed.), *Minimally Invasive and Robotic-Assisted Surgery in Pediatric Urology*, https://doi.org/10.1007/978-3-030-57219-8_27

movements allow for water-tight anastomoses during partial nephrectomies, features that are now provided by the robotic assisted laparoscopic system in ways conventional laparoscopy could not provide [4].

The current array of robotic platforms that participate in intra-abdominal surgeries is dominated by the da Vinci system and those that mirror the design. The main limitations of the da Vinci system are the size and cost, and new systems that are in development aim to address these shortcomings to continue to expand the robotic market. Breaking from the da Vinci design is a novel concept found in the MIRA system, which miniaturizes and internalizes the robotic working elements. Additional robotics work has been in developing endoscopic devices for natural orifice minimally invasive techniques. A summary of the principal robotic-assisted laparoscopic surgical platforms featured in this chapter are shown in Table 27.1.

Table 27.1 Current and developing robotic surgical systems for robotic-assisted laparoscopic surgery

Device	Developer	Status	Defining characteristics
da Vinci Xi	Intuitive Surgical (USA)	Commercially available	Articulating instruments, 3D HD visualization, tremor filtration, motion scaling, dual console
da Vinci SP	Intuitive Surgical (USA)	Commercially available	Single port access, flexible articulating instruments for triangulation
Senhance	TransEnterix (USA)	Commercially available	Eye-tracking camera control, haptic feedback, laparoscopic and articulating instrument options, individual robotic carts
Versius	CMR Surgical (UK)	Commercially available outside USA; FDA approval anticipated	Modular design, up to 5 robotic arms, multiuse instruments, laparoscopic and articulating instrument options
BITRACK	Rob Surgical (Spain)	FDA approval anticipated	Multiuse instruments for reduced costs, haptic feedback, laparoscopic and articulating instrument options
Revo-i	Meere Company (South Korea)	Commercially available outside USA	Multiuse instruments for reduced costs, haptic feedback
MiroSurge	German Aerospace Center, DLR (Germany)	Pre-clinical development	Modular, individual bed-mount robotic arms, dual-mode haptic feedback
SPORT	Tital Medical (USA)	FDA approval anticipated	Single port access, flexible articulating arms
Hugo	Medtronic (USA)	Pre-clinical development	N/A, still in early pre-clinical development
MIRA	Virtual Incision Corporation (USA)	FDA approval anticipated	Miniaturized, in vivo robotic components, reduced system size

da Vinci System

The da Vinci system is the market leader in robotic assisted laparoscopy. The fourth generation system, the da Vinci Xi (Fig. 27.1a), provides critical improvements compared to conventional laparoscopy. First, the complexity of the surgical instruments parallels the human hand, achieved with EndoWrist technology, which provides seven additional degrees of freedom, combined with the three degrees of freedom of the arms. Its console system provides high-definition (HD) 3D visualization, tremor filtration, motion scaling, and improved ergonomics. Another feature is the dual console system, which allows for a smooth transition from one surgeon to another, facilitating teaching and collaboration. Compared to the previous da Vinci generations, the da Vinci Xi was upgraded with a slimmer boom, more versatile camera, improved docking interface and increased instrument reach [5].

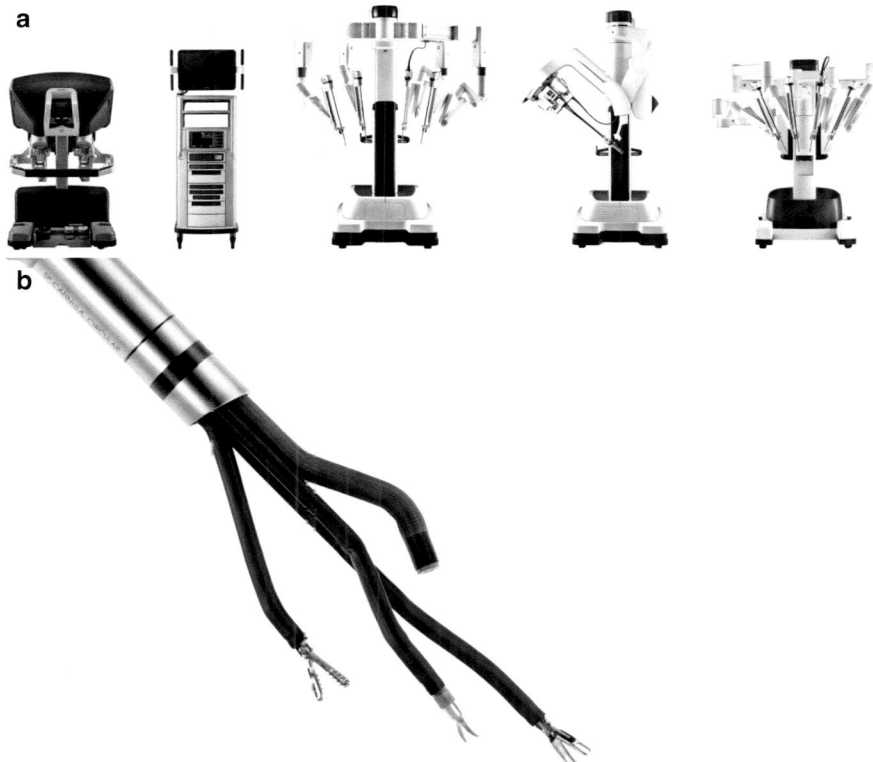

Fig. 27.1 The da Vinci surgical system. (**a**) From left to right, the surgeon console, vision tower, Xi patient cart, SP patient cart and X patient cart. (**b**) da Vinci SP single-port flexible articulating instruments. (© 2020 Intuitive Surgical, Inc. Reproduced with permission. https://www.intuitive.com/en-us/about-us/press/press-resources)

Intuitive Surgical has more recently entered the realm of single site surgery. The company first released a platform compatible with their current systems that used a multichannel port system through a single incision. They subsequently released an entirely separate system, the da Vinci SP, with a single cannula that contains flexible articulating instruments and a fully-wristed endoscope (Fig. 27.1b). Initial experience has shown that it is safe and effective [6–8]. Single incision surgery was introduced in conventional laparoscopy, but failed to achieve widespread popularity because of the added technical challenge of the procedure without sufficient benefits. The improvement in cosmesis was minor with the transition from multiple small incisions to one larger incision, though there were new concerns for port-site hernias [9] as well as the surgery itself being more challenging due to reduced triangulation and a tighter workspace [10].

As opposed to single site surgery in laparoscopy, further size reduction would further benefit the potential of robotic assisted single-port surgery as compared to standard robotic assisted surgery. While this aspect may be irrelevant in conventional laparoscopy, it is one of the reasons that development continues within the robotic realm, with a goal to increase access of robotic systems to a wider healthcare setting.

Senhance Surgical Robotic System

The only FDA-approved competitor of the da Vinci system for intra-abdominal surgeries is the Senhance robotic platform by TransEnterix, which entered the market in 2017, ending Intuitive Surgical's monopoly of the field. Initial experience in gynecological [11] and colorectal surgery [12] has shown it to be a safe and feasible system. Like the da Vinci, it is a large system with a stable platform and individually docking arms. Two critical features that distinguish this system from the da Vinci are haptic feedback and eye-sensing camera control.

One major shortcoming of a robotics systems is the reliance on visual clues during surgery to provide sensory substitution for tactile information. Haptic feedback provides the surgeon with tactile sensation of the force applied during a surgical maneuver to perceive the tissue consistency as well as the stress exerted by the instruments [13, 14]. The Senhance system rectifies the current lack of haptic feedback technology, which has been shown to be associated with poorer performance in ex-vivo models [15]. The haptic feedback of the Senhance is equivalent to that of laparoscopy, providing basic sensory information about the pressure on the instrument shaft to the console, though it is still inferior to natural tactile sensation [14].

The Senhance system also has a novel eye-tracking capability, delivered by an advanced eye-sensing camera that allows the laparoscopic camera to be controlled by the surgeon's eye movements, focusing it to where the surgeon is looking and using forward and backward head motions for magnification [14, 16]. This software simplifies the camera control, which is manually controlled on the da Vinci system and requires an assistant in conventional laparoscopy.

The use of separate carts for the robotic arms allows them to be independent, improving versatility in configuration of the robotic arm placement [17]. By using multi-use laparoscopic instruments, this system addresses the more prohibitive costs associated with the da Vinci system.

Versius Robotic System

The Versius Robotic System (CMR Surgical Ltd.) is a highly anticipated robotic system that has been approved for use within Europe and although its FDA approval is still pending, the first U.S. training program in Florida was launched in preparation for its debut in the United States (Fig. 27.2) [18]. The system has already been deployed in Galaxy Care Hospital, Prune, India, and has been utilized for transthoracic, hysterectomies and myomectomies [19].

The Versius system is a laparoscopic robotic hybrid system that has multiple advantageous features compared to the da Vinci system. Its advantages include a smaller, modular design, individual arm carts providing more versatility, competitive costs due to multiuse instruments, and a design that incorporates the best features of both laparoscopy and robotic arms [20]. For example, the system allows for the use of smaller, 5 mm laparoscopic instruments to provide smaller incisions, but also offers articulating instruments that move with seven degrees of freedom. Additional key features include haptic feedback, 3D HD visualization utilizing 3D glasses and an open console that can be used sitting or standing [16, 20].

BITRACK

The BITRACK system (Rob Surgical, Barcelona, Spain) is a robotic system modeled after the da Vinci system. It is distinct in that it only has three arms on a more versatile cart that allows for different positions around the patient. Similar to the

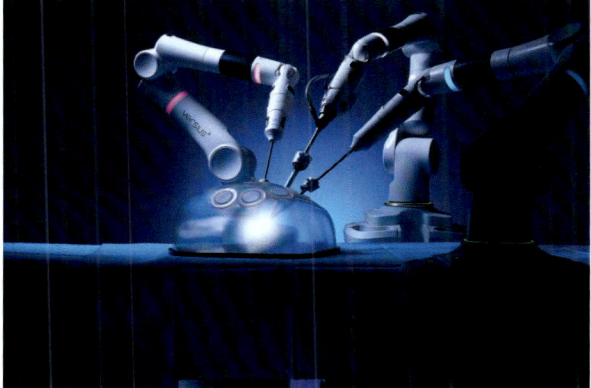

Fig. 27.2 Versius robotic system. (© 2020 CMR Surgical Ltd. Reproduced with permission)

Versius system, it offers both laparoscopic and robotic style instruments, haptic feedback and an HD 3D screen with an open console [21]. Animal models have proven successful and the company has applied for FDA approval, which is projected for next year [22].

Revo-i

The Revo-i robotic system (Meere Company, Seoul, South Korea) has been approved in Korea since 2017 and is modeled after the da Vinci system. It is essentially a replica of the da Vinci system, with additional benefits of haptic feedback and reusable instruments [23, 24].

MiroSurge

The MiroSurge (DLR, German Aerospace Center) system is a robotic system composed of individual robotic arms and a master console, similar to other systems capable of soft tissue, intra-abdominal surgeries (Fig. 27.3). The revolutionary feature of the MiroSurge system is the capability for mounting individual arms on the surgical bed [25]. This feature may be the key to overcoming the size-prohibitive aspect of the current robotic systems by eliminating the large, bulky carts. There is an added benefit of additional flexibility for arm placement and portability comparted to many of the systems [13, 25, 26]. Similar to other systems, the MiroSurge has an open console with 3D display and haptic feedback, which has a dual mode option. This system is still in pre-clinical development.

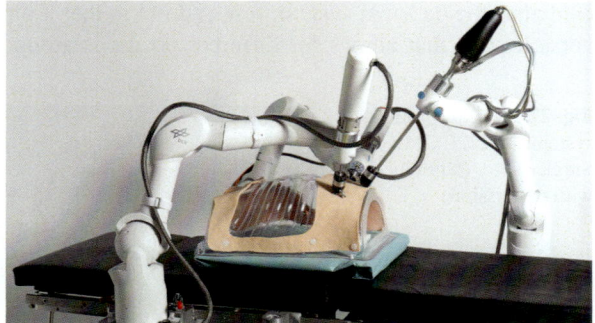

Fig. 27.3 The MiroSurge robotic system with endoscope and lightweight MIRO arms, allowing for direct attachment to the bed rails. (DLR, German Aerospace Center. Credit: DLR (CC-BY 3.0). Reproduced with permission)

Single Port Orifice Robotic Technology (SPORT) Surgical System

The SPORT (Titan Medical Inc.) system is a robotic assisted platform for laparoscopic surgery that gains access to the abdomen through a single incision, as small as 2.5 cm. Its working elements are concentrated into a multi-articulate device composed of a camera and instruments, which has provided a more compact design that facilitates use [4, 13].

As previously described, single-port surgery faces limitations that need to be overcome prior to gaining widespread popularity. SPORT's slim, portable design, however, addresses one of the fundamental difficulties that limits the current repertoire of surgical robots- their large size. It will be pertinent to see if this system, or other novel models, can address the current shortcomings of single-port surgery, such as inadequate triangulation, lack of instrument articulation, poor bedside assistant access, and clashing instruments [9, 27]. The company is preparing for FDA approval.

Hugo

Hugo is an intra-abdominal robotic system being developed by Medtronic, the largest medical device company in the United States, which utilizes a modular system loaded on wheels, allowing flexibility of placement and mobility. The system is interchangeable between their conventional and robotic assisted equipment and designed to be upgradeable, rather than requiring the purchase of an entirely new system when advances are made [28]. The company contends that their system will be more versatile and be available at a lower cost than the da Vinci. Hugo is still in the early stages of development, with information only unveiled at the end of 2019. The company plans to start experimenting with their system and gaining clinical insights outside the United States later this year [28].

Miniature In Vivo Robotic Assistant (MIRA) System

The MIRA system, developed by Virtual Incision Corporation, a company founded by a physician and mechanical engineer based out of the University of Nebraska, represents a novel design made to tackle the shortcomings of the current robotic systems (Fig. 27.4) [13, 29]. This system addresses current constraints in two ways: those related to working through the access port or across the abdominal wall and those related to size. As the name implies, the system has significantly reduced the size of the internal motors and pulleys, allowing the robotic arms to fit completely within the peritoneal cavity [29, 30].

Fig. 27.4 The MIRA robotic system with miniaturized robotic arms for complete in vivo use through a single site. (© 2020 Virtual Incision Corporation. Reproduced with permission)

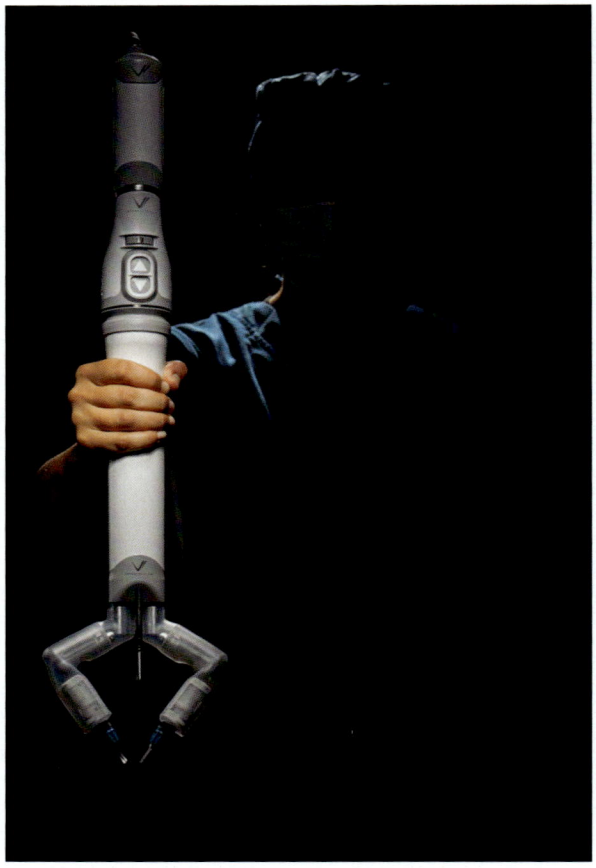

The system is introduced into the peritoneal cavity through a single incision and its two robotic arms are assembled and function within the cavity. The advantage of having the entire platform within the working field are the removal of the kinematic issues of working through a small single incision and the improved access to the peritoneal cavity [30].

Animal and human trials have proven its safety and feasibility and it is currently undergoing FDA clearance [29].

Medical Microinstruments

Medical Microinstruments (MMI, Paduletto, Italy) is not a robotic system itself, but an array of robotic instruments designed for open microsurgery. The instruments have a 3 mm diameter and incorporate wrist articulation and tremor reduction technology as well as use motion scaling to translate large movements into fine movements under the operating microscope [31]. Although the current application is for microsurgery, the implication of this technology could have impact in the field of pediatric surgery in the future.

Other Systems

The SurgiBot (Great Belief International Limited, Shantou, Guangdong, China) is a robotic system similar to the da Vinci SP system, developed for single port laparoscopic surgery with flexible instruments. The goal for this system was to reduce costs, expanding access to underserved populations as well as allowing for closer proximity of the surgeon and patient [13]. It was denied FDA approval, but is preparing to reapply. The platform on which SurgiBot was built, the SPIDER (Single-Port Instrument Delivery Extended Research) system, gained FDA approval in 2009 after studies demonstrated its feasibility as a smaller, less expensive system [13, 32].

The FDA-approved Flex Robotic system (Medrobotics Corporation) is designed for transoral endoscopic procedures, but has recently been expanded for additional indications in thoracic and abdominal procedures. The system uses a flexible endoscope with nearly 180° articulation to navigate through non-linear lumens to arrive at the target surgical site [4].

The MASTER (Master and Slave Transluminal Endoscopic Robotic) robotic system (Nanyang Technological University and National University Health System) was developed for natural orifice transluminal endoscopic surgery. This robotic system promises to facilitate intraluminal dissection of the gastrointestinal (GI) tract through a traditional flexible endoscope and provides a 3D reconstruction of the field, two effector arms, with adequate triangulation and haptic feedback [33, 34]. This system has not yet been approved by the FDA.

STRAS-iCUBE, a platform out of France, very similar to MASTER, which incorporates a robotic surgical system within a flexible endoscope, intended for more complex procedures within the GI tract than are currently feasible [32].

There are numerous additional endoscopic robotic systems in development that could expand their technology to the field of urology. For example, there are two FDA-approved robotic colonoscopes, the Invendoscopy E200 and NeoGuide colonoscope, which provide self-propulsion, 3D visualization and navigation [13, 32].

Multiple vascular devices that can navigate through the peripheral vasculature to the heart have been developed, including the FDA-approved Sensei X and CorPath systems [13, 32]. There are also robotic surgical systems for minimally invasive spine and brain surgery, as well as in orthopedic and ophthalmologic surgery that could represent relevant technology to the field of urology.

Overall, there are many systems that are progressing through the stages of development and there will be many more to come as the expiration of the da Vinci patents opens the field to competition.

What to Expect for the Future?

The field of robotics is exploding as new technologies flourish. Many robotic technologies that were mentioned above remain in the refinement phases, such as single-port surgery, haptic feedback, and un-linking the robotic elements from the external unit. Beyond the scope of these technologies there are new technologies that have potential to shape the longer-term future of surgery.

Single-port surgery is one technology that still requires substantial design improvements in order to gain widespread use. The main limitation of this technology remains the poor triangulation, which creates unnecessary difficulty performing the surgical procedure. Robotic technology has made some progress compared to its implementation in laparoscopy, by reducing tremor and easing ergonomics, but improvements are still vital. Because of the possibility of reducing the size of the surgical systems compared to the current multi-arm robotic design, there remains potential to pursue this technology. One of the design improvements was the transition from rigid to flexible, snake-like instruments. Further development of this technology could ultimately allow the single port systems to break past the triangulation shortcoming. There are multiple platforms that take advantage of flexible, snake-like tools, including the Flex system and the CorPath vascular catheter system, which can navigate peripheral vasculature with a robotic camera [32].

Haptic feedback is another topic undergoing significant study and development. One of the critical shortcomings of the da Vinci system is its lack of tactile feedback. A recent study found that participants performed worse in ex-vivo model with visual sensory substitution compared to one-dimensional haptic feedback (tactile force) and multi-dimensional haptic feedback (addition of vibratory feedback), which further emphasizes the benefits of haptic feedback [15].

Another concept on the horizon, which goes hand in hand with the miniaturization of robots, is the unlinking of the robotic elements from the external control component. This technology currently uses magnets to mount the robot to the interior abdominal wall [35]. Although there are limitations to this approach, such as identifying an adequate power source, the concept could provide even more flexibility.

Beyond the current developing technologies, themes are arising that will likely benefit the field of robotic surgery. First, the natural progression of robotics ultimately leads to the integration of data analytics and machine learning [36]. Some areas of robotics have seen great progression in this area, for example, with increasingly prevalent self-driving cars. Within surgery, this is far in the future, as we are currently still struggling with the master-slave relationship. The benefits of incorporating artificial intelligence and machine learning into surgery will be profound, potentially allowing for knowledge from millions of surgeries to be available at any surgeon's fingertips. Verb Surgical (Verb Surgical Inc., J&J/Alphabet) is a platform designed in collaboration between Johnson & Johnson subsidiary Ethicon and Google parent company Alphabet with a goal to eventually bring these concepts to robotic surgery. The overarching goal of the platform is to "democratize surgery" by increasing surgeon access to information through data-driven machine learning to create an autonomous surgical robot rather than just a surgeon controlled tool [4]. Although the day will likely arrive when this type of complexity is applied to surgical robotics, it remains far in the future at this point.

Another concept that could revolutionize surgery is microbots. One example of the potential application is for autonomous microbots, with the intrinsic ability to perform surgery with microinstruments, to be ingested by mouth and have the knowledge and capacity to perform a surgical procedure within the patient without any external guidance [32]. Currently, microbots remain basic and are used for passive purposes, such as capsule endoscopy [32], however, there is great potential for this technology to grow as robots continue to get smaller and less expensive.

A major motivator for the initial concept of robotic assisted surgery was the concept of telepresence, with the potential to expand surgical assistance overseas in war-injured patients. Despite a handful of successful robotic assisted procedures performed over long distances [37], this concept has not been capitalized on. Medicine has been slow to embrace telehealth implementation in general, and there remain many barriers to widespread implementation of telesurgery. However, this will likely become a reality as robotic technology becomes more integrated into our healthcare system and there is improved access to ultrafast, high bandwidth networks [36].

Overall the future of robotics is limited only to what the human mind can imagine. There are exciting developments on the horizon, as we continue to perfect technologies, and address the shortcomings of our current systems. As we develop new systems, new sets of challenges will arise, and we will continue to progress into uncharted territory.

References

1. Kwoh YS, Hou J, Jonckheere EA, Hayati S. A robot with improved absolute positioning accuracy for CT guided stereotactic brain surgery. IEEE Trans Biomed Eng. 1988;35(2):153–60.
2. Davies BL, Hibberd RD, Ng WS, Timoney AG, Wickham JE. The development of a surgeon robot for prostatectomies. Proc Inst Mech Eng H. 1991;205(1):35–8.
3. Lane T. A short history of robotic surgery. Ann R Coll Surg Engl. 2018;100(6_sup):5–7.
4. Sheth KR, Koh CJ. The future of robotic surgery in pediatric urology: upcoming technology and evolution within the field. Front Pediatr. 2019;7:259.
5. Ngu JC-Y, Tsang C3-S, Koh DC-S. The da Vinci Xi: a review of its capabilities, versatility, and potential role in robotic colorectal surgery. Robot Surg (Auckland). 2017;4:77–85.
6. Dobbs RW, Halgrimson WR, Madueke I, Vigneswaran HT, Wilson JO, Crivellaro S. Single port robot-assisted laparoscopic radical prostatectomy: initial experience and technique with the da Vinci SP platform. BJU Int. 2019;124:1022–7.
7. Kaouk J, Garisto J, Bertolo R. Robotic urologic surgical interventions performed with the single port dedicated platform: first clinical investigation. Eur Urol. 2019;75(4):684–91.
8. Maurice MJ, Ramirez D, Kaouk JH. Robotic laparoendoscopic single-site retroperitoneal renal surgery: initial investigation of a purpose-built single-port surgical system. Eur Urol. 2017;71(4):643–7.

9. Barrera K, Wang D, Sugiyama G. Robotic assisted single site surgery: a decade of innovation. Ann Laparosc Endosc Surg. 2020;5:4.
10. Kaouk JH, Haber G-P, Autorino R, Crouzet S, Ouzzane A, Flamand V, et al. A novel robotic system for single-port urologic surgery: first clinical investigation. Eur Urol. 2014;66(6):1033–43.
11. Fanfani F, Restaino S, Rossitto C, Gueli Alletti S, Costantini B, Monterossi G, et al. Total laparoscopic (S-LPS) versus TELELAP ALF-X robotic-assisted hysterectomy: a case-control study. J Minim Invasive Gynecol. 2016;23(6):933–8.
12. Spinelli A, David G, Gidaro S, Carvello M, Sacchi M, Montorsi M, et al. First experience in colorectal surgery with a new robotic platform with haptic feedback. Color Dis. 2017;20:228–35.
13. Peters BS, Armijo PR, Krause C, Choudhury SA, Oleynikov D. Review of emerging surgical robotic technology. Surg Endosc. 2018;32(4):1636–55.
14. Rassweiler JJ, Autorino R, Klein J, Mottrie A, Goezen AS, Stolzenburg JU, et al. Future of robotic surgery in urology. BJU Int. 2017;120(6):822–41.
15. Abiri A, Juo YY, Tao A, Askari SJ, Pensa J, Bisley JW, et al. Artificial palpation in robotic surgery using haptic feedback. Surg Endosc. 2019;33(4):1252–9.
16. Brodie A, Vasdev N. The future of robotic surgery. Ann R Coll Surg Engl. 2018;100(Suppl 7):4–13.
17. Gueli Alletti S, Rossitto C, Cianci S, Perrone E, Pizzacalla S, Monterossi G, et al. The Senhance surgical robotic system ("Senhance") for total hysterectomy in obese patients: a pilot study. J Robot Surg. 2018;12(2):229–34.
18. Medgadget Editors. Versius robotic surgical system coming to U.S. Medgadget [Internet]. 2020 Apr 24. Available from: https://www.medgadget.com/2018/12/versius-robotic-surgical-system-coming-to-u-s-via-nicholson-center-training-program.html.
19. RBR Staff. India hospital deploys CMR surgical versius robot [cited 2020 Apr 26]. Available from: https://www.roboticsbusinessreview.com/health-medical/india-hospital-deploys-cmr-surgical-versius-robot/.
20. Hares L, Roberts P, Marshall K, Slack M. Using end-user feedback to optimize the design of the Versius surgical system, a new robot-assisted device for use in minimal access surgery. BMJ Surg Interv Health Technol. 2019;1(1):e000019.
21. SURGROB. Bitrack from ROB surgical. 2019.
22. Rob Surgical. University research excellence for the patient 2020 [cited 2020 Apr 24]. Available from: https://www.robsurgical.com/story/.
23. Kang CM, Chong JU, Lim JH, Park DW, Park SJ, Gim S, et al. Robotic cholecystectomy using the newly developed Korean robotic surgical system, Revo-i: a preclinical experiment in a porcine model. Yonsei Med J. 2017;58(5):1075–7.
24. Chang KD, Abdel Raheem A, Alomair TA, Ahn HK, Rha KH. MP16-08 Revo-I; surgical robotic system: results of Korean FDA (KFDA) approved clinical trial. J Urol. 2018;199(4S):e200.
25. Hagn U, Konietschke R, Tobergte A, Nickl M, Jorg S, Kubler B, et al. DLR MiroSurge: a versatile system for research in endoscopic telesurgery. Int J Comput Assist Radiol Surg. 2010;5(2):183–93.
26. Beasley RA. Medical robots: current systems and research directions. J Robot. 2012;2012:14.
27. Seeliger B. Enabling single-site laparoscopy: the SPORT platform. Surg Endosc. 2019;33(11):3696–703.
28. Newmarker C. Medtronic finally unveils its new robot-assisted surgery system [cited 2020 Apr 24]. Available from: https://www.massdevice.com/medtronic-finally-unveils-its-new-robot-assisted-surgery-system/.
29. RBR Staff. Virtual Incision raises $20M for MIRA mini surgical robots [cited 2020 Apr 24]. Available from: https://www.roboticsbusinessreview.com/financial/virtual-incision-20m-mira-mini-surgical-robots/.
30. Wortman T. Design, analysis, and testing of in vivo surgical robots. Lincoln: University of Nebraska; 2011.

31. Medical Microinstruments (MMI). S.P.A. MMI's robotic platform for microsurgery [cited 2020 Apr 24]. Available from: http://www.mmimicro.com/solutions.
32. Khandalavala K, Shimon T, Flores L, Armijo PR, Oleynikov D. Emerging surgical robotic technology: a progression toward microbots. Ann Laparosc Endosc Surg. 2019;5:3.
33. Yeung BP, Gourlay T. A technical review of flexible endoscopic multitasking platforms. Int J Surg. 2012;10(7):345–54.
34. Lomanto D, Wijerathne S, Ho LK, Phee LS. Flexible endoscopic robot. Minim Invasive Ther Allied Technol. 2015;24(1):37–44.
35. Leong F, Garbin N, Natali CD, Mohammadi A, Thiruchelvam D, Oetomo D, et al. Magnetic surgical instruments for robotic abdominal surgery. IEEE Rev Biomed Eng. 2016;9:66–78.
36. Bary E. These companies are spending billions so robots can perform surgery without a doctor in the room. MarketWatch, 2020 [cited 2020 Apr 26]. Available from: https://www.marketwatch.com/story/these-companies-are-investing-billions-so-robots-can-perform-surgery-without-a-doctor-in-the-room-2020-02-19.
37. Marescaux J, Leroy J, Rubino F, Smith M, Vix M, Simone M, et al. Transcontinental robot-assisted remote telesurgery: feasibility and potential applications. Ann Surg. 2002;235(4):487–92.

Chapter 28
Education and Simulation in Minimally Invasive Surgery

Claudia Berrondo, Katie L. Canalichio, and Thomas S. Lendvay

Introduction

Advancements in technology to objectively assess skill and more rigorous education efforts to ensure skills competency and proficiency in trainees have led to a dramatic change away from the paradigm of 'see one, do one, teach one'. In an effort to improve the work and educational environments for trainees and promote patient-centered care, implementation of work-hour restrictions and the expectation of direct resident oversight in the operating room have been a forcing function to provide standard pre-clinical technical and cognitive skills training through simulation [1–3]. Surgical training programs are adapting to the change of education curricula and balancing both patient-centered care with learner-centered training is a work in progress. Given this goal, it is of utmost importance that programs have the tools necessary to implement a safe, efficient curriculum with an objective measure of trainees' technical skills [1, 4]. The Halsteadian apprenticeship education model has endured for over a century, yet this model has limitations, especially since it limits the ability of standardization of training experience. A 'train by opportunity' model is not inclusive and ensures that some trainees have different experiences than others. Urological training is currently assessed by a combination of the direct preceptor model, case logs, and the written and oral boards. With the introduction over the last two decades of minimally invasive surgery in the urological field, how to safely achieve these goals remains to be settled. Minimally invasive surgery lends itself well to defining metrics of skill through video capture and instrument/user movement tracking. These opportunities have enabled education experts to generalize and standardize training across large groups of learners. Because urology involves several technically challenging procedures, we must leverage these

C. Berrondo · K. L. Canalichio · T. S. Lendvay (✉)
Seattle Children's Hospital, Department of Pediatric Urology, Seattle, WA, USA
e-mail: katie.canalichio@seattlechildrens.org; thomas.lendvay@seattlechildrens.org

education technologies to advance trainees through a proficiency and competency model [1, 4]. Novel methods for objective skills assessment and skills transfer promise to place urology at the forefront of education among all surgical disciplines. Our aim in this chapter is to describe the current trends in education and simulation specifically in minimally invasive surgery within urology.

Needs Assessment: Why Simulation?

Upwards of 400,000 deaths annually are due to errors in medicine making medical errors the third leading cause of death in the United States behind cardiovascular disease and cancer and ahead of pulmonary disease and trauma [5, 6]. The U.S. has much higher reported errors compared to other developed countries, and unfortunately this is actually believed to be vastly underreported. Not every state in the U.S. requires reporting of medical errors, and due to this very low percentage of reported errors, interventions are unreliably initiated [7].

Furthermore, the technique of a surgeon has been directly related to patient outcomes [3, 8]. Surgical errors are common, but the majority are preventable with many attributable to surgical technique and communication failures [3]. The cost of a single surgical error is estimated to increase costs of a patient's care up to approximately $30,000 [3].

In addition to patient safety, another aspect to consider is the unseen costs of resident surgical training. By 2030 it is estimated that the cost to train enough surgeons to support the expected US population will be $37 billion dollars [9]. Some of the costs include increased operative time allotted to resident training, which have been estimated to incur sometimes more than $100,000 of cost per trainee. That is why shifting part of the education model into a simulated environment, decreasing the time to reach competency, and potentially decreasing the cost of training, is desirable. The Accreditation Council for Graduate Medical Education (ACGME) officially authorized simulation into the curriculum of surgical residency programs in 2008 [3]. Simulation affords educators with means of assessing and tracking skill adoption and transfer. The end goal is to decrease learning curves to enhance patient care.

Learning Curves in Minimally Invasive Surgery

A learning curve is a "theoretical concept that draws a surgeon's performance against time" and has been described as the plateau of some defined marker that is felt to demarcate competence in a procedure [10]. The concept was first described in laparoscopic cholecystectomy and has also been extensively studied in urological oncology [10]. As described in another eloquent way, "on the way to achieving mastery the (learning) curve represents the initial challenges in competence, and the change in technical proficiency and efficiency with increasing experience" [11]. Time in training does not necessarily reflect competency, and for difficult and invasive procedures it is important to understand when a surgeon in training has reached this important marker [12].

Endourology Learning Curves

Percutaneous nephrolithotomy (PCNL) is the operation of choice for challenging and/or large renal staghorns or calculi, and is therefore an important tool in the urologist's armory [10]. PCNL is a technically challenging procedure and a survey of urologists showed that only 11% obtained percutaneous access instead of relying on a radiologist [10, 13], suggesting that the training experience for percutaneous access is not adequate. Obtaining access is the most difficult and a critical step of the procedure. Watterson et al. showed fewer complications and better stone clearance rates were observed when the urologist performed this crucial step versus the radiologist [10, 13]

Allen et al. looked at three defined variables – operating time, fluoroscopic screening time and radiation dose – that were felt to reflect a surgeon's level of expertise [12]. Based on the time for a beginner surgeon to reach a plateau on these parameters, it was felt "competence" was reached after 60 cases and "excellence" after 115 cases. There was a plateau in operating time at 60 cases and another plateau observed in the fluoroscopic measures at 115 cases. The comparisons were drawn from a senior surgeon who had performed more than 1600 cases. This was done at a large tertiary referral center where both the novice and senior surgeons obtained their own access and performed the procedure in a similar fashion. The novice surgeon, although not familiar with PCNL, was otherwise already proficient in other endourological techniques and was observed for a defined period of time by the senior surgeon. This limits the applicability of predicted time to competence to a truly novice surgeon not experienced in any endourology and who is not in a similar supportive environment. Importantly, there were no major complications and the stone free rates were similar for both surgeons [12].

Ziaee et al. also looked to define the learning curve in PCNL [10]. A single surgeon was prospectively observed for his first 105 solo PCNL cases at a large tertiary referral center. Operation time plateaued at 45 cases. Only minor complications were observed, and these complications were all within the first 45 cases. Competence was therefore achieved at 45 cases. However, stone clearance continued to improve up to the final case, so excellence was felt to be achieved after 105 cases. Of note, the subject was an endourology fellow already adept at other endourological procedures. Applicability of this study to truly novice surgeons or residents remains to be seen [10].

Guiu-Souto et al. looked to break down fluoroscopic measures and apply this to the learning curve. Due to a deficit in radiological exposure training in the urologist, both urologist and patient are at risk for significant fluoroscopic exposure during the learning curve. Based on plateau achieved in procedure time and exposure time, competence was measured at 50 cases and excellence at 105 cases [14].

Song et al. assessed the learning curve in total ultrasound guided PCNL and found that the number of cases to achieve competency was similar to those of previous reported studies. They retrospectively reviewed the outcomes of a novice surgeon to that of a senior surgeon, who had more than 1000 cases under his belt. The study was done at a high-volume, tertiary referral center in China for complex stone disease where ultrasound guidance was performed for the entire procedure. Competency was felt to be obtained after 60 cases with no difference in stone free rates and complications. It is important to note that a surgeon can still safely and effectively perform the operation while still learning [15].

Laparoscopic Surgery Learning Curves

Ku et al. defined the learning curve in laparoscopic nephrectomy in children as 10 cases. Prior to this, laparoscopic nephrectomy had previously been shown to be a safe alternative to open surgery in children [16]. Ku et al. felt that the learning curve was defined by not only operating room time and case number, but also by the 'frequency' with which a surgeon performs a procedure. The experience of a single surgeon was retrospectively described over a 5-year time period in which he performed 20 consecutive cases. The first 10 cases were compared to the outcomes of the second 10 cases. In children aged 1–15 years, there was no statistical difference among the 2 groups in patient characteristics. The initial approach was transperitoneal, but with additional experience the retroperitoneal approach was employed. The time in the operating room statistically decreased – 181–125 min – and there was a significant decrease in median hospital stay – 5.4–2.5 days – between the two groups. Otherwise no major complications were seen and both had routine postoperative courses. The surgeon was already an expert in open surgery but had not specifically performed laparoscopy in children. It was unclear if the surgeon had performed laparoscopy in adults prior to this study. This should be taken into account when determining the true learning curve of a novice [16].

Robotic Surgery Learning Curves

Robot-assisted surgery has gained traction since the 1980's with its first use in neurosurgery, and since then has had increased utility in adult and pediatric surgery [17]. Unique features in robot-assisted laparoscopy, including 3-dimensional, enhanced (10X) vision and greater degree of rotational movement, lend towards an easier learning curve [17]. From prior studies that looked to define the learning curve in adult surgery, robot-assisted laparoscopic prostatectomy has a learning curve of 50 cases to achieve competency – with 150–200 cases needed to achieve more nuanced mastery over oncological margins [11]. In surgeons already adept at robotics, the learning curve for robot-assisted laparoscopic cystectomy was defined as 20 cases [11]. And for robot-assisted laparoscopic partial nephrectomy, competency was seen in 15–30 cases [11]. Abboudi et al. performed a systematic review of studies defining the learning curve in adult urological surgery [18].

A study in the Journal American College Surgeons assessed the anastomosis of a dismembered pyeloplasty using open, laparoscopic and robot-assisted surgery in a swine animal model [17]. The robotic arm had shorter anastomotic times and demonstrated an easier learning curve compared to the laparoscopic arm. Both the robotic and laparoscopic groups' procedural times improved with familiarity and approached those of the open arm. The adequacy of the repair was determined through a unique intraoperative design assessing pressure and volumetric measures to indicate patency. With experience, these parameters also approached those of the open arm. Histology taken from the robotic arm actually indicated a better profile (less collagen III deposition) than the open and laparoscopic arms [17].

Sorensen et al. completed a retrospective review of the first 33 consecutive children undergoing robot-assisted laparoscopic pyeloplasty when robot-assisted surgery was first introduced in 2006 at their institution [11]. The outcomes of two pediatric urologists performing these were compared to open controls. Both robotic and open groups had success of 97% at a mean of 1-year follow-up. The total operative time was used as a maker for defining a learning curve of 15–20 cases. The time for the pyeloplasty was examined separately from set-up time associated with positioning and other 'peripheral' time. The improvement in operative time seen in the robotic arm was mostly due to a decrease in the actual pyeloplasty versus this ancillary time. Early on there were 3 robotic failures that required conversion to laparoscopy for part or all of the remaining operation, but no conversion to open was necessary. There were no statistical differences in the postoperative complications between the two groups. However, there were more 'technical complications' that took place in the early learning period of the robotic arm. The authors highlighted that achieving excellency most likely takes more cases, but that a novice can safely and efficiently perform the procedure with this initial small learning curve. Other points of interest in establishing a robotic program at an institution, including training of the support staff and the authors describe what they believe to be a "synergistic effect, in that experienced robotic surgery staff may accelerate a novice surgeon…and vice versa." [11] Some advocate separating institution of a new technique, as seen in this study, from the learning curve of an already established procedure [18].

Tasian et al. performed a prospective cohort study at an academic institution comparing outcomes of pediatric urology fellows versus the attending surgeon [19]. The fellow cases were defined as the fellow performing >75% of the console time versus 100% of the console time being done be the attending. There were no failures as defined by postoperative imaging, and there were no intraoperative complications for either group. Median operative time was 58 min for the attending. The mean rate of fellow operative time decline was recorded and used to project a learning curve of 37 cases. Whether or not this is achievable during a 2-year fellowship depends on the program's "case volume and supervision" level. And it is not clear how this translates to post-training when a surgeon is operating independently. Other considerations include attendings performing the more difficult cases, defining the cost of obtaining proficiency in a robotic procedure, progressive involvement of the fellow in more difficult portions of the case (progression from renal dissection, to anterior anastomosis, to posterior anastomosis) [19].

Team Approach

Sim et al. assessed a unique team approach during introduction of robot-assisted laparoscopic prostatectomy at their institution [20]. A team of three urologists, progressing from bedside assistant to console surgeon, performed a total of 100 cases for organ confined prostatic adenocarcinoma. The first console surgeon had the most experience, however limited, and the other two acted as bedside assistants (one with more active involvement) [20].

Intra-Operative Assessment of Skills

Expert-Based Evaluation: Objective Structured Assessment of Technical Skills

The traditional model for evaluation of surgical skills has been through direct observation of the trainee at an individual level. This has obvious limitations, one of which is the subjective nature of the assessment and another is the irreproducibility [21]. Animal models have also been employed to measure surgical skill, which carries its own ethical implications. The development of bench models has been used as a more accessible and affordable avenue for the same purpose [21]. Bench models can represent inanimate simulations of tasks experienced in the operating room. The Objective Structured Assessment of Technical Skill (OSATS) was developed as an extension to a previous model designed to objectively assess clinical competency. Martin et al. showed the promise of this test by showing its feasibility in a group of general surgery residents at the University of Toronto. The authors were able to show that use of live and bench models were comparable. They used a three-prong scoring system: a procedure-specific checklist, a previously validated global rating scale, and a single pass or fail decree [21].

Kishore et al. took this format and applied it to endourology. A 14-point curriculum was developed to assess resident skills with cystoscopy and ureteroscopy [22]. This ranged from selection and assembly of instruments, troubleshooting common problems, to patient positioning. This model combined previous work that looked at these tasks individually [22–24]. The construct validity – whether a test measures what it purports to be measuring – was evaluated in this undertaking. In order to do this, it was necessary to show that the outcome was associated with experience or training level of the resident [22]. The authors believed that acquisition of the fundamental elements of the procedure was key to understanding the technique along with the manual skill required to complete that task. They also highlighted the importance of being accessible to the trainee – simply by occurring in a scheduled fashion separate from clinical duties at the start of the day. This initial phase of the study of this tool was done at a single institution. Resident feedback was utilized in the development of the final tool that took all of this into account [22].

Argun et al. went on to show the construct and internal validity of this tool in a multi-institutional setting [1]. Thirty urology residents at three institutions were enrolled in this study. Employing the same tool Kishore and colleagues used, cognitive and psychomotor skills were assessed. Anatomical models of the renal collecting system, reconstructed from CT scans, were used for the latter aspect of the test. Using this unique model, the trainee was asked to navigate, stone basket, perform laser lithotripsy and assemble equipment. A checklist was used to confirm each proposed step was performed, followed by a debriefing by the faculty examiner, and then resident feedback. Once again construct validity was similarly assessed. Internal validity was felt to be intact due to the correlation between the more subjective global assessment score and the total score for the psychomotor checklist [1].

Institutions are now employing these surgical assessment tools within their residency programs as a means to assess resident progress and provide feedback to the trainee [1]. The next step would be the ability to utilize this in competency assessments for trainee promotion. In order for a construct to be used in this fashion, it would need to be rigorously tested and validated at multiple institutions [1, 4].

Crowdsourced Assessment of Technical Skills

Novel models to use assessment tools in a more blinded and anonymous way have been developed to add objectivity to the process. Ghani et al. used a model created in Michigan to recruit urologists in the state to assess the video recorded performances of peers through blinded review as a means to coach one another – The Michigan Urologic Surgery Improvement Collaborative (MUSIC) [25]. This model has the advantage of providing a safe review forum free from politics of competing urology practices in part due to the common mission to improve the care of prostate cancer patients throughout the state. The group has even linked assessments to patient outcomes. These collaboratives are powerful assessment models, and require a significant amount of buy-in from the providers. The state of Michigan is also covered by one primary payer – Blue Cross and Blue Shield – which funds this endeavor and hires data abstractors to cull patient care outcomes data from each hospital. In many healthcare environments, this model is difficult to reproduce. Using the same assessment tools, Lendvay et al. has leveraged large groups of anonymous reviewers in a way that is scalable [26].

After validation in dry-lab settings, animate labs, and human surgery, Crowd-Sourced Assessment of Technical Skills (CSATS) has been shown to predict patient outcomes and correlates to expert reviews of providers' performances [27]. The technology leverages anonymous crowdworkers from an online platform that encompasses over a million reviewers. The reviewers need not be in the medical field, however, the large group of reviewers – 30–50 – who review each video provide an accurate assessment of the technique of a surgeon through video review. These numeric objective scores have been shown to correlate with the patient outcomes of the surgeons reviewed. The process takes only a few minutes to hours to review hundreds of surgical videos. The intention of this technology is to make an objective de-identified review process scalable and rapid so that the feedback provided can yield positive change before the next surgery is performed [27].

These methods to aggregate large numbers of either expert surgeons or crowdworkers all center on a theme of objectifying a process that for over a hundred years has been performed by one or two individuals always invested in the advancement or credentialing of the performer. It is imperative that our profession ensure public safety through iterative and reliable assessment methods.

Simulation Training in Surgery

Surgeon case volume is one of the most important factors in improving surgical outcomes and reducing surgical complications and improving morbidity and mortality. However, in our current environment of training, the question arises on whether or not it is ethical to train and practice in real life scenarios with live patients. Furthermore, the current residency paradigm is a 'train-by-opportunity' which means that if a certain disease is encountered within the rotation or residency experience, then the resident is fortunate to have seen the disease. But if the disease is not studied or seen in a patient, then the resident never sees that disease. Surgical simulation allows for development of technical and non-technical skills in surgery without risking patient safety and allows for every trainee to have similar experiences. These learner-centered education paradigms are increasingly incorporated into surgical training curricula, and surgeon credentialing mandates [28]. With the current technologies available, simulation training is become an important and emphasized part of surgical training. Additionally, simulation can be used at any stage of training, and even for maintenance of skills in surgeons who have completed their surgical training. A wide range of training platforms and curriculums have been utilized in surgical training with a focus on different aspects of surgical training. Surgical simulation by a variety of methods has been shown to improve surgeon performance in the operating room, suggesting that surgical simulation training contributes to acquiring and transfer of skills necessary to achieve surgical proficiency [18, 29].

Task-Based Simulation

Task-based simulation has traditionally been the most common platform that exists in surgical simulation. Task-based simulation is the simplest form of simulation in any platform for both reality-based and virtual reality simulation. Steigerwald et al. demonstrated that the surgical residents of all levels using either a reality-based laparoscopic trainer or a virtual reality laparoscopic trainer improved their scores in both the simulation setting and in the live operating room setting, but there was no significant difference in the performance of the residents using one system compared to the other [30]. Regardless of the type of simulation trainer, simulation correlates with improved operative performance in both the simulation and live operative setting in laparoscopy. Currently, there is no evidence that one method is superior to the other. The tasks themselves are not specific to operations, but rather tasks completed with inanimate objects focused on utilizing different surgical instruments and developing surgical skills. Some of the basic skills includes hand-eye and left-to-right-hand coordination, grasping, transferring, cutting, and suturing. These skills are acquired with a variety of common tasks including peg transfer, pattern cutting, ligating loop, clip application, needle driving, suturing, and knot tying [30].

Task Based Simulation: Reality-Based Simulation

In laparoscopic surgery, physical box or video trainers have been composed the majority of simulation surgery. One of the main advantages of this kind of training device, is that they utilize the actual laparoscopic instruments used in surgical procedures. This allows the trainee or user to familiarize themselves with the surgical instruments, and practice a variety of tasks using these instruments (Figs. 28.1 and 28.2). Simulation with these types of trainers have been established as an effective method of laparoscopic skills acquisition [30].

Several studies have been published evaluating the utility of laparoscopic surgical training platforms. A systematic review by Dawe et al. summarized the transferability of skills acquired from surgical simulation-based training to the live patient setting. This review included a total of 27 studies: 14 studies on laparoscopic simulation, 13 studies on endoscopic simulation and 7 studies on other procedures. The vast majority of studies reviewed demonstrated improved performance in the participants with simulation training compared to their peers without simulation training [28].

Task Based Simulation: Virtual Reality Simulation

In more recent years, virtual reality (VR) systems have become more widely available and have been integrated into some simulation curriculums. The virtual reality simulators utilize computer-generated environments to perform simulation tasks

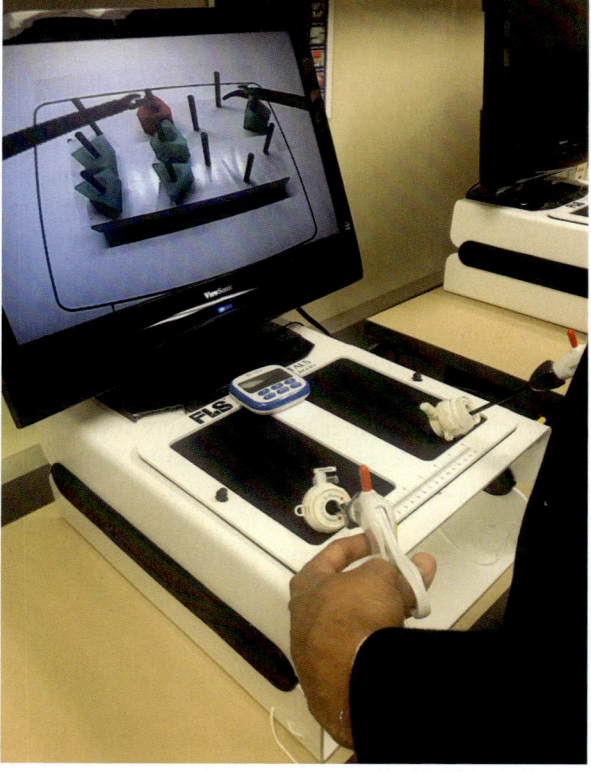

Fig. 28.1 Reality-based laparoscopic simulation. In this image, the operator is performing a task-based simulation commonly known as "peg transfer" using laparoscopic instruments to transfer objects from pegs on one side to pegs on the other side

(Figs. 28.3 and 28.4). Similar to the reality-based simulators, virtual reality simulation allows the trainee to perform specific tasks. A major advantage to VR simulation is that objective performance metrics beyond task time can be captured and used as feedback to the learner. Common metrics include path length, economy of motion, grasp forces, Cartesian coordinate data, velocities, object drops, etc. These metrics correlate with expertise [31]. One of the potential disadvantages of virtual reality simulators in laparoscopic surgery is the lack of haptic feedback to the user which is dissimilar to real surgery except in robotics where no haptic feedback exists.

Procedure-Based Simulation

Procedure-based simulation allows trainees to apply the fundamental skills in surgery that they have developed to perform more complex procedural tasks in the form of surgical procedures or steps of surgical procedures. Procedure-based models can include portions or specific steps of surgical procedures, or complete surgical procedures. One of the major challenges in procedure-based simulation is their

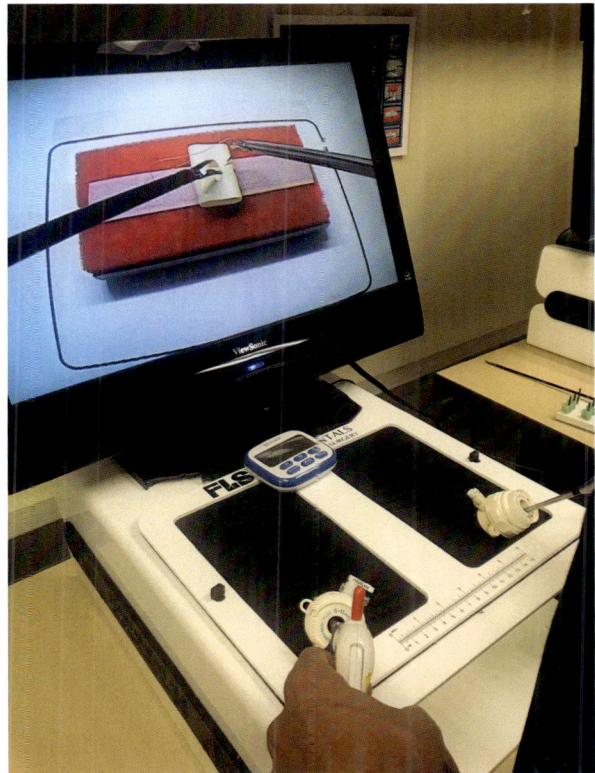

Fig. 28.2 Reality-based laparoscopic simulation. In this image, the operator is performing a task-based simulation for simple suturing and knot tying using laparoscopic instruments

ability to realistically represent the operative environment [32]. Santangelo et al. developed a carotid endarterectomy whole-task simulator which demonstrated high face-validity among experts and trainees [33]. Similarly, Ghazi et al. developed and tested a simulation model for PCNL [34]. The model included simulation of all steps of the procedure and was tested in experts and trainees. They were able to demonstrate excellent face and content validity of the model [34]. And most recently, Weiss et al. demonstrated excellent face and construct validity among experts and trainees in their cervical laminectomy simulator [35]. Future research will help delineate the role and utility of these and other procedure-based simulators in the training and assessment of surgical skills.

Procedure-Based Simulation: Reality Based Simulation

Procedure based simulation allows surgical trainees a safe and risk-free environment to practice specific portions of procedure or entire procedures. Millan et al. created a model laparoscopic ureteral reimplantation and found that use of the simulator increased technical performance in surgeons [36].

Fig. 28.3 A virtual reality simulator demonstrating a computer-generated image of a gallstone within a gallbladder. This simulator can be used for task-based and procedure-based simulation. In this this image, the operator can practice using laparoscopic instruments to touch and move the gallstone within the gall-bladder

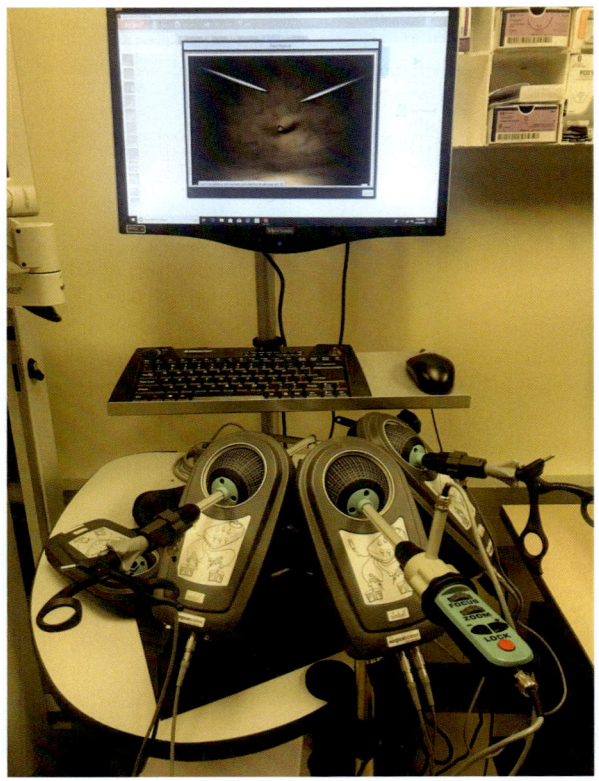

Procedure-Based Simulation: Virtual Reality Simulation

Virtual reality simulation training has been incorporated into some training curricula. Sethi et al. demonstrated face validity of a virtual reality simulator in 20 participants. Skilled surgeons, fellows and medical students performed several tasks using a robotic simulator. All participants found the simulator easy to use and realistic [37]. One study by Chowriappa et al. evaluated the use of virtual reality training in urology trainees. In this study, trainees were randomized to either a control group with typical training or the intervention group in which trainees were given procedure-based virtual reality training in a specific step of a robotic surgical procedure. They found that the virtual reality simulation group had overall higher scores and better performance compared to the control group. In addition, the majority of participants found that the simulation platform was similar to the real surgical procedure [32].

Whitehurst et al. conducted a randomized study to evaluate the use of virtual reality simulation compared to dry lab simulation in robot naive surgeons and trainees. In this study, participants were randomized to robotic training using either dry lab task completion using a surgical robot or virtual reality surgical simulation using

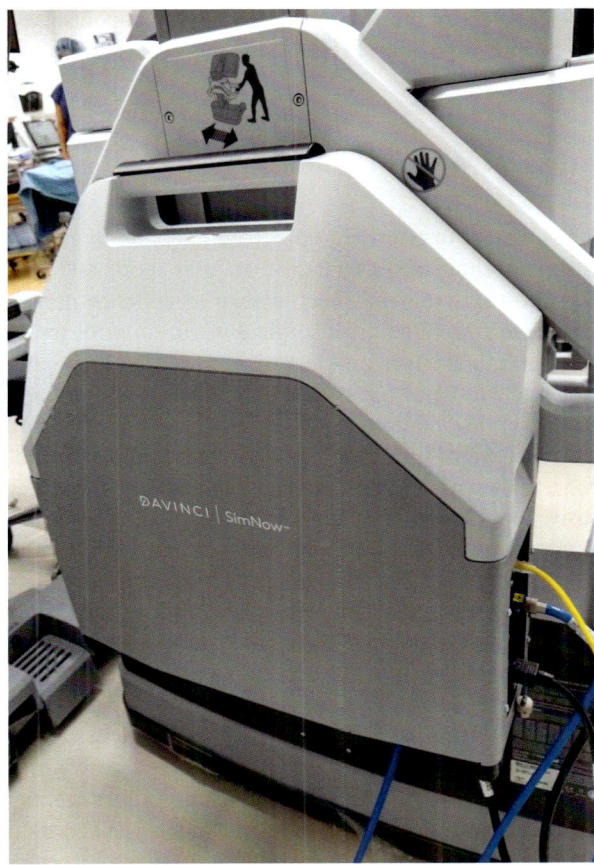

Fig. 28.4 A virtual-reality simulator designed for robot-assisted laparoscopic surgery simulation. This simulation system can be used for task-based and procedure-based simulation in robotic surgery

robotic surgery simulator. Performance was then assessed with procedure completion in a live animal model completed using the surgical robot. They found no difference in surgeon performance between the two groups and concluded that virtual reality simulation can be used for training in robotic surgery [38].

3D Simulation Models

3-dimensional model-based simulation training has recently emerged as another tool for surgical training. Ghazi et al. developed an anatomically correct 3-dimensional model for simulation of percutaneous nephrolithotomy. The model was tested in urology and interventional radiology trainees and experts and was found to have good validity [34]. Cheung et al. developed a 3-dimensional model of a kidney to be used as a model for laparoscopic pyeloplasty surgery. The model was tested using pediatric urology fellows and faculty members demonstrating usability

[39]. The use of these and other similar 3D models may allow for high-validity full-procedure simulation to be used in surgical training.

Surgical Warm-Up and Rehearsal

The concept of warming-up before is common and widely utilized across several disciplines outside of medicine, such as sports and performing arts. Warm-up prior to sports activities has been shown to enhance performance, reduces fatigue and reduce errors. In contrast surgical warm-up prior to operating remains a subject of debate among surgeons. The main concern among surgeons in the belief that this practice will delay or prolong surgical procedures and has not been widely adopted in the surgical community. Surgical warm-up can include both mental warm-up and physical warm-up. A variety of studies evaluating the utility of surgical warm-up have demonstrated improvements in intra-operative performance in technical, cognitive and psychomotor performance [40–42]. Lendvay et al. demonstrated that in a randomized controlled trial, expert surgeons performing robotic surgery tasks benefited from a brief VR warm-up session prior to doing ring transfer and intracorporeal suturing [43]. This has led to an on-going trial of expert surgeons in the operating room doing clinical cases and seeing if brief VR suturing tasks can prime the surgeons to perform better in the first 15–20 min of their robotic surgery.

Da Cruz et al. performed a study evaluating the performance of medical students utilizing warm-up prior to laparoscopic cholecystectomy in a porcine model compared to medical students completing the surgery without warm-up. The group participating in warm-up had significantly superior results compared to the group without warm-up. In this group of inexperienced medical students, pre-operative warm-up was effective in improving surgical performance [41].

Polterauer et al. performed a randomized controlled trial comparing the use of pre-operative warm-up training with a virtual reality simulator before laparoscopic salpingo-oophorectomy with no warm-up in experienced surgeons and residents. In this study, there was no statistically significant difference in the performance of surgeons in the warm-up group compared to the no warm-up group [44].

Pike et al. performed a systematic review of studies evaluating the effect of pre-operative simulation on surgical performance. The review included 13 studies: 5 randomized controlled trials, 4 randomized cross-over trials and 4 case series. Four studies were on real patients, and the remainder were on simulated outcome measures. All but one of the studies found that warm-up improves operative outcomes, although the specific measures of outcome varied among studies [42].

A systematic review by Abdalla et al. revealed that warming-up before an operative procedure improved trainee performance. This review included six randomized studies comparing the performance of trainees with and without warm-up on laparoscopic surgical performance. Improvement in intraoperative laparoscopic performance was observed with surgical warm-up pre-operatively in 5 of 6 studies [40].

In addition to physical warm-up, mental practice has also been demonstrated to be an important part of performance preparation. A randomized controlled study be Arora et al. evaluated the effect of mental practice on surgical performance of virtual reality laparoscopic cholecystectomy in novice surgeons. In this study of 18 participants, the group utilizing mental practice performed better compared to the group not using mental practice [45].

Similar to other fields, the use of pre-operative warm-up (both mental and physical) appears to be helpful in improving surgical performance. The positive effect of surgical warm-up appears to be present in novice surgeons, surgical trainees, and experienced surgeons.

Credentialing

Currently there is no standard US hospital credentialing guidelines for procedures. Hospitals turn to case currency (how many cases a surgeon has done), VR training, animate lab training, and residency/fellowship experience to drive credentialing decisions. With the increasing availability and diversity of surgical training tools, there is likely to be an increase in the demand for using these tools to demonstrate proficiency in training, and even for credentialing purposes. One current example is the Fundamentals of Laparoscopic Surgery (FLS) examination which is required by the American Board of Surgery for completion and Boarding of a General Surgery Diplomate. In robot-assisted surgery, Goh et al. developed a validated standard assessment tool for surgical skills. The Global Evaluative Assessment of Robotic Skills (GEARS) consists of 6 domains (depth perception, bimanual dexterity, efficiency, autonomy, force sensitivity and robotic control) with proficiency scored on a 5-point Likert scale [46]. This validated tool has been used by some institutions as part of an integrated robotic surgery training curriculum. Other similar simulation training curricula designed to teach surgical technique in different surgical subspecialties and proficiency benchmarks can be further implemented into surgical training programs. Eventually, demonstration of proficiency with simulation platforms may be required as part of formal credentialing by surgical governing bodies, or hospitals and institutions.

Conclusions

A recent focus on improved patient outcomes and safety has led to a shift in approach for medical education, particularly in surgical training. Simulation allows an opportunity for developing and maintaining surgical skills in a safe environment with no risk to patients (learner-centered). Surgical simulation has been implemented in several areas of surgical training over the past several decades. A variety of task-based, reality-based and VR simulation platforms have been utilized and have demonstrated validity and efficacy in improving surgical skills. Furthermore, several studies have demonstrated those skills acquired during surgical simulation translate to improvements in surgical performance in the live patient setting. More and more institutions are including simulation training as part of their formal surgical curricula and this trend is expected to continue. In addition, the use of simulation to demonstrate proficiency will likely have an increased role in surgical credentialing, and the use of patient specific rehearsal through simulation may help improve patient outcomes.

References

1. Argun OB, Chrouser K, Chauhan S, Monga M, Knudsen B, Box GN, et al. Multi-institutional validation of an OSATS for the assessment of cystoscopic and ureteroscopic skills. J Urol. 2015;194(4):1098–105.
2. Lendvay TS, Hannaford B, Satava RM. Future of robotic surgery. Cancer J. 2013;19(2):109–19.
3. Jabbour N, Snyderman CH. The economics of surgical simulation. Otolaryngol Clin N Am. 2017;50(5):1029–36.
4. Lendvay TS. Editorial comment. J Urol. 2015;194(4):1105–6.
5. James JT. A new, evidence-based estimate of patient harms associated with hospital care. J Patient Saf. 2013;9(3):122–8.
6. Heron M. Deaths: leading causes for 2016. Natl Vital Stat Rep. 2018;67(6):1–77.
7. Anderson JG, Abrahamson K. Your health care may kill you: medical errors. Stud Health Technol Inform. 2017;234:13–7.
8. Birkmeyer JD, Finks JF, O'Reilly A, Oerline M, Carlin AM, Nunn AR, et al. Surgical skill and complication rates after bariatric surgery. N Engl J Med. 2013;369(15):1434–42.
9. Williams TE, Satiani B, Thomas A, Ellison EC. The impending shortage and the estimated cost of training the future surgical workforce. Trans Meet Am Surg Assoc. 2009;127(4):221–8.
10. Ziaee SAM, Sichani MM, Kashi AH, Samzadeh M. Evaluation of the learning curve for percutaneous nephrolithotomy. Urol J. 2010;7(4):226–31.
11. Sorensen MD, Delostrinos C, Johnson MH, Grady RW, Lendvay TS. Comparison of the learning curve and outcomes of robotic assisted pediatric pyeloplasty. J Urol. 2011;185(6 SUPPL):2517–22.
12. Allen D, O'Brien T, Tiptaft R, Glass J. Defining the learning curve for percutaneous nephrolithotomy. J Endourol. 2005;19(3):279–82.
13. Watterson JD, Soon S, Jana K. Access related complications during percutaneous nephrolithotomy: urology versus radiology at a single academic institution. J Urol. 2006;176(1):142–5.
14. Guiu-Souto J, Otero C, Pérez-Fentes DA, Fernández-Baltar C, Francisco Sánchez-Garcia J, García-Freire C, et al. Characterising endourologist learning curve during percutaneous nephrolithotomy: implications on occupational dose and patients. J Radiol Prot. 2017;37(4):N49–54.
15. Song Y, Ma Y, Song Y, Fei X. Evaluating the learning curve for percutaneous nephrolithotomy under total ultrasound guidance. Hills RK, editor. PLoS One. 2015;10(8):e0132986.
16. Ku JH, Yeo WG, Kim HH, Choi H. Laparoscopic nephrectomy for renal diseases in children: is there a learning curve? J Pediatr Surg. 2005;40(7):1173–6.
17. Passerotti CC, Passerotti AMAMS, Dall'Oglio MF, Leite KRM, Nunes RLV, Srougi M, et al. Comparing the quality of the suture anastomosis and the learning curves associated with performing open, freehand, and robotic-assisted laparoscopic pyeloplasty in a swine animal model. J Am Coll Surg. 2009;208(4):576–86.
18. Abboudi H, Khan MS, Guru KA, Froghi S, De Win G, Van Poppel H, et al. Learning curves for urological procedures: a systematic review. BJU Int. 2014;114(4):617–29.

19. Tasian GE, Wiebe DJ, Casale P. Learning curve of robotic assisted pyeloplasty for pediatric urology fellows. J Urol. 2013;190(4 SUPPL):1622–6.
20. Sim HG, Yip SKH, Lau WKO, Tan YH, Wong MYC, Cheng CWS. Team-based approach reduces learning curve in robot-assisted laparoscopic radical prostatectomy. Int J Urol. 2006;13(5):560–4.
21. Martin JA, Regehr G, Reznick R, Macrae H, Murnaghan J, Hutchison C, et al. Objective structured assessment of technical skill (OSATS) for surgical residents. Br J Surg. 1997;84(2):273–8.
22. Kishore TA, Pedro RN, Monga M, Sweet RM. Assessment of validity of an OSATS for cystoscopic and ureteroscopic cognitive and psychomotor skills. J Endourol. 2008;22(12):2707–12.
23. Gallagher AG, Ritter EM, Champion H, Higgins G, Fried MP, Moses G, et al. Virtual reality simulation for the operating room: proficiency-based training as a paradigm shift in surgical skills training. Ann Surg. 2005;241(2):364–72.
24. McDougall EM, Clayman RV. Rapid communication: minimally invasive urologic surgery curricula. J Endourol. 2007;21(2):197–217.
25. Ghani KR, Miller DC, Linsell S, Brachulis A, Lane B, Sarle R, et al. Measuring to improve: peer and crowd-sourced assessments of technical skill with robot-assisted radical prostatectomy. Eur Urol. 2016 69(4):547–50.
26. Lendvay TS, White L, Kowalewski T. Crowdsourcing to assess surgical skill. JAMA Surg. 2015;150(11):1086.
27. Holst D, Kowalewski TM, White LW, Brand TC, Harper JD, Sorenson MD, et al. Crowd-sourced assessment of technical skills: an adjunct to urology resident surgical simulation training. J Endourol. 2015.29(5):604–9.
28. Dawe SR, Pena GN, Windsor JA, Broeders JAJL, Cregan PC, Hewett PJ, et al. Systematic review of skills transfer after surgical simulation-based training. Br J Surg. 2014;101(9):1063–76.
29. Brydges R, Farhat WA, El-Hout Y, Dubrowski A. Pediatric urology training: performance-based assessment using the fundamentals of laparoscopic surgery. J Surg Res. 2010;161(2):240–5.
30. Steigerwald SN, Park J, Hardy KM, Gillman LM, Vergis AS. Does laparoscopic simulation predict intraoperative performance? A comparison between the fundamentals of laparoscopic surgery and LapVR evaluation metrics. Am J Surg. 2015;209(1):34–9.
31. Gallagher AG, Satava RM. Surgical simulation. Ann Surg. 2015;262(2):e50–1.
32. Chowriappa A, Raza SJ, Fazili A, Field E, Malito C, Samarasekera D, et al. Augmented-reality-based skills training for robot-assisted urethrovesical anastomosis: a multi-institutional randomised controlled trial. BJU Int. 2015;115(2):336–45.
33. Santangelo G, Mix D, Ghazi A, Stoner M, Vates GE, Stone JJ. Development of a whole-task simulator for carotid endarterectomy. Oper Neurosurg. 2018;14(6):697–704.
34. Ghazi A, Campbell T, Melnyk R, Feng C, Andrusco A, Stone J, et al. Validation of a full-immersion simulation platform for percutaneous nephrolithotomy using three-dimensional printing technology. J Endourol. 2017;31(12):1314–20.
35. Weiss MY, Melnyk R, Mix D, Ghazi A, Vates GE, Stone JJ. Design and validation of a cervical laminectomy simulator using 3D printing and hydrogel phantoms. Oper Neurosurg. 2019;18:202–8.
36. Millán C, Rey M, Lopez M. LAParoscopic simulator for pediatric ureteral reimplantation (LAP-SPUR) following the Lich-Gregoir technique. J Pediatr Urol. 2018;14(2):137–43.
37. Sethi AS, Peine WJ, Mohammadi Y, Sundaram CP. Validation of a novel virtual reality robotic simulator. J Endourol. 2009;23(3):503–8.
38. Whitehurst SV, Lockrow EG, Lendvay TS, Propst AM, Dunlow SG, Rosemeyer CJ, et al. Comparison of two simulation systems to support robotic-assisted surgical training: a pilot study (Swine model). J Minim Invasive Gynecol. 2015;22(3):483–8.
39. Cheung CL, Looi T, Lendvay TS, Drake JM, Farhat WA. Use of 3-dimensional printing technology and silicone modeling in surgical simulation: development and face validation in pediatric laparoscopic pyeloplasty. J Surg Educ. 2014;71(5):762–7.
40. Abdalla G, Moran-Atkin E, Chen G, Schweitzer MA, Magnuson TH, Steele KE. The effect of warm-up on surgical performance: a systematic review. Surg Endosc. 2015;29(6):1259–69.

41. da Cruz JAS, dos Reis ST, Cunha Frati RM, Duarte RJ, Nguyen H, Srougi M, et al. Does warm-up training in a virtual reality simulator improve surgical performance? A prospective randomized analysis. J Surg Educ. 2016;73(6):974–8.
42. Pike TW, Pathak S, Mushtaq F, Wilkie RM, Mon-Williams M, Lodge JPA. A systematic examination of preoperative surgery warm-up routines. Surg Endosc. 2017;31(5):2202–14.
43. Lendvay TS, Brand TC, White L, Kowalewski T, Jonnadula S, Mercer LD, et al. Virtual reality robotic surgery warm-up improves task performance in a dry laboratory environment: a prospective randomized controlled study. J Am Coll Surg. 2013;216(6):1181–92.
44. Polterauer S, Husslein H, Kranawetter M, Schwameis R, Reinthaller A, Heinze G, et al. Effect of preoperative warm-up exercise before laparoscopic gynecological surgery: a randomized trial. J Surg Educ. 2016;73(3):429–32.
45. Arora S, Aggarwal R, Sirimanna P, Moran A, Grantcharov T, Kneebone R, et al. Mental practice enhances surgical technical skills: a randomized controlled study. Ann Surg. 2011;253(2):265–70.
46. Goh AC, Goldfarb DW, Sander JC, Miles BJ, Dunkin BJ. Global evaluative assessment of robotic skills: validation of a clinical assessment tool to measure robotic surgical skills. J Urol. 2012;187(1):247–52.

Index

A
Abdominal wall and umbilicus, 43, 44
ALF-X system, 58
Amplatz fascial dilators, 258
Antegrade ejaculation, 326
Anti-diuretic hormone (ADH), 25
Anti-Müllerian hormone, 188
Anti-reflux surgery, 149
Appendicovesicostomy (APV)
    anastomosis of appendix to bladder, 203–204
    anterior reimplantation, 202, 203
    anterior vs posterior implantation, 203
    appendix harvesting, 200–202
    bowel and antibiotic preparation 198
    catheters, 205
    detrusorotomy, 203
    distal configuration, 201
    hitch sutures, 204
    Mitrofanoff procedure, 197
    outcomes, 207
    patient positioning, 199
    port closure, 205
    port configuration, 199–200
    port placement and docking, 199, 200, 202
    posterior implantation 203
    postoperative care
        antibiotic prophylaxis, 206
        complications, 206–207
        diet, 206
        length of catheter duration, 205
    postoperative urodynamic changes 197–198
    preoperative systemic antibiotics, 198
    stoma location, 204–205
    testing for easy catheterization, 205
Arterial blood gas (ABG), 25, 27
Artery-sparing technique, 295
Augmentation ileocystoplasty
    appendiceal isolation
        and harvest, 226–227
    appendiceal mesentery and mobility, 227
    appendicovesicostomy, 229–231
    appendicovesicostomy anastomosis, 230
    complex reconstructive procedures, 223
    complications
        B12 deficiency, 236
        long term complications, 235
        metabolic deranagments, 236
        mucous production, 235
        neoplasia, 236
        outcomes, 236
        short term complications, 235
        stone formation, 235
        surgical complications, 234
    contraindications, 225
    cystotomy and patch ileoystoplasty, 231–232
    detrusorotomy, 229–231
    diagnostic peritonoscopy, 226
    electrocautery division, 228
    hand sewn bowel anastomosis, 229
    harmonic scalpel, 231, 232
    ileal detubulrization, 231
    ileal loop isolation and anastomosis, 227–229
    large bowel defect, 228
    leak test, 233
    maturation of APV stoma, 233
    patch ileocystoplasty, 232
    patient positioning, 226
    patient selection, 224
    port placement, 226
    post-operative management, 233
    preoperative preparation, 225
    pre-operative work up, 224

Augmentation ileocystoplasty (cont.)
  reducing operative time, 234
  robot docking, 226
  spatulation of appendix, 230

B
Bailez technique, 94, 95
Balloon-tipped trochars, 366
Bariatric length telescope, 343
Bilateral laparoscopic orchiopexy, 284–285
Bilateral RALUR, 150
Bilateral salpingo-oophorectomy, 58
Bilateral Wilms nephrectomy, 121
Biopsy-proven malignancy, 313
BITRACK system, 409
Bladder augmentation, 217, 218
Bladder diverticulae, 185–187
Bladder neck repair (BNR), 216–217
Bladder tumors, 187, 188
Bupivicaine, 74

C
Cambridge Endoscopic Devices, Inc, 63
Cerebral hemodynamics, 23, 24
Chorioamnionitis, 367
Clavien-Dindo classification, 264, 382
Clavien–Dindo grades I–III, 143
Clavien-Dindo scale, 386
Clavien grade I and II, 382, 388
Clavien grade III, 388
Clavien I/II complications, 175
Clavien system, 385
ClearPetra® nephrostomy tube system, 268
Cohen technique, 11
Complex bladder reconstruction
  abdominal access, 212–213
  augmentation, 209
  bladder augmentation, 217, 218
  bladder neck reconstruction, 209, 210
  BNR, 216–217
  bowel management, 220
  cholecystectomy and nephrectomy, 209
  complex bladder reconstruction, MItrofanoff, 213–215
  detrusor tunnel, 215
  dissected bladder neck, 217
  docking, 212–213
  ileo-vesicostomy and ileal conduit, 218, 219
  indications, 210, 211
  initial cystoscopy, 212
  intra-corporeal neobladder creation, 209
  Mitrofanoff, 209
  patient position, 212, 213
  patients with prior abdominal surgery, 219–220
  port position, 212–214
  post-operative, 220–221
  surgical techniques, 211–212
Complex upper tract reconstruction
  hydronephrotic lower pole, 142
  indications, 140
  laparoscopic ureterocalicostomy, 141
  magnetic resonance urogram, 142
  outcomes/complications, 143
  robot-assisted laparoscopic pyeloplasty, 141–143
  surgical principles, 140–141
  ureterocalicostomy, 139, 143
Congenital diaphragmatic hernia (CDH), 372
Congenital heart disease (CHD), 384
Contemporary laparoscopic surgery
  cardiopulmonary effects of positioning, 28
  cerebral blood flow, 26
  clinical decision-making, 26
  ergonomics and instrument articulation, 20
  first laparoscopic endeavor, 19
  gas absorption, 20
  indirect effects of
    cardiovascular, 24
    CNS, 26
    CO_2 pneumoperitoneum, 28
    renal, 25
    respiratory, 24, 25
  intraabdominal pressure, 20
  patient positioning, 20
  peritoneoscopy, 19
  pneumoperitoneum and direct effects
    cardiovascular effects, 20
    cerebral hemodynamics, 23, 24
    heart rate (HR), 21, 22
    renal, 23
    respiratory, 22
    stoke volume, 20, 21
  pre-existing renal dysfunction, 27
  venous air embolisms, 19
CorPath vascular catheter system, 414
Cosmesis, 301
Covidien SILS™, 339
Cowper's glands, 325
Credentialing, 433
Crowd-Sourced Assessment of Technical Skills (CSATS), 426
Cryptorchidism, 277
Cystoplasty procedures, 80

D
da Vinci instrumentation, 53
da Vinci® robotic surgical systems, 33, 37, 64
Da Vinci Si system, 76, 330

Da Vinci SP, 61
da Vinci surgical system, 51, 405, 407
Da Vinci system, 57, 58, 103, 407, 408
Da Vinci Xi system, 76, 94
Deep inguinal ring, 48–49
Desufflation, 69
Detrusor leak point pressure (DLPP), 197
Detrusorrhaphy, 159
Dextranomer - hyaluronic acid (Deflux), 6
Diagnostic laparoscopy, 3–9
Distal ureteral stump (DUS), 132
Double hydrodistention implantation technique method, 246
Duplex systems, 163
Duplication anomalies management
  absence of UTI, 167
  clinical presentation, 165, 166
  complications, 175–176
  dilated upper pole ureter, 173
  distal ureter, 173
  duplex kidneys, 163, 166
  duplication anomalies management
    pyeloureterostomy, 168
    ureteral reimplantations, 168
    ureteroureterostomy, 168
  dysplastic tissue, 167
  embryology of, 164–165
  hemi-nephrectomy, 168
  hidden incision port placement, 171
  high reconstructions, technique for, 172–174
  imaging, 166–167
  ipsilateral renal function, 168
  low reconstructions, technique for, 174–175
  low-grade VUR, 167
  monopolar wire electrode, 168
  pelvic procedures, 172
  positioning and port placement, 169–172
  post-operative care, 175
  reconstructive procedures, 169
  recurrent infections, 167
  robotic/laparoscopic approach, 169
  uncontrolled hypertension, 167
  ureteroceles, 165
  ureteroureterostomies, 168
  vesicoureteral reflux, 163
DynaCT, 266

E
End stage renal disease (ESRD), 130–131
EndoBags™, 347
Endoscopic Dx/HA injection, 247
Endothelin, 25
Endourology learning curves, 421–422
EndoWrist articulation of instruments, 52

Ethibond stitch, 286
Extracorporeal membrane oxygenation (ECMO), 372
Ex utero intrapartum therapy (EXIT), 373

F
FDA-approved Flex Robotic system, 413
Fetal cystoscopy, 371, 372
Fetal surgery
  anesthesia and monitoring, 363
  CDH, 372, 373
  complications
    fetal risks, 367
    maternal risks, 366–367
  dexterity, visualization and magnification, 359
  diagnosis, 361–362
  ECMO, 373
  fetal spina bifida dissection, 365
  fetoscopic access, 365, 366
  gastroschisis defect, 373
  history of, 360–361
  insufflation and amnioinfusion, 366
  LUTO, 370–372
  maternal-fetal anatomy and physiology, 362
  MMC repair, 374
  myelomeningocele, 364, 368–370
  open surgery, 364–365
  robot and instrument development, 374–375
  setup and positioning, 363
  simulation and training, 375
  staging criteria, 371
  team approach, 362–363
  telesurgery, 359, 375
  three-dimensional printed model, 376
  vesicoamniotic shunt procedure, 371
Fetoscopic access, 365, 366
Fetoscopic myelomeningocele, 369
Flank approach, 108–109
Flex system, 414
FlexDex, 64
Flexible 5 mm telescope, 342
Floseal®, 107
Fowler-Stephens procedure, 281, 284

G
Gartner's duct cyst, 164
GelPOINT device, 61, 350
Gerota's fascia, 104, 116–118, 316, 317, 319
Giusti's position, 254
Gonadectomy, 351–352
Guy's stone score, 252

H

Halsteadian apprenticeship education model, 419
Harmonic scalpel, 59
Harmonic® tools, 347
Hassan technique, 103, 212
Hasson open technique, 74, 87
Hasson technique, 286, 293
Heart rate (HR), 21, 22, 26
Hemi-nephrectomy, 10, 168, 348–349
Hidden incision endoscopic surgery (HIdES), 77–80, 121, 122, 152, 307
Hidden incision port placement, 171
Hitch sutures, 204
Holmium:yttrium-aluminum-garnet laser (Ho:YAG), 262
Horseshoe kidney, 122, 139, 141, 143
Hugo, 411
Hydrocele repair, 352
Hydrodistention, 244
Hydrodistention implantation technique (HIT), 245
Hydroxyl appetite, 6
Hysterotomy, 364, 367

I

Infant robotic surgery, 397–398
Inferior vena cava (IVC), 317
Inguinal hernia, 352
Internal inguinal ring, 285
International Society of Pediatric Oncology (SIOP) protocol, 125
Intra-abdominal pressure (IAP), 21, 26
Intravenous indocyanine green (ICG), 168
Intuitool device, 65
Invendoscopy E200, 413
Ioban™, 347

K

Kidneys, 44–46

L

Laparoendoscopic single-site (LESS) surgery, 60, 61, 132, 338, 396, 397
  ACE, 353
  cosmesis, 337
  cost of, 344
  crossing of instruments, 344
  flexible tip laparoscopes, 343
  grasper retraction, 344
  heminephrectomies, 339
  instrument clashing, 339
  lack of triangulation, 339
  multiple articulating instruments, 343
  multi-trocar single ports, 339
  needlescopic instruments, 342
  operating laparoscope, 338
  pelvic surgery
    gonadectomy, 351–352
    hydrocele repair, 352
    inguinal hernia, 352
    lower urinary tract surgery, 353
    orchiopexy, 351
    varicocelectomy, 350–351
  pyeloplasties, 339
  retrospective series, 345–346
  scissors/harmonic scalpel, 344
  upper urinary tract surgery, 339
    hemi-nephrectomy, 348–349
    nephrectomy, 347–348
    pyeloplasty, 349, 350
Laparoendoscopic single-site (LESS) pyeloplasty, 349, 350
Laparoscopic-assisted single incision (SILS), 317
Laparoscopic cholecystectomy, 420
Laparoscopic heminephrectomy
  complications and outcomes, 111–113
  ectopic ureter, 101
  equipment, 102, 108
  flank approach, 108–109
  laparoscopic heminephrectomy, upper pole, 106
  lower pole hilum, 106
  operating room set up, 105
  outcomes of, 112
  overzealous dissection, 102
  patient position and trocar placement, 104
  post operative care and pain relief, 111
  prone approach, 110
  retroperitoneoscopic paediatric heminephrectomy, 107
  3-dimensional magnified vision, 101
  transperitoneal approach
    dissection, 104–107
    patient position, 102–103
    placement of robot, 104
    vs. retroperitoneal approach, 110–111
    trocar placement, 103–104
  trocar placement for, 109
  upper pole parenchyma, 102
Laparoscopic nephrectomies (LN), 127, 128
Laparoscopic orchiopexy
  bilateral laparoscopic orchiopexy, 284–285
  complications, 286, 287
  first-stage Fowler-Stephens approach, 278
  internal inguinal ring, 285

Index 441

laparoscopic findings, 280–281
long-looping vas, 285
non-palpable testis, 277
one-stage orchiopexy, 281–282
outcomes, 287
outer sheath, 283
placement of laparoscopic ports, 279
positioning and trocar placement, 278–279
positioning of surgical bed, 278
single-site surgery, 279–280
traction orchiopexy, 285–286
two-stage orchiopexy, 282–284
ultrasound, 277
vascular supply, 281
Laparoscopic partial nephrectomy (LPN), 394
Laparoscopic pyeloplasties (LP), 10, 388, 389
Laparoscopic radical nephrectomy (LRN), 316–318
Laparoscopic retroperitoneal approach, 118–119
Laparoscopic RPLND (L-RPLND), 324
Laparoscopic surgery learning curves, 422
Laparoscopic transperitoneal approach, 119–120
Laparoscopic varicocelectomy
  closed camera trocar placement, 293
  complications, 295–296
  follow-up, 295–296
  laparoscopic approach, 291
  ligated cord vessels, 294
  open camera trocar placement, 293
  outcomes, 295–296
  patient selection/indications, 292
  spermatic cord, 294
  surgical technique, 292–295
  working port placement, 293
Laparoscopy
  ESRD, 130–131
  nonfunctioning kidney, 130–131
  renal cancer
    adequate lymph node sampling, 128
    indications of, 126
    transabdominal traction suture, 129
    large abdominal scar, 130
    local recurrence incidence, 128
    microscopic residual disease, 125
    neoadjuvant chemotherapy, 125, 126, 128
    non-syndromic patients, 127
    preopretavive chemotherapy, 125
    risk-benefit balance, 130
    suprapubic incision, 126
    TFE3 renal cell carcinoma, 126
    transperitoneal MIS total nephrectomies, 129
    tumoral rupture, 126
    vincristine - actinomycin D, 129
    Wilms tumor, 127, 128
  severe urinary tract infections, 131–133
Lich-Gregoir extravesical approach, 11
LigaSure™, 106, 347
Long-looping vas, 285
Lower urinary tract obstruction (LUTO), 370–372
Lower urinary tract surgery, 353

M
Macroplastique, 6
Magnetic resonance urography (MRU), 140, 142
MAK-NV system, 266
Market analysis, 33
Master and Slave Transluminal Endoscopic Robotic (MASTER) robotic system, 413
Mean arterial pressure (MAP), 24
Medical microinstruments, 412
Medtronic-Covidien SILS hand instruments, 63–64
Micro percutaneous nephrolithotomy, 259–260
Microbots, 415
MiFlex instrument, 65
Mini percutaneous nephrolithotomy, 258–259
Miniature In vivo Robotic Assistant (MIRA) System, 411–412
Minimally invasive pyeloplasties, 389
Minimally invasive surgery (MIS)
  bladder reconstructive surgery, 394–396
  Clavien-Dindo classification, 382
  credentialing, 433
  crowdsourced assessment of technical skills, 425–426
  dexterity, 383
  education model, 420
  expert-based evaluation, 424–425
  Halsteadian apprenticeship education model, 419
  infant robotic surgery, 397–398
  laparoscopy, 382–385
  learning curve
    endourology learning curves, 421–422
    laparoscopic surgery learning curves, 422
    robotic surgery learning curves, 422–424
  LESS, 396, 397
  lower pain scales, 381
  medical errors, 420
  national experience, 398–399

Minimally invasive surgery (MIS) (*cont.*)
   nephrectomies, 393–394
   partial nephrectomy, 382
   promote patient-centered care, 419
   pyeloplasties
      Clavien grade I and II, 388, 389
      Clavien grade III, 388
      Clavien IIIb, 389
      hydronephrosis, 389
      laparoscopic and open pyeloplasties, 387
      minimally invasive pyeloplasties, 388
      multivariate and comparative analysis, 388
      peritoneum and retroperitoneum, 387
      RALP, 387
   retroperitoneoscopic techniques, 382
   robotic surgery, 385–387
   robotic ureteral reimplantation, 382
   shorter hospitalizations, 381
   simulation training
      procedure-based simulation, 428–430
      stage of training, 426
      task-based simulation, 427, 428
      3-dimensional model-based simulation, 431, 432
      train-by-opportunity, 426
   surgical errors, 420
   surgical warm-up and rehearsal, 432–433
   team approach, 424
   ureteral reimplantations
      Clavien grade I and II complications, 391
      Clavien grade III complications, 391
      extravesical approach, 390
      extravesical reimplantation, 391
      extravesical ureteral reimplantation, 391, 392
      febrile UTI, 391
      ileus, 391
      intravesical and extravesical ureteral reimplantations, 390
      intravesical approach, 390
      extravesical robotic reimplantation, 392
      nerve sparing reimplantation, 393
      NSQIP Peds, 393
      open ureteral reimplantation, 392
      perinephric fluid collection, 391
      renal injury, 390
      ureteral obstruction, 391
      urinary retention, 390, 391
      UTIs, 390

Minimally invasive surgical (MIS) techniques
   anatomy in
      abdominal wall and umbilicus, 43, 44
      bladder, 47, 48
      deep inguinal ring, 48–49
      inferior epigastric vessels, 48
      kidneys, 44–46
      transmesenteric access, 45
      urachus, 47
      ureter, 46, 47
   augmentation cystoplasty, 13
   bowel reconfiguration, 13
   clinical care of, 4
   costs of, 3
   DaVinci system, 12
   deflux, interventions, 4
   diagnostic laparoscopy, 8–9
   endoscopic treatment of VUR, 5–6
   future evolution of, 13, 14
   intravesical robotic ureteral reimplantation, 11
   laparoscopic pyeloplasty, 10
   metrics of length, 5
   narcotic dosages, 5
   non-palpable testis, 3, 8
   open and laparoscopic methods, 4
   operative intervention, 4
   operative laparoscopy, 9–11
   post-operative cystography, 13
   pyeloplasty and ureteral reimplantation, 13
   retroperitoneal laparoscopic nephrectomy, 9
   roboskeptics, 12
   robotically assisted pyelolithotomy, 7
   stone disease, 6–8
   VUR and UPJ obstruction, 4
   Zeus (Computer Motion) system, 12
MiroSurge robotic system, 410
Mission statement, 32
Mitrofanoff, 197, 212–215, 220
Mitrofanoff appendicovesicostomy (MAPV), 233
MOMS protocol, 361
Myelomeningocele (MMC), 361, 368–370

N

National Inpatient Sample (NIS) database, 311
National Surgical Quality Improvement Program (NSQIP) Peds, 393
Near infrared fluorescence (NIRF), 168
NeoGuide colonoscope, 413
Nephrectomy, 347–348, 393–394

Nephrogenic adenoma, 188
Nerve-sparing technique, 326
Nissen fundoplication, 54
Non-orthotopic kidneys, 122
Novare Surgical Systems Inc, 63
Novel robotic systems
    BITRACK system, 409
    conventional open surgery, 405
    da Vinci system, 405, 407, 408
    data analytics and machine learning, 414
    democratize surgery, 414
    FDA-approved Flex Robotic system, 413
    haptic feedback, 414
    Hugo, 411
    intra-abdominal surgeries, 406
    MASTER system, 413
    medical microinstruments, 412
    MIRA system, 411, 412
    MiroSurge system, 410
    Revo-i robotic system, 410
    ROBODOC system, 405
    Senhance Surgical Robotic System, 408–409
    single-port surgery, 414
    SPORT system, 411
    STRAS-iCUBE, 413
    SurgiBot, 413
    Versius robotic system, 409

O

Olympus TriPort©, 340, 350
One-port umbilical surgery (OPUS), 338
One-stage orchiopexy, 281–282
Open Hasson technique, 74, 87
Open pyeloplasties (OPN), 32, 387
Open radical nephrectomy (ORN), 127
Operative laparoscopy, 9–11
Orchiopexy, 351

P

Page-kidneys, 23
Palomo varicocelectomy, 295
Para-testicular rhabdomyosarcoma (PT-RMS)
    benefits of, 332, 333
    complications, 332, 333
    left-sided RPLND sequence, 331
    local and hematogenous spread, 323
    lymphatic drainage, 326
    multi-modal approaches, 324
    nerve sparing, 332
    outcomes, 332, 333
    para-testicular rhabdomyosarcoma (PT-RMS), embryonal histologic subtype, 323
    post-operative tachycardia, 332
    robotic port placement, 328
    RPLND
        bilateral dissection, 330, 331
        indications for, 324–325
        left-sided dissection, 330
        lymphatic drainage, 325
        operative planning, 327–328
        para-aortic pathway, 325
        patient positioning and port placement, 328–329
        right-sided dissection, 329–330
        spermatic cord dissection, 329
        sympathetic nervous system, 326
        testicular germ cell tumors, 324
        traditional approach, 324
Partial nephrectomy, 10, 314
Pediatric nephrectomy, 394
    bilateral procedures, 120
    bilateral Wilms nephrectomy, 121
    clear cell sarcoma, 127
    horseshoe kidney, 122
    indication and outcome
        laparoscopy (*see* Laparoscopy)
        robot-assisted, 133
    kidney retrieval, 123–124
    laparoscopic and robotic approaches, 115
    laparoscopic retroperitoneal approach, 118–119
    laparoscopic transperitoneal approach, 119–120
    ligation of ureter, 123
    long-standing infection, 120
    lymph node dissection, 124–125
    partial nephrectomy, 120
    patient positioning, 120
    patient preparation, 115, 116
    pelvic kidneys, 122, 123
    port placement, 122
    prophylactic antibiotics, 124
    pyeloplasty, 120
    renal access
        retroperitoneal, 116–117
        single-site access, 118
        transperitoneal, 117–118
    retroperitoneal approach, 121
    TFE3 renal cell carcinoma, 127
    transabdominal approach, 121, 122
    transperitoneal fashion, 121
    transverse incision, 121
    ureteroureterostmy, 120
    Wilms' tumor, 127

Pediatric robotic surgery program
  articulated instruments, 31
  business plan
    cost analysis, 33–34
    cost efficient, 32
    market analysis, 33
    overcome learning curves, 32
  complex reconstructive procedures, 31
  dedicated OR space, 34
  dedicated OR team, 34–35
  documentation and review, 37
  education and expansion, 38
  intraoperative checklist, 35–37
  Intraoperative Safety Checklist, 36
  list of metrics, 38
  minimum requirements for launching, 33
  mission statement, 32
  non-palpable testis, 31
  operator-controlled camera movement, 31
  personal preparation, 35
  positioning, 37
  removal of fulcrum effect, 31
  three dimensional vision, 31
  tremor filtration, 31
Pelvic kidneys, 123
Percutaneous nephrostolithotomy (PCNL), 421
  adjacent organ injury, 265
  antegrade pyelography, 266
  antegrade ureteral stents, 268
  bleeding, 264, 265
  ClearPetra® nephrostomy tube system, 268
  CROES nomogram, 252, 253
  DynaCT, 266
  Guy's stone score, 252
  imaging
    Bull's eye technique, 255
    cone-beam CT, 256
    cross-table lateral Bull's eye technique, 256
    eye of needle, 255
    hybrid technique, 255
    lower pole posterior calyx, 254
    risk from fluoroscopy, 257
    triangulation technique, 255
    ultrasound-guided access, 256
  infection, 265
  instrumentation and tract size
    micro PCNL, 259–260
    mini and ultramini PCNL, 258–259
    standard PCNL, 257, 258
  MAK-NV system, 266
  management of complications, 264
  outcomes, 264
  patient positioning, 253, 254
  pediatric anesthesiologists, 252
  post-operative drainage and hemostasis, 262–264
  probabilities, 264
  renal pelvis and collecting system, 266
  risks, 264
  skin-to-stone distance, 251
  spina bifida, 251
  spinal dysraphism, 251
  stone fragmentation, energy sources for
    combined pneumatic and ultrasonic lithotripsy, 261
    electrohydraulic, 260
    laser lithotripsy, 262
    pneumatic lithotripsy, 261
    TFL, 262
    ultrasonic lithotripsy, 260, 261
  STONE nephrolithometry score, 252
Peritoneoscopy, 19
Persistent Müllerian duct syndrome (PMDS), 188
Pfannenstiel incision, 152, 153, 318
Pneumatic lithotripsy, 261
Pneumoperitoneum, 158
Polydioxanone (PDS), 169, 172
Polyglactin (Vicryl) poliglecaprone (Monocryl), 172
Positive end expiratory pressure (PEEP), 22, 26
Post-Anesthesia Care Unit (PACU), 152
Posterior bladder lesions and urachal anomalies, 183
  bladder diverticulae, 185–187
  Bladder diverticulae, 185
  bladder diverticulum, 181, 186
  bladder tumors, 187, 188
  complex lesions, 191–193
  complications, 190, 193, 194
  female pelvic structures, 182
  follow up, 194
  lesions posterior, 188–189
  management, 184–185
  MDR, symptoms of, 189
  port placement for laparoscopic, 191
  postoperative care, 194
  simple lesions, 190
  surgical techniques, 190
  three-dimensional imaging, 181
  umbilical-urachal sinus, 183
  urachal adenocarcinoma, 183
  urachal anomalies, 181

Index 445

Urachal anomalies and posterior
    bladder lesions
    vesicourachal diverticulum, 183
urachal cyst, 183
vesicourachal diverticulum, 184
Posterior prone retroperitoneoscopic (PRP)
    approach, 131
Prenatal ultrasound, 360, 361
Procedure-based simulation, 428–430
Prone approach, 110
Pulse oximetry, 363
Pyeloplasty, 12, 382
Pyeloureteral stents, 94

R
Radiation reducing gloves (RRGs), 257
Radical nephrectomy (RRN), 318
Radius surgical system, 64
RealHand, 63
Reality-based laparoscopic simulation,
    428, 429
Reality-based simulation, 427
Renal hilum, 45
Renal malignancies
    antibiotic prophylaxis measures, 316
    foley catheter placement, 316
    Gerota's fascia, 319
    indications for
        MIS nephrectomy, 313–314
        partial nephrectomy, 313–314
    intravenous mannitol, 320
    laparoscopic fundoplication, 311
    LPN and RPN, 319
    LRN, 316–318
    NIS analysis, 311
    open radical nephrectomy, 312
    open vs. laparoscopic vs. robotic
        approaches, 315
    partial nephrectomy, 314
    pediatric and adolescent tumors, 316
    postoperative outcomes, 312
    pre-procedural care, 315–316
    radical nephrectomy, 314, 316
    renal artery and vein, 317
    renorrhaphy and capsulotomy repair, 320
    RRN, 318
    surgical armamentarium, 312
    tumor spillage, 311
    ureter and gonadal vein, 317
Renin-angiotensin-aldosterone system
    (RAAS), 23, 25
Retrograde intrarenal surgery (RIRS), 265
Retroperitoneal lymph node dissection
    (RPLND), 323–324

Retroperitoneal partial nephrectomy
    (RPN), 394
Retroperitoneoscopic nephrectomy for
    nephrotic syndrome, 123
Retroperitoneoscopic paediatric
    heminephrectomy, 107
Retroperitoneoscopic pyeloplasty, 302
Revo-i robotic system, 59, 410
Rhabdomyosarcoma, 187
ROBODOC system, 405
Robot-assisted laparoscopic
    pyeloplasty, 141–143
Robot-assisted laparoscopic surgery (RALS),
    185, 406
    anesthetic and physiologic
        considerations, 301–302
    complication, 302
    cosmesis, 299, 301
    docked robot configuration, 305
    ergonomics and visualization, 299
    extravesical, 300
    intra-abdominal space, 299
    mean operative time, 300
    open pyeloplasty, 300
    operative time, 300
    patient padding, 304
    pure-laparoscopic pyeloplasties, 300
    pyeloplasties, 299
    troubleshooting robotic surgery
        orogastric tube and urethral
            catheter, 303
        patient and robot positioning, 303–304
        patient selection, 302–303
        trocar placement and
            instrumentation, 304–307
Robot-assisted laparoscopic
    ureterocalicostomy, 141
Robot-assisted surgery (RAS), 54, 139
Robotically-assisted laparoscopic ureteral
    reimplantation (RALUR), 390
Robotic and laparoscopic instrumentation
    abdominal wall laxity, 55
    advantages of Da Vinci Xi, 53–54
    anterior superior iliac spines, 54
    da Vinci instrumentation, 53
    Da Vinci SP, 61
    energy instruments, 52
    handle-controlled mechanism, 64
    history and iteration, 51–52
    instrument diameter, 52
    instrumentation development, 53–54
    intuitive surgical systems, 54
    learning curve, 64
    LESS, 65
    LESS surgery, 60, 61

Robotic and laparoscopic instrumentation (*cont.*)
   8mm vs. 5mm instrumentation, 55–57
   Nissen fundoplication, 54
   REVO-I, 59
   Senhance (Transenterix, USA), 57–59
   size and length of, 54
   standard laparoscopic instruments, 52
   thumb-controlled mechanism, 64
   UPJ obstruction, 54
   wrist articulation axes, 64
   wristed laparoscopic instruments, 62–65
Robotic assisted laparoscopic appendicovesicostomy (RALMA), 395
Robotic assisted laparoscopic pyeloplasties (RALP), 387
Robotic-assisted radical nephrectomy, 319
Robotic-assisted RLPND (RA-RPLND), 324
Robotic-assisted RPLND (RA-RPLND), 327
Robotic assisted transvesical antireflux surgery, 81
Robotic laparoendoscopic single-site (R-LESS), 60
Robotic pyeloplasty, 32, 92
Robotic surgery learning curves, 422–424
Robot oriented surgery (ROS)
   complications
      patient positioning, 86
      patient-related factors, 86
      port placement and access, 86–87
   CO_2 working pressure and flow rate, 75
   da Vinci Si and Xi system, 85
   docking process with da Vinci Si device, 82–85
   lateral decubitus position, 73
   lower urinary tract procedures
      accessory and assistant trocars, 80
      docking, 80
      positioning, 80
   magnified 3-dimensional view, 69
   nuances of MIS, 70
   partial and complete nephrectomy, 69
   patient positioning, 70–72
   port placement, 69, 70, 81
   pyeloplasty for ureteropelvic junction obstruction, 69
   retroperitoneal access, 81, 82
   robotic assisted transvesical antireflux surgery, 81
   robot oriented retroperitoneal pyeloplasty, 82
   room setup, 70
   simplification of suturing, 69
   transition to Da Vinci Xi model, 85
   transperitoneal approach
      accessory and assistant trocars, 74
      docking, 76–80
      HIdES, 77–80
      patient positioning, 72
      port placement, 74
   trocar placement in HIdES procedure, 78
   umbilical port insertion technique, 75
   upper urinary tract procedures, 72
   ureteral reimplantation, 69

S

Seldinger technique, 366
Senhance surgical robotic system, 58, 408–409
Shanfield technique, 203
Shanfield's anastomosis, 204
SILSTM Clinch, 64
SILSTM Dissect, 64
SILSTM Shears, 64
SILSTMHook, 64
Single-incision laparoscopic surgery (SILS), 60, 317, 350
Single-port-access nephrectomy, 118
Single-port surgery, 414
Single Port Orifice Robotic Technology (SPORT) Surgical System, 411
Single-site laparoscopic percutaneous extra-peritoneal closure (SLPEC), 352
Single-site robotic surgery, 60
Single-site surgery, 279–280
Spina bifida, 368
Standard PCNL, 257, 258
STING technique, 245
Stomal stenosis, 206
Stone disease, 6–8
Stone free rates (SFR), 258
STONE nephrolithometry score, 252
Stone scoring systems, 252
Stroke volume (SV), 20–21
SurgiBot, 413
Surgicel®, 107
Systemic vascular resistance (SVR), 21, 26

T

Task-based simulation, 427, 428
Team approach, 424

Index   447

Teleflex Minilap™, 342
Telesurgery, 375
3-dimensional model-based simulation, 431, 432
Thulium fiber laser (TFL), 262
Thulium fiber laser lithotripters, 268
Tocolysis, 360, 363
Tracheal Occlusion to Accelerate Lung Growth (TOTAL), 373
Traction orchiopexy, 285–286
Traditional laparoscopic instruments, 62
Transabdominal preperitoneal (TAPP), 58
Transperitoneal nephrectomy (TP), 132
Transvesical partial prostatectomy (TVPP), 61
Trendelenburg, 191
Trendelenburg positioning, 28
Tuebungen Scientific, 64
Twin-twin transfusion syndrome (TTTS), 367, 373
Two-stage orchiopexy, 282–284

U
Ultramini percutaneous nephrolithotomy, 258–259
Ultrasonic lithotripsy, 260, 261
Urachal anomalies, 181, 183, 184
    bladder diverticulae, 181, 185–187
    bladder tumors, 187, 188
    complex lesions, 191–193
    complications, 190, 193, 194
    female pelvic structures, 182
    follow up, 194
    lesions posterior, 188–189
    management, 184–185
    MDR, symptoms of, 189
    port placement for laparoscopic, 191
    postoperative care, 194
    simple lesions, 190
    surgical techniques, 190
    three-dimensional imaging, 181
    umbilical-urachal sinus, 183
    urachal adenocarcinoma, 183
    urachal cyst, 183
    vesicourachal diverticulum, 183, 184
Ureter, 46, 47
Ureteral injury, 391
Ureteral reimplantation
    bowel and bladder dysfunction, 150
    complications, 153
    cosmesis, 152–153
    cost, 152

    DMSA scans, 149
    dysfunctional voiding, 150
    extravesical LUR, 150
    extravesical RALUR, 150
    grades I-IV VUR, 150
    length of stay, 151–152
    operative success, 153–158
    operative technique, 158–159
    outcomes and surgical complications, 154–157
    pain control, 151
    platform's 3D vision, 150
    transvesical RALUR, 150
    vesicoureteral reflux, 151
    VUR, 149, 150
Ureterocalicostomy, 139, 140, 143
Ureteroceles, 165
Ureteropelvic junction obstruction (UPJO), 139, 387
    accessing abdomen, 93–94
    complications, 98
    congenital/acquired, 91
    diagnostic evaluation, 92
    endoscopic management, 93
    excising aperistaltic segment, 97
    hydronephrosis, 91
    internal *vs* external pyeloureteral stenting, 95
    intrinsic/extrinsic etiology, 91
    patient positioning, 93–94
    patient presentation, 92
    pelvicalyceal system, 91
    port placement, 94
    proximal ureter, 97
    pyeloplasty procedure, 95–96
    treatment of, 91
    trocar placement, 93–94
Ureteroureterostomies (UU), 300
Urinary tract infection (UTI), 92, 143, 163, 243
Urothelial carcinoma, 187

V
Varicocelectomy, 350–351
Varicoceles, 291
Velcro straps, 93
Ventriculoperitoneal (VP), 224
Veress needle, 74, 87, 95, 158, 293, 328
VersaStep® sheath, 81
Versius Robotic System, 409
Vesicoamniotic shunting (VAS), 360, 370

Vesicoureteral reflux (VUR), 149, 166, 224
    complications, 247, 248
    continuous antibiotic prophylaxis, 243
    endoscopic therapy, 243
    HIT and double HIT methods, 245–247
    hydrodistention grading, 245
    indications, 244
    outcomes, 247, 248
    recurrent pyelonephritis, 243
    STING technique, 245
    surgical principles, 244–245
Vicryl/polydioxanone (PDS), 231
Videourodynamics, 224
Virtual reality simulation, 427–428
Virtual-reality simulator, 430, 431
VisiPort©, 117
Voiding cystourethrogram (VCUG), 186, 245

W
Weck® Hem-o-Lok® clips, 329
Weigert-Meyer rule, 47
Wiegert-Meyer rule, 164
Wilms tumor (WT), 128, 311
Wolffian duct, 164
Wrist deflection, 64

X
Xanthogranulomatous pyelonephritis (XGP), 131

Z
Zeus (Computer Motion) system, 12

Printed by Books on Demand, Germany